D1348309

A General Textbook of Nursing

*Dedicated to the nurses of
today and tomorrow*

EVELYN PEARCE

State Registered General and Fever Nursing. State Registered
Sister Tutor. State Certified Midwife. Teacher's Certificate
Chartered Society Physiotherapy. For many years Member of
the General Nursing Council for England and Wales, and
Examiner in Nursing to the Council; Senior Nursing Tutor,
The Middlesex Hospital; Examiner in Fever Nursing and
Epidemiology for the Diploma in Nursing, London Uni-
versity; and in General Nursing, Leeds University; Pioneer
research in the establishment of a Course in Social Science for
Indian Students at the Institute of Social Service, Bombay.

other books by the author

MEDICAL AND NURSING DICTIONARY AND ENCYCLOPAEDIA

ANATOMY AND PHYSIOLOGY FOR NURSES

INSTRUMENTS, APPLIANCES AND THEATRE TECHNIQUE

NURSE AND PATIENT: Human Relations in Nursing

A General Textbook of
NURSING
a compendium of nursing knowledge

by EVELYN PEARCE
in collaboration with consultants,
specialists and other experts

NINETEENTH EDITION

FABER AND FABER
3 Queen Square, London

First published 1937
Second edition, 1938
Third edition, 1939
Fourth edition, 1940
Fifth edition, 1941
Sixth edition, January 1942
Seventh edition, September 1942
Eighth edition, 1943
Ninth edition, 1945
Reprinted 1945, 1946 and 1947
Tenth edition, 1949
Eleventh edition, 1950
Twelfth edition, 1952
Thirteenth edition, 1953
Fourteenth edition, 1956
Fifteenth edition, 1960
Sixteenth edition, 1963
Seventeenth edition, 1967
Eighteenth edition, 1971
Nineteenth edition, 1975
by Faber and Faber, Limited
3 Queen Square, London WC1
Printed in Great Britain by
Jarrold & Sons Ltd, Norwich
All rights reserved

ISBN 0 571 04855 2

Author's Note

I express my thanks and gratitude to all those who have collaborated with me in compiling this compendium of nursing knowledge. They have given their time, thought and interest, which are so liberally displayed in the individual chapters. I do thank them all most sincerely and I am particularly indebted to Dr A. B. Christie, who has helped with the preparation of this book over the years, for writing the entire Section 5 on Communicable Diseases and to Mr Michael Hobsley, who has written a number of chapters in the Surgical Section 6, assembled this entire section and in addition has been at all times readily available to help with my many problems and to find answers to my numerous queries.

I have found much interest and pleasure in writing the first fifteen chapters related to nursing practice and procedure as an introduction to the excellent contributions based on current specialist subjects, and in carefully correlating the function of nursing throughout the book. Many references to the importance of good nursing care and observation will be found in the text demonstrating the vital role of the nurse in the team.

E.P.

Publisher's Note

We publish this nineteenth edition as a tribute to the late Evelyn Pearce who died in October 1971 just before the publication of the eighteenth edition.

She herself handled that entirely new edition when thirty-eight contributors wrote chapters on their specialities and the book appeared with a new format and new illustrations.

We have asked all the contributors to revise their chapters for this nineteenth edition and all have brought their chapters up to date. Dr Ann Miller, M.R.C.P., has kindly revised the preliminary chapters written by Miss Pearce.

We know that this very comprehensive textbook now caters even more fully for every nurse whether trained or in training.

January 1974
P. Jean Cunningham
B.A., S.R.N., S.C.M. H.V.Cert.
Editor of Nursing and Medical Books

Contributors

Contributors	*Subject contributed*
P. E. Baldry Esq., **M.B., B.S.**(Lond.), **F.R.C.P.**(Lond.) Consultant Physician Ashford Hospital Middlesex	Disorders of Respiration
W. T. C. Berry Esq., **M.A., M.D.,** **D.T.M. and H.** Principal Medical Officer (Nutrition) Department of Health and Social Security London S.E.1	Understanding Nutrition
Professor N. M. Bleehen, **M.R.C.P., F.F.R.** Professor of Radiotherapy The Middlesex Hospital Medical School London W1N 8AA	The Treatment of Cancer
A. E. Booth Esq., **M.B., B.Chir.,** **F.R.C.S.**(Eng.) Senior Neurosurgical Registrar The Middlesex Hospital London W1N 8AA	A Brief Account of Some Neurosurgical Conditions Neurological and Neurosurgical Investigation
A. C. Boyle Esq., **M.D., F.R.C.P.**(Lond.) Director, Department of Rheumatology and Physical Medicine The Middlesex Hospital London W1N 8AA	The Chronic Rheumatic Diseases
A. J. E. Brafield Esq., **M.B., B.S.,** **F.R.C.Path., D.C.P., D.Path.** Consultant Haematologist Whipps Cross Hospital London E.11	Diseases of the Blood and Lymphatic System Blood Transfusion

Contributors	*Subject contributed*
G. Bryan Esq., F.P.S. Chief Pharmacist The Middlesex Hospital London W1N 8AA	*Section 3. Pharmaceutical* *Preparations* The Administration of Drugs Drugs and Their Presentation for Use
*J. L. Burn Esq., M.D., D.Hy., D.P.H., General Practitioner Recently Medical Officer of Health, Salford Lecturer in Public Health University of Manchester	Health and Environment
Miss B. E. Chadney, S.R.N., R.S.C.N. Chief Nursing Officer The Hospital for Sick Children (Great Ormond St) London and Associate Hospitals	The Feeding of Infants up to Two Years
T. M. Chalmers Esq., M.A., M.D., F.R.C.P., F.R.C.P.E. Consultant Physician United Cambridge Hospitals	Disorders of the Heart and Circulation
A. B. Christie Esq., M.A., M.D., D.P.H., D.C.H. Physician Superintendent Fazakerley Hospital, Liverpool Head of the Department of Infectious Diseases University of Liverpool	*Section 5. Communicable* *Diseases, Treatment and* *Nursing Care* Introduction Epidemiology Food-borne Infections Some Acute Infections (three chapters) Some Tropical Infections Tuberculosis Prevention and Treatment of Acute Infections
Miss Mary Craig, *O.B.E.*, Hon. F.S.R., S.R.N. Superintendent Sister, Department of Radiotherapy The Middlesex Hospital London W1N 8AA	The Nursing of Patients Receiving Radiotherapy

* Died after publication of the eighteenth edition of this book.

Contributors	Subject contributed
Miss Marion Frank, F.S.R. Group Superintendent Radiographer and Principal of the School of Radiography The Middlesex Hospital London W1N 8AA	Nursing Duties in the Preparation of Patients for X-Ray Examination
L. C. L. Gonet Esq., M.B., B.S., F.R.C.S. Consultant Orthopaedic Surgeon Westminster Group of Teaching Hospitals and the Chelsea and Kensington Group	Orthopaedic Surgery Part 1. The Use of Splints, Plaster of Paris and Traction Part 2. Common Injuries to Bone and Joint, Outline of Treatment Part 3. Examples of Orthopaedic Conditions
Roy Goulding Esq., B.Sc., M.D., F.R.C.P. Director, Poisons Reference Service Guy's Hospital London S.E.1	Poisoning and its Treatment
Desmond P. Greaves Esq., B.Sc., M.B., Ch.B., F.R.C.S., D.O.M.S. Senior Consultant Ophthalmic Surgeon University College Hospital Consultant Surgeon, Moorfields Eye Hospital London	The Nursing of Patients with Diseases of the Eye
John Greene Esq., O.B.E., S.R.N., R.M.N. Area Nursing Officer Gloucestershire Area Health Authority	An Introduction to Psychiatric Conditions Treatment and Nursing Care
David I. Hamilton Esq., M.B., B.S., F.R.C.S. Consultant Cardiac Surgeon to the Liverpool Regional Hospital Board at Broadgreen and Sefton General Hospitals and to the Royal Liverpool Children's Hospital	Surgery of the Heart and Great Vessels, Treatment and Nursing

Contributors	*Subject contributed*
Michael Hobsley Esq., *T.D.*, M.A., Ph.D.(Lond.), M.Chir.(Cantab.), F.R.C.S.(Eng.) Reader in Surgical Science, London University Honorary Consultant Surgeon The Middlesex Hospital London W1N 8AA	Introduction to Surgical Nursing Life-Threatening Conditions Damage to Tissues Postoperative Care, Complications of Surgical Operations Surgery of the Alimentary Tract (excluding disorders of the large bowel) Surgery of Peripheral Vascular Disease Operations on the Thyroid, Breast and Adrenal Glands
Quentin J. G. Hobson Esq., M.A.(Oxon.), D.M.(Oxon.), F.R.C.P.(Lond.) Consultant Physician West Middlesex Hospital Isleworth Middlesex	Diseases and Disorders of the Endocrine Glands
Peter F. Jones Esq., M.A., M.Chir., F.R.C.S.(Eng.), F.R.C.S.(Edin.) Consultant Surgeon Aberdeen General Hospitals and Royal Aberdeen Hospital for Sick Children Honorary Reader in Surgical Paediatrics University of Aberdeen	Surgical Conditions of the Colon, Rectum and Anal Canal, and Their Nursing Care
Ambrose King Esq., *T.D.*, M.B., B.S.(Lond.), F.R.C.S.(Eng.) Hon. Consulting Venereologist to the London Hospital Acting Consultant Venereologist to the Moorfields Eye Hospital, London Member of the Expert Advisory Panel on Venereal Infections and Treponematoses, W.H.O. Formerly Consultant Adviser in Venereology to the Ministry of Health	A Short Outline of Venereal Diseases and Their Management
G. M. Levene Esq., M.B., M.R.C.P. Senior Lecturer, Institute of Dermatology Honorary Consultant Dermatologist St John's Hospital for Diseases of the Skin and Hackney Hospital, London	Diseases and Disorders of the Skin

Contributors	*Subject contributed*
John Maddison Esq., M.D., D.P.H. Recently Director Maddison Clinic for Research in Preventive Medicine for Older People, Teddington, Middlesex	Care of the Elderly
Miss A. Marjorie Matthias, S.R.N., Diploma Clinical Instruction, University of Toronto Senior Nursing Officer—Theatres Redhill and Netherne Hospitals Lecturer in Surgical and Theatre Techniques	Some Points in Surgical Technique
Mrs Ruth McKay, S.R.N., S.C.M., M.T.D. Senior Midwife Teacher Duchess of Kent Maternity Wing Hillingdon Hospital Middlesex Examiner for the Central Midwives Board	*Section 7A. A Brief* *Introduction to* *Obstetrical Nursing* An Outline of the Physiology of the Female Organs of Reproduction Pregnancy and Prenatal Care Labour and the Puerperium Care of a Newly Born Baby
Miss Marjorie McLaughlin, S.R.D. Chief Dietician The Middlesex Hospital London W1N 8AA	Samples of Normal and Therapeutic Diets
John Meadows Esq., M.D., M.R.C.P. Neurological Registrar The Middlesex Hospital London WIN 8AA	Disorders of the Nervous System
I. F. K. Muir Esq., *M.B.E.*, V.R.D., M.B., M.S., F.R.C.S. Hon. Senior Lecturer in Clinical Surgery University of Aberdeen Consultant in Plastic and Reconstructive Surgery, North East Regional Hospital Board, Scotland	Plastic and Reconstructive Surgery and the Nursing Care
L. F. W. Salmon Esq., *M.B.E.*, M.S., F.R.C.S. Consultant Surgeon, The Throat and Ear Department Guy's Hospital London S.E.1	Diseases of the Ears, Nose and Throat, and Nursing Care

Contributors	*Subject contributed*
Miss Mary P. Shepherd, M.B., B.S., F.R.C.S.(Eng.), F.R.C.S.(Edin.) Consultant Thoracic Surgeon Harefield and Clare Hall Hospitals	An Outline of Thoracic Surgery
W. K. Slack Esq., M.R.C.S., L.R.C.P., D.A. Consultant Anaesthetist and Consultant in Charge of the Hyperbaric Oxygen Unit Whipps Cross Hospital London E.11	Anaesthesia—Basic Principles and the Duties of the Nurse Oxygen and Hyperbaric Oxygen Therapy— Indications and hazards in relation to nursing care
James G. Sommerville Esq., M.D., M.R.C.P. Medical Director, Medical Rehabilitation Centre 152 Camden Road London N.W.1 Consultant, Wolfson Medical Rehabilitation Centre Atkinson Morley Hospital London S.W.20	Medical Rehabilitation
*G. A. Stephens Esq., M.P.S. Professional Services Department B.D.H. Pharmaceuticals Ltd London E2 6LA Author *Hormones and Vitamins*, George Newnes	Some Side-Effects of Endocrinological Preparations— Appendix ii
James S. Stewart Esq., M.D., M.R.C.P. Consultant Physician West Middlesex Hospital Isleworth Middlesex	Diseases of the Digestive System
J. E. A. Wickham Esq., B.Sc.(Hons.), M.S., F.R.C.S. Consultant Urological Surgeon St Bartholomew's Hospital and St Peter's Group Hospitals, London Senior Lecturer, the Institute of Urology, London	Diseases of the Urinary System Surgical Conditions of the Genito-Urinary Tract

* Died before publication of the eighteenth edition of this book.

Contributors

Subject contributed

Miss P. A. M. White, S.R.N., S.C.M.
Administrative Sister—Gynaecology,
Hospital for Women, Soho Square
(The Middlesex Hospital)
London W.1

Section 7B.
Gynaecological
Conditions, Their
Treatment and Nursing
Care
Inflammatory
Conditions, Diseases
and Disorders of the
Female Generative
Organs
Some Gynaecological
Operations, Pre- and
Postoperative Care

Acknowledgements

I find it impossible to make a comprehensive list of all those I should like to thank, as this embraces not only nurses and doctors but almost every grade of staff engaged in the care of patients in hospital and in the community. They are comparable to the background men and women who form part of every scientific and human achievement in the world today.

No scientist, individual nurse or doctor works in isolation but as part of a great research and working team. Team-work, or, to coin a term, 'team thinking', has been the basis of this new edition and the co-operation received from so many may well be unique. I ask them all to accept this expression of my gratitude, whilst mentioning a few individuals and groups who have helped me personally in some special way.

Mrs Bethina A. Bennett, *O.B.E.*, S.R.N., D.N. (Leeds Univ.), formerly Principal Nursing Officer, the Ministry of Labour, Chairman, Scholarships Committee, British Commonwealth Nurses' War Memorial Fund, for her help and encouragement throughout.

Miss Valerie Paull, S.R.N., who during her training as a student nurse made helpful observations in regard to basic nursing.

Miss Dorothy M. Sykes, S.R.N., R.N.T., Group Director of Education, Whipps Cross and Forest Hospitals, London E.11, for her interest and help in maintaining, together with her staff and the background of her nursing school, a modern approach in basic nursing.

I also express my thanks to:

Miss Kathleen M. Biggin, B.A., S.R.N., R.N.T., D.N.(Lond.), and Chief Nursing Officer, the Middlesex Hospital, London W1N 8AA

Miss Eirlyn Rees, S.R.N., S.C.M., Dip.N.A., R.C.N., Matron, Whipps Cross and Forest Hospitals, London E. 11

Miss Susan Camerloher, S.R.N., S.C.M., M.T.D.

Miss P. J. Colwell, S.R.N.

Miss Lois Dyer, M.C.S.P.

Miss J. Elise Gordon, *O.B.E.*, M.A.

Miss Gladys E. Ludbrook, S.R.N., S.C.M., R.N.T.

Miss R. C. Perkes, S.R.N., S.C.M., M.T.D.

Miss Anna M. Reid, S.R.N., S.C.M., R.N.T.

Miss Anne M. Toumey, S.R.N., R.C.N.T.

Miss Jean Watson, S.R.N., S.E.N.

Russell Grant Esq., M.A., M.R.C.S., L.R.C.P., Dip.Phys.Medicine.

Brian D. Johnson Esq., F.F.A.R.C.S., M.R.C.S., L.R.C.P., D.A., for his great interest and useful help.

F. X. Keene Esq., M.D.

Arthur Naylor Esq., M.B., Ch.B., F.R.C.S.

I am indebted to the Controller of Her Majesty's Stationery Office for permission to reproduce Appendix II of the *Report on the Control of Dangerous Drugs and Poisons in Hospitals* and for permission to use an abridged version of Table I from the *Report on Public Health and Medical Subjects*, no. 120—Recommended Intakes of Nutrients for the United Kingdom.

The International Council of Nurses for permission to reprint the Code of Ethics as applied to nurses.

The General Nursing Council for England and Wales for permission to reprint Examination Question Papers.

The following Departments of Medical Illustration: The Middlesex Hospital, London W1N 8AA; The Institute of Child Health, London W.C.1 (The Hospital for Sick Children); The Institute of Orthopaedics, London W.1 (Royal National Orthopaedic Hospital); The Department of Audio-visual Aids, The Institute of Ophthalmology, London.

To a number of firms for material for illustrations and/or information, including: Air Shields, Shoeburyness; Ames Company Division of Miles Laboratory; British Schering Chemicals Ltd; Down Bros. and Meyer and Phelps Ltd; Glaxo Laboratories Ltd; Henley's Medical Supplies Ltd; Johnson and Johnson Ltd; Riker Laboratories Ltd; Roussel Laboratories Ltd; Scholl Mfg. Co. Ltd; Smith and Nephew Ltd.

To: Mrs Lesley Bardrick and Miss Thelma Misquitta for their patience and care in typing manuscripts; Mrs Audrey Besterman for her excellent drawings; and Maurice Turney Esq., F.R.P.S. for his careful photography.

Finally I thank the publishers Messrs Faber and Faber for their courteous assistance, and in particular Miss P. Jean Cunningham, B.A., S.R.N., S.C.M., H.V. Cert., Editor Nursing and Medical Textbooks, for her expert help and great interest in seeing the 18th edition through the press, and in this connection I also thank Mrs Jill White, her editorial assistant.

Contents

Section 2
NUTRITION

Section 3
PHARMACEUTICAL PREPARATIONS

Section 4

MEDICAL CONDITIONS, TREATMENT AND CARE

Section 5

COMMUNICABLE DISEASES—TREATMENT AND
NURSING CARE

Illustrations

Section 1

Some General Nursing Measures and Procedures

Introduction

Those of you who have known previous issues of my textbook may wonder why the eighteenth edition was different. Changes in the content and format were necessary but the text contains all the basic nursing presented in previous issues. In addition, progress in treatment necessitated the inclusion of newer aspects of nursing, consequently many more formal nursing procedures will be found in the individual sections. Although an occasional example may be given, it is assumed that the nurse in training will follow the customary practice of her nursing school, consulting the procedure sheets available to her for detailed methods of nursing.

New chapters by consultants, specialists and other experts enhance the usefulness of the book. This 'combined operation' reflects the modern outlook in total patient care, in which you are involved, and emphasizes the increasing co-operation and partnership between doctor and nurse. My collaborators and I have had the greatest satisfaction in compiling this book. And I, as a nurse, can wish you nothing better than that you may find in its pages not only the means of extending your knowledge of nursing but also of achieving fulfilment in your chosen profession.

EVELYN PEARCE

In describing a nurse, the pronoun *she* is used throughout, but with the increasing number of male nurses it would be equally accurate to write *he*. For the sake of brevity common usage over the years has been followed.

Chapter 1

The Patient

Approach to the care of patients—the influence of environment on health—the patient in the community

Twenty years ago a nurse tended to a patient's needs, making him comfortable, inspiring confidence and calmness in creating an environment which gave him the best possible chance of recovery. Advances in medical science and particularly in technology during the past two decades have in no way diminished this valuable function of a nurse but have made nursing more, not less, important. Nursing is a most essential service. There can scarcely be a more satisfying profession.

THE MODERN NURSE

The present generation of nurses has grown up entirely in the technological age of this century. The modern nurse, like the modern doctor, is the product of an evolutionary process, but one where, nevertheless, her compassionate approach to patients remains unchanged; she is developing a new role in order to assist physicians and surgeons in a closely knit patient-centred team. Those with sufficient education and a liking for the work are assuming increasing responsibilities for tasks hitherto carried out by doctors in the various branches of the National Health Service. Nurses are part of a new world-wide student movement but, unlike many others, the student of nursing enters an environment which provides reasonable stability and tremendous interest in a two-fold challenge:

A highly scientific and technical one with opportunities of participating in medical progress in the prevention and cure of disease.

A philosophical field in a satisfying life of service adapted to the circumstances and needs of each patient. Whether a patient is in a hospital bed, in a chair, in a hostel visiting the clinician regularly, in an intensive care unit or passing from one department or hospital to another; whether he is conscious or not, dangerously ill, oblivious to his surroundings, delirious or disorientated, on a slow or rapid road to recovery or happily ambulant, *his basic human needs must be supplied.*

The patient as a member of the curative team is the most important one; he is the central figure—a fact which should never be forgotten. Without a patient's collaboration, and that of his relatives, complete cure and rehabilitation may be impossible. A patient should be listened to.

Patients come from many income groups and from different cultures in the changing social pattern and according to their ability will desire and be able to co-operate with physicians and surgeons who, sitting beside a patient, will endeavour to explain what has gone wrong, how this can be dealt with and approximately how long it may take.

The nurse is almost exclusively the interpreter of the hospital. She will explain every treatment, its purpose, result anticipated and the value of the patient's collaboration. Her explanations must carry the weight of her responsibility as a nurse whose function *vis-à-vis* the patient is unique in the team. Her training fits her for making decisions and using discretional power in providing, with the other members of the curative team, the best possible care of the patient.

Nurses soon learn to realize the value of a pleasing professional approach and that the occasional glance in passing, nod of the head or smile takes no time and makes a valuable contribution to good relations. Communication need not always be verbal, and the nurse by the exercise of her skill can convey sympathy and assurance to a patient who may be too weary or ill to listen to much conversation, or who speaks no English.

TRAINING IS ARDUOUS

The training of a nurse is an exacting one and her calling demands the utmost she can give. She has to acquire scientific knowledge, exercise the exquisite judgement only achieved by experience, and develop her skill to the highest degree. This is only obtained by practice. Above all she has to give these services not at any self-chosen moment but daily at the needs of others.

An alert, observant nurse may notice a change in a patient and avoid a crisis by summoning medical help and instituting immediate treatment in an endeavour to safeguard his life through vital minutes until help comes. She must remain calm and collected in any emergency, with a calmness which is communicable. In less dramatic circumstances a nurse by simple intuition may realize the pressing needs of a patient; she may take her place, as it were, in his mind in order to interpret his needs.

A patient's relatives and sometimes his friends should whenever possible be integrated into the programme of his care and treatment. The relations of a nurse with the patient's family should always be generous; a very high degree of sensitivity to the needs of these people is required.

It is useful to talk with the relatives of a patient just as a good hostess would do. Both sides are helped: the nurse can learn many things about a patient which may assist in her care of him; the relatives are put at ease by a nurse who will keep them informed of his progress and his needs. However, this depends entirely on the doctor taking the nurse fully into his confidence as to what it would be wise for the relatives to know and the best way of conveying it.

The attraction of nursing to young people demonstrates a worthwhile desire to help which does not depend on social status, nationality or creed, but on a temperamental suitability for the work. Most of those who decide on nursing as a career possess a fairly consistent attitude towards life; they have made an evaluation of themselves and considered all aspects of the work. They realize that the nature of illness may alter a patient's attitude and that this can give rise to abnormal behaviour, that they will find some patients trying and many nursing duties unpleasant. Not all stay the course, but those who do will have a life-long interest.

Nursing, though full of thrilling opportunities, is primarily a simple life where one is brought face to face with sickness and suffering. There must be kindness and emphasis on many personal qualities. These include sincerity, integrity, tolerance, sympathy, understanding, tact and, above all, a real liking for people.

THE DIGNITY OF MAN

The most precious possession any human being has is his spirit—his will to live, his sense of dignity and his individuality. As nursing becomes increasingly technical, more than ever we need men and women who are concerned with people and *who accept the challenge of the whole person.* With all the scientific progress and new techniques in medicine *it is essential always to remember that patients are people.* Those who tend a patient must recognize the dignity of this human person and the consideration due to him, and respect his wishes. When a patient is unconscious or lacking in some of his mental faculties, as the result of illness, age or disability, it is even more essential to remember the respect due to him.

Nursing is for all times, adaptable to all ages, selecting what is good and resisting what is not. Our professional Code of Ethics (see Appendix iii, p. 759), passed on to us traditionally, can only be preserved by nurses who will administer it in the much wider field of the services expected of them in the seventies.

HEALTH AND ENVIRONMENT

Life and health are greatly affected by the influence of the *environment*, that is, all the surroundings and circumstances of our lives, which includes everything except the physical and mental qualities we have inherited from our parents through the genes. Much disease is the consequence of the interaction of the body and mind with the *total* environment—the physical, mental and social aspects of our surroundings.

The physical factors in the environment are of basic importance. They include the quality of the air we breathe, the food we eat, the home and neighbourhood in which we live. If these factors are of good quality, they will help us to health and well-being. If they are bad, they tend to foster disease, disability and discontent.

For example, the *air* may contain smoky particles. In *crowded urban areas and where domestic and industrial air pollution is high* tarry particles which contain chemicals such as the carcinogens (cancer-producing substances, e.g. 3,4 benzpyrene) may exist. Gases such as petrol exhaust fumes and the oxides of sulphur and nitrogen, together with a host of harmful substances, act as abrasive irritants to the tissues of the respiratory tract, from the nasal mucous membrane to the alveoli in the lungs. Added to these are the very real dangers of cigarette smoking—a form of personal air pollution. Many patients have been brought up from babyhood breathing a heavily polluted atmosphere. Some suffer from chronic respiratory disease, unable to work fully or even at all, and are not able to get reasonable satisfaction in living.

Many other environmental factors may also contribute to the chronic illnesses of patients.

Bad housing. The lack of modern facilities such as the provision of ample hot water and adequate facilities for the preparation, storage and cooking of food is a serious hindrance to health. Foodstuffs should be kept cool, clean, covered and free from contamination. It is a sad fact that *at least 2 million houses in England and Wales do not fulfil these elementary requirements.*

INDUSTRIALIZATION AND URBANIZATION

Environmental health has been greatly affected by the rapid growth of industrialization and increase in the number of people living in towns. This in turn has brought new stresses of noise, transport difficulties, traffic fumes, rush and bustle, more crowds and yet sometimes greater loneliness. Recent studies have shown that these circumstances may lead to a greater incidence of mental disorder.

Noise can produce alterations in respiration and circulation, in basal metabolic rate and in muscle tension. Mental and physical work and efficiency are endangered. Disturbance of sleep is one of the most frequent ill-effects on the well-being of infants and older people and night workers who are obliged to get sleep during the day.

Climate. The adverse environmental influences of climate and geography in places where there are extremes of cold and heat must not be forgotten. In *warm climates* there is increased danger to health from insect vectors (such as the mosquito in transmission of the malarial parasite).

Pest-control is thus an important means of improving environmental health. At the same time the use of chemical pesticides and certain organic compounds has brought about a new danger of contamination of water and of soil and consequently of food products.

In many parts of the world, and particularly in some tropical countries, many infestations cause diseases which impair health and reduce energy and ability to work. *This can form a vicious circle of disease* (see Fig. 1/1), leading to unemployment, which in turn leads to poverty, thence to malnutrition and misery. One harmful condition leads to another and sometimes with the addition of ignorance and squalor.

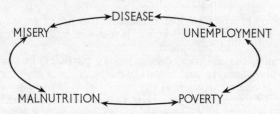

Fig. 1/1 The vicious circle of disease.

ENVIRONMENT AND THE FAMILY

Psychological influences of the surroundings may make or mar bodily as well as mental health. One need only compare a baby who receives loving attention from mother and father with high standards of health and care with the unfavourable fate of an unwanted baby born in a household where there is poor parenthood and low standards of living. In such a house there is more danger to the baby from accidents, infections, dirt and disease.

It is fair to say that *his mother is the baby's environment* during the first few months of life, and a good mother provides a good environment. A baby's well-being depends greatly on her capability and her knowledge of standards of hygiene, particularly in the field of infant feeding.

Even before birth, the fetus may be affected by outside influences—by infection of the mother from rubella or syphilis, or harmful drugs used by the mother from the fourth to sixteenth week of pregnancy.

Conclusion. Environment in its true and wide sense has a very great influence on health, but it must not be forgotten that medical and nursing care can do much to modify the harmful effects of an adverse environment. Even more important, man can control his environment and thus not only prevent it from being a hindrance to a state of well-being, but alter it for the provision of a full, healthy life.

J. L. Burn, M.D.

THE PATIENT IN THE COMMUNITY

Every hospital patient is a person who is part of the community and he is subject in his social environment to many influences for good or ill—in his home, at his work and in his leisure. In order to help him, any seemingly important factors which have led to his breakdown should be considered.

A patient should occupy a hospital bed for as short a time as is absolutely necessary. The needs of others awaiting admission, the rising accident rate, the number of beds needed for psychiatric and geriatric cases, and the shortage of hospital resources make this imperative. The patient will pass from the care of the medical and nursing staff in hospital into the care of the family doctor and, when necessary, the staff of the health authority.

In close co-operation the chief nursing officer and her staff can take a *decisive part in the health education of the patient and also in guiding the relatives to help the patient towards better health.* The family's capacity to cope with health and social problems and to prevent the breakdown of the family unit, with the sad result of broken homes and deprived children, should be strengthened.

Health education (including marriage guidance and sex education) is essential for suitable housing, conditions of work favourable to health and facilities for adequate recreation which ensure that mind and personality as well as body are catered for.

Protection against special hazards to health. This embraces immunization against some infections, protection against accidents in the home and at work, and from harmful substances in the air we breathe. These will include allergenic and carcinogenic substances.

Personnel Concerned with Physical and Mental Care in the Community at present include:

The **health visitor** is a State Registered Nurse with some obstetric experience who has taken a further year's course in a wide range of subjects, including family and community relationships, the physical and emotional development of people at all ages, preparation for parenthood and factors which place people at risk, either physically or emotionally.

She or he detects early deviation from normal and is aware of the resources available to help in both urgent and long-term difficulties. She can discuss problems and persuade people to seek help or permit others to arrange help by referral. For the elderly she assesses needs and mobilizes resources.

She does not offer a service of practical nursing and will not normally expect to undertake nursing duties or other work which does not require the additional training she possesses. Her role is basically an educational one, her primary object is to promote health and she has chosen to use her nursing knowledge and experience of the effects of illness to enable her better to fulfil this role.

The **home nurse**, who is also a State Registered or State Enrolled general trained nurse with special training in district nursing, gives skilled nursing care in the home. Her work becomes increasingly varied as so many more patients, of all ages—some consider it to be 90 per cent—are nursed at home.

In addition to her general care of the patient's toilet and the prevention of pressure sores, the administration of injections, suppositories and enemas, see Chapters 4, 9 and 10, the home nurse attends to the improvement of the patient's immediate environment, to his nutritional and social needs and, in collaboration with the family doctor, to his medical care. Because of his early discharge from hospital, she performs many other duties: to mention only a few, surgical dressings, removal of stitches, catheterization, changing in-dwelling catheters, the early care of ileostomies and colostomies, the use of respirators and dialysis units. She also has the care of the elderly and disabled people domiciled at home.

The **home help** assists by cleaning, cooking and shopping and other forms of domestic work, when there is an elderly person needing help, illness, an emergency or grave disability.

The **Public Health Inspector** carries out the task of lessening the environmental evils such as bad housing, dirty air, unsafe food. Pest-control and sometimes refuse disposal come under his care. Noise control, an increasing health hazard, may also be within his province.

The **physiotherapist** makes an increasingly important contribution to rehabilitation both in the home and in the schools for physically handicapped children.

The **chiropodist** gives skilled care, working either from a clinic or in the home. The elderly, the disabled, and those patients, e.g. diabetics, in need of special chiropodial care should be able to rely on his services.

The social worker for mentally ill and subnormal patients. He is available for advice and support for the family of the mentally disordered.

Brief mention may be made of the *Social Security service* which provides financial assistance in time of need. It includes sickness, unemployment, maternity benefits and family allowances and a graduated pension scheme in addition to the present pension. Supplementary allowances can be made to meet special needs such as those for the blind.

Welfare Services locally provide special facilities and accommodation for the aged and disabled. Lastly, the voluntary services, including the numbers of young people who throw themselves with interest and zeal into any work needed, greatly assist in social services not provided by official bodies, particularly with the housebound and lonely.

Problems of health today are far wider and more difficult than formerly, and the help of the psychologist and sociologist is increasingly needed. For example, addiction to drugs, to alcohol and to cigarettes and the excessive consumption of carbohydrates are largely preventable personal problems when when established need medico-socio-economic measures for their relief.

WITHIN THE NATIONAL HEALTH SERVICE

This is the present position. When the National Health Service started it was thought that everyone would have access to the most modern treatment and that all would be healthier. Perhaps this is the case, but other diseases now preoccupy us. The infections causing the deaths of infants and young children and the middle-aged have been brought under control by comparatively inexpensive methods, whereas heart disease, cancer and cerebro-vascular accidents are present problems in the Western world and to cope with them is much more expensive, demands a large team of specialists and very complex equipment.

The costs of patient hospital treatment are rising and may reach a figure which resources would be unable to support. This has already given rise to *five-day wards* and *day hospitals* and we are on the way to the provision of a comprehensive health centre serving an area. *That brings the patient back into the community.*

A patient who has experienced the benefits of the Welfare State is at present demanding much more help and attention from his doctor. A man who would have been content with aspirin and hot lemon for a febrile condition 10 years ago now expects either antibiotics or other drugs on prescription. 'Medicine is news'; people everywhere are reading, listening and watching television; they have knowledge and are capable of criticism and will press towards a high standard of care. A patient operated on as a 'day case' and sent home the same evening will expect the community to provide the expert care he might have had in hospital.

All this needs new thinking, first towards a unified health and nursing service which may mean considerable changes in the preparation of doctors and nurses and the training also of other groups for work in the community. Already more nurses are attracted to the community health and social services, a field which is increasingly varied as surgical patients are discharged from hospital earlier, more children are being nursed at home and the teaching of health is being correlated throughout the world.

The establishment of conferences and congresses at national and international level, where a number of disciplines meet to pool experience and consider ways and means of providing comprehensive nursing and social care, is most encouraging. When the same problems are ventilated in different parts of the world at the same time, progress is made and provision should follow.

Chapter 2

Reception and Admission of a Patient

Reception and admission—taking a history—observations—the religion of the patient—preparation for initial examination—discharge and transfer of patients—convalescence—the needs of a child in hospital

---

The nurse as hostess. The courtesy with which every patient is received, a courtesy which must be maintained throughout his stay, cannot be overestimated.

The apprehension of many patients coming into hospital cannot be exaggerated. There is always fear of the unknown and of what the immediate future may hold, but the nurse who receives a patient can dispel most of his fears and change a somewhat formal situation into a less upsetting informal one.

The admission card which has been made out at his initial interview will give sufficient details to guide the nurse in her dealings with this patient:

His name   The diagnosis
   address   reason for admission
   general practitioner   religion

Glancing at the details and addressing him by name and prefix she might ask what sort of journey he had, whether he has had to wait, when he last had some food or a drink, and act according to the information she receives.

Observing his condition without appearing to do so, the nurse will note:

His general appearance and condition.
The attitude he adopts in sitting or standing, whether he seems comfortable or in pain.
His mental attitude, cheerful or depressed.
Does he look cold? He may be trembling or shivering.
The character of his breathing, any difficulty or cough.
The colour of his skin and the condition of his eyes and lips.

These observations are developed on pp 14–15.

All this has taken only a matter of seconds. Most patients admitted do not go to bed immediately; he and his relatives can see the plan of the ward, the position of his bed, the accommodation for his personal possessions and clothing, the situation of the bathrooms, toilet and day rooms.

They should be told of the arrangements for visiting, the postal arrangements, visits of barber and hairdresser, supply of daily papers, library facilities and so on.

Questions will be asked and the opportunity should be taken to make sure that the relatives are at the address on the admission slip, or to obtain their address, give them the telephone number of the hospital and the ward extension number.

The relatives may like a private word with the nurse, when she can learn of any likes and dislikes the patient has, how many pillows he is used to sleeping on; they will be glad to know what fruit or food they may bring in for the patient and, if some of his outdoor clothes are taken home, it is as well to have a list so that everyone may know which articles he has with him in hospital. Any money and valuables he wishes to have with him can be similarly listed and if desired can be sent to a safe room and a receipt be given for them.

Depending entirely on the reason for hospitalization, and indeed on the type of hospital, the nurse's responsibilities may vary. She may be required to take the initial case history or alternatively she may accompany the medical officer concerned with admission. Whether the nurse takes the history or not, she must be conversant with its details in order to collaborate fully in the care of the patient. The following details will be required:

> The patient's previous illnesses.
> Whether the relatives consider that his present condition may be associated with any of these illnesses.
> Any distressing symptoms of the present illness, and any measures which seem to give relief.
> The diet the patient has been having.
> The normality of micturition.
> His bowel habit and any laxatives he has been taking.
> Whether he has ever had any tendency to a nervous illness, fainting or fits.
> How long he has been away from work and what his reactions have been.

Talking over with the nurse the history of his illness and what he is complaining of and what he thinks about it all go far to making a patient realize that the nurse is interested and that she *cares*.

In taking the history of the present illness, the following points have to be considered.

Present complaints, i.e. of what symptoms the patient complains.

How the illness began, and whether the patient has been completely in bed, or getting up for sanitary purposes. Questions regarding the condition of his *appetite, bowels* and *urine*; the quantity and character of the *sleep* he usually obtains.

If the patient complains of coughing and pain in the chest, inquiries should be made regarding the character of the cough, whether paroxysmal, whether the patient coughs more first thing in the morning, or after exertion, or after eating. The existence of any expectoration, character of it, including the colour and quantity, whether it is difficult to bring up, and if it has an unpleasant taste or smell.

Having asked questions on the points about which a patient has complained, the nurse should then proceed to discover any other symptoms and, in order to elicit fairly accurate and comprehensive information, she might consider the different systems of the body, taking them each in turn and running through them in her mind.

At the same time it is important to avoid putting questions in such a way as to suggest that the patient had any particular symptom.

Nervous system. Headache, drowsiness, sleeplessness, any wanderings of the mind or delirium, fits of twitchings, pain, hyperaesthesia or anaesthesia and any other sensory symptoms such as tingling and profuse sweatings.

Respiratory system. Cough, sputum, breathlessness, and blood-spitting.

Circulatory system. Palpitation, pain over the heart, swelling of the ankles or other parts of the body, attacks of faintness or fatigue, coldness of extremities, pallor or blueness, any sense of fullness in the neck, pulsation or throbbing of the blood vessels.

Alimentary system. Loss of appetite, nausea, vomiting, diarrhoea, constipation, abdominal pain or indigestion. Blood loss from mouth or anus and occurrence of jaundice.

Renal system. Character of urine, regarding quantity, whether scanty or copious, the colour and any deposit. Any difficulty in passing urine, including any pain on passing it, having to get up in the night to pass urine, frequent micturition during the day, the presence of any blood in the urine and whether there is any offensive odour. She should also inquire whether there is any pain in the loins, or over the bladder, whether the ankles swell at night or whether the patient wakens with puffiness of the face or under the eyes. Symptoms such as nausea or headache may accompany renal disorder.

In admitting women patients, the nurse should inquire regarding the regularity of menstruation, its character, including the number of pads used, any discomfort experienced, and whether this is sufficient to incapacitate the patient; also the presence of any vaginal discharge; and she should obtain a brief outline of the history of any pregnancies, abortions or miscarriages.

In admitting a child, all particulars must be obtained from those who bring him and, in order to do this effectively, the nurse should make it her business to receive the full confidence of the person who may be, and probably is, the mother of the child.

History of birth. It may be possible for the nurse to say, 'What a lovely baby—did he have a normal birth?', and having thus gained the mother's heart she will hear the full story of this and can then interpose questions which will elicit any history of abnormality at the time of birth.

Breast feeding. Whether this was carried out and was satisfactory, or, if the child had to be artificially fed, the type of food used and the results obtained.

Normal childhood. Whether the child had any infectious diseases; if so, at what age, and whether he was nursed in hospital or at home, and any complications which occurred.

Convulsions. Without actually mentioning this terrifying word, the nurse in a casual way may say, 'I suppose the child has never had any fits when teething', and this again will elicit the history as to whether the eruption of the teeth was normal or irregular.

School life. The health when at school, and the regularity of attendance —irregularity of attendance usually means defective health, either mental or physical.

Appetite, condition of *bowels,* and *sleep,* particularly whether the child sleeps all night; particulars of any *night fears* or *bedwetting.*

The *history of the present illness* will next be elicited on the lines indicated in the case of an adult.

It is usual to ask if the child has been immunized, vaccinated and christened. In the event of christening having been omitted, find out the wishes of the parents should the child become suddenly dangerously ill.

If the child is being admitted for operation, consent for the operation should be obtained from the parents.

In admitting immigrants, one may need an interpreter when the history is taken. It is essential to ascertain which of the accompanying friends are the nearest relatives and the address where they can be found. Any dietary details due to religious customs should be taken and referred to the dietitian.

OBSERVATIONS ON A PATIENT'S CONDITION

Nursing observations are necessary from the moment a patient enters a ward until his discharge. The keenness and interest which a student displays when she first enters the hospital should never be permitted to lapse into routine. She should always be on the look-out for something new and she will never be disappointed.

The first observations made have been noted at the initial interview, see p. 11. These are now further developed as time and opportunity permit.

The *condition of the hair,* whether lank and damp, dull or bright, and the presence of nits or lice; the hair may be separated in order to ascertain the condition of the scalp.

The *expression of the face,* particularly whether drawn as in pain; the condition of the *eyes,* any discharge from them; whether the pupils are uneven, normal size; whether the sclerae are white, or too bluish-white which indicates anaemia; whether jaundiced or bloodshot; whether the eyes are sunken or prominent; is there any squint, ptosis, or other abnormality of the eyelids, such as oedema, ulcers, deformed eyelashes? Is the patient wearing an artificial eye?

The *nose,* whether it moves in breathing, indicating dyspnoea, whether pinched and blue, the presence of beads of perspiration on it, whether the edge of the nostrils are sore, or covered with crusts, and the presence of any herpes.

The *lips,* their colour, whether steady or trembling, whether dry or moist, the presence of any sores, cracks or sordes.

The *mouth* is carefully inspected when it is cleansed; but at this point the nurse might ask the patient to open his mouth, in order to get a general impression of the condition of his teeth, and to put out his tongue so that she may notice whether it is dry or moist, red or grey, furred, cracked, smooth or oedematous, whether it is marked by the impression of the teeth round its margins, and whether it is steady or trembling.

The *colour of the cheeks* should be observed as to whether a malar flush is present, whether the capillaries are prominent in this region and, in this case, whether they appear red or bluish, whether both sides of the face are even in contour and the presence of any facial paralysis.

The presence of any rash. See types of skin lesions, p. 311.

The position a patient adopts, whether he lies limply on his back, taking no apparent interest in his surroundings, or is raising himself on his pillows, apparently anxious as to what is to happen next; which side he is lying on, whether he objects to facing the light, and whether his knees are curled up, which would indicate either that he was extremely cold or perhaps in abdominal pain.

Notice also where he places his arms, particularly if he raises them above his head, which would indicate an attempt to assist the movements of the chest in breathing.

Then observe any pulsation of the veins, or any enlargement of the thyroid or lymphatic glands in the neck, and note whether the patient moves his head easily or not.

The *skin* of the trunk and limbs should be inspected for the presence of rash, abrasion, wounds, scars or swelling.

The *colour* should be noted and the *general condition of the skin*, as to whether it is dry and harsh, normally soft and flexible, or abnormally wet and sticky.

The nurse should feel the limbs, and notice whether they are hot, cold, limp, firm, whether there is any tremor, whether both sides of the body are equally developed, and whether the muscles feel limp and wasted, normally firm, or whether they are abnormally spastic and rigid.

She should be on the look-out all the time for any indication of twitching or convulsion, either local or general, and she should investigate every part, particularly the abdomen, and the back, each side of the vertebral column, for the presence of tender spots.

Any odour from the patient's body should be noted.

The *conditions of hands and feet* are deserving of special observation, since much can be learnt from them.

The *development* will perhaps suggest the type of work, and in some cases be a guide to the temperament of the individual, as to whether he is energetic or lethargic.

The *age of the patient* is often indicated by his hands, and by this is meant the physiological age rather than the actual age in years.

The *ends of the fingers and toes* should be observed for the presence of clubbing, and the *nails* as regards colour, character, particularly whether cracked and brittle or deformed—the state of these is often an indication of the amount of interest the patient takes in his personal appearance.

The nurse should observe his mode of speech, and by talking to him a little about his condition she may elicit very valuable information (see also details of taking a history, p. 12) such as the condition of his appetite, his likes and dislikes in regard to food. She should find out when he last had his bowels open and any specially troublesome symptoms he may be suffering from, such as coughing, vomiting or insomnia.

All these considerations serve to demonstrate the attitude of the nurse in her care for the patient's welfare.

THE RELIGIOUS NEEDS OF A PATIENT

It is fundamental that a nurse has the right attitude to Ministers of Religion to whom she should be kindly and courteous as she would be to members of the medical staff. In the early part of her training a nurse soon learns how to deal with patients and members of the medical team; but she may be diffident in her relations with Ministers of Religion and may not understand that they are attending to a patient's needs from a different aspect.

Considerable stress is laid at present on nursing the total patient and this is important, for the patient is not merely a sick body, but a human being—a person. His needs are more than bodily and mental (psychiatric), they are spiritual as well. It is therefore of great importance that the nurse, no matter what her own convictions may be, should be aware of the spiritual needs of her patients and should cultivate the correct attitude to those equipped and appointed to deal with this aspect of patient-care.

Great influence is exercised on the health of a patient by his religious beliefs and practices. *He does not abdicate his right to spiritual attention by entering hospital.* A nurse is not competent to supply his spiritual needs and must never impede a patient's right to have these needs attended to.

The Minister of Religion is the competent authority in this case and has the right to attend to his patients, he is a member of the hospital staff appointed by the regional health authority or Management Committee to perform his special function in the therapeutic team. Sometimes a patient will wish to see a Minister of Religion who is a friend rather than the official chaplain of the hospital. Any failure to afford a Minister of Religion the facilities he requires can cause great distress to a patient and to his relatives. Thus two points should be kept in mind:

The patient's right to spiritual attention.
The right of the Minister of Religion to attend to his patients.

The details of the requirements when attending to any patient should be sought from the appropriate Minister of Religion. If a nurse is requested to do anything which troubles her conscience she should consult her own Minister of Religion.

In danger of death, even though not immediate, the religion of the patient should be ascertained if not already known, and the Minister of Religion should be informed immediately of the condition of the patient.

PREPARATION FOR THE EXAMINATION OF A PATIENT

A nurse should have some knowledge of the routine examination of a patient so that she may be able to prepare what is needed and anticipate the wishes of the doctor whom she is assisting.

The physical examination is carried out as follows:

By inspection. The light must be good, the room warm and the patient comfortable, and not unduly exposed. Inspection provides information regarding the general condition of the patient's body.

Palpation. By touching and handling different parts of the body, alterations and variations in development are found. For example, in diseases of the lungs, palpation would discover that there was less movement on one side of the chest than on the other. Palpation of a tumour would provide information regarding its character and size.

Percussion. By tapping an area of the body over different organs, the note obtained will suggest the presence of air, when this is *resonant*; and of some fluid or other cause of solidity when the note obtained is *dull*.

Auscultation. This means listening to the sounds of the heart and lungs, usually by means of a stethoscope. It is very important that friction rub between clothing should not be permitted to take place during auscultation.

Preparation of the patient for any definite form of examination. The patient should be told of the nature of the examination unless he is too ill, or for some reason incapable of taking any interest in the matter. The following points should be taken into consideration.

The light should be good, whether it is artificial or natural. The patient should be placed in such a position that shadow does not fall on the part under examination.

Absolute quiet is essential—the patient should not talk and the nurses should move as quietly as possible. The bedclothes should be handled quietly and gently, as even the rustling of these may make it difficult for the doctor to detect the sound he is listening for, or the note he is trying to elicit in percussion.

The bed and personal clothing should be conveniently arranged so that different parts of the body can be exposed with comparative ease, without undue movement and unnecessary exposure of the patient's body, as the examination progresses.

For examination of the chest the patient may be lying in the semi-recumbent position or sitting. If he is sitting, support should be supplied for the lower part of the back so that his lumbar region does not ache. As separate sides of the chest are examined the nurse should turn the patient's head from side to side so that he does not breathe directly into the doctor's face.

When the *back of the chest* is to be examined, the personal clothing should either be removed or drawn well up to the root of the neck, and well forward on each side, so that the area of the axillae is clearly visible. The patient may sit up leaning forward, or lie forward on one side in a semi-prone position. When the former posture is used, draw the pillows down to the small of the back as the patient sits, to give support there; and support the patient from the front by putting one arm across his chest, unless the doctor prefers that he should lean forward—in this case see that the patient's arms are resting on his knees in front of him, and not held stiffly at his sides.

Examination of the abdomen. It is important that the bladder be empty, otherwise the patient is anxious about this. The patient should lie on his back quite straight and flat with his arms down by the sides of his body. The doctor may require his knees to be either straight or slightly flexed. The shoulders and chest should be protected by a small jacket, or by a covering folded round, shawl fashion. The bedclothes should be folded down to below the pubes as the patient lies ready. The lower part of the trunk may be covered by a blanket, towel or sheet which can easily be moved about during the examination.

It is a good plan to tuck one of the coverings, which has been folded down, under the patient's buttocks; this prevents the clothes slipping, and gives a sense of confidence that exposure will be avoided, for which the patient will be exceedingly grateful.

When the *pubic region* is included in the examination it is usual to place a disposable towel over the folded bedclothes, as the nurse will find it easier to manipulate this small article during the doctor's movements.

Examination of the legs and feet. For examination of this region of the body, the bedclothes should be untucked at the sides and bottom of the bed, and turned up to above the knees, leaving one covering over the legs. Both legs ought to be exposed. The sheet can be turned back onto the other bedclothes, or pleated up in folds to lie between the legs, so that it can be in readiness to cover one leg when one is finished with.

EXAMINATION OF THE DIFFERENT CAVITIES OF THE BODY

Examination of the mouth. In order to be able to report upon its condition, the nurse should ask the patient to open his mouth, and observe the condition of his *tongue*, whether it is clean or furred; the presence of any cracks or fissures, and whether the patient moves it easily or not.

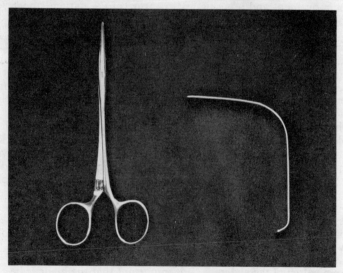

Fig. 2/1 One example of a tongue depressor and a pair of artery forceps in which swabs can be held securely. *In addition* there will be needed a good light, Anglepoise lamp or torch, swabs, several wooden spatulae, a disposable towel to put under the patient's chin, and a disposable bag for all disposable used articles. A receiver should also be supplied for any non-disposable instruments. A mouth wash should be supplied if the patient can use one.

The *teeth and gums* should be observed regarding their colour, whether they are healthy or pale and spongy, and the presence of any sordes on the teeth.

The *condition of the lips* should be inspected to see whether they are cracked or fissured; whether there are any little ulcers or sores on the inside of the lips; the presence of herpes, and the colour of the lips should also be noted.

In order **to inspect the throat**, the nurse should ask the patient to put his tongue out and say 'ah'. This will permit examination of the upper part of the pharynx. She should then take a spatula, place it gently on the tongue, as the tongue lies in the mouth, not protruded. She should place the spatula about halfway along the tongue and press gently, and again ask the patient to say 'ah', when the soft palate and uvula, the posterior pharyngeal wall and tonsil area can be seen. She will notice whether these tissues are normal, pale, injected or congested, whether there is any exudate or any membrane, whether any deposit is present in the follicles of the tonsils, or whether the whole area is covered with an exudate.

As the mouth and throat are examined, the odour of the breath should be noted.

Rectal examination

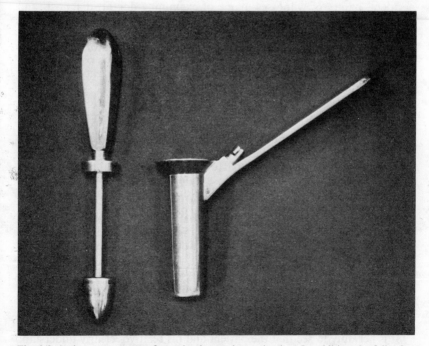

Fig. 2/2 A short proctoscope for a simple rectal examination. In addition the following articles will be required for a patient to be examined on a bed or couch: a disposable glove; paper towel; swabs and lubricant; disposable bag.

Other articles sometimes needed include: sterile laboratory swabs and pathology forms; an Anglepoise lamp.

Preparation. The patient should empty his bladder before the examination, which is generally carried out with him in the left lateral position (see Chapter 8, p. 79).

For a more extensive examination carried out in a rectal clinic see Chapter 51, p. 488.

For examination of: the ear, nose and throat, see p. 612; the eye, see p. 636; neurological conditions, see p. 257; the vagina, see p. 744.

ACCIDENTS TO PATIENTS IN HOSPITAL

The incidence of accidents occurring to patients has increased in recent years. Those most often sustained include:

> Falling out of bed.
> Falling in the ward because of unsuitable slippers.
> Tripping over unnoticed objects when unsteady after sedation.
> Slipping and falling in the bathroom.
> Burns from a heat pad or hot-water bottle.
> Scalds from spilling a cup of tea or other beverage; spilling an inhaler.
> Fainting.

Most hospitals have an accident form which includes description of accident, names of witnesses, name of examining doctor, diagnosis and nature of injury.

However minor an accident it must be reported to the charge nurse or ward sister and the form filled in. The doctor must be informed and the patient seen within 24 hours, but in a serious accident the patient is seen immediately. The examining doctor completes the accident form which is then filed.

DISCHARGE AND TRANSFER OF PATIENTS

The discharge of a patient, either to his home or to some other hospital or to an institution, is a very important undertaking. Everything therefore should be done to make his departure easy and as free from anxiety as possible, and he should also be given an opportunity to express his opinion as to whether he has been comfortable during his time in hospital and whether there is anything he would like to say regarding this.

A day or two before the date of discharge the relatives or friends are informed that they may come for the patient at a given time on a stated day and, if they have taken any of his outdoor clothes home, they are asked to bring them when they come.

The ward sister or *head nurse* sees that the patient is ready to go home, that he is recently bathed, that his head is clean and that he has safely in his own custody, if he is capable of this, any articles of his own which he has been using and, at the last minute, any valuables which have been kept safely locked up for him.

It is her duty to see that the patient and his relatives clearly understand the nature of any treatment which is to be carried out at home—and that he knows whether he is to come to the hospital to be seen again and, if so, that he is quite clear about the date and time of his visit.

When the friends arrive and the patient is ready dressed, the ward sister sees that they are given all the patient's belongings, or alternatively, a porter may come to the ward for the patient and he will take care of them.

Transfer to another hospital or institution. Should a patient have to be transferred to another hospital, it is usual to inform the relatives of this first; if the transfer has to be made quickly, it may proceed before they have received the information, but the nurse, while making arrangements for it, must try to get in touch with the relatives. If, however, they have not arrived by the time the patient departs, she must see the driver of the ambulance or other person who comes to take the patient away, and obtain the address of the place to which the patient is going, in order to give or send this to the relatives at the earliest opportunity.

As a rule all the patient's belongings will be sent with him—if not, they are given to the relatives when they call and a receipt is obtained.

Case sheet. Immediately on the discharge of a patient the ward sister examines the bed card, sees that it is complete, removes any unused sheets and sends it to the department where records are kept; unless the patient has been transferred to another ward or department, in which case she sees that the bed card accompanies the patient to his new ward.

Treatment of the bed, sheets, etc., after discharge of a patient. The bed is stripped, all linen sent to the laundry, waterproofs washed and disinfected, or, if disposable, destroyed; the furniture, including the bed, washed, disinfected and polished.

Charts and bed cards are placed ready for the next patient; also visiting cards, to be given to the relatives on admission of the patient who is next to occupy the bed.

The **discharge of a patient with a communicable disease**, or one who has been suffering from some infective condition, is rather more complicated.

After any infection, however slight, the mattress, pillows, bedding and both the bed linen and patient's personal linen, should all be treated as is customary in the hospital, and all the utensils which have been used for the patient should be sterilized. The soap and washcloths should be burnt. The bed and other furniture, the area of the floor around the bed, and between it and the adjacent beds and wall space behind this area, should be well washed with soap and water.

If the patient has been occupying a separate room or small isolation ward, it will probably be fumigated with one of the disinfectant aerosol preparations.

CONVALESCENCE

Convalescence is recovery from illness and a return to health. When a person falls ill he wonders what may happen to him and whether he will recover completely. From that moment he is convalescent, and everything contributes to his recovery.

First aid given in any emergency.
Medical, surgical and nursing care and physiotherapy.
Visits from relatives and friends.

Whatever a patient does, whether he reads, talks, writes, puts a puzzle together, does a crossword or is engaged in some planned occupation such as carpentry, painting or handwork; all these incidents, rightly used, help in his recovery.

In a hospital ward the sister is responsible for the convalescence. She will ensure that a patient is not exposed to the sight of others dangerously ill, or recovering from operation.

If he, himself, has been operated on, she will position him so that he feels better, give him a drink as soon as possible, which indicates that all is going well.

If any apparatus has been brought to the bedside, e.g. for blood transfusion, it will be cleared away immediately and thus produce the atmosphere of reassurance he needs.

Recovery. *Patients need a warm welcome to the place where they will spend this period*; and any treatment, any precautions they should take, and the routine of the establishment should be clearly explained.

Those in charge should do all they can to provide a happy social environment.

Good food, rest, acceptable companionship and some occupation adapted to the interests and ability of the individual, and to his state of health should be provided. Patients should follow a planned routine in order to re-adapt to a normal disciplined life.

Any source of irritation, tension and anxiety should be avoided. For example, a mother cannot relax unless she is sure her home and children are cared for; a child should be aware that his parents will visit, and if possible his mother should accompany him to the recovery home and see him settled in.

Nurses should be capable, but also tactful and sympathetic. They must never forget that for full and complete recovery the patient's co-operation is essential, and that he needs to have confidence, hope and courage. Getting better is not easy; it can be depressing and difficult, but these factors can be offset by a good environment and help from the nurse.

THE NEEDS OF A CHILD IN HOSPITAL

The nursing of sick children, *paediatric nursing*, is a specialized field, but nurses in any type of hospital may well have children as patients and be glad of some guidance (apart from the medical and surgical conditions) in the care of them.

A few principles are outlined here. It is important to understand the healthy as well as the sick child, and to understand the prevention of disease and accidents. The essentials of child nursing are the same as when caring for an adult but adaptations are necessary because of differences in understanding, sensitivity, size, interest, etc. It is vital to work with and through the child's parents or guardians and essential to be able to interest and comfort the child, to inspire courage and to gain the child's confidence and co-operation. The aim of hospital care should be to change the child's routine as little as possible and to make his environment as pleasant as the ward permits. If a child is very ill or apprehensive the mother should stay in the hospital. If this is not possible, she might remain to tuck the child up for the night. Telephone messages, the occasional postcard or a little letter can give great pleasure and help to reassure the child more than is realized. Frequent visits by the parents make their comings and goings acceptable to the child as routine, and their departures less disturbing.

A child's basic needs are *security*, *love* and *play* and the nurse acting as mother-substitute should do her best in the interest of the normal development of the child to provide these.

Security. The *residence* of the mother and *her visits* have been mentioned. Her help in caring for her child at mealtimes and bedtime and the extra attention she can give play a real part in the care of a sick child.

The nurse as mother-substitute. The first contact with the nurse is most important, as she must become a friend to be trusted in this strange environment. The nurse might suggest he keeps a favourite toy, and discuss with the mother his food likes and dislikes, and ascertain his toilet habits, which will give him a feeling of security. It brings confidence if the nurse is there during any unpleasant treatment, with some petting and spoiling afterwards and praise for his courage.

An older boy or girl might be brought to look upon any treatment and operation as an adventure, thus providing something to explore and overcome.

A child should never, even unknowingly, be deceived. His questions should be answered honestly. If he is given medicine he should know it is medicine; if it is disguised in a spoonful of jam, he should be told why, otherwise if he is unable to trust the nurse his sense of security will diminish.

Preparation for sleep. It is a good plan to learn from the parents how the child is settled down for the night, which toy he likes to have beside him and any prayers he says which the nurse should go over with him.

Love. The emotional development of a child depends on the love of a mother (or her substitute) and contact with her body, in which love is demonstrated. This is particularly so in the case of infants and toddlers. Physical contact with the nurse will supply the infant's needs in his mother's absence. A child expects to find harmony in his environment. He expects to be accepted, loved and liked.

Play. A baby plays with his toes and fingers; as he develops he explores and plays with his body, and as he grows everything he handles becomes a plaything. The nurse can make all his little activities savour of play: washing, dressing, changing clothes, preparing for and eating his meals, getting up and so on. This may take longer but is time well spent as it contributes to his psychological development.

Play is an essential part of children's lives, as through it they can temporarily forget their fears, can learn, explore, develop and grow. It is essential that during their stay in hospital children should be as occupied and as happy as at home.

The inclusion of 'play ladies', who are preferably nurses or nursery nurses specializing in play therapy, or alternatively a young occupational therapist, is of great value in preventing boredom when a child is getting better, and even when he is ill there will be intervals which can be filled with interest and occupation. 'Play ladies' are part of the ward team, and each day should be carefully informed of the children's medical progress and the need for any special observations or restrictions. No child is kept in bed longer than is necessary, the majority are up and dressed so that all types of play and games can be introduced. Praise for good accomplishment should be liberal. A child will be happy doing things he enjoys at home.

There is a great deal to consider when dealing with children, who are easily pleased and easily hurt. One's gestures, voice and attention should all be considered. A child may not comprehend words, but he understands tone and attitude. Most mothers are careful, they seem to have an intuition where their own children are concerned. Nurses have to acquire this knowledge, but a real love for children will help them to avoid the numerous pitfalls which may distress their little charges.

Little ears hear everything and put their own construction on what they hear. Therefore careless gossip should not be indulged in within the hearing of a child. Even a bad weather report should not be discussed in front of a child; it may so dismay him that he is afraid to go to sleep.

Listening. Children are naturally truthful, even though they have not reached the age of reason but may live in a phantasy world, like the child who will say, 'I've got a friend at the bottom of the garden. I tell him everything.' Another will tell his toy everything. He may say, 'My head hurts', 'My ear hurts', and he may tell a nurse. Never neglect the complaint of a child. It is true and the ache he speaks of may have some real significance. Report it to sister or head nurse. Never belittle what a child says, as he may not speak of that subject again and it may be most important.

Sometimes a child does not accommodate easily to being in hospital. He may be unhappy, crying, distrustful, suspicious or even apparently hostile. He is not naughty, only frightened. The nurse may seem to fail in all attempts to console him, but thinking of this child as a child she must not resent him, neither should she press her attentions on him. By doing her work in the ward calmly, being courteous to his relatives and visitors, noting towards whom he looks, whether he seems to regard a certain toy with desire, she may begin to know him. Her interest and love will win through, otherwise there will just be a little child, like a wild bird in a cage, fed and watered but not happy. One day a smile will reveal his dawning trust and only then will the child be ready to respond to her affection.

Sudden and dramatic changes can take place in the condition of sick children which may be most alarming. A child may be prostrate and listless, with a high temperature and all the indications of acute illness; and yet within an hour or two, or less, he may be sitting up playing with his toys. This tendency demands constant, intelligent observation, as prompt and correct attention given during an acute phase can result in stimulating the remarkable recuperative powers children possess. All changes should be noted, including the time factor, as only a physician can decide the significance of any untoward symptom or group of symptoms.

Chapter 3

Temperature, Pulse and Respiration

Temperature: the variations of temperature in health and disease—the clinical thermometer—methods of taking the body temperature— charting—the stages of rigor. Pulse: the variations of the pulse in health and disease—abnormal pulses. Blood pressure, taking and charting. Respiration: variations of respiration in health and disease— abnormal respirations—dyspnoea and cyanosis

The **normal body temperature** is 36·9 °C or 98·4 °F, having a diurnal range from 36·3 to 37·2 °C, or 97·4 to 99 °F. The temperature is taken by means of a clinical thermometer, which registers from 95° to 110° on the Fahrenheit scale. It is so constructed that it retains its reading even when removed from the patient. The mercury rises up the tube from the bulb in response to heat, but is prevented from falling, until it is shaken down, by a slight constriction above the bulb of mercury. For comparison of the Centigrade and Fahrenheit scales, see Fig. 3/1.

In health very little variation of temperature occurs. The degree recorded depends on the part of the body in which the temperature is taken. A *rectal* temperature gives the highest reading, probably two degrees higher than the *skin* temperature and one degree higher than a temperature taken in the *mouth*.

In conditions of starvation and after exposure to cold and during sleep the temperature is a little lower. It may be slightly increased by muscular activity, by mental excitement or any other form of nervous tension and also by taking a hot bath or sitting closely over a fire or by exposure to an abnormally humid atmosphere; but these variations are slight and usually only temporary.

The body temperature is higher in the evening than in the morning.

Variation in disease. The temperature is *decreased* in all conditions which produce dehydration, as in vomiting and diarrhoea, severe haemorrhage, marked toxaemia and in conditions of shock and collapse. It is also depressed in certain conditions of auto-intoxication as in jaundice. The temperature is *increased* in all febrile conditions, of which there are many causes, including infective conditions, metabolic disorders, and derangements of the heat-regulating centre such as occur in certain nervous conditions.

It is very important for a nurse to realize that a condition of fever,

pyrexia or temperature—all these terms being used synonymously to indicate a rise in temperature—is *protective in function* because the increased
temperature is generally antagonistic to the growth of the organisms
causing the disease.

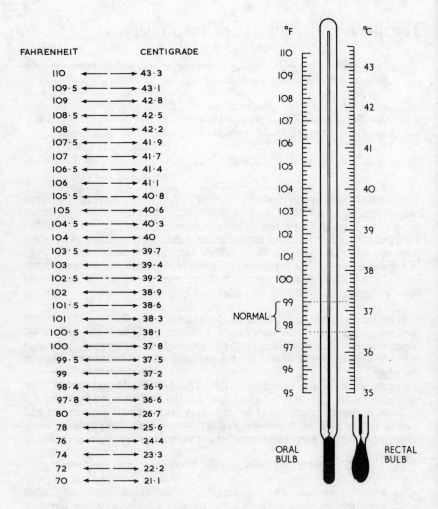

Fig. 3/1 Comparative scale between Fahrenheit and Centigrade. Low-registering
thermometers recording temperatures
down to 21 °C or 70 °F are available (see
text, p. 28. A high-registering thermometer recording figures above 43·3 °C or
110 °F may be required in certain circumstances, e.g. illness due to heat, generally in
tropical countries.

Fig. 3/2 A clinical thermometer. One registering 35 to 43·5 °C is shown.

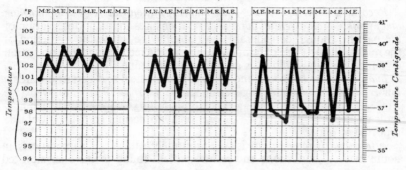

Fig. 3/3 Types of pyrexia (constant, remittent and intermittent).

Degrees of temperature (Centigrade and Fahrenheit scale):

Hyperpyrexia, over 40·6 °C or 105 °F.

Pyrexia, High: 39·4 to 40·6 °C or 103 to 105 °F.

Moderate: 38·3 to 39·4 °C or 101 to 103 °F.

Low: 37·2 to 38·3 °C or 99 to 101 °F.

Normal, 36·9 °C (ranging from 36·3 to 37·2 °C) or 98·4 °F (97·4 to 99 °F).

Subnormal, 35 to 36·1 °C or 95 to 97 °F.

Collapse, below 35 °C or 95 °F.

Types of fever (temperature or pyrexia) (see Fig. 3/3).

Constant, when the fever, remaining high, varies not more than two degrees between night and morning.

Remittent, a fever characterized by variations of more than two degrees between night and morning, but which does not reach normal during the 24 hours.

Intermittent. This is also described as *hectic*, or *swinging*, because the range of temperature varies from normal or subnormal to high fever at intervals varying from 24 hours to two or three days, but whatever the duration, the changes occur with a fair amount of regularity.

Irregular. A fever not corresponding to any of the above three groups, but manifesting characteristics of some or all of them at one time or another.

Inverse. In this type the highest range of temperature is recorded in the morning hours, and the lowest in the evening, which is contrary to that found in the normal.

Apyretic. Sometimes an infectious disease, e.g. typhoid fever will run its course without any increase in temperature. This is described as an apyretic type.

THE CLINICAL THERMOMETER

Those in use are mercury filled, with a constricting bore, fitted with a magnifying lens and short temperature range.

Before taking a patient's temperature, the level of the mercury should be below 35·5 °C (96 °F); if not it must be shaken down by a flicking movement of the wrist. The bulb varies in shape as indicated in Fig. 3/2.

Recording the temperature, pulse and respiration rate regularly, morning and evening, is an essential nursing duty. It ensures frequent observation of the patient, though considerable latitude may be left to the discretion of the nurse. The first rise of temperature in adults recovering from operation or during a medical illness is an important warning sign.

In a premature baby unit and generally in medical and geriatric wards *a low-reading thermometer* registering 21 °C and 70 °F is employed (see Fig. 3/1). In debilitated and aged persons a falling temperature which may indicate hypothyroidism (see p. 292) or hypothermia (p. 342) should be reported at once.

A four-hourly temperature is taken routinely after surgical operations, in acute medical conditions and in any patient found to have an elevated temperature.

Nurses working in intensive care units or nursing patients with vascular disease of the limbs will learn the use of skin thermometers based on the traditional glass bulb system, the thermo-couple, or the newer electronic devices.

The temperature may be taken most conveniently in the mouth, rectum, or on the skin of the axilla, groin or popliteal space. A thermometer should never come in contact with a diseased part. Each patient should have his individual thermometer fitted to the wall at his bedside, or kept in a suitable container. Small disposable medicated swabs are used for wiping the thermometer, and are placed after use in a disposal bag.

The mouth. The temperature may be taken in the mouth, except in the case of infants, unconscious, delirious or insane patients, or where keeping the mouth closed would inconvenience the patient as in conditions characterized by cough, dyspnoea, or obstructed nasal breathing.

In taking the temperature in the mouth, the patient is asked to open his mouth, then the thermometer is placed under the tongue, and he is told to close the lips but not the teeth on it. The nurse should then consider whether it is necessary for her to hold the thermometer or not. It should be stated on the temperature chart if the recorded temperature was taken other than in the mouth.

After taking the temperature, read the thermometer carefully, make a note of it, then shake the mercury down below 35·6 °C (96 °F), wipe or wash the thermometer and replace it in the disinfectant.

To shake a thermometer down take hold of it between the thumb and two fingers of one hand, grasping the lower third of the thermometer just above the bulb, hold it away from the body, supinate and extend the forearm and wrist, and then sharply pronate and flex the wrist.

The rectum. A special thermometer should be kept for this, and it should have a short blunt bulb. In many hospitals quite distinctive thermometers are used, filled with alcohol instead of mercury, and having a coloured bulb.

Before insertion the thermometer bulb should be evenly lubricated for about two inches of its length, care being taken not to lubricate it too heavily lest the lubricant by forming a coating should make reading unreliable.

In the case of infants the patient should either be held face downwards on the lap for the insertion of the thermometer; or, if lying in the cot, the legs may be held up with one hand and the thermometer passed into the rectum with the other.

In older children and adults the thermometer can be inserted while the patient is in almost any position.

In all cases it is very important that the patient should keep still or be held steady while the thermometer is in the rectum, and it should be inserted for quite two inches.

Skin reading. Whether the temperature is taken in the axilla, groin or popliteal space, it is important to see that the skin surfaces are dry, and that the thermometer bulb is closely in contact with two skin surfaces in order to exclude air, since upon this the accurate recording of the temperature depends.

The *time required to obtain an accurate reading* varies according to the area where the temperature is taken, and with the type of thermometer used—some thermometers are supposed to record a temperature in half a minute, one minute, two minutes and so on, but *to obtain an absolutely accurate reading five minutes should be allowed.*

The mercury will rise most rapidly in the rectum because in the interior of the body the surfaces are very close together, and air is excluded.

The next quickest record will be obtained in the mouth, and it will take longest when the skin surface is used.

It has been found by experience that a thermometer marked to record a temperature in half a minute will usually do so if the patient is suffering from a fairly high degree of fever; but, in cases where there is a low degree of pyrexia, an accurate reading will usually not be obtained under five minutes as already mentioned.

If the nurse is at all in doubt as to the reading she has obtained and thinks it does not conform to what she knows the patient's condition might lead her to expect, she should take the temperature a second time. If she doubts the accuracy of the thermometer, she should use a second one and test the first by placing it in a little water not over 37·8 °C (100 °F).

In a few instances a nurse may have to be on the look-out for *the registering of a false temperature* either accidentally, or intentionally assisted by the patient. It may be that the patient has recently had a hot drink, or has been smoking, which might alter the temperature of the mouth locally for about half an hour. If a hot-water bottle has been near the axilla or other skin surface used, the same thing might happen there.

A temperature should not be taken within half an hour of having a bath.

Specially made thermometers are necessary in certain cases. The use of a low-registering one is mentioned on p. 28. On rare occasions a patient acutely ill may run a temperature above 43·3 °C (110 °F), in which case a high-registering thermometer will have to be used.

Mode of onset and decline of a temperature. A disease characterized by a rise in temperature may have a *rapid* or a *gradual onset*. In the former a very high temperature is reached in a few hours, frequently being ushered in by an attack of shivering which may be severe enough to be a rigor; in children convulsions more often occur.

In the case of a *gradual onset* the temperature rises a little each day until, at the end of several days or a week, it has reached its maximum degree.

Crisis. The fever may *decline suddenly* when the temperature falls in a few hours, within 24 at most; provided that there is a corresponding, though perhaps not such a complete, drop in the pulse and respiration rate.

Lysis is the term used to describe a more *gradual decline* of fever when it takes from 2 to 10 days or longer to return to normal. A *short lysis* occupies about 3 days; a *long lysis* may take from 7 to 10 days.

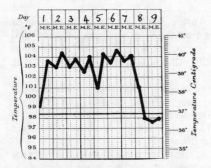

Fig. 3/4 Example of abrupt rise of temperature and rapid decline by crisis in untreated lobar pneumonia.

Fig. 3/5 Example of rapid onset and decline by lysis in a case of untreated scarlet fever.

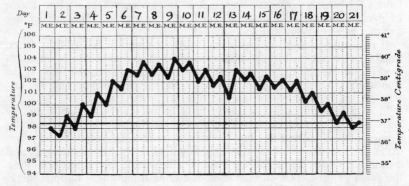

Fig. 3/6 Temperature chart in a case of untreated typhoid fever. Note gradual onset and gradual decline.

Reduction of a temperature. A rise in temperature is regarded as one of the protective mechanisms of the body, and drugs are not given as a general rule, in order to reduce it.

It is considered inadvisable to permit a patient to sustain a temperature of over 40·6 °C (105 °F), or in some instances over 39·4 °C (103 °F), for long at a time, as this leads to prostration often accompanied by delirium, which lowers the resistance of the patient and retards his recovery.

Sponging with tepid or cold water, once, twice or at regular intervals will usually give relief (see Chapter 12, p. 107). Anti-pyretic drugs may be used in some cases—aspirin is a useful one.

RIGOR

A rigor is a severe attack of shivering which may occur at the onset of disease characterized by a rise in temperature, such as pneumonia. It may also arise during the course of infective diseases and conditions. A rigor is marked by three stages which are fairly distinct one from another:

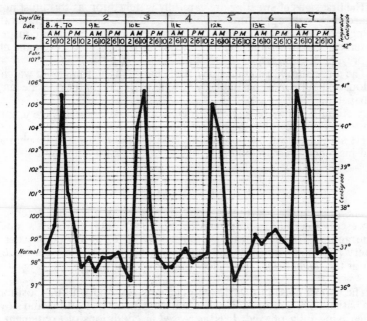

Fig. 3/7 Example of rigors occurring in benign tertian malaria (see text and Chapter 40, p. 389).

The *first* or *cold stage* in which the patient shivers uncontrollably. The skin is cold, the face pinched and blue and the pulse rapid and small. The temperature is rising rapidly and may reach 40 °C (104 °F), whilst the patient still feels cold.

The *second* or *hot stage* follows immediately. The patient is now uncomfortably hot, his skin hot and dry, and he suffers thirst and headache and tosses about in bed in an agony of restlessness. The pulse becomes full. The temperature may continue to rise.

The *third* or *stage of sweating* sets in. The skin acts, the patient sweats profusely, the temperature falls, the pulse improves and the former acute discomfort abates, though the patient is now conscious of his dripping skin and if not well cared for will get very cold and may collapse.

Nursing. A patient should not be left alone during a rigor. The different stages require appropriate treatment.

During the shivering attack the patient must be given hot drinks and have hot blankets put around him until he begins to feel warm.

During the hot stage he is given cool drinks, cool compresses are applied to his forehead or an ice-bag to his head to relieve the sensation of head congestion and pain.

The patient's temperature is carefully recorded every 10 to 15 minutes throughout the rigor, and should it rise to 40·6 °C (105 °F) or over, *cold sponging may be necessary.*

The first signs of sweating are carefully watched for, as this must not be retarded by cold applications which should then cease, the temperature being recorded as before so that the rate at which it is falling is constantly observed. The sweat must be wiped from the patient's face, neck and chest to prevent discomfort.

The nurse should rub him down and change his clothing, and watch his colour and pulse most particularly now, as at the end of the rigor he may be exhausted.

A stimulant may have been ordered which can now be given, and if made very comfortable the patient may sleep.

He should be watched constantly and his pulse rate and its character and his blood pressure noted at regular intervals for some hours.

THE ARTERIAL PULSE

The pulse is the heartbeat—conveniently felt at the wrist. Each pulse represents a cardiac cycle. A cardiac cycle includes a period of *systole* or contraction, *diastole* or rest. The pulse may be felt at any point where an artery passes superficially and lies over a bone. It is most conveniently felt at the *radial artery* just below the root of the thumb.

The normal pulse rate varies with age and sex, and with the position of the patient, being more rapid when standing than when sitting, and slowest when lying fully relaxed. It is *increased* in conditions of excitement, including anger, fear and anxiety. It is *decreased* during sleep, and to a lesser extent during rest and relaxation.

> *Pulse rate. In a newborn infant*—120 to 140 beats per minute.
> At 12 months—110 to 120.
> From 2 to 5—about 100.
> From 5 to 10—about 90.
> *Adults*—from 65 to 80 beats per minute, being five beats quicker in a woman than in a man.
> *In old age*, the pulse usually becomes slower.
> *In extreme old age*, it may quicken again. This depends on the general condition.

As a rule the *ratio of the pulse* to the respiration rate is four pulse beats to every respiration. Its ratio compared with temperature suggests that, others things being equal, the pulse will rise five beats with every degree Centigrade of temperature over 37·8 °C (or 10 beats with every degree Fahrenheit over 100 °F).

A normal pulse should show the following characteristics:

> Its *rate* should correspond with the age of the person.
> The *rhythm* should be regular.

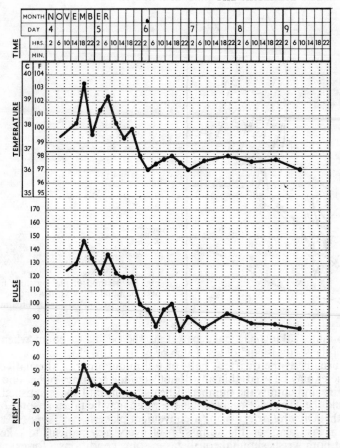

Fig. 3/8 One method of charting temperature, pulse and respiration.

The *volume* moderate.
The pulse should not be too easily compressed.

In taking a pulse the patient's hand and arm should be supported, and the muscles on the anterior aspect relaxed; this may be obtained by flexing elbow and wrist as the limb lies on the bed. If there is no indication to the contrary the arm might be laid across the patient's chest or abdomen. If this is not possible, then it should be supported on a pillow as in the accompanying figure.

The nurse gently places three fingers of one hand on the anterior surface of the forearm, just above the wrist, and feels the pulsation of the radial artery there. She notes the *rate, rhythm, volume, tension* and *degree of compressibility* and *the condition of the artery*. When familiar with the general character of the pulse the nurse is feeling, she begins to count, and counts

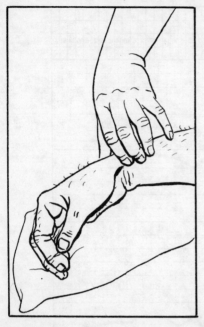

Fig. 3/9 Method of placing three fingers over the radial artery when taking the pulse. Note the patient's relaxed forearm and hand.

for a minute, taking particular care that she begins to count when the finger of the second-hand of her watch or of the ward clock is on a definite figure, usually at the quarter-, half- or full minute mark. Alternatively a pulsometer may be used. If in any doubt as to the accuracy of her findings she begins and counts the number of beats again until she is satisfied.

Should the wrists not be available the pulse may be taken at some other part—the *temporal artery* being a convenient place.

It is a wise plan, on the admission of every new patient, to take the pulse at both wrists simultaneously, as in some conditions—for example, an aneurysm of the blood vessels of one side—the pulse would be slightly delayed on the affected side and this observation by a nurse might be the first means of detecting the abnormality.

ABNORMAL PULSES

The pulse may vary in its different characteristics:

Rate. A rapid pulse may be anything up to 140—above that it is difficult to count. A term used to describe any rate above 100 is *tachycardia*, and this state may be continuous or paroxysmal. It may be functional in character or due to organic disease. A slow pulse is described as *brady-cardia*. It may be due to the fact that the cardiac contractions are not strong enough to reach the radial artery.

The **cardiac impulse** starts in the sino-atrial node near where the inferior vena cava joins the atrium. From here it is transmitted through the atrium to the *bundle of His*, which is a highly specialized neuro-muscular bundle which picks up the atrial impulses and as it were stabilizes them, acting as a *pacemaker* (which it is frequently called), and passing them on to the ventricle.

The ventricle contracts in order to force blood into the arteries, and this contraction transmitted along these vessels becomes the *pulse wave*.

A second wave, due to closure of the aortic valve, is described as a *dicrotic wave*.

In conditions of *heartblock*, a condition which may be partial or complete, impulses do not reach the ventricle. If partial, a ventricular beat, and consequently a pulse beat, may be missed at regular or irregular intervals. In complete heartblock, when no impulses pass, the ventricle contracts independently of any control from the atrium, and this results in a very slow pulse, usually below 40, and is always a serious condition.

Variation in rhythm. By rhythm is meant that beats occur at regular intervals, any interference with this results in a state of *arrhythmia*.

A pulse is described as *intermittent*, when beats are missed—for example, every third or fifth beat may be missed, or the pulse may be irregularly intermittent.

In *taking such a pulse* the nurse should count the cardiac impulses by placing her fingers over the apex beat of the heart which she will find a little to the left of the nipple line and just below it, or she might use a stethoscope, in order to enable an accurate report of cardiac beat and pulse beat to be made.

A pulse is *irregular* when the intervals between the beats are of varying length. Beats are not missed, they simply run together at one time and are widely separated at another. This condition is seen in cases of *extrasystole*, when some of the cardiac contractions occur prematurely, that is, before they are normally due in the cardiac cycle. This is caused by irritability of the muscle. The premature beat occurring before the heart is quite ready for it, is weak in character and unable to transmit the impulse to the arteries.

Auricular fibrillation is a condition in which the atria, being very irritable, are quivering rather than contracting. The bundle of His deals with this as best it can, but the result is a rapid and irregular pulse.

The prognosis of this condition is always grave though it may persist for a number of years. The patient may complain of palpitation, difficulty in breathing and swelling of the ankles.

In **sinus arrhythmia** the pulse is rapid during inspiration and slower during expiration. This is comparatively unimportant and occurs most commonly in children and, if the child is asked to hold his breath, the irregularity will disappear.

Strength. A pulse contraction should be strong enough not to be too easily compressed. This is intimately bound up with the condition of *volume*, that is, the amount of blood in the artery. The pulse is described as full, or large, or small, according to its volume.

Pulsus alternans occurs when the contraction of the ventricle varies and results in alternately weak and strong pulse beats; this is usually serious.

Another point that the nurse must be very careful to observe when taking the pulse, is the condition of the artery as it lies under her examining finger. Normally it would be soft and pliant. She should note whether it is flabby and lacking in tone, or wiry, hard and tortuous.

Dicrotic pulse. In conditions where prostration has been very marked, or grave toxaemia has been present for some time, the muscles become toneless; when this happens to the muscles of the blood vessels, the flabbiness permits the dicrotic wave, spoken of on p. 35, to be felt. This is experienced by the nurse as if she were feeling a pulse beat followed by an echo of a beat. She is really feeling a true pulse wave and also the dicrotic wave, present normally, but not normally perceptible. She should therefore take the cardiac contraction rate at the apex beat and compare the two.

Corrigan's pulse. This is named after the doctor who first described it. It is also described as a *collapsing pulse*, and *waterhammer pulse*. It is present in cases of *aortic incompetence* (see Chapter 59, p. 604).
Read also Nursing Considerations in Heart Disease, p. 128.

BLOOD PRESSURE

The **factors maintaining the blood pressure** are:

1. *The pumping force* of the heart.
2. *The quantity of circulating blood* (loss of blood lowers the pressure, giving intravenous fluid will cause it to rise again).
3. *The viscosity of the blood* derived from plasma proteins and the number of blood cells.
4. *The elasticity of the blood vessel walls* (pressure in the arteries is highest).
5. *The peripheral resistance.* This is the resistance offered to the blood passing through the vessels.

Nurses are frequently required to keep records of a patient's blood pressure. This can only be done by means of a sphygmomanometer (see p. 37).

The **normal arterial blood pressure** is estimated as being 100 plus the age in years. In a man of 20 the systolic pressure is estimated as being 120, the diastolic pressure will be fairly constant at 70. Systolic pressure varies with excitement, exercise, rest, etc., but diastolic pressure remains constant.

Increased peripheral resistance, *hypertension*, throws a greater load on the heart muscle, which becomes thickened and more powerful and this produces a pulse which is hard, full in volume and difficult to compress. The pulse in a person with low blood pressure, or *hypotension*, is low in volume, soft in character and easily compressed by the examining finger.

Persistent hypertension eventually leads to *cardiac dilatation* with weakening of the heart muscle and results in a pulse which is described as *wiry*, which means that it is hard but not of large volume. Cardiac dilatation in a person with normal blood pressure would give rise to a *weak, thready pulse*.

To take a blood pressure reading the patient lies on a bed or couch with his arm outstretched. The *sphygmomanometer* (Fig. 3/10) is placed beside his arm and on the same level; it consists of a mercury manometer, the tube calibrated in millimetres, and a collapsible bag in a cuff or armlet for encircling the arm or limb used. A pump attached to the bag has a valve which when closed retains the air pumped into the bag, and when open releases it.

This pneumatic band is wound round the arm above the elbow; it is inflated by pumping and the operator palpating the radial artery at the

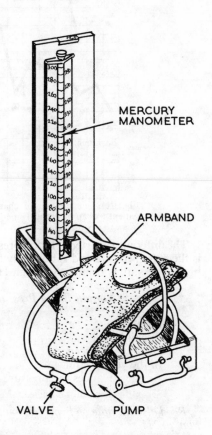

MERCURY
MANOMETER

ARMBAND

Fig. 3/10 Sphygmomanometer. A desk model is shown with arm band. Many recent models have a rigid cuff for ease of manipulation.

VALVE   PUMP

wrist notes the level of the mercury at which the pulse disappears. He then releases slightly the pressure on the arm, places his stethoscope (see Fig. 3/12) on the radial artery just below or at the bend of the elbow, and inflates the bag until the mercury registers 5 millimetres above the figure noted at the first reading.

The flow of blood into the artery is obliterated and the air in the bag is then slowly released until the first sound is heard—this is the *systolic sound* and the level of the mercury at this point gives the systolic pressure. The operator continues to release the pressure, listening carefully, the sound increases in intensity, reaches a maximum and then a first soft sound is heard followed by a second soft sound—the *diastolic sound*. The level of the mercury gives the diastolic pressure.

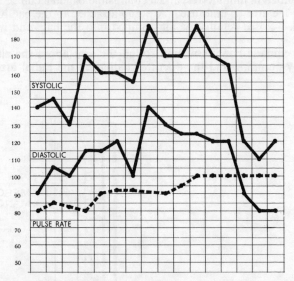

Fig. 3/11 One method of charting the blood pressure. This patient was an obstetrical emergency.

The difference in arterial blood pressure between the systole and diastole is the **pulse pressure** and is normally from 30 to 50 mm Hg. In women the blood pressure is from 5 to 10 mm Hg lower than in men.

Normal Blood Pressure Range (in mm Hg)

	DIASTOLIC	SYSTOLIC
In infancy	50	70–90
In childhood	60	80–100
During adolescence	60	90–110
In the young adult	60–70	110–125
As age advances the pressure increases .	80–90	130–150
		average—140

Read also the note on hypertension in Disorders of the Heart and Circulation, p. 211.

The **stethoscope** is an instrument for performing direct auscultation of respiratory, cardiac, pleural, arterial, venous, uterine, fetal, intestinal and other sounds. Nurses use one principally in taking a patient's blood pressure, which may under special circumstances be recorded every few minutes, and in some instances when the pulse cannot be counted accurately at the wrist (see p. 33). The nurse must be able to count the apex beats and also determine bowel sounds.

The ear pieces must fit well; in taking up a stethoscope clasp the ear pieces between finger and thumb and look at the chest piece. The bell or diaphragm must face towards the patient or the ear pieces will not fit properly and sound fails to come through. The adapter piece may need turning so that the instrument is turned in. Apply the bell or diaphragm firmly over the area concerned, with no raised edges, and listen.

The first stethoscope was a monaural one invented by a French physician, Laënnec, and monaural auscultation is still used by obstetricians and midwives in monitoring the fetal heart sounds.

The most sensitive stethoscopes are electronic, and nurses who work in intensive care units will learn how to use them.

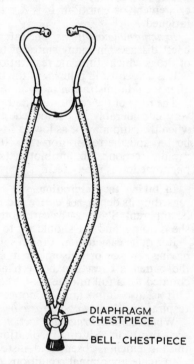

DIAPHRAGM CHESTPIECE

BELL CHESTPIECE

Fig. 3/12 Stethoscope. A model is shown having both a bell end and a diaphragm.

RESPIRATION

Respiration consists of an *inspiration, expiration* and *pause*. By means of respiration oxygen is taken round the body, carbon dioxide is collected and excreted.

Respiration is involuntarily performed. It is brought about by stimulation of the respiratory centre in the medulla oblongata due to the presence of carbon dioxide in the blood, representing the need of the body for oxygen. The centre thus stimulated causes impulses to be passed out by the phrenic and intercostal nerves to stimulate the diaphragm and intercostal muscles, and this results in a rhythmical rise and fall of the chest walls accompanied by descent and ascent of the diaphragm, alternately enlarging and decreasing the size of the chest as air passes in and out.

Normal respiration is rhythmical, quiet, regular and comfortable. The rate varies with age, and sex.

> *Rate per minute*
> A newborn infant—40.
> At 12 months—30.
> From 2 to 5—24 to 28.
> An adult—rate from 16 to 18, slightly quicker in a woman than in a man.

The *rate* may be *increased* in a normal person by exercise, and by any excitement or emotion. It is *decreased* during rest and sleep and when fatigued.

In abnormal conditions. The rate is *increased* in most febrile states, in all chest diseases, in many states of toxaemia, and after the administration of drugs which stimulate respiration such as atropine.

It is *decreased* in injuries to the brain, in most conditions of coma, and after the administration of hypnotics, particularly opium.

The *ratio* of the respiration and pulse rate is normally 1 to 4. This alters very considerably in certain chest diseases, particularly in pneumonia, when the ratio may be as low as 1 to 2; for example, a patient's pulse may be 100 and the respiration rate 50 in an untreated case, but pneumonia rapidly responds to antibiotics (see Chapter 21, p. 201), so that this phenomenon is rarely seen.

In taking the respiration, the nurse should note the *rate*, *character* regarding its depth, *regularity* and *rhythm*, and any discomfort which may be apparent. She must be careful that the patient is not conscious of what she is doing, and she should try to divert his attention from himself.

It is quite easy to count the respiration rate with the hand on the pulse, having a watch or pulsometer in such a position that the movements of the patient's chest can be seen at the same time. The rate should be counted for a full minute.

It is also important to notice where the movements occur during respiration. *Abdomino-thoracic breathing is the normal.*

When the *diaphragmatic action predominates*, the epigastrium will be seen protruding during inspiration. In cases of diaphragmatic paralysis this movement is absent, and, instead of protrusion, recession occurs here.

In acute abdominal conditions *thoracic movement* will predominate as the abdomen is held rigid; and conversely, in painful conditions of the chest, *abdominal movement* predominates. A nurse may be of great assistance to the physician by observing and reporting on all these points.

For further information read a thoracic surgeon's note on the mechanics of respiration, p. 582; a physician's note on applied physiology, p. 193; a further note on common symptoms in diseases of the lung, p. 194; and finally the brief note on nursing care in respiratory disease, p. 127.

Abnormal respirations. The rate may be abnormally quick or slow. As a rule rapid respirations are shallow, and slow respirations are deep in character.

The *rhythm* may also vary. *Sighing* is manifested by long, slow inspiration followed by rapid expiration. It occurs in shock, collapse, and in certain emotional states. *Yawning* indicates a condition of syncope.

In *Cheyne-Stokes* breathing the rhythm is very irregular. The respiration begins fairly normally and increases in depth and vigour until a maximum is reached, then gradually fades until a period of apnoea occurs, after which the cycle commences again. See page 194 for description and graph.

Inverse. In this type of breathing, which is most frequently met with in children, a pause occurs between inspiration and expiration, instead of, as in the normal, after expiration.

DYSPNOEA

In dyspnoea the breathing is difficult and noisy and in most instances it is painful or at least uncomfortable. The difficulty may affect inspiration or expiration, or both acts may be difficult.

In *orthopnoea* the difficulty is usually relieved when the patient sits up.

Apnoea is a feature of some types of dyspnoea and indicates that there is absence of breathing for a short period.

Inspiratory dyspnoea occurs when there is obstruction of the respiratory passages, breathing is *stridulant*, resulting in a high-pitched shrill whistling, and sometimes in crowing sounds characteristic of croup.

Expiratory dyspnoea is often accompanied by a grunt, particularly marked in asthma and emphysema.

Combined inspiratory and expiratory dyspnoea is the most usual form, seen in most chest disorders and in coma.

Stertorous breathing; *stertor* or *sonorous* breathing is noisy and the cheeks are puffed out and in with each breath taken.

Wheezing and rattling noises occur when the air is forced through fluid as in severe bronchitis.

(Cheyne-Stokes and the inverse type of breathing have been mentioned under disorders of rhythm above.)

Causes. Dyspnoea may be due to a variety of causes, including *pressure or obstruction in the respiratory passages* such as a tumour, the membrane present in laryngeal diphtheria, blood, mucus or a foreign body, the occurrence of oedema in congestion (for example, of the larynx), and stricture which may follow an injury.

The obstruction may be due to pressure on the trachea or larynx as in hanging or strangling, the presence of a mediastinal tumour, an aneurysm of the aorta or an enlarged thyroid gland. Dyspnoea may also be due to *paralysis of the respiratory muscles*; to *diminished lung capacity* as in emphysema, bronchiectasis and advanced pulmonary tuberculosis; to *cardiac failure* for any cause, most often seen in diseases of the heart and acute disease of the lung.

COUGH

A cough is a reflex act primarily to protect the air passages from the entry of a foreign body. It is produced by a violent expiratory effort preceded by a preliminary inspiration. The glottis is partially closed, the extraordinary muscles of respiration are brought into action, and the air is noisily expelled. There are a number of varieties (see Disorders of Respiration, Chapter 21, p. 194).

The therapeutic value of coughing in order to expand the lungs is instanced in patients confined to bed. To teach deep breathing and coughing pre-operatively and after operation is a valuable physiotherapeutic measure, in order to avoid respiratory and circulatory complications.

Read also the nursing care in Disorders of Respiration, p. 127.

CYANOSIS

This condition is due to defective oxygenation of the blood which can be central or peripheral. It occurs in most heart and lung diseases, in cardiac failure, congenital malformation of the heart (blue baby, see Chapter 59, p. 601), in obstruction of the air passages or in embarrassment of respiration.

Cyanosis may be marked, the patient being lividly blue or it may be slight and first seen in the lips, at the tips of the lobes of the ears or at the ends of the fingers or toes.

A local cyanosis occurs in some diseases and disorders of the blood vessels, as in Raynaud's disease when the digits may be pale or blue, and red when reaction sets in and peripheral changes occur.

Read also the comprehensive note on cyanosis by a surgeon, p. 412.

Chapter 4

The Toilet of the Patient

Bathing adult patients and children—care of the mouth—care of the head and hair—prevention of pressure sores—giving bedpans and urinals—the use of Sani-chairs

BATHING

Most patients who come into hospital can bathe in the bathroom, some who are confined to bed can wash themselves, a few will need help. Others again in geriatric or long-stay hospitals will require *bed bathing*. A trolley on the lines indicated in Fig. 4/1 may well be necessary; it is more convenient to have everything collected in this way rather than attempting to cope with an overcrowded tray or locker.

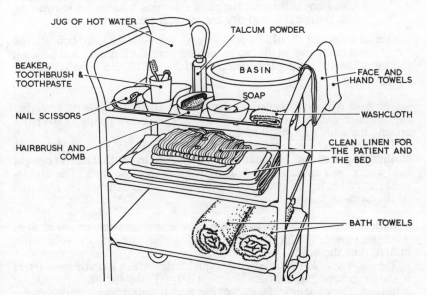

JUG OF HOT WATER

TALCUM POWDER

BEAKER,
TOOTHBRUSH &
TOOTHPASTE

BASIN

FACE AND
HAND TOWELS

SOAP

NAIL SCISSORS

WASHCLOTH

HAIRBRUSH AND
COMB

CLEAN LINEN FOR
THE PATIENT AND
THE BED

BATH TOWELS

Fig. 4/1 Articles assembled for bed bathing: towels for the patient; clean linen for the bed and for the patient; basin for washing water and jug of hot water and soap and washcloths, face and hand towels for the patient; talcum powder; nail scissors in receiver; beaker, toothbrush and paste and brush and comb in receiver. In addition provide pail on nearby side for used water and a soiled-linen carrier.

It is important to work firmly, steadily and evenly when washing and drying a patient; a light touch is apt to be irritating; a patient likes to feel that he has been washed and he likes to be well dried.

Method. Inform the patient that he is to have a bed bath, offer a bedpan or urinal, close any windows near the bed, draw the bed curtains or screen the bed. Remove the top bedclothing as in making a bed and then place one of the bath towels over the patient, rolling the second beneath him, and remove his personal clothing.

The washing is performed in the following order:

A face towel is placed across the neck and chest.

The *face, neck and ears* are washed and dried.

The *chest and arms* are next washed, one arm being exposed at a time, and the patient is allowed to swill the soap off his hands by dabbling them in a basin of water which the nurse holds conveniently near him. The water is then changed and kept hot.

The *lower part of the chest and abdomen and sides of the body* are best done by working under the bath sheet without exposing the patient.

The *umbilicus* must be cleansed and carefully dried.

The *lower limbs* are washed separately.

The patient is turned and *his back* thoroughly washed and dried.

The *genital region* is most easily washed from this aspect. If the patient is well enough, he does this for himself, if possible, and is then handed a well-soaped washing cloth and finally a clean rinsed one; otherwise the nurse does this, taking care to rinse the area thoroughly and dry and powder the groins.

Special attention should be paid to any creases in the skin, beneath the breasts, the mubilicus, in the groins, and between the buttocks and between the toes. Careful drying is necessary and a little talcum powder may be lightly applied.

The *nails* may be attended to during the bath, cutting them, receiving the scraps of nail onto a paper towel, and if necessary cleansing the parts around the nails with small moist swabs.

The *mouth and hair* are next attended to (see p. 45–7). The patient's clean clothing is put on, the bed made, he is inspected to see that he has not got cold and is well covered up. A drink is given in most cases. The articles used should be cleared away, the windows opened and the screens removed or the curtains drawn back.

Bathing a patient in the bathroom. The room must be prepared first, windows closed, the bath half filled with water, running the cold water in first, then the hot.

The *water* should be well stirred up and tested with a bath thermometer; it should not be hotter than 37·8 °C (100 °F); the bath mat should be arranged, the patient's clean clothing and towels placed ready on the radiators, and the soap, washing cloths, nailbrush and towels put comfortably within reach.

A *bell* must be within reach of the patient and it should not be possible for the bathroom to be locked or bolted from the inside, though a screen may be placed round the bath for the comfort and convenience of the patient.

The nurse will bathe a female patient, paying attention to the points described in giving a bed bath. For a male patient a male nurse will be required unless the ward sister considers this unnecessary, in which case he bathes himself.

The bathing of children needs great care. Many can be taken to the bathroom. A child's temperature should always be taken before bathing as the temperature of a child can rise so quickly. He should pass urine. A child may like to have a floating toy to amuse him.

The water should be comfortably warm, but never hot. The head and face, eyes, ears and neck should be washed and dried.

The crevices, creases and hollows of the body and the skin between fingers and toes and of the umbilicus should be carefully washed and dried. Most children will clean their own teeth.

Care should be taken that the child is warmly wrapped up and not chilled after a bath.

A very sick infant or child may be washed in his cot, or on the nurse's lap, if quite small. Very great gentleness is essential, the skin should be carefully handled and dabbed or blotted dry.

Bathing affords an excellent opportunity to observe how well, or how ill, a small child is. His apathy, listlessness, lack of normal reaction to being handled, any crying or whimpering as well as his general condition should be most carefully noted.

The *bathing of a baby* is described in Chapter 72, p. 731.

THE CARE OF THE MOUTH

The care of the mouth is an important nursing service as most patients who are in the least dehydrated have dry mouths. The *object of cleansing* is to remove sordes and prevent their formation and to stimulate the flow of saliva.

Mouth washes are refreshing, especially for patients not taking a normal diet and for those who may be vomiting. Citrus fruit drinks are useful in stimulating the flow of saliva, or citrus fruit drops may be liked.

Patients who are able *to clean their own teeth* are given a beaker of warm water and a bowl when washing.

Dentures are removed from the mouths of unconscious patients and before the administration of a general anaesthetic. They are cleansed and put into an individual disposable denture container, labelled and left in the patient's locker.

To *clean dentures*, use warm water and a denture cleaning powder—or alternatively sodium bicarbonate solution 1 in 60. Debris is removed with the patient's dental brush. The dentures are thoroughly rinsed before returning them to the patient or putting them into his dental container.

To **cleanse a patient's mouth** who is unable to do so. The bed is screened, the procedure explained to the patient, and the nurse then washes and dries her hands.

The *articles* required are assembled on a tray.

A pre-sterilized mouth pack would contain swabs, linen squares or dental napkins, gallipots, a pair each of artery forceps and dissecting forceps and possibly some orange sticks.

A paper towel to place under the patient's chin.

A disposable bag for used swabs, used towel and forceps (if disposable).

A solution of sodium bicarbonate 1 in 60 and glycerin of thymol Co. B.P.C. 1 in 4 or any other lotion suitable.

A lubricant and a small wooden spatula.

Procedure. Having protected the bed if considered necessary, the mouth should be inspected and the treatment begun in some definite order.

Dentures will be removed first and carefully cleansed with the patient's dental brush, ready for his use again (see above).

It is very comforting if the mouth is rinsed or at least swabbed with a liquid preparation before the cleansing by rubbing is commenced.

In preparing the swabs, see that they are firmly gripped by the forceps; moisten the lips and tongue with the first solution, clean the teeth with an up and down movement, paying special attention to the insides, using the orange stick to remove particles from between the teeth.

The insides of the cheek should receive careful attention, as also the gums, tongue and roof of the mouth, taking care when touching the two last named parts not to make the patient 'gag'. If this should happen, allow him to rinse his mouth out if possible and thus obtain a little rest for fear he should be made sick.

Precautions. Care must be taken to remove all sordes and crusts gently as sometimes there is a tendency for parts underneath to bleed. Each swab should only be used once. It should be dipped in the solution and then pressed against the side of the gallipot to prevent its being dripping wet.

After the treatment the patient should be given a drink, either water or weak lemonade or other fruit drink.

In the case of *a patient on milk feedings*, the mouth will be cleansed before the feeding and a small drink of water given after the feeding in order to prevent milky particles remaining in the mouth, remembering that sordes consist of dry mucus and saliva and decomposing food, which form a favourable collecting ground for micro-organisms.

In cleansing the mouth the nurse should note carefully *the condition of the patient's tongue*. When thickly furred, it is a good plan to smear it with a little lubricant before cleansing, as this helps to soften it. The same precaution might be taken with regard to the lips if they are dry and cracked.

In some cases of insane and delirious patients a mouth gag may have to be inserted whilst the mouth is cleansed.

The **nose** should receive attention at the same time as the mouth, as it frequently becomes full of crusts and dried secretion. It is very important to keep the nose clear. It should always be kept free of discharge, and the edges of the mucous membrane smeared with a bland ointment to prevent soreness.

In cleansing a baby's mouth, it is very important to remember that in the normal baby it does not require cleansing, as the baby should be given enough water to drink to keep the mouth clean. In the case of very ill babies, it may be necessary to make some attempt at cleansing by using a little glycerin, but rubbing or friction should be avoided.

A common oral infection in babies is *thrush*, in which small white flakes appear on the mucous surfaces of the mouth. This will generally respond to cleanliness, both of the mouth and the utensils used. In a few instances mild antiseptic applications, preferably nystatin, may be used, or alternatively a weak solution of gentian violet, but this stains clothing.

Complications which may occur if the mouth is neglected. The first is the collection of sordes and crusts on the lips and teeth, cracking of the lips and furring of the tongue, and the occurrence of herpes at the corners of the mouth.

A condition of dirty mouth, which will invariably have an odious taste, unless it has destroyed the sense of taste altogether, leads to nausea and the refusal of food.

As the mouth communicates with so many other parts of the body infection may spread, for example:

To the stomach, giving rise to gastritis.
To the lungs, causing inhalation pneumonia.
By the spread of infection to the middle ear, otitis media may arise.
By the posterior nares, rhinitis may be set up and infection, spreading from this part to the meninges, may cause meningitis.
Sepsis may travel by Stensen's duct and infect the parotid glands, or by way of the local lymphatics and bloodstream, giving rise to adenitis and tonsillitis.

CARE OF HEAD AND HAIR

On the admission of every patient a nurse looks over the head to see that it is clean and free from nits and lice.

In routine care of the hair, it is brushed and combed twice a day. In doing this the nurse must avoid giving pain; the hair should be held firmly at the roots and the ends combed first; when all tangles have been removed the hair may be combed from root to end. If hair is badly tangled, moistening it helps and the tangled part should be gently teased with a comb until the individual hairs are loosened and it is free.

Long hair may be arranged in two plaits if the patient wishes, one each side, so that she does not lie on it.

A nurse should notice if the scalp is clean and free from dandruff. It is of great importance in surgery of the head to keep the scalp quite free from any scurf or scales. If the head is badly covered with dandruff, the application of a weak solution of Cetavlon or a preparation containing tar well rubbed into the scalp before washing may be effective in removing it, or a special lotion may be used.

TREATING A VERMINOUS HEAD
The following requirements are assembled on a tray:

A measure containing the application of choice, e.g. Dicophane Application B.P.C. 15 ml is sufficient for most patients, alternatively one of the proprietary preparations may be preferred.
A pipette in a small receiver.
A waterproof pillowcase and a shoulder cape in a large receiver.
The patient's comb.

Method. The curtains are drawn and the procedure is explained to the patient. The waterproof pillowcase is placed on the top pillow, beneath the pillow slip and the cape is placed round the patient's shoulders.

The hair is parted in six to eight places and the application applied to the roots of the hair, near the scalp, distributing it as evenly as possible. Using the fingers, gentle massage is employed to spread it over the scalp. The hair is then arranged in the customary fashion, the patient is made comfortable and the equipment removed, washed, dried and put away.

Not less than 24 hours later, the hair is washed to remove dead pediculi. Enough of the application remains on the hair to kill further pediculi as they hatch and the hair should be shampooed again in 10 days' time, to complete the treatment. Vermin may be found in the long-hair styles of some men.

Nits
Dicophane applied to the head will persist long enough to kill larvae. The nit cases can then be removed from the hair by using a Sacker's nit comb.

The use of hospital barber and/or hairdresser. *Men* generally present no difficulty, a barber is available to trim and arrange their hair style if necessary. *Women* need a hair style which is attractive and comfortable if they are obliged to lie in bed. Most hospitals provide the services of a hairdresser, if not the nurse must do her best to set the hair attractively. A hair shampoo is necessary for all but short-term patients who have had the hair dressed before admission—moreover, it is a great stimulant to morale, as is all good grooming.

Washing a patient's hair in bed is only necessary when it is quite impossible for the patient to be taken to the bathroom where the hair can be washed over a basin. If a patient cannot be moved the head of the bed (which is usually adjustable and movable) is lifted out, the patient's shoulders are protected by a waterproof cape and towel, the pillows and mattress are similarly protected and the hair is washed just as it would be at any hairdressing establishment, alternatively the mattress may be folded under.

The hair is first well soaked, the shampoo is applied, the scalp firmly rubbed and finally the hair is well rinsed and wrapped in a towel to squeeze out the water. The patient is then settled comfortably in bed on pillows, the hair of a woman patient is set and dried by an electric dryer and then dressed.

PRESSURE SORES AND THEIR PREVENTION

Pressure sores may occur while lying long in bed; they are the result of pressure on the tissues and depend on the intensity and duration of the pressure. The skin does support great pressure, but only for short periods, and most modern research into the prevention of pressure sores has been directed towards providing relief from and distribution of pressure (see p. 50).

The causes of pressure sores have been divided into local or *external causes* contributing to pressure (see below) and predisposing or *internal causes*, i.e. the general health of the patient, including serious illness, old age, immobility, lowered tissue resistance to pressure, diminished ability to appreciate the sensation of pressure, mental apathy, and muscle weakness particularly in paraplegic and quadriplegic patients.

External sources or causes which contribute to pressure sores include:
Friction when the patient either drags himself or is dragged and not lifted over a surface which may be uneven, described as the 'wet and dry sandpaper type'.
Shearing due to blood vessels being torn owing to laxity of the sub-cutaneous tissues when patients are slid along a surface (again instead of being lifted).
Pressure from bony areas (see parts liable to pressure) against the bed or other unyielding surface which is certain to kill tissues, muscles being the first to suffer. In these *deep sores*, erythema over the area may be the only early evidence, but where there is considerable necrosis of muscle and fascia extending to the surface a quite serious degree of pressure sore may be expected. Maceration of the skin from prolonged contact with moisture, from sweat, urine and faeces are contributory factors.
In considering sources of pressure, the length of time patients, some of whom may be elderly, lie on an operating theatre table cannot be ignored. Returned to bed semi-conscious they continue to lie heavily; sedated for the first night the pressure continues. Thus many patients having a hip prosthesis, for example, develop pressure sores.

Areas liable to pressure:
The *back of the head* may become sore, particularly in the case of infants and children who continually rub their heads or who are given to head banging.
The *shoulder blades*, which are prominent, particularly in emaciated people.
The *vertebral spines* throughout the entire extent of the column and over the sacrum.
The *back of the heels* as they lie heavily on the bed. All or any of the protuberant parts of a patient who lies long in bed may become liable to pressure sores.
In patients who lie on their side, sores only too readily occur over the *great trochanters*, on the *outer aspect of the knees, between the knees* or *ankles* as they may rub together. Soreness *over the knees* has already been mentioned. The *elbows* are apt to become sore in people who lie on the back or who lean on their elbows for reading and eating.

Factors which are of importance in the care of patients liable to sustain pressure include:

> Prevention of pressure.
> Early detection.
> Attention to nutrition by a well-balanced diet with good protein content.
> Relief of anaemia, as those with a haemoglobin blood content below 80 need correction and tend to get pressure sores.

The avoidance of protein loss in the exposed dermis in burns, in wound secretions and discharges, in diarrhoea and in ulcerative colitis, for example, are all important and need attention to improve the general state of health.

Turning the patient at regular intervals of two hours often proves effective, provided the patient's general condition is good and that any anaemia has been treated. This method, however, is time-consuming and needs adequate, well-instructed helpers.

Routine treatment of pressure areas include attention to the hygiene of the skin, thorough washing, massaging it with circular and kneading movements to *move the underlying tissues*. Careful drying is absolutely essential, followed by a light application of smooth, fine powder. When the skin is liable to moisture or contamination the use of a silicone cream or spray is a good protection. This must be washed off and the skin dried before another application is made. No specific rules can be laid down, nurses should follow the customary treatment of their hospital.

The use of sheepskins is helpful provided too much reliance is not placed on them. The patient lies on a sheepskin, woolly side up. The dense fleece provides a resilient, springy surface, and allows some circulation of air and evaporation. Moreover, the wool absorbs an appreciable amount of moisture before it feels damp. The skins used are specially prepared; they are kept clean and hygienic by a prescribed method of washing. It is advisable to have two skins per patient, to wear and wash, without interrupting the treatment. In addition to their use for bed patients, specially shaped skins are used as cushions in chairs, wheelchairs, and as heel pads, elbow pads and slippers.

Considerable research into the prevention and treatment, principally directed to avoiding or distributing pressure, and the use of devices in minimizing pressure has been and is being undertaken. A number of specialized beds have been brought into use, including the Ripple bed with its alternating pressure-point pad providing regular, frequent, automatic redistribution of body pressure which is useful provided the large-celled type of bed is employed and, as in the use of sheepskins, not too much reliance is placed on it and that the hygiene of the skin is not neglected.

The experimental stage of the *water-immersion bed* has been completed and a six-bedded unit has been opened in Wessex. The patient literally lies in water but is separated from it by a loose, impermeable, waterproof covering and, because the water moves freely within the covering, he is subject to its natural buoyancy and is not exposed to any pressure. This bed is used principally for the healing of pressure sores and proves most effective. When a sore is present a thin ventilated polythene film is the only dressing used.

It should be realized that this is not a water bed (water mattress) in the sense usually understood in which the water is encapsulated so that its natural buoyancy (a feature of the water-immersion bed) is lost.

Sterilization after cleaning the bed is easily effected by one of the hypochlorites.

The essential features are:

A water container or tank which provides a buoyant surface on which the patient lies.
A film of waterproof material.
A method of heating the water plus a thermostat keeping it within a degree or less of body heat.
A method of circulating the water.

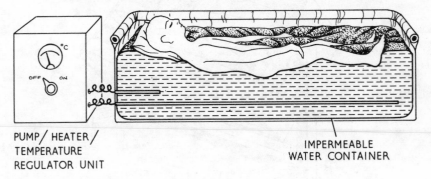

PUMP/ HEATER /
TEMPERATURE
REGULATOR UNIT

IMPERMEABLE
WATER CONTAINER

Fig. 4/2 Water immersion bed, for description see text.

From the nursing point of view it is quite easy to insert a bedpan under the patient; much easier than lifting him. All that is needed is to press the bedpan down on the waterproof cover on the water.

For other nursing procedures it is simple to slide a Terylene-covered foam mattress under the patient; for the short time needed for treatment the temporary increase in pressure does not do harm.

The Keane Rota-Rest Bed (see Fig. 4/3) has proved its *value in preventing pressure sores during long periods of immobilization* in the treatment of paralytic conditions—paraplegia, quadriplegia, following spinal injury. The bed is covered with a non-toxic plastic; the bedsides and the leg abduction pack are adjustable. Full instructions are issued with each bed. By means of a motor the bed rotates from the horizontal to either side to an angle of 45 degrees, thus the patient's weight inclines first to one and then to the other side, for a determined period or continuously so that pressure on any one area is avoided. The oscillatory movements can be regulated to a gentle, rhythmical, rocking movement so that sleep is not interrupted.

The movement of the patient's body exerts intermittent pressure on muscles, blood vessels and lymphatics, thus improving the circulation and preventing venous stagnation in the lower limbs and pelvic veins so that thrombosis is avoided. The contents of the thorax and abdomen are similarly affected by the movements of the bed so that pulmonary congestion is avoided, constipation does not occur as bowel action is stimulated. The constant movement keeps the urine in the bladder well mixed so that deposits do not settle and bladder stone does not form. Urethral drainage into a plastic bag beneath the bed keeps the bladder empty when necessary. A padded window over the sacral region is removable for the insertion of the bedpan. A patient can be nursed in this bed in his home; he may be up in a wheel chair by day and have the advantages provided by this bed at night and for rest periods.

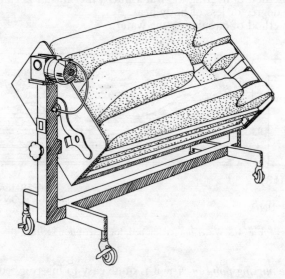

Fig. 4/3 Keane Rota-Rest Bed, which rotates to either side to an angle of 45 degrees. For importance of this movement see text.

A further use of this bed is to provide full immobilization in order to facilitate the healing of pressure sores over the sacrum and femoral trochanters in geriatric cases or otherwise bed-fast patients, the sores being dressed through the removable window mentioned above.

Treatment of pressure sores. Once the skin is abraded every care must be taken to prevent the entry of micro-organisms. Such a lesion is therefore treated with all aseptic precautions, using the non-touch dressing technique. There are many local applications in use which will be prescribed and which may include antibiotics. The nurses should observe and report on the effect of the treatment.

It is exceptional to find a patient with pressure sores who is not anaemic and who may not also be very short of serum iron. The physician will attend to this but the nurse may be the first to notice either that the patient gets breathless on exertion or is easily tired and wearied. It may be that he is not interested in his food and not getting enough nourishment; the nurse will observe this and arrange for his diet to be supplemented in some way.

GIVING BEDPANS AND URINALS

In most hospitals the ward is 'closed' at regular stated times for the purposes of the *sanitary round*, by placing a screen in front of the ward door, thus indicating to visitors, including the doctors and clergy, that they may not enter without first inquiring if this is convenient.

A request for a bedpan (or a urinal) *at any time* should be answered with alacrity as most patients will have experienced discomfort before asking.

When **giving a patient a bedpan** it should be warm and dry, and be carried to the bedside covered. If the patient can help himself, that is, get himself onto the bedpan, the nurse should turn the bedclothes back and slip it under his buttocks, generally from the right side.

To **place a patient on a bedpan** who is unable to do much to help himself, the nurse should turn the quilt and blanket down to the foot of the bed, leaving the patient covered by a sheet and blanket; and then, standing on one side of the bed, by placing one hand under the lower part of the patient's back, raise him sufficiently to slip the bedpan under his buttocks with her free hand. She should then feel that the pan is in a convenient position, neither too high nor too low, and arrange the patient's pillows so that he is propped comfortably on it. For *helpless patients*, two nurses will be required, one at each side of the bed.

To **cleanse the patient**. Either soft toilet paper tissues or moist swabs may be used. If he particularly wishes to do so and is able he may perform this himself; otherwise the nurse will do it.

If moist swabs are used the patient's skin should either be dried with dry swabs or with a paper towel. The used swabs are put into a disposal bag.

A patient who has cleansed himself should always be able to wash his hands.

When a woman is menstruating a receiver should be provided for the sanitary pad. She will appreciate the opportunity of washing her genital region frequently.

To empty a bedpan. The contents should be inspected; any bits of material not suitable for emptying into a bedpan flush should be removed by forceps and put into a disposal bag.

After flushing the pan should be looked over to see that it is clean, as it may be necessary to use a mop on the interior before the pan is disinfected (or sterilized), dried and put away.

Urinals are made of glass or stainless steel and many are disposable. A urinal is taken to the bedside under a suitable cover. It should be emptied immediately after use and disinfected or sterilized and placed upside-down to drain.

In the routine care of bedpans and urinals, means are taken to keep them clean and quite free from any deposit, such as may be the result of highly concentrated urines depositing urates or phosphates. Sterilization after use is the ideal; alternatively disinfection may be employed.

To keep urinals free from deposit, washing with water containing washing soda and using a bottle brush to help remove any deposit may be adequate; in some cases of marked phosphaturia a urinal may become crusted in a very short time, when one of the cleansing materials specially recommended for removing any deposit from the glazed surfaces of sanitary pans may be used. *Disposable utensils* are available.

A nurse should always make sure *whether a specimen of urine or stool is to be saved* and should observe the character of these in every instance and also any untoward symptoms, such as frequency, variations in quantity and so on (see Chapter 5).

A Sani-chair may be used at the bedside with a device for fitting a bedpan, which can be removed; or Sani-chairs may be wheeled to the toilet where the opening fits over the lavatory pan. In both cases a disposable seat cover is available.

Chapter 5

Observations on Excreta and Secretions and Collection of Specimens

The characteristics of normal urine and its variations in health and disease—the testing of urine—characteristics of normal faeces with variations in health and disease—handling and disposal of sputum and observations—the collection of specimens of urine, faeces, sputum and vomit; of pus, fluid and secretions, and of blood

---

Urine normally contains the by-products of metabolism except carbon dioxide which is mainly excreted by the lungs. It is composed of:

Water 96 per cent, urea 2 per cent and other metabolic products 2 per cent.

Products not normally present in urine, but present in certain metabolic disorders, include glucose in diabetes mellitus, and products of inflammation such as blood and pus in infective conditions of the urinary tract.

The normal characteristics of urine are:

Colour, amber, dark when concentrated, pale when diluted.
Odour, aromatic, not unpleasant.
Reaction, slightly acid, turning blue litmus paper red.
Specific gravity, urine is denser than water, from 1·010 to 1·025.
Quantity, in the adult 1,500 ml in 24 hours, varying with the fluid intake and the external temperature (see below).

VARIATIONS IN HEALTH AND DISEASE

The quantity is decreased in health when the amount of fluid taken is limited, or when sweating is heavy as the result of exercise or excessive clothing and in hot weather. When the quantity is much diminished the colour becomes deeper, the specific gravity higher, and there may be a deposit of urates on cooling.

The quantity is increased in opposite conditions, as when sweating is decreased as in cool weather, in conditions of fear and nervousness, when little exercise is taken, and when the fluid intake is increased. In these circumstances the colour is paler and the specific gravity is lower.

The normal odour varies very little during health, and the **variation in the reaction** is also slight—for example, it may be found to be alkaline after a meal rich in carbohydrates.

The characteristics vary more considerably under conditions of disease. The quantity is decreased in febrile conditions, heart disease, acute nephritis; in some cases of chronic nephritis; in some surgical diseases of the kidneys; after the administration of certain drugs, and in all cases in which fluid is lost to the body as in haemorrhage, vomiting and diarrhoea, and in many conditions of toxaemia, and also when there is marked oedema.

The quantity is increased in diabetes, in some disorders of the pituitary gland, in hysteria and other functional nervous conditions, in most cases of chronic nephritis, by the administration of diuretic drugs, and when the intake of fluid is increased.

The colour varies with the quantity as previously mentioned. *Bile* colours the urine deep orange to olive-green, *blood* renders it smoky or red. *Certain drugs also alter the colour of urine.*
The *urine is rendered cloudy or opaque* by the presence of blood, pus, excessive mucus, and also by phosphates and urates until these have been deposited.

The deposits normally seen in urine are urates, which may be pink or white; *phosphates*, usually whitish grey, but sometimes slightly tinged by pink; *pus*, which is very dense, lying heavily at the bottom of the glass; *blood* may be present in clots; *crystals of uric acid* suggest a sprinkling of cayenne pepper over the specimen glass; *excess of mucus* may form a gelatinous mass.

The odour is slightly fishy when decomposition is commencing; when very marked the odour becomes ammoniacal. The presence of acetone bodies gives a scented urine which recalls the smell of new-mown hay.

The reaction may vary very considerably in disease. A concentrated urine is usually highly acid, and consequently irritating; urine containing phosphates is generally neutral or alkaline, and urates give an acid urine.

As a general rule, **the specific gravity** is low when the quantity is increased and high when decreased; in diabetes mellitus, however, the presence of sugar in the urine results in the passing of large quantities of pale urine with a characteristically high specific gravity.

Certain abnormalities particularly relating to the amount of urine secreted and passed can usefully be mentioned:

Polyuria is an increased output which occurs in diabetes mellitus and also in diabetes insipidus.

Oliguria is a decreased output occurring in acute nephritis, congestive heart failure, in starvation and in dehydration. It also occurs during the first 24 hours after major surgery, and after any serious injury owing to increased output of the anti-diuretic hormone following physical stress. This is why observation of the amount of urine passed is important during these hours (see also Chapter 44, p. 421).

Suppression of urine or **anuria** is cessation of urinary excretion; at first the amount may be markedly reduced even to 30 to 60 ml (a dangerous sign), then cease altogether. This state may occur in a number of medical and surgical conditions involving the urinary tract, in eclampsia and in incompatible blood transfusion. Anuria will be fatal unless it can be relieved.
Read Chapter 25, p. 245, for full information.

Retention of urine. Urine is secreted and it reaches the bladder but is not passed. The causes are numerous:

> *Nervousness* may cause spasm of the urethral sphincters which fail to relax.
> A lesion of the brain or spinal cord may have the same effect.
> The condition may follow operation on the abdominal and pelvic organs.
> Certain sedative drugs may inhibit micturition.
> It occurs in shock when vital centres are depressed.
> Pain, as in urethritis and cystitis, causes the patient to inhibit micturition.

Dysuria or difficulty in micturition may be due to pain and spasm when the act is attempted.
Read also Disorders of Micturition for a fuller description, p. 533.

Abnormal constituents of urine. The substances for which urine may be chemically examined by a nurse are protein, sugar, acetone bodies, bile, blood, pus, urates and phosphates, the presence and quantity of chlorides. In addition, urine may be examined for uric acid, the presence of red blood cells and pus cells, casts and bacteria, and for the quantity of urea, albumin and sugar; but these tests are not usually performed by a nurse, and are therefore not described here. The modern trend, however, is that most urine testing should be carried out in a laboratory, apart from the initial screening for which Ames Stix are so admirably suited (see below).

COMPREHENSIVE URINE TESTING USING AMES METHODS

The Ames range of standardized strips and tablets has greatly increased the simplicity and efficiency of urinalysis, but, like any laboratory method, correct results can only be obtained if the reagents are stored correctly and used according to the manufacturer's instructions, and if reasonably fresh samples are used.

When performing any of the 'Ames Tests' keep the test instructions nearby, together with the colour chart for comparison when reading off results.

Do not acidify urine before carrying out the tests.

Strip tests

Wherever possible the impregnated reagent areas have been grouped together to form a complete test system on one plastic strip. The technique for most of the strip tests is identical:

1. Dip the strip into *fresh*, well-mixed, uncentrifuged urine, so that all the reagent areas are covered. Remove immediately.
2. Tap the edge of the strip against the side of the urine container to remove excess urine.
3. Compare the test areas closely with the corresponding colour charts on the bottle, at the stated times. *Hold the strip close to the colour blocks and match quickly.*

The reading time interval for each test is given on the package leaflet and on the bottle label for each product.

Reading times for the test areas of multiple or single test strips

Strip tests on urine	*Reading interval*
pH	Read immediately
Protein	Read next
Glucose	Read at 10 seconds precisely
Ketones	Read at 15 seconds precisely
Bile	Read at 20 seconds precisely
Blood	Read at 30 seconds precisely
Urobilinogen	Read at 60 seconds precisely
Phenylpyruvic acid	Read at 30 seconds precisely
P.A.S. and aspirin	

Strip tests on blood	
Dextrostix* for blood glucose	After exactly 60 seconds, quickly wash off the blood with water and
Azostix* for blood urea	read immediately.

Tablet tests with urine	
Sugar (Clinitest*)	Read 15 seconds after the reaction has stopped. Remember to shake the contents of the test-tube before comparing with the colour chart.
Ketones (Acetest*)	Compare with the colour chart at 30 seconds.
Bilirubin (Ictotest*)	Observe colour on the mat around the tablet, exactly 30 seconds after flowing water over the tablet.

General notes

Collection of specimen:

1. Fresh specimens of urine should be used for all tests as changes in the composition occur when the urine is allowed to stand. This is especially important if the urine is known to be infected. The complete specimen should be mixed well before taking a sample for testing. If urine has been chilled it should be returned to room temperature before testing.
2. The specimen container must be absolutely clean and free from contaminants such as antiseptic or detergents.

3. Do not acidify, centrifuge or filter specimen before testing.
4. When using Ames strip tests, they should be dipped into the urine cleanly and quickly and removed immediately.
5. The tests must be compared with colour blocks at the stated time.
6. Testing instructions must be carefully followed particularly when using blood-testing systems.
7. Recap bottles tightly after removing a test strip. Store the bottles in a cool, dry place away from excessive heat, moisture or direct sunlight. Do not refrigerate.

Multistix* Reagent strip test for pH, protein, glucose, ketones, bilirubin, blood and urobilinogen in urine.

Bili-Labstix* Reagent strip test for pH, protein, glucose, ketones, bilirubin and blood in urine.

N-Labstix* Reagent strip test for pH, protein, glucose, ketones, blood and nitrite in urine.

Labstix* Reagent strip test for pH, protein, glucose, ketones and blood in urine.

Urobilistix* Reagent strip test for urinary urobilinogen.

Phenistix* Reagent strip test for phenylketones in urine and as a check for the presence of P.A.S. or other salicylates.
   All the test portions are available as single test strips, and in different combinations, but, when used alone, they do not form a total routine urinalysis picture.

Interpretation and comments

1. *pH*—Values for the pH may be interpreted to one half unit.
2. *Protein*—A colour which matches any block marked with + signs indicates significant proteinuria. Clinical judgment must determine the significance of 'trace' results.
3. *Glucose*—'Light' generally indicates ¼ per cent or less. 'Dark' generally indicates ½ per cent or more. 'Medium' indicates that glucose is present but does not denote amount.
4. *Ketones*—'Small', 'Moderate' and 'Large' concentrations of ketones may be recorded.
5. *Bilirubin*—'Small', 'Moderate' and 'Large' colour blocks indicate increasing concentrations of urinary bilirubin.
6. *Blood*—The shade of blue developed at 30 seconds indicates 'Small', 'Moderate' or 'Large' urinary concentrations of blood.
7. *Urobilinogen*—Results are given in Ehrlich units because the test is not specific for urobilinogen. Urobilinogen is the commonest urinary constituent which will produce a colour with *Urobilistix** strips, but small amounts of other substances may contribute to the final colour produced.
   1 Ehrlich unit is equivalent to 1 mg of urobilinogen.

N.B. 1. A high pH value may indicate that the specimen is 'stale'.

2. It is not uncommon to record a positive test for blood on a specimen which gives a negative reaction to the protein test area. This is because the minimum pathological concentration in urine of red blood cells is much lower than that of proteins, therefore a test for haematuria must be more sensitive than a test for proteinuria.
3. In paediatric wards and departments, additional tests for sugar must be made with *Clinitest** reagent tablets (whether the strip test is positive or negative) to exclude galactosaemia, etc.
4. *Ictotest** reagent tablets are four to eight times more sensitive than the bilirubin portions of the strip tests.

Diabetic information systems

Two different patterns of testing are recommended for insulin-dependent and non-insulin-dependent diabetics. Insulin-dependent diabetics are best monitored with *Clinitest** reagent tablets which provide a semi-quantitative estimation of urinary sugar.

Acetest* reagent tablets provide a complementary test for ketonuria. Many non-insulin-dependent diabetics enjoy long periods of good control. In these cases, the more easily performed strip tests using *Clinistix**, *Diastix**, or *Keto-Diastix** are recommended for routine monitoring, to keep the patient just free of glycosuria.

Two tests sometimes carried out in the wards, not yet covered by the Ames series, are the Fantus test for chlorides and Esbach's quantitative test for albumin, set out below.

A. Fantus test for approximate estimation of chlorides

Place 10 drops of urine in a test-tube, using a pipette. Wash the pipette with *distilled water*; using the same pipette add one drop only of a 20 per cent solution of potassium chromate. Wash the pipette again in distilled water. Add a solution of 2·9 per cent silver nitrate drop by drop, holding the pipette upright, counting the number of drops and stopping at the first sign of a permanent red colour which indicates that all the chlorides have been precipitated from the solution. (The same pipette is used for each solution to ensure that the drops are of the same size, but it *must* be rinsed in distilled water between each solution.) The number of drops of silver nitrate needed is the number of grams per litre of chloride.

B. Esbach's quantitative test for albumin

The quantity of albumin may be approximately ascertained by using Esbach's albuminometer which is a graduated stoppered test-tube.

Method. Filter the urine if not clear and if alkaline render it slightly acid by the addition of acetic acid. If the specific gravity is 1·010 or more, dilute the urine sufficiently to reduce the specific gravity to below that level.

Fill the tube with urine, up to the mark 'U'. Add Esbach's reagent (a mixture of picric acid and acetic acid) up to the mark 'R'; the tube is then inverted several times to allow these fluids to mix, labelled with the patient's name, date and the *time the test was put up*, and kept standing upright for 24 hours. The albumin is deposited and is read off on the

---

* Can be obtained from Ames Company (London) Ltd.

graduated marks as representing grams of dried albumin per litre of urine. The percentage of albumin present is obtained by dividing by 10. Allowance must be made if the urine has been diluted before the estimation was undertaken; when diluted by equal parts of water divide the final reading by 2.

If a more delicate test is required, which applies equally to all urine testing, this can only be carried out in a laboratory.

The Tests of Renal Function could now be read with advantage, p. 245.

STOOLS

The normal stool varies in health, according to age and to some extent with the diet. A *fluid diet* produces soft stools, a *dry diet* gives a hard stool. A *heavy protein diet* will make a stool offensive and dry, a *milk diet* will render it dry and crumbly and pale in colour. *Certain vegetables may alter the colour*, spinach producing a greenish stool and carrots a reddish colour.

Certain drugs taken may affect the stools; astringents, such as tannic acid contained in tea, will decrease the quantity, iron and bismuth will render the stool greyish black; laxatives and purgatives are intended to increase the quantity and the fluidity.

The characteristics of a normal stool are:

> *Frequency*—one or two a day.
> *Quantity*—in the adult about four ounces (120 g).
> *Consistency*—soft solid.
> *Colour*—light brown.
> *Odour*—characteristic but inoffensive.

Variations in disease. The *quantity is increased* in intestinal catarrh, diarrhoea, and whenever peristalsis is stimulated. It is *decreased* when peristalsis is sluggish, as in constipation, and in conditions in which fluid is being lost, as in sweating, vomiting and excessive bleeding.

The *consistency* is always in relation to the quantity: increased quantity produces fluidity, decreased quantity renders the stool hard and solid, as water has been excessively absorbed. Very hard stools are described as *scybala*. Gritty particles occur when faecal collections have formed as in diverticulitis. The term 'sheep droppings' is used to describe little hard round knobbly bits of faeces which have probably been passed through a spastic colon. *Ribbonlike* stools are those which have been passed through a constricted colon, which may be due to spastic constipation or may indicate the presence of a growth. A soft solid stool may sometimes be grooved as it is pressed past a prominence in the wall of the rectum.

Ricewater stools are a special type of fluid stool which has a turbid appearance with little flecks of mucus in it, characteristic of cholera.

Odour. Sour-smelling stools occur in digestive disorders, and the stools are offensive whenever there is excessive decomposition or tissue destruction as in ulcerative enteritis and jaundice.

The *colour* varies rather more considerably. Bile, which normally colours the stool brown, is absent in jaundice, and so the stools are *clay* or *putty coloured*.

Green stools suggest digestive disorder.

The more common abnormal constituents which are occasionally present in faeces are:

> *Blood*, which alters the colour of the stools, may be red blood, clots or melaena which gives tarry black stools and which can only be demonstrated by laboratory tests.
> *Mucus*, which may be in flakes or shreds, or as epithelial casts.
> *Pus.*
> *Sloughs*, usually indicating separation of ulcers, as in typhoid fever.
> *Gallstones*, little grey particles, usually searched for after an attack of biliary colic.
> *Undigested food*, fat as globules; curds, from undigested milk; and substances such as fruit stones, skins, fish bones, etc.
> *Intestinal worms.*

The stools of an infant. During the early days, *meconium* is passed, which is a dark green fluid; during the first two months of life, the stools are like beaten-up egg in colour and consistency, slightly sour and numbering three to four a day. They then gradually become slightly faeculent, and at the age of about six months have become of a fairly thick consistency and slightly brown in colour.

SPUTUM

Sputum or expectoration is coughed up from the lungs, though in many instances it contains a lot of saliva.

Observations. It is important that a nurse should observe the *amount* of sputum, its *colour, odour, tenacity*—that is, whether or not it is clinging to the patient's lips, and difficult to spit up. It is important to note the time when most of the expectoration is brought up, whether it is early morning, after a meal or after exertion.

Character. Sputum is described according to its character.

> It may be *abundant* or *scanty, clear* or *opaque.*
> If opaque it may be *mucoid, muco-purulent, purulent, albuminoid, bloodstained* or *rusty.*
> It may also be *frothy, deposited in layers or nummular.*
> It may be *blue-black* in colour in gangrene and abscess of the lung.

Certain diseases have very characteristic sputa. In *pneumonia* it begins by being mucoid, then becomes tenacious and if the disease is untreated will progress to the rusty coloured sputum characteristic of pneumonia.

In *bronchiectasis*, the sputum is fetid, having a deposit of pus, a layer of brown fluid on top of this surmounted by froth.

In *pulmonary tuberculosis* the sputum is described as *glairy*, when it looks like seed grains. It is *nummular*, which means that it comes up in coin-shaped masses lying on the bottom of the vessel into which it is expectorated. This occurs when cavities are present. When the disease is advanced, and there is a good deal of destruction of lung tissue, the sputum is greenish grey and purulent.

In *asthma*, the sputum is scanty, frequently brought up in pellet-shaped masses, described as *Laennec's pearls*.

Precautions in handling sputum. Waxed-paper disposable sputum cups are generally supplied. When a specimen is needed a sterile container is provided.

Ambulant patients carry the waxed cup in their pockets; there are types available which are almost non-spillable. Patients with less copious sputum might manage with paper handkerchiefs, but it is important to ensure that before taking a clean one the used one is disposed of adequately.

Disposal of sputum. Non-infectious sputum may be emptied down the sluice or lavatory pan, care being taken to avoid soiling the sides of the basin. *Infectious sputum* and *sputum from all tuberculous persons* should either be rendered innocuous by boiling or disinfecting, or may be disposed of by burning.

COLLECTION OF SPECIMENS

A nurse will be called upon to collect specimens of the excretions and more rarely of the secretions of the body from time to time. Most commonly specimens of urine, faeces, sputum and vomit will be required.

The examination of such specimens may be necessary for a variety of reasons:

In order to arrive at a *diagnosis*.
To note the *progress* of the disease.
To observe the effect of any special treatment or drug.
Before the administration of a general anaesthetic.

A specimen required for bacteriological examination may be rendered useless by being carelessly collected.

Specimens that have been in contact with disinfectants are of little or no value.

Proper labelling of specimens is as important as careful handling.

Urine

An ordinary specimen—that is, the routine specimen collected either on admission or daily, or twice weekly, in the routine administration of a ward—may be taken first thing in the morning or last thing at night.

To collect this, the nurse gives the patient a clean bedpan or urinal, and saves 150 ml of the quantity passed in a specimen glass, which should then be covered and labelled with the name of the patient, the ward, and the date on which it was collected.

A woman should be asked not to have her bowels moved at the same time if she can avoid this. Should she be menstruating the nurse should swab the vulva and place a pad of absorbent wool into the vaginal orifice over which the urine trickles into the bedpan and, with care, mixing of the menstrual flow can be avoided. A note that the woman, from whom the specimen was obtained, is menstruating should be made.

A *sterile specimen* can only be obtained by means of catheterization and then it is put up in a sterile specimen bottle provided by the laboratory and the word 'sterile' added to the label.

A mid-stream specimen. The principles for collecting this type of specimen are:

1. The *first stream* is passed into a vessel or the lavatory pan; this flushes the urethra—the flow is arrested
2. The *mid-stream* is passed into a sterile receiver or into a sterile container supplied by the laboratory and again arrested
3. The *remainder of the stream* is voided

A procedure sheet is supplied by some authorities for preliminary cleansing and drying. In women the labia are cleansed and held apart as the mid-stream specimen must pass from the urethra into the sterile receiver without being contaminated.

In an apprehensive patient unable to arrest the flow as directed, the sterile container may be inserted to collect the specimen at mid-stream and then withdrawn. The outside of the container is then cleansed, dried and labelled for transmission to the laboratory.

To collect a 24-hour specimen. At a given time the urine passed is discarded, then all the urine passed during the next 24 hours is collected. Label a large bottle into which this urine is poured, noting on a label each time of collection and the amount passed.

Sometimes the whole quantity is sent for examination; sometimes only a specimen from it which should be obtained after slowly inverting the bottle once to ensure thorough mixing of the contents.

To collect a specimen from a baby. There are special disposable polythene urine collecting bags which can be used for both sexes.

Alternatively, in the case of a girl, use a sterile napkin, place a pad of wool in front and below the vulva, and when the baby has passed urine the nurse places this wool in a sterile wringer by means of forceps and squeezes the urine into a clean glass.

If the infant is a boy the penis may be placed in a sterile test-tube provided the sharp edges of the top are covered by stretching a piece of rubber or polythene from a finger cot over it, or by means of wool.

Faeces

A 'suitable container' supplied by the laboratory ready sterilized is used. This is never glass since the whole container and contents are usually incinerated after examination. This should be labelled, and the specimen sent to the laboratory as soon as possible after it is passed, the hour it was collected being added to the information on the label. The specimen should not contain any disinfectant. When collecting it, choose the soft solid portion of the stool, removing this from the bedpan by means of a sterile spatula or scoop specially provided for the purpose; add to the specimen anything that looks abnormal in the stool and take great care not to contaminate the outside of the container. See that it is securely sealed.

Wrap it in a piece of clean white paper, or enclose it in an envelope or paper bag marked 'faecal specimen'.

If a specimen of faeces is to be examined for the presence of amoebae, the whole stool should be poured into a receptacle warmed by standing it in water at a temperature of 37·8 °C (100 °F) and sent to the laboratory while still warm from the patient's body.

When a specimen of faeces is needed for examination to detect the presence of *occult blood* it is important for the nurse to see that the diet has not included red meat during the previous 48 hours.

She should also warn the patient to try to avoid injuring his gums when cleaning his teeth, and she should also ask him to let her know if by any chance he swallows a little blood from the back of his nose, mouth or throat, as this would render the test useless.

Any abnormal stool should be saved intact for inspection at the doctor's next visit, either in the vessel in which it is received or in a shallow bowl. It should be covered and placed in an air cupboard if one is available.

Sputum

In collecting a specimen of sputum it is best to get this first thing in the morning, before the patient has had his breakfast. He should be told that such a specimen will be required. A small screw-topped container (see above under containers for faeces), ready labelled, is provided standing on a receiver at his bedside, and he is told that he is to expectorate the secretion that comes up from his lungs into this without moving it about in his mouth or collecting a lot of saliva. It is important that saliva should not form the bulk of the specimen.

Vomit

As a general rule vomit is kept in the bowl in which it is received, which should be covered as it is moved about the ward or conveyed to a laboratory for examination (see also pp. 130–1).

Specimens from the throat

These are usually collected on sterile cotton swabs and taken immediately to the laboratory. The laboratory supplies the glass test-tubes ready sterilized containing cotton wool swabs. The neck of the tube is plugged with sterile wool. In taking a swab from the throat, or elsewhere, the specimen is obtained from the affected area and the swab replaced in the tube without contaminating it. Some specimens are placed directly onto culture media ready in the culture tubes.

In taking a swab from the throat, the specimen should be taken from the affected area, taking care not to touch any other part of the mouth.

The same precautions apply to specimens taken from the *ear, nose* and *naso-pharynx.*

Specimens of cerebrospinal fluid, or fluid from the serous cavities are usually collected in sterile test-tubes or bottles. When handling the receptacle the nurse must be careful to see that the outside is not contaminated, and that the rubber bung, which is also sterile, is replaced as quickly as possible, without touching the sides of the container.

Pus or fluid from wounds and abscesses may be collected in the same way.

A *specimen of the secretion* from the eye or other mucus-lined cavity is usually taken by means of a sterile swab. The specimen is obtained by gently touching the part affected, so that secretion is received onto the cotton wool; the swab is then immediately replaced in the test-tube.

In all cases the label conveying the necessary information should be attached immediately.

Containers for all specimens will be supplied by the laboratory. It is a matter of convenience, to the laboratory, which container is used.

A nurse may be expected to provide for the accommodation of a specimen of blood, cerebrospinal fluid, fluid from one of the serous cavities such as may be obtained on aspiration of the chest or pericardial sac, or of the peritoneum, or specimens from any of the body cavities such as the nose, conjunctival sac, throat or vagina, or the pus or other contents from any wound or abscess.

Specimens of blood. These may be obtained in small quantities by simply puncturing a finger pad, or ear lobe (capillary blood) or in larger amounts by withdrawing blood from a vein with a syringe.

Capillary puncture is performed with a Hagedorn needle or some other suitable instrument, and the blood collected into one of a variety of pipettes or micro-containers depending on the needs of the laboratory. The procedure is always carried out entirely by the laboratory staff and no assistance is required beyond, perhaps, the provision of a swab and antiseptic for cleansing the skin.

A nurse may, however, be required to assist in the collection of *venous blood*. Requirements are:

A dry syringe and needle (20 gauge).
Articles for cleansing the skin.
Sphygmomanometer cuff or piece of tubing with which to compress the veins.
Towels to protect the bed.

The skin over a vein (at the bend of the elbow or, alternatively, when veins are very collapsed, those on the dorsum of the hand are used) is cleansed and the vein rendered prominent by pressure on the upper arm with the sphygmomanometer cuff. The needle is introduced into the vein, the pressure on the upper arm released, and 5 to 10 ml blood is withdrawn. After withdrawing the needle a swab is pressed over the puncture wound for 2 to 3 minutes. Meanwhile the needle should be detached from the syringe and the blood introduced *gently* into a suitable container which should be closed with a bung. Never squirt the blood vigorously through the needle; it causes frothing, and sometimes haemolysis.

Containers for blood. There are a large number of these available for a great variety of tests. When clotted blood is needed, as for cross matching, a plain empty bottle is used. For other tests various anticoagulants are added to prevent the blood clotting, e.g. heparin, Sequestrene, citrate or fluoride. These containers are generally identified by a variety of coloured labels, and a list is usually obtainable from the laboratory indicating which container should be used for each test.

Sedimentation rate. The rate at which the *red blood cells* sink in plasma is increased in cases of tissue breakdown due to infection and toxaemia. The rate is related to the levels of the different plasma proteins, particularly fibrinogen.

Estimation of the sedimentation rate is valuable only as an indication of the progress a patient is making. By observation of the sedimentation rate at weekly intervals variations can be noted. The rate is increased in pleural effusion, tuberculosis, in practically all true febrile conditions and in rheumatism.

Two methods of estimation are employed: *Wintrobe's* and *Westergren's*. In each case an anticoagulant is added to the blood.

Requirements:

      Sterile 2 ml syringe and No. 1 needle.
      Sodium citrate solution, 3·8 per cent.
      Dry gallipot.
      Tube of the required pattern and stand.
      Articles for cleansing the skin.

(Alternatively 2 ml of blood is sent to the laboratory in a Sequestrene container.)

Chapter 6

Beds and Bedding and other Equipment

Materials used for beds and bedding—care of linen—adjuncts to hospital beds, bed tables, cradles, bed elevators—bed-strippers—rubber and plastic foam beds and cushions—hot-water bottles—disposable equipment

Hospital beds. For general purposes the ordinary *bedstead* is 26 in. high, 6 ft. 6 in. long and 3 ft. wide. The framework is enamelled steel or iron, the castors are well made and move easily without jarring. The bottom legs are solid; by means of a lever the bedstead is raised on to a central castor when it is to be moved and lowered to rest on the solid blocked ends. The spring mattress is of stout wire. There are many adaptations of this bedstead:

> The *high-low or variable height bed* is adjustable between 15 and 27 in. high, so that a patient sitting on the edge of his bed can have his feet on the floor.
> A *movable back* is supplied with most beds. This can be brought forward to act as a back rest; or removed for any treatment when necessary.
> The *head or foot of the bedstead* may be raised or lowered by levers. Many other modifications are available.

Mattresses. Many of these have interior springs; others are rubber foam, plastic foam, 'Sorbo' and 'Dunlopillo'.

Protection of mattresses is essential. The commonest type of cover is polythene, which is disposable. It has one open end so that the mattress is ventilated. It is hygienic as a new cover is supplied for each patient.

Plastic mattress covers are also available but they are more expensive. Some firms are producing mattresses made with a plastic cover; the surface is washed and dried when necessary and always on the discharge of a patient.

According to the type of mattress it may require brushing, or washing, and it may also require disinfecting or sterilizing.

Pillows may be filled with down, feather or kapok and should be inspected occasionally to see that they are comfortably filled; they can be steam disinfected. This type requires a plastic or polythene cover (beneath the cotton pillow case) which can be changed on the discharge of a patient.

Other pillows are of rubber foam, plastic foam, 'Sorbo' or 'Dunlopillo'; these can usually be surface washed or disinfected; they are covered by a cotton pillow case.

Blankets. *Terry blankets* and *cellular cotton blankets* have almost entirely replaced woollen ones. They have the advantage of being smoother, so that less fluff and dust is raised; they can be washed and sterilized repeatedly and though not as warm as woollen blankets they are reasonably warm and light.

Woollen blankets are warm but are injured by repeated washing and sterilizing and they need protection from moth during storage.

Linen. Sheets, drawsheets and pillow cases may be made of linen or cotton material. *Sheets* must be long enough and wide enough for the type of bed employed.

Drawsheets are generally supplied in a slightly thicker, more absorbent and warmer cotton than bed sheets. They may be of single or double material and should be long enough to be drawn through so that a patient may lie on a cool uncreased part of the drawsheet. Soiled or wet drawsheets may never be 'drawn through'; they must always be changed immediately. Disposable drawsheets are available.

Alternatively *disposable incontinence pads* are employed, but many patients complain that these are less comfortable than lying on a drawsheet.

A drawsheet may never be patched or darned; a patient's buttocks lie heavily upon it and any unevenness of the surface will predispose to pressure sores.

Pillow cases are generally of cotton material.

Waterproof sheeting. There are many varieties; rubber sheeting has largely given place to plastic and polythene materials. The latter, as already mentioned, is used as a mattress cover; it is also used as a waterproof beneath the drawsheet and has proved to be smooth and comfortable; moreover it is disposable.

Quilts are usually made of an easily washable cotton material.

Care of linen. A central linen store is generally available where the linen is inspected before it is put away for re-issue to the wards, so that there should never be any question of torn linen being put on the beds.

Old linen can be obtained from the linen store for use in the dressing of certain skin conditions and for any other purposes.

Removing stains. As a rule the linen-store staff will deal with the removal of stains from linen, but in emergencies the nurse in the ward may have to deal with this matter.

The application of some absorptive substance, such as salt, will prevent the staining agent from spreading.

> *Detergents* will dissolve most substances.
> *Blood stains* should be soaked in cold water and then washed.
> *Stains from medicines* may be treated by water or methylated spirit, as many medicines are soluble in water and others in spirit.

Iodine stains can be washed out if treated immediately.

Coffee, tea and *fruit stains* generally respond to soaking in water. Alternatively stretching the stained material over a basin and pouring hot water through it may be effective. If the stains do not respond to this treatment rubbing with a little lemon juice may help.

Inkstains respond most quickly to soaking the linen in milk. 'Biro' ink can be removed from any material by methylated spirit.

Precaution. Bleaching agents used to whiten linen should not be used by an amateur as they are destructive to materials.

Adjuncts to hospital beds include the following:

Bed tables should be of a suitable height (some are adjustable) so that a patient can take his meals comfortably, lean his arms on it when resting, and his book when reading. As a rule only two legs have castors, the back or the front, in order that the table may be moved as required but is quite stable.

Bed cradles may be of the usual semicircular shape or of the Harboro make, when one limb passes beneath the mattress which gives stability and the other lies over the part to be protected from pressure.

Bed elevators. Some beds are so adapted that the head or foot may be raised. Alternatively a *metal bed elevator* which is very stable may be used, or occasionally *bed blocks* which are much less stable are employed.

Bed-strippers are metal stands to be placed at the foot of a bed over which the bed clothing is draped.

Rings, cushions and air beds. The air ring or bed is not often employed; it needs inflating and the air pressure needs maintaining.

Any of the rubber materials employed for mattresses or pillows, e.g. rubber or plastic foam, may be obtained as circular or more conveniently horse-shoe shaped cushions.

In the prevention and treatment of pressure sores one of the special beds is increasingly used (mentioned in Chapter 4, pp. 50–2).

Hot-water bottles. Many authorities do not permit the use of a hot-water bottle under any circumstances. Generally speaking the *rubber hot-water bottle* is most commonly used; it should be filled three parts full, the air expelled, the screw cap firmly applied, the bottle inverted to test the stopper for leakage and covered with an adequate cover.

Precautions. Patients can easily be injured by the proximity of a hot-water bottle. It is definitely contra-indicated in unconscious patients, in those who have paralysis or any anaesthesia of the skin, in children and in irresponsible or restless persons.

DISPOSABLE EQUIPMENT

Never has nursing received a greater impact than from the use of products colloquially known as 'disposables'. The field is wide; the advantages include, first and foremost, the prevention of cross-infection by articles used once only, and commercially pre-sterilized. The syringe, which has received such spontaneous reception in the hospital world, is an outstanding example. An inexhaustible list of items include:

forceps	catheters
scissors	tubing
razors	connections
scalpels	clamps
transfusion	pre-packed
and infusion sets	enemas and
gloves	other equipment

Much time is saved as the nurse does not have to pack and cleanse many items. The *reduction of noise* in and near the ward, in the preparation and assembling of equipment because of the materials from which disposables are made, is very important. *In the field of textiles* most bed clothing is available, also towels, dressing gowns, examination-couch covers, surgeons' robes and nurses' caps and gowns.

Paper garments already produced by the fashion houses will no doubt influence the hospital field in the use of disposable garments.

The cost of all disposables is high at the present time but, as commercial possibilities increase, the cost may decrease because of competition between different manufacturers.

Many hardware items are available, including:

Surgical tape	Sputum cups
Bowls	Bath mats
Tooth mugs	Bed pans and urinals
Denture containers	

All types of receivers and bins are replaced by paper bags or plastic sacks.

As far as nurses are concerned disposables must be used with economy. The most important factor, however, is that by using them nurses are relieved of much time-consuming work and are thus freed for the care of patients.

Chapter 7

Bedmaking

The principles of bedmaking—lifting and moving patients in bed—special types of bed

---

Certain principles have to be considered, and certain points remembered, in making beds: (*a*) in order that the patient's comfort may be enhanced, and (*b*) that due economy may be observed in the use of equipment.

The locker or bedside table should be cleared and either a bed-stripper or two chairs placed back to back should be arranged near the bottom of the bed, on which the bedclothes can be neatly laid whilst the bed is being made, so that they will not drag along or touch the floor.

All articles likely to be required, such as the linen, a receptacle for soiled linen, a bedbrush or duster, should be collected. If the bed is occupied it should be inspected to see what clean linen may be necessary, and also as to whether clean bed attire is needed for the patient, and these should then be provided.

For a helpless patient, two nurses would be required to make the bed: as far as possible one should take the lead and stand on the right of the patient and the other follow, so that they work together in harmony. Their work should be quietly and quickly performed. The nurses should be opposite one another, at each side of the bed; needless journeys up and down the bedside should be avoided; the whole of the arm from the shoulder should be employed in the necessary movements, which should not be limited to the forearm, as this is poor economy of energy and leads to clumsiness of movement. All patting of bedclothes and jarring of the bed should be most carefully avoided. The bedclothes, including the bottom sheet, should be untucked all round before beginning to make or strip a bed.

The bedclothes should be placed ready at the bedside; they should be arranged in the order in which they will be used; linen articles will be folded by the laundry and the folds will make creases; as everything ought to be put on the bed straight, the crease down the centre of a sheet may be used as a guide to straightness.

The bottom bedclothes, waterproof, if used, and the sheet should be taut; the latter should be tucked over the mattress at the top, then pulled taut and tucked in at the bottom of the bed, then across the middle where the patient's buttocks will rest, then at the top and from side to side across the bottom part of the bed which is tightened last.

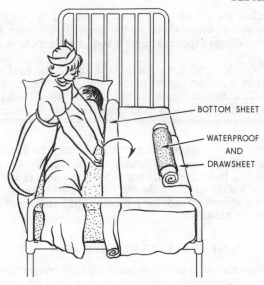

BOTTOM SHEET

WATERPROOF
AND
DRAWSHEET

Fig. 7/1 Changing the bottom sheet when the patient may be turned onto one or both sides. The short waterproof sheeting and the drawsheet are being changed at the same time.

This order of handling the bedclothes is also adhered to when making a bed with a patient in it.

A short polythene sheet and drawsheet are supplied to prevent soiling of the bottom sheets by excreta when sanitary utensils have to be used in bed.

A patient's face should never be covered by a sheet whilst making the bed. If the clothes are turned up, they should be folded under his chin and not placed over his face. The bedclothes should not be drawn tightly over the patient's body, nor taut over his feet. They must be comfortable, and the patient should always be able to dorsiflex his feet quite easily and freely and move his legs up and down in bed, and turn over as he wishes.

A patient must always be warned when movement is expected or is about to be carried out; if he is unable to help himself or this is inadvisable, he should be properly helped and well supported during movement.

Making a bed with a patient in it is so essentially practical that it should always be taught at the bedside.

LIFTING AND MOVING PATIENTS IN BED

Certain principles have to be considered when about to move a patient in his bed. It is essential to have a plan, which should be explained to the assistant so that she may thoroughly understand what is about to happen and that any jerky uncomfortable movements may be avoided. The one in charge should give the commands throughout.

The bedclothes should be rearranged so that their weight does not impede movement of the patient. In the majority of cases all top bed-clothes are removed as in the making of a bed, and the patient lies beneath one covering.

The nurses should bend from the hips, keeping the back straight; in this way a maximum effort can be made with the minimum discomfort.

The arms of the nurses handling the patient should pass fairly well round his body, and in lifting him from the bed should be passed well under the patient, and as far to the other side as possible, in order to give adequate support.

Nurses should never attempt to move a patient who is too heavy for them to lift, as this will not only be uncomfortable for the patient but probably mean that he loses confidence in his nurse and, in addition, cause undue and unnecessary strain on the nurse. The use of hoists and a variety of equipment for lifting and moving patients in bed and out of bed relieves nurses of considerable strain.

SPECIAL TYPES OF BED

Beds may be modified in different ways for the convenience of nursing a variety of cases. Some of the commonest modifications include:

Operation bed. A bed for a patient who has had an anaesthetic (see Fig. 7/2). Certain points require consideration in the preparation of this bed:

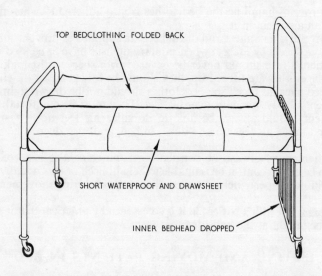

TOP BEDCLOTHING FOLDED BACK

SHORT WATERPROOF AND DRAWSHEET

INNER BEDHEAD DROPPED

Fig. 7/2 Bed for reception of patient after general anaesthesia. The top bedclothing is folded back, a short waterproof and drawsheet are in position. The inner bed head is dropped. Towel and receiver for vomit are always supplied. Tongue spatula, sponge holders (one with gauze), spare swabs and a pair of tongue forceps may be required should the airway become obstructed.

Generally it may be warmed, but for a patient who is hot, such as one having had thyroidectomy, for thyrotoxicosis, a cool bed should be prepared and a sheet may be adequate covering; any external application of heat is likely to cause sweating and loss of body fluid which is undesirable.

The bottom of the bed and any pillows likely to be used should be protected by waterproof sheet and covers. Articles for giving blood transfusion or fluid infusion should be at hand. Oxygen and/or carbon dioxide may be required.

Reception of the patient. When the patient is brought to the ward the nurse should see that there is a clear gangway from the ward door to the bedside. If the bed has not been prepared as in Fig. 7/2 the upper bedclothes should be removed and the patient placed gently on the bed in the position in which he is to lie until he has recovered from the effects of the anaesthetic. In the majority of cases he will be placed on his back or side.

The head should be turned to one side. The towel provided should be tucked round the patient's neck, and under his chin, and spread out on to the bed and so arranged that the patient's cheek rests on it; in this way the bedclothes would be saved should a little vomiting occur before the nurse can reach the bedside.

The nurse should notice whether:

> The patient's colour is good.
> His breathing is deep and regular.
> His pulse is satisfactory.
> The state of his blood pressure.

As far as possible a patient recovering from an anaesthetic should be screened from the view of other patients in the ward, but the screens or bed curtains should be so arranged that the nurses passing backwards and forwards up and down the ward can see the patient. If the patient is inclined to vomit or is at all restless the bedside should not be left.

Divided bed. The upper bedclothes are divided—usually about the middle. It may be used when an examination of the lower part of the abdomen or pelvis is necessary, or when a dressing, or other treatment of this area, has to be carried out. It is also used for amputation of the lower limb above the knee.

To prepare. For the purpose of making a divided bed the lower bedclothes are put on as usual, but for making the top of the bed two sheets will be required and two cotton cellular blankets.

To arrange the lower half of the top bedclothes, a sheet is placed lengthways over the patient and tucked in at the bottom; one blanket is laid on this, folded over so that it reaches to the level of the patient's pelvis. The upper part of the sheet is folded down over this blanket.

A *second sheet is taken*, also placed lengthways on the bed, and a blanket is placed on top of this sheet to cover the upper part of the patient's body. The lower part of this sheet is then folded up, over the lower edge of the doubled blanket, and the upper part of the sheet brought down over it to look like an ordinary sheet overlay. This part of the bedclothing is then tucked in at the sides.

It is important to arrange for the bedclothes to overlap from eight to twelve inches where they meet in the middle; unless contra-indicated the lower part should overlap the upper part, so that as the patient moves when a little separation of the bedclothes may occur he does not feel that he is exposed to the gaze of persons in the room—this arrangement is also neater.

The bedclothes can easily be separated for purposes of examination, inspection or treatment without unduly exposing or uncovering the patient, and this type of bed is particularly useful when treatment to the lower part of the abdomen, perineal area, or upper part of the thighs requires to be frequently repeated. Moreover, the necessity of making the bed each time, which proves not only trying to the patient, but exhausting to the nurse, is obviated.

Should this form of bed be utilized **in the case of an amputation of a lower limb above the knee**, a small bedcradle should be placed over the stump and the divided bedclothes arranged around the stump but not over it. Two sandbags should be supplied and a length of strong calico or, alternatively, a strong roller towel to keep the limb from flexing.

Fracture bed. A bed in which a case of fracture is to be nursed, particularly of the spine, pelvis or femur, must provide a firm unyielding surface on which the broken bone is to lie. For this purpose fracture boards may be used, either one large lathed board, or several small boards with holes bored in them.

Plaster bed. *As in the case of a bed for a fracture,* this also requires to be *firm and unyielding,* particularly when the trunk is encased in plaster or when a plaster spica of the hip has been applied. In both these cases any sagging of the bed before the plaster was completely dry would be likely to cause cracking.

Plaster of Paris is applied wet, and although the patient is not moved until it has set, even after this, considerable evaporation of moisture must take place before it can be considered satisfactorily dry and hard. Arrangements should therefore be made so that the part encased in plaster is *exposed to the air for evaporation and drying* (see Chapter 55, p. 542).

In the case of *a trunk in plaster,* for example, a divided bed might be utilized, with bedcradles over the patient's trunk, and one or two inlets arranged to allow air to circulate freely around the body.

In the case of *a leg in plaster,* having first wrapped the foot, if exposed, in a leg wrap to prevent its getting cold, the bedclothes might be turned back so that the entire limb is exposed, but a cellular blanket should be placed next to the patient so that he is not chilled by this process.

Heat is an aid to the drying of plaster of Paris; the bed may be drawn up near a fire or radiator; an electric cradle may be placed over it. Heat assists drying, as warming the air increases convection and evaporation of moisture from the damp plaster.

Blanket bed. The old-fashioned blanket bed is rarely used, though patients with some chronic conditions do occasionally prefer to sleep between some form of cellular or flannelette blankets or cotton twill sheets.

When patients, such as those with acute rheumatism, need protection from chilling, wrapping in a light absorbent cellular woollen blanket or simply wearing light woollen personal clothing which can be changed frequently is generally preferable.

Rheumatism bed. The bed should be firm but comfortable and steady so that it does not move easily; every movement causes pain. Bedcradles may be required to take the weight of the bedclothes from the aching limbs, and pillows or sandbags to support them steadily in as comfortable a position as possible.

Renal bed. *A bed for a patient with renal disease should be warm.* The number of pillows he needs will depend on whether there is oedema—a patient with swollen legs will generally be more comfortable sitting up.

Heart bed. *A bed prepared for a patient with heart disease* is described as a heart or *cardiac bed.* The position in which the patient will be nursed depends entirely on the condition of his heart.

In *acute heart disease*, with fair compensation, patients are best nursed flat; in this position the greatest rest is obtained.

In *chronic heart disease* in which pulmonary symptoms, including dyspnoea, have developed, or in the case where decompensation is marked, the patient may have to be propped up in order to breathe comfortably.

The bed for a patient with chronic mitral disease will, for example, require:

> A backrest, and several pillows, to support the patient's head and back.
>
> A rubber, foam or air ring pillow to protect the bottom of his back from pressure.
>
> A footrest to prevent him slipping down the bed.
>
> A bedtable or armrest in case he wishes to lean forward, as he may do when dyspnoea is so marked that the accessory muscles of respiration are continually in action, as this position, by fixing the shoulder girdle, makes movement easier.

Chapter 8

Positions Used in Nursing

The positions described are: supine—prone—semirecumbent—erect sitting—left lateral—Sims's semiprone—genu-pectoral—orthopnoeic —coma position or exaggerated semiprone for unconscious patients

The positions used in nursing vary with the needs of the patient—as a rule patients are nursed in *recumbent, semirecumbent* or *erect sitting positions*.

The best position is, if possible, the one the patient finds most comfortable; otherwise it must be one which will enable a patient's limb or limbs or organs to function to their maximum capacity and, if feasible, to be restored with complete function.

The dorsal recumbent or supine position is lying flat on the back with one soft pillow, the knees being straight or very slightly flexed.

This position provides for full relaxation and is the one in which many acutely ill patients are nursed.

It is contra-indicated in elderly persons, or any who may be subject to bronchitis, or liable to contract hypostatic congestion of the lungs; also in all surgical abdominal cases where drainage is necessary, and after operations on the breast or thorax, and in a great many other conditions.

It is also contra-indicated in most long-standing illnesses and in neurological conditions, as it is apt to become depressing—partly because of the difficulty of carrying on any little occupation in this position, and partly because the patient is not able to see and take an interest in the life which is going on around him.

This position is also used for examination of the front of the trunk and for examination of the abdomen. It is sometimes used for examination of the rectum and vagina provided the thighs are flexed and outwardly rotated.

Prone recumbent position. In this position the patient lies on the front of the body. A pillow is placed beneath the chest, and usually one arm lies beneath the body in a hollow below this pillow. A second pillow is provided on which to rest the side of the face, the arm on the side to which the face is turned lying flexed beside this pillow.

This position is not very often employed; it is useful when there is danger that pressure sores may form on the back, and it also prevents and relieves flatulent distension; it is occasionally used to facilitate drainage from the front of the body or after an operation on the spine.

Dorsal elevated or semirecumbent position. The patient lies on his back with his chest raised on several pillows. It can also be maintained by elevating the top of the bed on blocks so that the patient lies on an incline. This position is freely used, both in medical and surgical nursing. It is the one in which most gastric cases are nursed; most chronic and subacute and some acute chest conditions; many patients after a general anaesthetic and after abdominal or pelvic operations, except when the erect sitting position is indicated. In the **erect sitting position**, the patient must be supported by a bed rest. This has entirely replaced Fowler's position. Practically all convalescent patients favour this position, but there is a tendency for patients to slip down. A foot rest can be provided, this will help, but a better plan is to elevate the foot of the bed six inches from the floor which will not only prevent a patient from slipping down, but will help the circulation in the lower limbs. This not only reduces the tendency to thrombosis but by aiding the circulation lessens the liability to pressure sores.

Left lateral position. This must not be confused with Sims's position (see Fig. 8/2). The left lateral position is used when a patient is turned onto his side for purposes of washing and rubbing his back as in the routine treatment for the prevention of pressure sores. It is also frequently used for giving any form of enema, for the insertion of a suppository, the taking of the temperature by the rectum, or for any treatment to, or examination of, the perineal region.

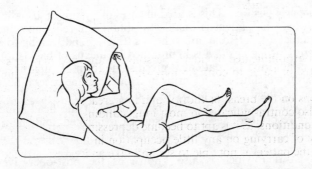

Fig. 8/1 The left lateral position, as would be used for examination or treatment of the rectum.

Sims's semiprone position is one in which the patient lies partly prone, and on her left side. Her right arm lies on the bed in front of her and the left is behind her, lying on the bed on which she lies (see Fig. 8/2).

Both knees are drawn up, *the right being rather more flexed than the left*, and lying on the bed in front of it, thus rendering the position fairly steady.

The left side of the face rests on a small pillow placed under the cheek.

This position is used for examination of the vagina; the effect of it is to cause ballooning of the vagina when a Sims's speculum is introduced, thus facilitating examination of the vaginal walls. It is also useful when a rectal treatment is to be undertaken, should it be considered necessary for the anus to be more clearly visible than is possible in the left lateral position.

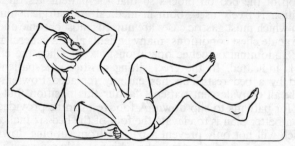

Fig. 8/2 Sims's semiprone position, as used for vaginal examination.

Genu-pectoral (knee chest) position. The patient rests on his knees, arms and chest. To obtain it, he is asked to kneel on the bed and, keeping his thighs upright, to bend forward until his chest rests on the bed; he then places his arms in front on each side of his head. His head is turned to one side and his face rests on a small pillow. This position is used when the effect of gravity is employed as in the administration of high colonic lavage in some cases; and also as a position in which sigmoidoscopy may be performed on male patients.

Orthopnoeic position. This is used in cases of dyspnoea, usually in heart disease, when the patient is unable to obtain any relief and finds it extremely difficult to breathe unless he is sitting up and leaning forward.

This *erect sitting position* is maintained by means of back support and pillows. In addition the patient is given some form of support, such as a bedtable, on which to rest his arms in front. In some cases a headrest on which the forehead can be placed is also provided.

Nurses will notice the nodding movements of the head which occur with every respiratory act when dyspnoea is marked, and the provision of a headrest in such cases adds considerably to the patient's comfort.

Coma position which is also known as the post-operative 'tonsil' position is *an exaggerated semiprone position used for patients who are unconscious.* The trunk is practically prone, the right arm flexed, the left lying beside his body. The right leg is flexed and lying on the bed or couch in front of the patient to give him stability (see Fig, 8/3).

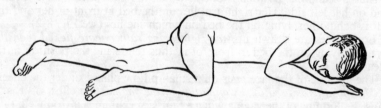

Fig. 8/3 Patient in semiprone position, suitable for the unconscious (see text, above).

Chapter 9

The Administration of Medicines and Drugs

Method of checking drugs—modes of administering drugs—giving medicines by mouth—the use of special drug identity cards—parenteral administration—inhalations—Croupaire air humidifier—use of therapeutic and pressurized aerosols

It is most important to recognize that the patient's treatment card (or bed card or prescription sheet, as it is sometimes known) is the focal point from which all actions stem. Except in extreme emergencies, no drug should be administered to a patient unless it is prescribed by a doctor on the treatment card. This applies to any drug whether or not it is a poison because sometimes an apparently harmless drug can produce an unwanted effect by interaction with another drug which the patient is taking.

Every medicine whether or not it is poison should be checked *against the prescription on the treatment card at the bedside immediately before administration*. The method of checking drugs given below should be followed whenever possible.

A METHOD FOR CHECKING DRUGS ADMINISTERED BY THE NURSING STAFF

1. Read the prescription carefully
2. Ascertain that the prescribed dose has not already been administered
3. Select the drug required and check the label with the prescription
4. Prepare the drug in the presence of a witness who should check with the prescription:
    - (*a*) the drug
    - (*b*) the calculation if any
    - (*c*) the measured dose and
    - (*d*) the name of the patient
5. Take the measured dose and the prescription to the bedside, check the identity of the patient and administer the drug in the presence of the witness
6. Enter the details of the administration in the appropriate ward record book, which should never be a loose-leaf book. In the case of Controlled Drugs the details should be entered in the Ward Controlled Drugs Record Book. Both these records should be signed in full by both donor and witness.

Knowledge of dosage and usage. A trained nurse should be familiar with the customary dose of the drugs in constant use. If in doubt, she should verify the dose, and she must query a dose if she considers it excessive in amount, though such a query should of course be made with tact. A nurse should never be afraid to ask questions about the dosage and action of drugs. The number of dangerous drugs on the market is so varied and they are so often made up in different strengths that no one need ever be ashamed to show ignorance on this matter.

The *British National Formulary*, published annually, provides useful information on the action and uses of most commonly used drugs, and if possible a copy should be provided in every ward for use on the ward medicine trolley or medicine cupboard, for the information of nurses.

MODES OF ADMINISTERING DRUGS

By *way of the alimentary canal*, either by mouth, which is by far the most common route used, or by means of the rectum. Rectal doses are sometimes, though not invariably, larger than oral doses.

By *hypodermic* or *subcutaneous injection*. By this route drugs enter the circulation through absorption by means of the lymphatics.

By *intramuscular injection* more rapid action is made possible.

Intrathecally, or by means of the cerebrospinal fluid route. This method is chosen in the treatment of some forms of meningitis (for mode of administration see lumbar puncture, p. 120).

Intravenous (for mode of administration see p. 458).

By the skin by inunction and ionization.

By inhalation, p. 87.

GIVING MEDICINES BY MOUTH

Medicines must be given punctually at stated hours, such as 10, 2, and 6; or 11, 3, and 7, unless the medicine is specially required to be given in relation to food. A gastric irritant, such as ferrous sulphate tablets, should be given after food. Medicines employed to increase weight are also given after food.

Medicines given to allay spasm, such as chalk, and bismuth; to inhibit secretion, such as belladonna, atropine and olive oil; to affect the reaction of the gastric juices, such as hydrochloric acid or alkalis, and bitters, which are given to stimulate the gastric secretion, are given before food; but alkalis used in the treatment of peptic ulcer, with the object of reducing the acidity of the gastric juice are given after meals.

Aperients are usually given on an empty stomach, last thing at night, especially when the drug employed is laxative in its effect and acts slowly, taking from 10 to 12 hours to produce its effect. Aperients which have a rapid action, such as the saline aperients, are given on a fasting stomach first thing in the morning, half an hour before the first drink of tea is taken.

A nurse should have a good working knowledge of the time an aperient she may be asked to give will take to act, and she should administer the medicine at a time which will allow the patient to be as little disturbed as possible.

The administration of medicines requires the greatest possible care and thoughtfulness, as well as undivided attention.

Whilst pouring out and delivering medicines at the bedside, when possible, a nurse should not attend to any other matter; there should be no general conversation or chatter; the nurse engaged in giving medicines should not be spoken to, or otherwise interrupted, except in a case of emergency. The directions on the medicine bottle label should be read carefully, before and after pouring out the dose of liquid medicine.

In **pouring out a dose of medicine**, the bottle should be held with the label uppermost, and the fluid should be poured out from the side away from the label, any drips being caught with a swab before replacing the screw cap.

The marked medicine glass or measure should be held with the marks against the light, just above the level of the eye, so that the person pouring out the medicine has to raise her head slightly to look at the level of the fluid in the glass. The surface of fluid in a small measure is not flat, it has a curve—the *meniscus*—which is lowest at the centre so that, if the measure is held just above the level of the eye, the lowest point of the curve of the meniscus may be considered to be on a level with the marking on the medicine glass. It is important to remember that liquid mixtures which contain an insoluble solid will not provide accurate dosage for the patient unless the bottle is well shaken before each dose is measured. Vigorous shaking of the bottle is essential: gentle inversion of the bottle once or twice is not sufficient to distribute evenly throughout the liquid all the insoluble material suspended in it. Before pouring the dose of a liquid medicine containing a sediment, the bottle should be inverted after shaking and no impacted powder should be seen adhering to the bottom of the bottle. If it is, then the shaking has been inadequate.

In **giving tablets, pills, cachets** and **capsules**, they should be delivered in a spoon and accompanied by a fairly long drink of water. *Cachets* may be softened by placing them in a spoonful of water before swallowing. *Powders*, which are rarely used, should be unfolded, collected to the middle of the packet and poured onto the centre of the protruded tongue. The patient should be given water sufficient to swallow the powder. If he objects to this mode of administration, the powder may be buried in a spoonful of jelly or jam, provided they form part of the patient's diet.

Effervescent powders should be dissolved in half a tumbler of water and drunk whilst effervescing.

Giving medicines to children. The formulated paediatric preparations are pleasant to take. In the event of these not being available a child can usually be persuaded to swallow his medicine by having a sweet, a pleasant drink or a little fruit or other similar treat after it.

The Use of Special Drug Identity Cards

Many patients who are to be treated with certain drugs as out-patients or by their own family doctors are provided with Drug Identity Cards which they are instructed to carry wherever they go. These drugs include the following:

Anticoagulants.
Corticosteroids.

Corticotrophin (A.C.T.H.).

Insulin and oral hypoglycaemic drugs.

Monoamine oxidase inhibitor anti-depressant drugs.

The reason for this is that in the case of some of these drugs a sudden withdrawal can result in serious or even fatal consequences and in others the concurrent administration of other drugs may produce a toxic interaction. Patients who are taking these drugs are at risk if for any reason they lose consciousness or require medical treatment in an emergency.

Thus, as far as the nurse is concerned, it is important that when admitting a patient either to a ward or to the Casualty Department, she should attempt to discover whether or not the patient is carrying a Drug Identity Card and advise the doctor accordingly.

PARENTERAL ADMINISTRATION

The intracutaneous or intradermal route

The injection of a small amount of fluid, 0·1 ml, is made into the substance of the skin and not beneath it. It is employed for diagnostic purposes; pollen extracts and certain proteins are prepared for injection by this route to enable the physician to diagnose the cause of allergic reactions. The result of the test is read after a prescribed interval; a positive result is usually denoted by an area of redness or inflammation or by the appearance of an indurated area or weal. The Mantoux test (see p. 403), is another example.

Subcutaneous or hypodermic administration or injection

By this means drugs reach the bloodstream more rapidly than when given by mouth. It is also employed in many instances where the drug does not remain potent when it is administered by the mouth, owing to its action being affected by the digestive juices. About 1 to 2 ml is an average amount of fluid for this injection. Having charged the syringe the air is expelled by holding it, needle pointing upwards, and slowly pressing the piston into the barrel until all air bubbles have been expressed and a drop of the solution is seen at the end of the needle. Having explained the procedure to the patient the skin over the triceps on the outer aspect of the arm or on the exterior aspect of forearm over the brachio-radialis muscle is chosen as these areas are fairly well-covered with subcutaneous fat; the skin is cleansed with a medicated swab and either stretched by pressure of the thumb and forefinger of the left hand or the tissue may be grasped.

The needle is then inserted beneath the skin *parallel with the surface*, the grasp of the tissue is relaxed and the solution gently, but not too slowly, flows out of the barrel of the syringe by gentle pressure on the end of the piston, either with the thumb or the palm of the hand.

The needle is withdrawn and as it leaves the skin a swab is placed over the puncture and held there for a few moments. If a tumour of fluid is visible, gentle massage in an upward direction away from the puncture should be used to disperse it.

All subcutaneous injections should be given in an upward direction as this corresponds with the flow of the lymphatic stream by which the drug is carried into the blood. An injection should not be made over a joint or over any part in which the fascia is taut as this would be painful.

Care should be taken to avoid injecting the fluid into a vein *by withdrawing the plunger slightly prior to injecting.*

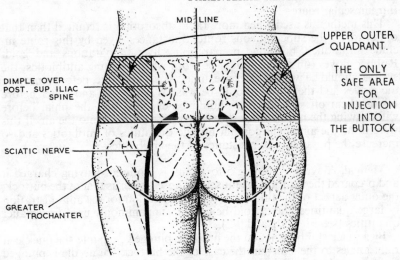

Fig. 9/1 Area of buttock for intramuscular injection. Note the upper outer quadrant as the correct site.

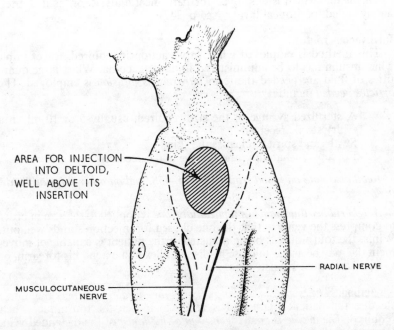

Fig. 9/2 Deltoid area for intramuscular injection.

Intramuscular route

This method is used when more rapid absorption is required than that obtained by the subcutaneous route. Substances given by this route include antibiotics, hormone preparations, liver preparations and gold. Rubber gloves (unsterile) should be worn when injecting antibiotics; the syringe should be washed after use, unless it is disposable, before removing the gloves and the gloves should be washed with soap and water before taking them off. Air bubbles should be expelled into the phial before withdrawing the needle; they should never be expelled into the air. If this were done the air might contain minute quantities of antibiotics and so increase the possibility of resistance to the antibiotics.

Method. A syringe holding 5 to 10 ml is required. Having charged it and prepared the skin, a large muscle is chosen, such as that of the buttock, the outer aspect of the thigh or the scapular region for the administration of large quantities, the deltoid being the site commonly used for smaller quantities (see Figs. 9/1 and 9/2).

By a quick stabbing action the needle is plunged deep into the muscle at right angles to the skin—in the case of the buttock the needle is plunged right up to the hilt, the nurse steadying its passage through the skin by a forefinger placed on the hilt of the needle. The plunger is withdrawn slightly, about a quarter of an inch, to make sure the needle is not lying in a vein; the injection should then be steadily made. On withdrawing the needle the puncture is covered by a small adhesive dressing.

Intraperitoneal route

This is one which is employed for peritoneal dialysis, or, as it is alternately called, peritoneal lavage (see p. 247).

Intravenous route

This method is employed when rapid action is required, for example when insulin has to be administered in diabetic coma. When large quantities of fluid are needed the term *intravenous infusion* is employed. The *articles needed* include:

> A sterilized syringe of the size required, usually 5 or 10 ml, in a dry sterile receiver.
> Swabs and spirit to cleanse the skin.
> Forceps for handling the syringe and a receiver.

Read also note on blood transfusion, p. 458, and on other infusion fluids, p. 460.

A light rubber tourniquet or a *pneumatic one* is applied to the arm in order to compress the veins so that the one chosen for injection stands well out. Whilst the tourniquet is being adjusted, if the patient is capable of movement, he may be asked to close his fist and flex and extend his forearm, or to open and close his fist.

Method. *The syringe is charged and the needle adjusted,* the nurse steadies the patient's arm and is ready to loosen the tourniquet when required. *The needle is passed gently into the lumen* of the distended vein, taking care that it is not passed through it.

The *tourniquet is now loosened*, the operator withdraws the piston slightly and a little blood enters the barrel of the syringe, *which proves* that the needle is in the vein.

The injection is made slowly and evenly and the needle gently withdrawn. The nurse now puts a dry sterile swab over the puncture, flexes the arm on to this and holds it steady for a few moments. The slight oozing will cease and no further dressing is needed.

INHALATIONS

Gases, vapours and the fumes of drugs may be inhaled:

(a) In order to produce a direct effect on the upper respiratory passages through which the vapour passes.

(b) To influence the circulation in the lungs and so either increase or decrease the bronchial secretions.

(c) To allay spasm by effecting alteration in the vasomotor control of the bronchial blood vessels.

(d) To produce a systemic effect by absorption through the lungs.

Ammonia, which is inhaled in cases of fainting and syncope, irritates the mucous membrane and also reflexly stimulates the respiratory, cardiac and vasomotor centres, thus improving the circulation. It should be applied to the nostrils with caution, the eyes being kept closed, otherwise the conjunctiva would be irritated by it.

Amyl nitrite is used in the treatment of some forms of angina pectoris. Capsules containing 0·1 to 0·2 ml of the drug crushed in gauze are held to the nose for the patient to inhale. The immediate effect produced is flushing of the face, head and neck, as the drug causes dilation of the arterioles and capillaries, and its effect on the spasmodically contracted coronary blood vessels is thereby demonstrated.

Steam inhalations are used in tracheitis, bronchitis and sinusitis to clear the air passages and give relief. Even steam from hot water may give relief but the use of medicated inhalations is more effective. These should be added to hot, not boiling, water, a temperature of 70 °C (160 °F) is a safe guide. The substances mentioned in the *British National Formulary*, p. 82 and also p. 183 are:

Menthol and Benzoin Inhalation, B.P.C.
Menthol and Eucalyptus Inhalation B.P.C.

Nelson's inhaler is supplied in various sizes, the average being a one-litre capacity. *The air inlet should never be covered*, as if air cannot reach the fluid in the vessel the vapour cannot rise.

The *mouthpiece*, generally made of glass, passes through a bung which fits the inhaler; it should be placed in a direction opposite to the air inlet (see Fig. 9/3).

The patient places his lips to the mouthpiece, which should be protected by a piece of gauze as it tends to get hot and patients have had their lips blistered by it. Breathing in, the patient inhales the steam; if he breathes out into the inhaler, steam will escape from the outlet; it is better for him to remove his lips from the mouthpiece whilst breathing out.

In many instances the nurse must stand by a patient steadying the

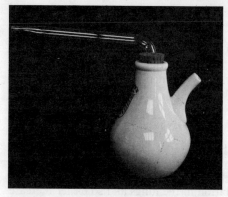

Fig. 9/3 Nelson's inhaler.

inhaler for him. To inhale the steam which will rise from one litre of water will take about 15 to 20 minutes.

Patients with breathlessness and painful chests find stooping over a short mouthpiece distressing—a long mouthpiece (Fig. 9/3) has been designed so that the inhaler can be placed on a bedtable with the patient sitting upright against his pillows; alternatively the inhaler may be placed on a table, the patient sitting beside it on a chair. The use of the long mouthpiece results in the water vapour cooling a little by the time it has reached the patient. A disadvantage is that the long stem becomes hot to touch without protection.

Jug inhalation. Any ordinary jug or a large stone jam jar, or the base of Nelson's inhaler may be used. The opening is draped turban-fashion with a towel and the patient applies his nose and mouth to this opening inhaling the steam, raising his head to breathe out and continuing the process as long as steam rises.

Paper handkerchiefs and a disposal bag and/or a sputum carton should always be within reach of a patient who is having an inhalation.

A *steam kettle* may be used when it is desirable to maintain a constantly moist atmosphere.

The Croupaire

The need to humidify the atmosphere more continuously is met by the Croupaire which provides a directional cool vapour mist delivering water droplets in correct particle size to a distance of 3 feet or more and at a temperature several degrees lower than the room.

This cool soothing mixture prevents dryness, loosens bronchial exudate and eases breathing. It is safe and simple to use, driven by electricity and with a reservoir capacity of 3,000 ml.

The piece of equipment shown in Fig. 9/4 is directed towards a child's bed but is equally of value in acute and chronic chest infections in any age group.

As a rule water only is used to provide liquid for the 'mist'. The Croupaire, whilst functioning like other aerosols, is not in any way a pharmaceutical preparation. Its main purpose is to humidify the air where formerly steam inhalations were used, but more comfortably and more effectively.

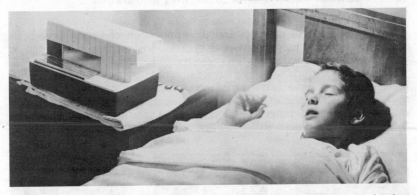

Fig. 9/4 Croupaire air humidifier which provides a directional cool vapour mist that prevents dryness, loosens bronchial exudate and eases breathing.

THERAPEUTIC AEROSOLS

An aerosol may contain plain water, as in the Croupaire shown above, or some medium which can be atomized into a fine mist for application to:

> *A body cavity*, such as the ear, nose, mouth, throat, vagina and rectum; or specifically to *a wound* to promote healing and as a *protective skin* covering for surgical stitches.

Aerosols are used:

> In the prevention and care of *pressure sores* and *napkin rashes*.
>
> As a silicone or balsam preparation for application to any surface areas likely to be contaminated by sweat, urine, faeces or discharges.
>
> For *inhalation therapy*, e.g. in asthma and bronchitis to liquefy mucus and make breathing easier, and to bring a decongestant like ephedrine into contact with the respiratory tract. *Inhalation therapy is also employed in place of a subcutaneous injection as absorption through the blood in the lungs is transmitted rapidly into the general circulation. This method is considered useful for children and ambulant patients.*
>
> As *nose sniffs* to relieve nasal congestion when a combination of ingredients—menthol, thymol, camphor, etc.—may be employed as a decongestant.
>
> To produce local anaesthesia to the skin and underlying tissues and in dentistry. *Intranasal anaesthetic and astringent aerosols are replacing packing the nasal cavity with gauze soaked in a mixture of adrenaline and cocaine prior to a nasal operation.*

Aerosols which lower the bacterial content of the air and act as *space disinfectants* are employed in intensive care units, in wards and annexes and to treat rooms, buildings, and transport vehicles, including aircraft.

Pressurized aerosols

The insufflation of powders and the application of sprays have been constantly in use in medicine over the years. Most were bulb-operated or driven by compressed oxygen or electric power. More recently *pressurized aerosols* which contain a suspension of finely powdered drug in an inert propellant have been introduced. Release of the valve allows a measured dose of the drug to be expelled. This is directed through a mouthpiece to the lungs of the patient. The illustration shows the 'Medihaler' (Fig. 9/5), a Riker Laboratories preparation, in use.

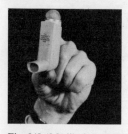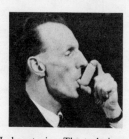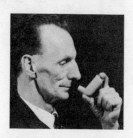

Fig. 9/5 'Medihaler', Riker's Laboratories. The technique which we advise is as follows: (*a*) With the adapter dust cap removed, the 'Medihaler' should be shaken to disperse the particles of medicament in the propellant. (*b*) The mouthpiece should then be placed well into the mouth and the lips closed firmly around it. (When the adapter is held at the correct angle, the spray will go right to the back of the throat and down into the lungs.) The patient should now breathe out fully through the adapter. As soon as the patient starts to breathe in, the vial should be pressed firmly down into the adapter. This actuates the 'Medihaler' and a dose is released. (*c*) The adapter should now be taken from the mouth and the inspired breath held for as long as possible to avoid exhaling particles of medicament. Before taking a further inhalation, the patient should wait for at least one minute to allow the full effect of the puff to become apparent.

'The self-propelled aerosol'. There are many preparations and a number of drugs are available. Clear warning as to the dangers of misuse or overdosage is included on instruction cards from the makers.

In using aerosols for inhalation therapy the patient is subject to the same therapeutic effects as in intravenous therapy. A nurse must be aware of this, as a patient's natural desire to obtain relief from frightening symptoms of breathlessness must be dealt with by adequate instruction and discipline to ensure that the prescribed dosage is not exceeded. Each puff from 'Medihaler' delivers a measured dose. One to three puffs should be sufficient to provide relief in most cases. It should not be necessary for the patient to take further treatment for at least thirty minutes, or more than eight treatments a day.

Chapter 10

The Use of Enemas and Suppositories

Evacuant enemas, disposable, water, saline or soap solution—olive oil—olive oil and glycerin—arachis oil—magnesium sulphate—Veripaque—retention—to pass a flatus tube—suppositories, evacuant, retention

---

An enema is an injection into the lower bowel. It is given for several reasons:

> *To empty the bowel* in some cases of constipation, before an operation, in elderly people or paraplegics in whom large quantities of faecal matter may be retained, even impacted.
>
> *To give drugs in solution* when, as these must be *retained*, less than 300 ml should be given (see Retention Enemas, p. 94).
>
> *To inject a radio-opaque solution*, as when a barium enema (see p. 689) is given.

EVACUANT ENEMAS

A disposable enema may be given which does not usually contain more than 150 ml. of solution; other articles required include:

> A lubricant on a swab.
> A disposable (paper) towel.
> A paper bag for the used enema, swab and towel.

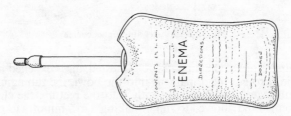

Fig. 10/1 A disposable enema.

Method 1. The procedure is explained to the patient who lies in the left lateral position, covered and so arranged that only the buttocks are exposed, the paper towel is placed beneath the buttocks, the stopper is removed, or the end of the enema container is cut, a little lubricant is applied to the nozzle which is gently inserted into the rectum for about 8 cm (3 in.). The plastic envelope is rolled up to expel the contents through the tube, the tube is withdrawn and any lubricant remaining around the anus is removed using the paper towel. The patient may move or be moved into a more comfortable position and retains the enema for a time—after he has used the bedpan or commode, if he attends to his own toilet, he is given water in which to wash his hands.

Method 2. Using water, saline or a soap solution, a litre or less is prepared. The articles to be assembled include:

A bowl containing a funnel with about 25 cm of tubing.
Glass or plastic connection.
A Jaques' catheter, size 10 to 14 E.G.
A spring clip.
A lotion thermometer.
Lubricant for catheter.
Either paper towels or a small incontinence pad to place under the buttocks.
A bedpan.
Cellulose tissue for the anal toilet.

The approach to the patient, who may wish to empty his bladder, and the position adopted is as for a disposable enema.

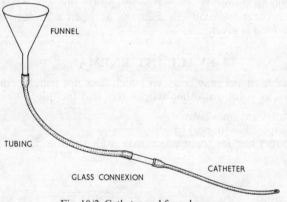

FUNNEL

TUBING

GLASS CONNEXION

CATHETER

Fig. 10/2 Catheter and funnel enema.

The temperature of the fluid (38 °C) is tested, air is expelled by running a little fluid through the apparatus into the bowl, the tubing clip closed, catheter lubricated and inserted gently into the rectum, the clip released and the enema fluid allowed to run in, taking 3 to 5 minutes to give a litre.

If discomfort is experienced the tubing clip should be closed for a few minutes while the patient, breathing through his mouth, rests and relaxes.

On completion the catheter is withdrawn, placed in a receiver, putting the remaining apparatus into the bowl. The patient is encouraged to retain the enema for a few minutes, he is then given a bedpan or, if allowed out of bed, helped to a commode.

The articles may be removed from the bedside but the nurse should remain within call and observe the condition of the patient. His condition before and after the enema should be noted and reported.

Observation. The condition of the returned enema should be inspected and a report on the character of the result made.

> Whether it is merely coloured fluid, contains only particles of faeces or is a good action.
> The character of the stool should be stated.
> The presence of any abnormal constituents or abnormalities of shape, colour, etc.
> The passage of flatus should be noted.

When an enema is given to relieve retention of urine it is important to discover whether urine is passed, and for this purpose the returned enema must be measured and compared with the quantity given, unless evidence from some other source is obtained.

Olive-oil enema. A quantity of 180 to 600 ml of warmed olive oil constitutes an olive-oil enema, although many authorities advocate the mixing of olive oil with equal quantities of warm water. This enema is given slowly, with a large catheter, or a rectal tube and glass funnel. The apparatus should be prepared in hot water to keep the tubing as pliable as possible and so facilitate the passage of the warmed oil.

Olive-oil-and-glycerin enema. Equal parts of olive oil and glycerin may be administered in the same way as the enema described above.

Arachis-oil enema. This is 60 to 120 ml given in hot water, taking 10 to 15 minutes. Alternatively *a disposable arachis-oil enema* is available. Both are employed for softening impacted faeces.

A magnesium sulphate enema is made by mixing 30 to 60 g in 120 to 240 ml of warm water. Alternatively a 25 per cent solution of magnesium sulphate is available in a disposable container.

This enema is hygroscopic, producing a watery stool, and is sometimes used to relieve intracranial pressure but its place has been largely taken by suitable drugs (see p. 660).

Veripaque enema

This enema contains a substance which activates the colon; it may be given in combination with barium or before a barium enema. A phial of Veripaque is dissolved in 2 litres of water at a temperature of 38 °C. It is given with catheter and funnel or by other gravitational method; the lubricated catheter is passed about 12 cm into the rectum with the patient in the lateral position. The enema is given slowly and the patient should be able to hold at least 1 litre for some minutes before it is evacuated into pan or commode. The patient may feel weak and faint and his general condition should be watched. If not effective this enema should not be repeated under two hours.

Most hospitals have their method of using Veripaque, some adopt the following procedure:

Wash out the colon thoroughly with water or some bland solution, using 4 to 5 litres.

Give the Veripaque enema.

A straight X-ray may be taken to determine that the colon is empty.

A barium enema is then given in the usual way (see p. 689).

RETENTION ENEMAS

The solution usually contains prednisolone sodium phosphate, 20 mg in 100 ml of buffered solution. This enema is also available as a proprietary product, Predsol Retention Enema, prepacked ready for immediate use, a convenient means for self-administration. It is used each night, and/or morning. Lying on the left side with knees drawn up, the stopper is removed, the nozzle lubricated and gently inserted for half its length into the rectum, the plastic bag is slowly rolled up like a tube of toothpaste taking a minute or two, the contents of the enema being injected; the nozzle is removed after ensuring that no solution flows back into the bag which is discarded. The patient then rolls into any comfortable position and rests. These enemas are valuable in some forms of ulcerative colitis.

TO PASS A FLATUS TUBE

A flatus tube may be passed:

> To relieve abdominal distension.
> Before giving an enema which is to be retained.
> Occasionally before giving an evacuant enema.

Method. The anal region should be swabbed clean, the tube lubricated and passed (for about 12 cm) into the rectum. The free end of the tube is attached by a connection to a piece of tubing long enough to be passed into a bowl of antiseptic lotion, e.g. Sudol, so that the amount of gas bubbling through the fluid may be observed and reported.

The effect may be enhanced by giving the patient a hot drink or a carminative such as peppermint water or by a light application of heat, e.g. an electric pad to the abdomen.

SUPPOSITORIES

These are usually cone-shaped solidified preparations containing a lubricant or drug. They may be divided into:

> Evacuant suppositories.
> Retention suppositories (a flatus tube should be passed before inserting one to be retained).

Composition. *A glycerin suppository* is of glycerin solidified with gelatin; those containing drugs are composed of oil of theobroma, except in hot climates where this would melt, when purified beeswax is employed.

To insert a suppository, if possible have the patient in the left lateral position though this is not essential. The lubricated or moistened suppository should be inserted well beyond the anal canal, into the rectum, slowly and carefully in order to avoid injury to the mucous surfaces.

Types of suppositories. There are several well-known *evacuant suppositories:*

> *Glycerin* which, acting as a hygroscopic agent, causes evacuation by withdrawing fluid from the tissues.
>
> *Bisacodyl suppositories* B.P.C. (proprietary product Dulcolax) act as an aid to evacuation by increasing the mucous secretion of the membranes with which they are in contact.
>
> *Beogex* (proprietary preparation liberating CO_2). One to be inserted half an hour before evacuation expected.

Suppositories given to be retained include:

> *Aminophylline* suppositories B.P.C. in specially prescribed dosage for adults and children are used in the treatment of bronchial spasm as in chronic asthma.
>
> *Anaesthetic. Thiopentone* given to children as an alternative to the intravenous route.
>
> *Medicinal steroids.* Hydrocortisone or prednisolone used as local treatment in proctitis, and ulcerative colitis.
>
> An *analgesic*, such as aspirin 300 mg.

Precautions. After the insertion of a suppository which is to be retained the patient should be placed to lie in a position in which he can be comfortable and relaxed. He may read.

When giving a suppository to a child very great care is needed and it would be wise to hold the buttocks pressed together for a few minutes, otherwise it may be ejected immediately. If the child is interested in some pleasure he will soon relax.

Chapter 11

Bandages and Bandaging

Types of bandages—material used in bandaging—examples of bandages and bandaging—crêpe, Kling, Netelast, Tubegauz

There are varieties of bandage, examples including the *roller bandage* made from strips of material of convenient lengths and from half an inch to eight inches wide. These bandages should be prepared without selvedge; in many cases raw edges are used; in the woven bandages the edges are firm but not hard. A roller bandage should be closely and firmly rolled, with all the edges even.

Special bandages include the T-shaped bandage, plain and many-tailed binders and the four-tailed binders. A *T-bandage* is made by taking two strips of material, about 5 in. (12 cm) wide, and stitching them together in form of the letter T. It is used to retain dressings on the perineum. In the case of a male patient the strip of material carried up in front of the pubes is divided into two, one being placed on each side of the scrotum.

A *plain binder* is made by stitching two strips of material together, so forming a double layer.

A *many-tailed binder* or bandage, the bandage of Scultetus, is made by stitching strips of material together in the middle third of their length, leaving the ends on either side free, in tail formation. A many-tailed bandage can be made in an emergency by tearing a piece of material into shape; the bandage, with the tails at one side rolled or folded up, can be slipped under a limb by pressing down on the pillow or mattress on which it lies; then, by taking the tails across in front of the limb, a dressing may be retained in position and changed without movement of the limb.

The *four-tailed bandage* for the jaw is made by taking a piece of material of the desired length and width, about $3\frac{1}{2}$ in. (9 cm) wide, and shaping it as shown above. The wide part is placed over the chin, the upper tails which are 40 in. long are taken round, below the ear, to the occiput where the ends are crossed and carried obliquely across the side of the head, to be fastened over the forehead in front. The lower tails are carried up the side of the head and fastened on top.

Materials used for bandages. *Cotton, linen, muslin, gauze, calico* and *net* are fairly light materials. *Flannel, flannelette* and *domette* are warmer than cotton, and a little firmer. *Crêpe* material is used where slight elasticity is required, and *elastic* and *rubber* bandages where firm support is needed.

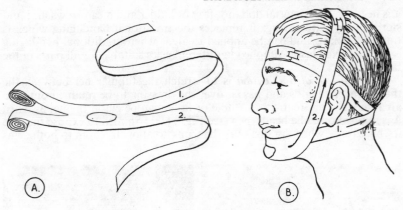

Fig. 11/1 Method of cutting and applying a simple four-tailed jaw bandage.

For warmth and protection, *lint* or *cotton wool* bandages are used. *Plaster of Paris* bandages are employed where a very firm surface is required to act as a splint (see p. 542).

Application of a roller bandage. The operator should stand facing the patient, generally with the bandage in the right hand if a right arm or leg is to be bandaged. Application is made from within outwards and below upwards though this is not invariable and depends on the effect which is desired. When *circular turns* are taken as round the neck, over the wrist or ankle they should be adequately firm without being tight. Pressure should always be even. Readers are referred to the excellent manuals of the British Red Cross and St John Ambulance Association for the illustrated and descriptive accounts of roller bandaging.

A crêpe bandage is a many-purpose one; it has a one-way stretch. The bandage is purchased rolled with a certain degree of tension but many prefer to re-roll it in order to regulate the tension to any particular need before applying it. A crêpe bandage should be unrolled close to the limb, the hands controlling discharge of the bandage; it should never be drawn tightly around a limb as this would create unevenness and result in tight strands which could interfere with the circulation.

A Kling conforming bandage is a crêped gauze bandage with a two-way stretch. Its surface texture enables adjacent layers of the bandage to cling together. This bandage is particularly suitable for the head in neuro-surgery, the face in plastic surgery and in stump bandaging as well as for universal use. It is cool and comfortable to wear, adapting well, and does not slip; its soft finished edges make it valuable, too, when applied over an inflamed or oedematous surface.

Netelast bandaging system. An elasticated net of cellular cotton and elastic in a wide-mesh tubular net is a recent advance in a material provided to secure a dressing quickly, easily, comfortably and firmly wherever it is needed. The material does not fray or ladder and it can be washed and sterilized by autoclaving. It replaces the traditional bandaging which is time-consuming and can be applied to areas where traditional bandaging is difficult. Netelast is supplied in different sizes suitable for all parts of the body.

The principle of application is to stretch the tubular net between the the operator's hands and pass it over the dressing to be retained onto the area undergoing treatment. A hole or holes can be cut in the net as when it is applied over the head, then (see Fig. 11/2) trimmed to expose the face in this case or when applied over the trunk to allow freedom to both arms or legs.

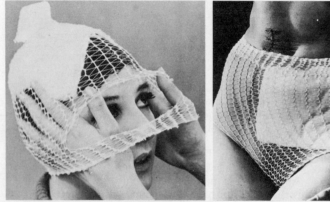
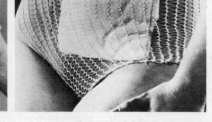

Fig. 11/2 (*a*) Half the Netelast length is drawn over the head, covering the dressing. (*b*) Colostomy night belt with Netelast.

Patient manoeuvring is lessened considerably during re-dressing, as wounds can be exposed by folding back the Netelast, which can secure successive clean dressings provided that the Netelast is not contaminated. A comfortable dressing can be retained on the perineum, affording support and security to the patient; a girdle round the waist can be fashioned in such a way that a 'tail' of Netelast hangs from the waistband—either at the front or back. This 'tail' can be brought through the legs and fastened to the original girdle. Scrotal support can be achieved by a similar technique.

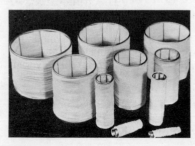

Fig. 11/3 Tubegauz applicators.

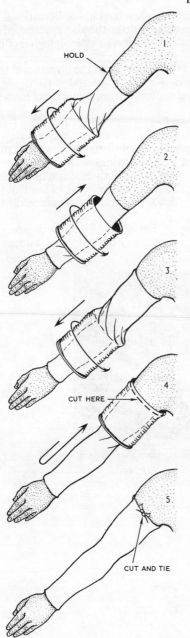

Fig. 11/4 Tubegauz applied to retain a dressing on the arm. Load a suitable size of applicator with Tubegauz. With the channelled rim foremost, slide applicator over the limb and half-way along the dressing. Take off bandage onto the dressing and hold bandage and dressing. Carry the applicator down the limb, at the same time rotating the applicator (1). Continue this rotating movement while carrying the applicator backwards and forwards over the dressing area (2 and 3). Finish bandage by cutting round the channelled rim of applicator, then split the edge of the bandage and tie, or pleat the edge of the bandage and secure with zinc oxide plaster (4 and 5).

The use of the word 'rotating' is deliberate to emphasize that there is no need to twist the applicator repeatedly to obtain an efficient bandage. The action is a simple rotating movement, which obviates the likelihood of tightness at any point.

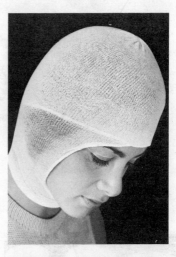

Fig. 11/5 Tubegauz applied to the head as an alternative to a capeline bandage.

Bandaging with Tubegauz has replaced roller bandaging because of its simplicity and comfort. Seamless circular cotton tubular material, fine yet strong enough to withstand reasonable tension as in applying traction, is supplied.

Tubegauz is adaptable to all parts of the body, from the fingers and toes to the trunk. It is easily applied, gives even pressure and is particularly useful in out-patient departments and minor ailment clinics and first-aid units in industry and elsewhere.

Applicators, which range in sizes (see Fig. 11/3) are supplied; the Tubegauz is slightly stretched over the applicator in order to facilitate the elastic-like grip which makes the application comfortable to wear. Tubegauz can be washed and sterilized and may be used more than once. These bandages are suitable for use on any part of the body and are obtainable in many sizes. When applying it the hands should be used to control the discharge of the bandage which should not be permitted to come off the applicator too readily.

Fig. 11/4 shows the method of applying Tubegauz to retain a dressing in position on the arm. Other figures show a variety of completed Tubegauz bandages.

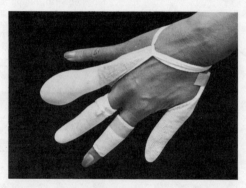

Fig. 11/6 Tubegauz applied to thumb and fingers.

Chapter 12

Applications, Local and General

Local, *of heat, dry and moist—cold icebag, compress, evaporating dressing—poultices, kaolin, starch, linseed—plasters, e.g. belladonna—creams, ointments, liniments, lotions—glycerins—counter-irritants, mustard leaf, cupping*
General—*measures to reduce temperature, tepid and cold sponging, fanning—applications of ice packs—hot applications, baths and hot sponging—radiant heat cradles, electric blankets—warm baths and medicated baths*

LOCAL APPLICATIONS

Local applications are applied for many purposes—they may be hot or cold; contain antiseptic, sedative, stimulating, soothing or antispasmodic substances.

HOT APPLICATIONS

Local applications of heat may be applied dry, or moist. The most commonly used form of dry heat is an *electrically heated pad* made of flexible material which can be adapted to the surface of the body. It is fitted with a heat-regulating switch on the wall-plug adjustment.

A hot moist application can be made by wringing out any soft absorbent material in very hot water, shaking it to allow steam to escape, applying it to unbroken skin and changing it as soon as it becomes cool. When applied every few minutes there is no need to cover this dressing, but if it is only changed every two hours, for example, it should then be covered with a piece of cotton wool lightly bandaged on. Waterproof material may alternatively be used but this would tend to make the skin sodden and this ought to be avoided. One example of a hot moist application is spoon bathing an eye (see p. 644).

An alkaline or soda hot dressing is sometimes considered in the treatment of painful rheumatic conditions; but here again dry heat is preferable to moist heat. A teaspoonful of sodium bicarbonate is sprinkled over the soft absorbent material before the hot water is added, and it is wrung out.

A hypertonic saline hot dressing or compress may be applied for the relief of tension of the tissues when congestion and swelling are causing pain. Two teaspoonfuls either of salt or of magnesium sulphate are added to each 300 ml or half pint of hot water. As the skin is tense it should be smeared with olive oil before making this application, which must not be too hot.

Saline soaks are other moist, warm applications used to soften and separate an encrusted area as in impetigo. Several layers of gauze, soaked in normal saline are applied over the area and kept moist by sprinkling or dabbing with saline. When applied to the head the dressing may be kept in position by a Kling bandage or by Netelast or any open-weave bandage through which the dressing can be kept moist.

COLD APPLICATIONS

Local applications of cold are employed:

> To limit inflammation, especially when of non-bacterial origin, and in the early stages of injury.
> Cold is also useful in limiting the effusion which rapidly follows on injury, especially injury to a joint.
> It is also effective in reducing bleeding when applied over a bleeding part.
> It is sometimes used for the relief of pain.

Ice is fairly often used in nursing, either as an application of cold, or for patients to suck if they especially wish to have it, although this is not always advisable as it tends to crack the lips.

Icebags, or *icecaps* as they are most often called, are made of rubber, and are of different shapes and sizes though generally round or oval (see Fig. 12/1). The *ice is prepared* by chopping it into convenient pieces about the size of a walnut, and if allowed to stand a moment or two any sharp corners which might injure the bag will disappear. Sprinkling salt over the pile of prepared ice makes a better freezing mixture. The ice is then put into the bag until the latter is half full, the air expelled and the stopper screwed on. The surface of the bag should be wiped dry, and it is then put into a flannel bag which should fit well, or it may be wrapped in a piece of towelling and applied to the part ordered.

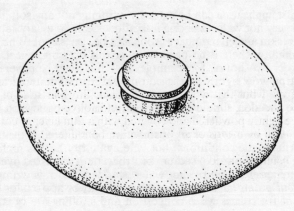

Fig. 12/1 Icecap.

Any mottling of the skin would indicate that the cold application should be removed and replaced by a piece of cotton wool.

For *larger applications ice crushed or flaked by machine* is tilted into a bag of varying size, often made of turkish towelling, for application to the area undergoing treatment, as for the relief of effusion, spasm or pain.

Precautions. One result of an application of ice is to produce an erythema. This occurs quite quickly and particularly when treating fair-skinned patients; the skin should be inspected every minute or two for the first five minutes for removal of the application if necessary.

Occasionally an 'ice burn', which is presumably a form of frostbite, can occur. This may happen when the application is too prolonged. Treatment should then be discontinued. The patient will complain of skin soreness and pain, the skin will be red but this should all disappear within a few days with no ill effects.

Compress. Two types of compress are employed: one, described here as a cold compress, and the other as a moist dressing because it is not always kept cold.

Cold compress. A single layer of material which permits of evaporation is essential for the application of a *cold* compress. This is a means of keeping a part cool by evaporation of water from the material used.

Evaporating dressing. Evaporation and consequent chilling is more rapid when spirit is applied to water—a mixture of one part of spirit to three parts of water being used. Methylated spirit is frequently added, but as this has an unpleasant odour a little lavender water or eau-de-Cologne might be added (see also lotions, p. 105).

POULTICES AND PLASTERS

A *poultice*, or *cataplasm*, is a hot application of moist, soft consistency.

Kaolin Poultice B.P. contains heavy kaolin, boric acid, methyl salicylate, peppermint oil, thymol and glycerin. It is kept in air-tight containers.

Requirements for application. A *poultice board and material* on which to spread the heated poultice (the margins should not be turned in as this makes uncomfortable hard ridges), cotton wool to cover, and bandage or binder and safety pins.

Alternatively the heated poultice may be applied directly to the skin, which should be free from cuts and abrasions, and covered with a thin layer of cotton wool; this is a comfortable method provided that the poultice is *not too hot*.

When the poultice is removed the skin should be washed and gently dried, or wiped over with a little warmed olive oil; any particles of poultice adhering to the skin should be removed with olive-oil swabs. The skin may then be lightly powdered and covered with a thin layer of cotton wool kept in position by means of an open-weave bandage.

A starch poultice is used to soften and remove dried crusts in some skin conditions. *To prepare it take four tablespoonsful of starch flour* from maize, rice, wheat or potato, add *a teaspoonful of boric acid* and mix to a smooth paste with a little cold water. Now pour on a pint (600 ml) of boiling water, stirring slowly at first, then as the mixture thickens stir quickly until it is of a suitable consistency. A stiffer mixture can be obtained by boiling the poultice. The thickness of the poultice required depends on the depth of the crusts. The mixture should be spread between two layers of soft muslin and applied when cool; it can be kept in position by means of a triangular piece of muslin or an open-weave roller bandage.

This poultice should be carefully removed, easing slowly and gently any crusts which have been loosened, detaching any portions (using dissecting forceps and olive-oil swabs) which will come away and mopping with sterile swabs any bleeding points. A soothing non-adhesive dressing may be required.

A linseed poultice made of linseed which contains a good deal of oil is applied hot. It is mixed with hot water until a soft consistency which leaves the sides of the basin is reached, and then spread about a quarter of an inch thick on lint or linen, the edges are turned over and the poultice is applied. It must not be too hot and by gently holding it over the area to which it is to be applied, the patient will decide when he can bear it on his skin. It may be covered with cotton wool and lightly retained in position.

Because a linseed poultice is rather messy and heavy and soon gets cold its place has been taken by an application of kaolin, easier to apply and more comfortable to wear (see p. 103).

Plasters. A belladonna plaster is sometimes used to relieve muscular pain, spasm and rigidity as in low backache. If it is warmed by holding the back of the plaster against a jug of hot water or some other form of heat such as a radiator, it will become slightly tacky and adhere more easily. It may be necessary to snip the edges in order to make the plaster fit without creasing. As a rule this plaster is left on until the edges begin to curl up, though sometimes it is ordered for a specified time.

APPLICATIONS OF CREAMS, OINTMENTS, LINIMENTS, LOTIONS AND PASTES

The terms are well defined in Chapter 20, p. 186. With regard to the use and mode of application, **creams** are prescribed in subacute dermatological conditions to cool, moisten and soothe. As a rule they are gently smeared over to cover as wide an area as possible.

Ointments are applied to dry skins to make a supple protective layer. Zinc and castor oil, for example, is used to protect the perineal area, groins and buttocks from maceration such as may occur in incontinent patients. It is very important to remove ointment thoroughly by washing before making another application. When an ointment contains an analgesic substance it should be well rubbed in to obtain the maximum effect.

Liniments should never be applied to abraded skin surfaces. The method of application varies, those which contain soothing substances should be gently applied but those containing an ingredient intended to stimulate and redden the skin should be vigorously rubbed in until the area is well reddened.

Lotions are generally soothing applications. *Watery lotions* such as calamine may be freshly applied cold to an area of sunburn or any irritating inflamed or erythematous area. This application acts by evaporation and should be re-applied frequently.

Lead and opium lotion is applied to a congested or bruised area. Depending on the degree of congestion it may be cold to act as an evaporating dressing, or either warm or hot to act as a moist dressing or compress, when it should be replenished before it dries.

Shake lotions are used for dry lesions; they cool by evaporation and deposit an inert powder on the surface and are renewed as required.

Pastes are protective and emollient. They usually contain zinc oxide, starch and soft paraffin and are used in circumscribed skin lesions. They should be applied liberally, with a palette knife. They are not removed at every dressing, more paste being applied to fill any gaps.

OTHER APPLICATIONS

Glycerins. The preparations most commonly employed are:

Glycerin of borax, used in cleansing the mouth.

Glycerin of belladonna, which is used to relieve pain in neuritis and rheumatism, phlebitis and thrombosis.

Glycerin of ichthyol, an antiseptic substance prepared from fossilized fish. It is used for the treatment of many forms of local inflammation provided the skin is not broken.

Leeches are bloodsucking parasites which are occasionally used to relieve congestion and pain in eye surgery. They are used on the continent of Europe to relieve cyanosis when applied to the chest in cases of cardiac congestion and in the same situation for the relief of pain in pneumonia, but not generally in the United Kingdom.

Counter-irritants are means of producing superficial irritation or inflammation with the object of relieving a symptom arising in the deeper tissues—such as pain—or with the object, by bringing blood to the surface, of relieving a more deeply seated congestion. They act thus by producing a condition of hyperaemia, and by this means they alter the blood supply of the part to which they are applied though this is not invariable.

Rubefacients cause local reddening of the skin. Any means which produces hyperaemia can be included, such as the brisk rubbing of a part, as for example when a liniment is rubbed in, and if the liniment should contain a substance stimulating to the circulation, such as camphor, the effect is enhanced.

A number of proprietary *rubefacient preparations* are available. They all contain, amongst other ingredients, *nicotinic acid esters* which are vasodilators. Many of these preparations are supplied as a cream to be rubbed in, 'Algipan' is one.

Iodine may be painted on the skin to produce a counter-irritant effect.

A *mustard leaf* or plaster is another example of a rubefacient, rarely employed in hospital but occasionally recommended by a family doctor for use in the home. It is simply a sheet of paper with a tacky mixture of flour and mustard in suitable proportions applied to one side and allowed to dry. It can generally be obtained from a pharmacist.

To apply, it is dipped in tepid water, shaken gently to remove free fluid and applied to the skin of the area to be treated by reddening, in some cases to the chest to relieve pain in pleurisy. The skin to which it is applied must be free from rash, abrasion or other blemish.

Effects. Soon after application the skin begins to feel hot, the patient may say it is burning. Someone should be near him and, lifting a corner of the plaster, note the degree of reddening. The plaster should be removed when the skin is red, *but before it is deeply or angrily red as this indicates a pre-blistering stage and blistering must be avoided.*

After this application the skin should be inspected, wiped over gently with olive oil, lightly dusted with baby powder and covered, for protection, by a layer of cotton wool.

CUPPING

Cupping is a form of counter-irritation by which the dilation of the subcutaneous blood vessels is effected. Heated glass cups are used to create a partial vacuum; the prepared cup or glass is applied to the selected area, consequently the superficial tissues are attracted to it to fill the partial vacuum, bringing a good deal of blood, in the vessels, to the surface.

Cupping is rarely, if ever, used in the United Kingdom. In countries where it is employed in treatment of the inflammatory diseases of the chest as in bronchitis and pleurisy, in lumbago and other forms of fibrositis, every member of a family is expert in its application.

APPLICATIONS OF COLD

Measures for the reduction of temperature. It is generally inadvisable to allow a patient to maintain a temperature of 38·3 °C (101 °F) to 39·4 °C (105 °F) for long. Reduction of a raised temperature is invaluable in making a patient comfortable, relieving his headache, inducing sleep, avoiding mental confusion and delirium when acting as an adjunct to antibiotic therapy in acute infections. In these instances the method chosen should be one which will disturb the patient as little as possible. In certain cases, as in head injuries and in heat stroke where the patient may already be semi-conscious, more drastic measures are employed where they can be life saving.

Methods which are available include:

> Exposure of the whole body, with a covering only over the loins.
> Fanning the body.
> Fanning over ice.
> Cold sponging.
> Cold sponging accompanied by fanning.
> Applications of ice.

Note Fanning is more likely to cause shivering than any other application but once arrested the shivering generally ceases. Even when using cold sponging under fanning, shivering may cease when the fanning is turned off and the cold sponging can then proceed without interruption. In a few resistant cases of severe shivering chlorpromazine (Largactil), which has a pronounced effect, may be ordered.

Sponging may be by tepid or cold water. *In cold sponging* the water should be about 21 °C (70 °F), the temperature of the water being regulated by the addition of ice as necessary. A *bath thermometer* kept in the water will ensure accurate observation. The patient lies between bath sheets or towelling. Several sponges are necessary, at least four, some nurses recommend six, so that two are in use, two cooling in the water and two placed at intervals in the axillae or groins (see below).

A conscious patient has his face sponged and dried first, the only part that is to be dried; he may hold a sponge in his hands or dabble his hands in the cool water.

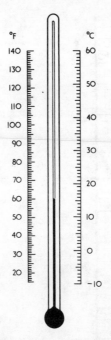

Fig. 12/2 Bath (or lotion) thermometer.

Sponging cools by evaporation of moisture from the surface of the body, therefore long sweeping strokes should be made by sponges as full of water as possible so that beads of moisture rest on the skin. Each sponge should be used once, returned to the water for cooling and a fresh cool sponge taken for the next stroke. Marine sponges are preferable but alternatively Sorbo may have to be used.

There should be some order in the procedure such as sponging each arm first, giving three minutes to each; the front and sides of the body, spending four to five minutes; each lower limb, four to five minutes; and, if the patient may be turned, the back, taking care to pay particular attention to the thick muscles on each side of the spine. In order to save movement the lower part of the back might be subject to routine treatment for the prevention of pressure sores (see p. 50). Then the towel on which the patient is lying is removed and his bed made comfortable.

Careful attention should be paid to the axillae, groins, the inner aspect of the thighs and the popliteal spaces; hot spots are frequent in these areas and judicious treatment materially assists cooling of the body. Throughout the treatment, whenever possible, a cold compress should be applied to the patient's forehead and changed as often as necessary to keep it really cool.

A more drastic method of cold sponging is made by the application of ice and some methylated spirit in the water, which enhances evaporation. Alternatively see General Applications of Ice, p. 109.

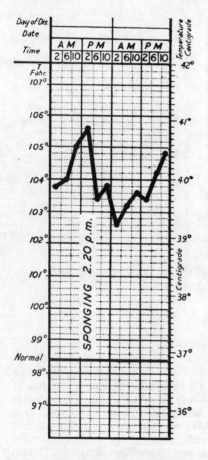

Fig. 12/3 Method of charting a drop in temperature following tepid or cold sponging, or any other method employed for the reduction of body temperature.

Recording the temperature. The temperature is taken ten minutes after the sponging and the result charted—a fall of between two and three degrees being considered satisfactory. The temperature obtained by sponging a patient or reducing fever by any similar method is charted as described on the accompanying illustration.

Observation of patient's condition. The general condition of the patient should be very carefully watched for any signs which would suggest that the reaction expected might be retarded or absent. Untoward signs include weakness and irregularity of the pulse, pallor or cyanosis, anxiety of facial expression, the appearance of perspiration on the face; complaints of palpitation and sighing or irregularity of respiration. Such signs are comparatively rare.

GENERAL APPLICATIONS OF ICE

Hyperpyrexia, which may occur in head injuries and in heat strokes, needs more drastic cooling. The danger of hyperpyrexia is that irreversible damage to the brain may arise from the increase of intracranial pressure which accompanies it. Applications may take the form of ice-packing, or the patient may be wrapped in turkish towelling rung out in water and ice and rubbed down with slabs of ice, which must be kept moving to avoid the ice trauma, mentioned on p. 103 of this chapter. In the case of heat stroke, the treatment may have to be vigorous in order to reduce a temperature of 41 to 42 °C (106 to 107 °F).

The treatment may last for 15 to 20 minutes, *the temperature is taken rectally every 5 minutes*. The fall may be rapid and the blood pressure also may fall, so that the patient needs watching carefully for early signs of collapse. When the temperature has been reduced to 38·8 °C (101 °F) the treatment should cease as the temperature will continue to fall and must be taken every 5 minutes until it becomes stabilized.

GENERAL APPLICATIONS OF HEAT

The immediate result of a hot application is to stimulate the nerve endings in the skin and, as this increases the activity of the central nervous system, the pulse rate also is increased. In certain conditions some degree of congestion of the internal organs, particularly of the brain, occurs, and it is to prevent the discomforts associated with this—such as headache and throbbing of the veins of the head—that a cold compress is applied to the head during the administration of any general application of heat.

This effect is soon followed by relaxation; the patient begins to feel drowsy and comfortable.

HOT BATHS AND HOT SPONGING

Apart from cleansing baths, hot baths and hot spongings may be employed:

(*a*) As a prophylactic to possible infection, and for the relief of shivering in persons who have been exposed to severe wetting and chilling.

(*b*) At the outset of a severe cold in order to promote sweating and to stimulate the subcutaneous circulation.

(*c*) For the relief of fatigue following physical strain.

(*d*) In spastic conditions, as when employed for the relief of muscular rigidity in convulsions, and for the relief of restlessness in chorea.

For an adult patient unable to bathe himself, a bath should be filled half full of water at a temperature of 37·8 °C (100 °F) which may be increased to 40·6 °C (105 °F) or even higher.

The patient should be watched carefully for any signs of distress such as change in colour, anxiety and restlessness.

The *duration of the bath* should not exceed 5 or 10 minutes. At the end of this time the patient, wrapped in a bath sheet, should be taken back to bed, gently dabbed dry and given a warm drink.

RADIANT HEAT CRADLES AND ELECTRIC BLANKETS

A *radiant heat cradle* is a convenient and easy method of warming a patient who is cold, but as in all applications of heat it is important to note when the patient is comfortably warm and remove the heat. There is no advantage in overheating a patient, it only induces sweating which causes loss of fluid and body salts (electrolytes).

An *electric blanket* is a large heating pad in which heat is generated by an electric current. In hospital a transformer is used, so that the current does not come from the main. It is important to make sure that every blanket used carries the approval mark of the British Electrical Approvals Board (B.E.A.B.).

WARM BATHS AND MEDICATED BATHS

Warm baths at a temperature of 35 to 38 °C (95 to 100 °F) are used for a variety of conditions. Possibly their most important use is in the treatment of insomnia, when lying in warm water soothes the circulation generally and results in relaxation of muscle and a reduction of the activity of the brain, so probably helping to induce sleep.

Warm baths are also used to soak off adherent dressings and so avoid trauma.

Emollient baths. *Saline*, 120 g (4 oz.) of common salt to a bath is soothing to sensitive skins.

Starch, 480 g (1 lb.) made into a mucilage, like laundry starch; or *borax*, 240 g (½ lb.) added to a bath is soothing.

Antiseptic baths. *Permanganate of potash*, a 2 per cent solution is made by adding a few drops to the water until it is pink, not red. It should not be put into the bath first as it would stain the surface.

Tar added to a bath relieves irritation in pruritus and urticaria and potentiates the effect of ultra-violet light in the treatment of psoriasis.

Stimulating baths are employed to improve the circulation in the subcutaneous tissues and are considered to have a general tonic effect. Examples include:

A *cold bath* followed by brisk rubbing.

A *sea-water bath* when several kilograms of sea salt is added.

A *mustard bath* by adding 240 to 480 g (½ to 1 lb.) of mustard to a bath. The mustard must first be mixed to a smooth paste with cold water and then carefully mixed well into the bath.

Chapter 13

Selected Procedures which Need the Attention of a Nurse

Artificial feeding, naso-gastric, gastrostomy—fluid infusion (sub-cutaneous), rectal infusion—lavage and irrigation, gastric, rectal, colonic—aspiration and drainage of body cavities, stomach, pleural, pericardial sac—acupuncture—lumbar and cisternal puncture

ARTIFICIAL FEEDING

Food may be introduced into the body in artificial feeding in the following ways:

> By the nose in *naso-gastric feeding.*
> It may also be administered by means of openings artificially made, as when food is introduced into the oesophagus by *oesophagostomy*, into the stomach by *gastrostomy*, and into the small intestine by *duodenostomy* or *jejunostomy*.

General rules, applicable in most cases:

> Only liquid food can be used.
> The temperature of food should be 35 to 37·8 °C (95 to 100 °F).
> The amount given must be measured and recorded.
> In most cases the liquid should be strained, otherwise the tube through which it is passed may become blocked.

If the patient is capable of knowing what is being carried out, the treatment should be explained to him and the character of the feeding described.

Naso-gastric. A fine catheter is passed through the nose and on into the oesophagus for about 50 cm or 20 inches.

The following articles should be assembled:

> Disposable waterproof and towel.
> Swabs and lotion for cleansing the nostril.
> A *lubricant* may be needed.
> Catheter or tube with funnel, glass connection and rubber tubing (a much finer nasal tube would be required for a child).

Litmus paper to test whether the tube is in the stomach.

Thermometer to test the feeding and a glass measure to hold the prepared fluid food.

Disposable bag for all disposable articles, swabs, etc.

Method. When possible have the patient propped up, cleanse the nostril that is to be used, choosing the one seen to provide the clearest passage, lubricate and insert the tube gently but quickly, passing it in a backward *not* an upward direction.

See that it has not come forward and curled up in the mouth, listen with the ear against the funnel as the movement of air may be heard if the tube is in the trachea. Look at the patient and see if he is at all cyanosed, whether he is coughing, and note if he appears to be quite comfortable. If in doubt withdraw the tube, rinse it, and try again.

When satisfied that the tube is in the stomach, pour a little sterile water into the funnel and allow it to trickle down, checking the flow by constricting the tubing—the absence of distress will confirm that the tube is not in the trachea. Give the feeding, then pour a little water down to clear the tube, pinch the tube close up to the nostril and withdraw it gently but rapidly.

When a patient is having naso-gastric feeding at frequent intervals, the tube may be left in position. It should then be closed at the end of the feeding either by spigot or clamp and fastened up onto the side of the temple by means of a piece of strapping.

Continuous milk feeding (by the 'drip' method). Sometimes, not often, milk is run continuously into the stomach from a vacolitre, drip chamber and indwelling intranasal tube. It is used in the treatment of acute peptic ulcer when it is desirable to control the gastric hyperacidity and the pain which it is causing. The temperature of the feeding should be about 37·8 °C (100 °F).

The 'drip' may be given continuously or simply overnight, at about 20 drops a minute, or by giving at the rate of a litre in 10 hours.

The usual precautions in passing an intra-gastric tube nasally are taken (see naso-gastric feeding above). There is no objection to the patient taking whatever diet he is having as well if the physician allows it.

Gastrostomy feeding. It is important that these feedings are given separately from the surgical care of the wound.

The following articles should be assembled on a covered tray:

A jug containing the feed at 37·8 °C (100 °F) standing in a basin of hot water.

A glass measure containing warm water.

A bowl containing a Jaques' catheter, clip, tubing connection and funnel which may be of glass or plastic.

Method. The apparatus is connected and a little warm water run through it to test patency; the catheter is passed into the tubing in the stomach, the feeding is given, more water is poured in to leave the tubing quite clear, the spigot is replaced and the area covered. The amount given is recorded on the feeding chart.

FLUID INFUSION

Subcutaneous injection of fluids, *hypodermoclysis.* By means of this method fluid is absorbed principally by the lymphatics. The addition of the enzyme hyaluronidase, *Hyalase,* promotes diffusion of the fluid. All the apparatus used must be sterile and the skin into which the needles are to be inserted should be cleansed.

The *injection is made* into some part where the tissue is loose, such as the skin of abdomen, axillae or thighs.

The *apparatus* consists of one or two special needles attached to rubber tubing. If two needles are used, a Y-shaped connection is employed.

The skin is prepared, the fluid is allowed to run through the apparatus to expel air, the tubing is clamped, the needles inserted as in the administration of a hypodermic injection and the flow regulated.

Some means should be taken to prevent the needles from either slipping out or being pulled out by any tension on the tubing. As a rule a small piece of Elastoplast placed across the blunt end of the needle is sufficient support.

Rectal infusion of fluid, *proctoclysis.* To supply fluid to a dehydrated patient by rectum is a useful emergency nursing measure pending intravenous infusion (see Chapter 48, p. 460). Tap water or saline solution may be injected slowly, with the patient in the left lateral position. The bladder should be empty lest the desire to micturate should stimulate return of the rectal infusion. A small amount, not more than 300 ml, may be given at intervals by means of a catheter and funnel taking 5 to 6 minutes. Alternatively a continuous drip infusion described below can be given.

The following articles should be assembled:

A vacolitre of the fluid ordered on an infusion stand.
A drip connection.
18 to 24 in. or 45 to 60 cm of tubing.
A screw clip to regulate the drip.
A graduated connecting tube to attach the tubing to a Jaques' catheter size 6–8 E.G.
A lubricant.
An incontinence pad.

The rectal catheter is inserted either with the patient in the left lateral position or lying on his back. If in the former, he is then helped over on to his back and the incontinence pad placed beneath his buttocks in case of leakage of the infusion fluid.

The rate of flow averaging 20 drops a minute is achieved by adjusting the screw clip. The quantity of fluid infused is entered on the 'input and output chart'.

LAVAGE AND IRRIGATION

For bladder irrigation, see Chapter 25, p. 254, and for vaginal douching, Chapter 74, p. 749.

Gastric lavage. The washing out of the stomach is performed for the removal of poison which has been swallowed, and sometimes to cleanse the stomach before an operation or afterwards when the patient is vomiting large quantities of fluid, though aspiration of the stomach is more usually performed in these instances (see p. 117).

The apparatus to be assembled includes:

> Materials (disposable) to protect bed and patient's clothing.
> A sufficiency of the solution ordered at a temperature of 37·8 °C (100 °F).
> A lotion thermometer.
> A funnel, connecting tube, and an oesophageal tube.
> A lubricant.

In special cases when a patient may resist the treatment a mouth gag, tongue forceps and spatula may be needed. A mouth wash should be supplied for use after the oesophageal tube has been withdrawn, if the patient can use one.

Method. When large quantities of fluid are to be used the patient should be lying prone on a couch, with his head supported over the end or on a tilted table. In these positions there is no danger that the fluid regurgitating around the tube in the pharynx will fall into the trachea, which happens in unconscious patients when the cough reflex is absent, but a cuffed endotracheal tube is passed in an unconscious patient in order to avoid this danger.

When the patient is in position his dentures are removed and, if he is unconscious, a mouth gag is inserted. The tube is lubricated and passed into the mouth, slight pressure on the tube as it reaches the posterior wall of the pharynx will direct it into the oesophagus; it is then passed quickly on, until the mark on the tube (20 in. or 50 cm from the end in the case of an adult and 10 in. or 25 cm for a child) is at the level of the lips—the tube is now in the stomach.

300 ml, about half a pint, of lotion is poured in and siphoned back into a receiver—in a case of poisoning plain water is used—this specimen is kept for examination. Washing out of the stomach is then continued, using 600 ml at a time until the fluid begins to return clear and odourless. Anything up to 10 litres may be required.

When the treatment is over, the tube is withdrawn and either the mouth is cleansed or the patient given a mouth wash. The soiled tube should be washed in tepid water, and sterilized after use. The nurse's report should include the condition of the patient during and after treatment, the amount of lotion used, the state in which it was returned and the presence of any blood, mucus and bile, and the odour. It may be necessary to save all the fluid for the inspection of the doctor.

Rectal lavage (Alternatively rectal wash-out). By this method fluid is run into the rectum, and before it is distended, the funnel is inverted and the fluid siphoned out. It is used to ensure cleansing in order to remove mucus, blood or debris before some rectal operations.

The articles to be assembled include:

> A bowl containing a funnel, 12 to 14 in. or 30 to 35 cm of rubber tubing attached, a spring clip, straight connection and a Jacques' catheter, No. 14–16 E.G.
> A lubricant.
> Several litres of warmed tap water or other fluid.
> A lotion thermometer.
> Paper towels and a disposable waterproof sheet.
> A bag for soiled disposables.
> A pail for the returned fluid.

This procedure is not an enema, it is simply for cleansing the rectum, and an evacuant enema may be necessary before this treatment is possible. The patient should empty the bladder before the procedure commences. The temperature of the fluid should be about 37·8 °C (100 °F). The end of the catheter is lubricated and a little fluid allowed to run through it to expel air. The catheter is inserted gently for about 6 cm (2 to 3 in.) into the rectum, the clip released and fluid allowed to run in. The patient should be warned to describe any discomfort he may have. As a rule it is possible to refill the funnel three or four times and then by inverting it over the pail at the bedside return it by siphonage. This is repeated until the fluid returned is clear or a reasonable amount has been used. The apparatus is then removed, the anal area dried and the patient made comfortable.

Colonic irrigation and lavage. In the treatment of diverticulosis, and sometimes in preparation for X-ray examination of the colon by a barium enema, and in preparation for operation on the rectum or colon, irrigation or lavage may be ordered to cleanse the colon. *Read also the preparation for operation described by a rectal surgeon, p. 495.*

The fluid employed may be tap water, a solution of sodium bicarbonate, saline solution or any other non-irritating fluid of the surgeon's choice. The temperature of the fluid should not be above 37·8 °C (100 °F). The nurse should work from the right side of the bed. The rectal catheter is inserted with great care and gentleness after being well lubricated, with the patient lying in the left lateral position, and the treatment is given with the patient lying supine.

Apparatus. The most suitable apparatus is the *Dierker therapeutic apparatus* by which tap water or other solution may be delivered and the temperature kept under constant observation.

The *pressure of the flow* can be regulated; not more than a quarter-pound pressure is advisable, and when it is desirable to empty the colon, a vacuum, measured in inches (average 1½ in. or 4 cm), can be created.

The *returning fluid*, which can be observed through large glass tubes acting as windows, passes directly into the soil pipe.

Alternatively any apparatus suitable for giving a rectal injection may be used, such as a rectal catheter, tubing and funnel, or an irrigation can.

It is more difficult, however, to regulate the pressure by this method and a patient may soon experience some discomfort.

The *condition of the patient* must be most carefully noted before treatment and observed throughout the treatment; questions as to discomfort should be asked, and the fluid should be siphoned back or returned by creating a slight vacuum, according to the type of apparatus in use whenever there is any discomfort. The patient must be kept warm.

The *duration of the treatment* and the amount of fluid used will depend on the condition of the patient. It will vary from 4 to 5 litres to as many as 20.

Report on the result. The colour of the faeces, amount and appearance, whether loose, normal, impacted, constipated, and the presence of undigested food should be noted. If the faeces are red, green or black the patient should be questioned about any medicine he is taking. The presence of mucus should be noted. The amount of gas evacuated should be noted.

The condition of the patient during treatment should be reported in adequate detail: whether nausea was experienced, discomfort or pain. As a rule, a patient is requested to evacuate the bowel immediately after the treatment; if he can use a W.C. he must be requested not to pull the plug so that the amount of faeces and its character can be observed.

ASPIRATION AND TAPPING

The nurse will be expected to prepare both patient and apparatus for the performance of different forms of aspiration and paracentesis, or tapping, in order to remove fluid from the various cavities of the body. She should know the effects that are expected from any investigation made, and should be familiar beforehand with any untoward symptoms which may arise during the performance of it.

The nurse must watch both the patient and the physician or surgeon, and be able to anticipate the wants of both. She should supply the necessary specimen bottles with bungs to fit, and have the appropriate pathological labels ready at hand.

Paracentesis consists of passing a hollow needle into the cavity from which the fluid is to be taken; the fluid, being under pressure in the cavity, will then run out as when a beer barrel is tapped.

Aspiration describes the evacuation of a cavity when the fluid will not run out in the same way, and where some form of suction has to be employed in order to draw it out, as in the case of the stomach and the pleural cavity.

Aspiration of the stomach is carried out when it is advisable to keep the stomach empty as:

Before an operation on the stomach when there may be some initial bleeding into the organ.

In gastric dilation.
In persistent vomiting.

After an operation on the stomach, when aspiration begins immediately, the amounts recovered are measured and charted. Aspiration is repeated at short intervals and, when the patient begins to take fluid, immediately before a drink. For full details of this treatment read Chapter 49, p. 464.
The following articles should be assembled:

Ryle's tube.
Syringe for aspirating.
Measure for fluid withdrawn.
Litmus paper to test reaction.
Test-tubes if specimens required.
Saline or other bland fluid which may be first injected, then withdrawn, in order to cleanse the stomach of blood, bile, gastric fluid and debris.

In *paralytic ileus* when bowel sounds are absent, by keeping the stomach empty of fluid the alimentary tract is rested and the temporary paralysis from which the patient is suffering can be relieved. The patient is kept at rest, and given whatever fluid his body needs, such as blood, plasma or one of the plasma substitutes by intravenous infusion until he can take enough fluid by mouth.

Aspiration of the pleural cavity, *or thoracentesis.* This operation is performed for the relief of symptoms in cases of pleural effusion, and also in some instances in order to collect a specimen of fluid for examination.
Preparation of the patient. Having told the patient the nature of the operation, and allowed him, if it seems at all reasonable, to see the apparatus that is to be used, he is placed in position, either leaning forwards over a bedtable or pillow on his knees, with his arm on the side to be treated carried well forward across his chest in order to separate the intercostal spaces and keep the scapula well up out of the way.
Alternatively he may be lying on the unaffected side with a firm pillow under his chest so that he lies with his trunk flexed laterally over the pillow. The arm on the affected side is carried up over his head and the patient may grasp the rail at the bedhead, or clutch the mattress, or have his hand held in this position.
The *skin is then prepared,* the bedclothes re-arranged and towels are placed around the area of injection.
The physician gives the local anaesthetic and passes the needle into the chest. When the operation is completed the needle is withdrawn, the puncture covered by the dressing provided and the patient made comfortable in his usual position in bed and given a warm drink. The nurse has already inquired what is to be done with the fluid, and collected a specimen if necessary; the remainder of the fluid should be measured and inspected for colour, odour and any abnormal appearance, and then thrown away.
For a fuller description of examination of structures in the chest, see under Thoracic Surgical Procedures, p. 585.

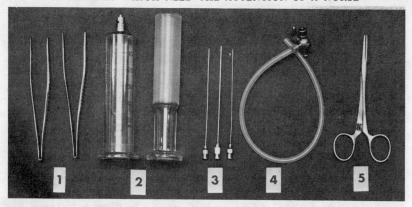

Fig. 13/1 Articles for aspiration of the chest: 1. Two five-inch plain dissecting forceps. 2. One 50 ml all-glass Luer Lok syringe. 3. Three four-inch aspirating needles, sizes 16, 18, 20. 4. One Luer Lok tap with twelve inches of 3·2 mm tubing which remains patent. 5. One five-inch Spencer Wells' forceps. The following are also included in the Central Sterile Supplies Department (C.S.S.D.) pack: two gallipots and wool balls, ten gauze swabs, four folded paper towels and two pairs of five-inch dissecting forceps.

Aspiration of the pericardial sac. The same apparatus as previously described may be employed, but, as the amount of fluid withdrawn from the pericardial cavity is small compared with that from the thoracic cavity, a 5 or 10 ml syringe and needle are usually found to be adequate.

The front of the patient's chest is exposed, and he may either lie on his back, or be propped up with pillows.

As considerable shock may attend this operation the nurse should watch the patient very carefully for changes of colour and irregularities of pulse.

PARACENTESIS ABDOMINIS

Tapping the peritoneal cavity or paracentesis abdominis for the removal of fluid is usually undertaken for the relief of troublesome symptoms produced by ascites: *It is important for the nurse to realize that the removal of a large quantity of fluid will decrease the intra-abdominal pressure, and may give rise to considerable shock* (see below).

Preparation of the patient. The patient will be propped up as well as possible in a sitting posture. As the puncture is made in the midline *it is essential for the bladder to be empty*, and when collecting the apparatus the nurse must provide a suitable bedpan or urinal, and also have ready at hand the articles for catheterizing the patient.

An abdominal binder should be placed ready behind the patient in case it is necessary to tighten it to prevent too rapid a decrease of intra-abdominal pressure as the fluid drains away which would cause shock and collapse unless carefully graduated. It is very important to watch the patient's pulse carefully, and the nurse should stand at his side with her hand on the pulse and if it loses volume and tone she should at once tighten the binder and give the patient any stimulant ordered or a warm drink.

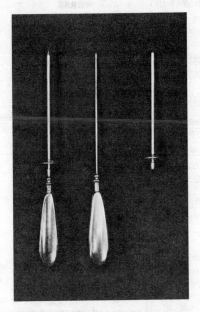

Fig. 13/2 Trocar and cannula (with shield attached) for abdominal paracentesis. The assembled instrument is shown on the left and a dismantled one on the right. After the puncture is made the trocar is withdrawn leaving in the abdominal cavity the cannula to which rubber tubing is attached, and the fluid is drained into a pail at the bedside. In addition a pack usually contains ten 4×4 inch gauze swabs, two gallipots, a scalpel handle and blade in case a small incision is to be made in the skin to facilitate the passage of the trocar and cannula, a skin needle and suture and two pairs of dissecting forceps. An abdominal binder and safety pins should also be supplied (see text).

At the termination of the treatment the cannula is removed. If an initial incision was made, a local anaesthetic is used and the wound sutured; a suitable dressing is applied, the binder firmly adjusted and secured in position by safety pins. The patient should be made comfortable in his bed, but should be moved as little as possible, since the movement of a patient who has just undergone any operation is liable to induce shock. *The patient must be very carefully watched for some hours, and the binder, which must not be allowed to get slack, should be readjusted from time to time.*

Drainage of the subcutaneous tissue may be carried out by means of *acupuncture*—when minute punctures are made in the skin by means of a sharp sterile scalpel, the fluid which runs out being collected in large pads of sterile gauze and wool; or *Southey's tubes* may alternatively be employed.

The limbs that are being drained should be *kept warm by being wrapped* in cotton wool. When possible the patient should be sitting up with his legs over the side or over the foot of the bed or be sitting on a chair with his feet on a footstool, as, by having the limbs hanging down, drainage proves most effective.

LUMBAR AND CISTERNAL PUNCTURE

Lumbar puncture is performed to tap the fluid in the subarachnoid space for a number of reasons:

(a) To obtain a specimen of cerebrospinal fluid.
(b) To remove fluid preliminary to the introduction of drugs, saline or serum, etc.

(c) To ascertain the pressure of the cerebrospinal fluid, in which case a manometer is fitted to the apparatus used (Greenfield's apparatus).

(d) To remove fluid for the relief of intracranial pressure in a variety of cases including meningitis and conditions of oedema of the brain.

(e) For the administration of drugs in therapy.

(f) For investigations such as myelography (see Chapter 63, p. 675.

In, infective conditions—meningitis and encephalitis—the number of white blood cells in the fluid may be increased and it may be possible to grow the causative organism on culture. *In intracranial tumour* the pressure may be grossly raised and the protein content of the fluid (normally less than 40 mg per 100 ml) may be raised. In *subarachnoid haemorrhage* there is blood in the fluid whilst the fluid itself is stained yellow (xanthochromia) by the disintegrating red cells.

As a child develops, the rate of growth of the bony spine exceeds that of the spinal cord. In the embryo the cord extends down into the sacrum. At birth it reaches the lower border of the 3rd lumbar vertebra, whilst in the adult the bottom of the cord reaches only to the lower margin of the 1st lumbar vertebra. Below this level, the spinal canal still lined by dura and arachnoid membranes contains only the elongated nerve roots running down from the cord to their exits from the canal at the intervertebral foramina. Thus if a lumbar puncture needle is passed between the spines of two adjacent lumbar vertebrae (usually the 4th and 5th) and through the dura and arachnoid membranes, cerebrospinal fluid (C.S.F.) may be withdrawn or substances injected without fear of damaging the spinal cord. The slack nerve roots will be pushed out of the way of the advancing needle and are unlikely to be damaged.

In certain special circumstances it may be necessary to take cerebrospinal fluid from a higher level than in a lumbar puncture (see cisternal puncture below).

Preparation of the patient. This procedure is usually performed with *the patient lying in the left lateral position with his thighs flexed on the abdomen, the knees flexed on the thighs and the head and shoulders drawn forward onto the front of the chest, so that the spine is as thoroughly flexed as possible, and therefore, the vertebral spines will be comparatively well separated,* thus facilitating the passage of the needle between them.

The skin is cleansed over the area to be treated. As a rule the interval between the 2nd and 3rd or 4th and 5th lumbar vertebrae is punctured. If the nurse is in doubt as to the position of these bones, she can determine the level of the 2nd or 3rd lumbar vertebra by drawing a line with a skin pencil from the top of the crest of the ilium to the middle of the patient's back. She should hold the patient in the curled-up, flexed position while the puncture is made.

Another position in which this operation is sometimes carried out is to have *the patient seated on a stool* and leaning forward on some support placed in front of him, or, if he can manage it, with his hands clasped round his knees. The nurse stands in front of him and places her hands on the

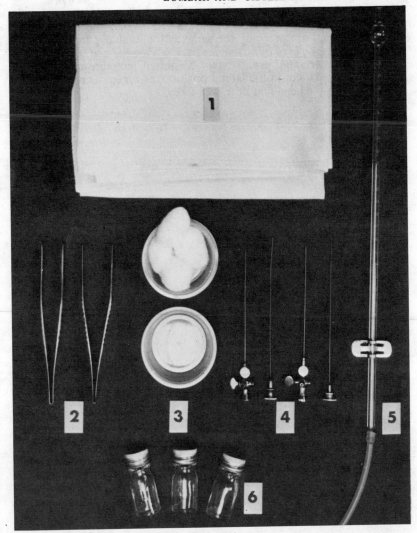

Fig. 13/3 Lumbar puncture set. The articles to be assembled are generally obtained from a C.S.S.D. 1. Sterile towel. 2. Forceps for holding skin cleansing swabs. 3. Gallipots for lotion. 4. Two sizes of Greenfield needles. 5. Manometer which may be attached to the needle to record C.S.F. pressure. 6. Specimen bottles for the C.S.F. In addition, the nurse must provide a local anaesthetic (usually 1 per cent Xylocaine) and disposable syringes and needles for its injection.

posterior aspect of his shoulders and keeps the trunk flexed, allowing him to rest his head against her side.

In **cisternal puncture** the needle is passed from behind, between the base of the skull and the atlas (the 1st cervical vertebra), until its tip lies in the subarachnoid space just below the cerebellum. At this point the space is relatively wide and is called the *cisterna magna*. The technique and instruments used are precisely the same as for lumbar puncture *but the patient must be prepared by having the back of the head and neck shaved up to the external occipital protuberance.* Cisternal puncture may be made either with the patient in the lateral position, as for lumbar puncture, or sitting up with the head and neck well flexed.

Chapter 14

Some Special Aspects in Nursing

*The apprehensive, anxious patient—the delirious patient—sleepless-
ness and pain—nursing in disorders of respiration—nursing considerations in heart disease—vomiting and diarrhoea—fits and convulsions—
paralysis—unconsciousness—incontinence—high dependency patients
—intensive care—patients with communicable diseases*

THE APPREHENSIVE, ANXIOUS PATIENT

All patients are anxious, some more than others and each in a different
way. A suggestion of admission to hospital may bring about physical
changes, a rapid pulse, dry mouth and lips, trembling, flushing, perspiration and inability to talk, but once the patient knows nothing is wrong
these manifestations of anxiety disappear. He had expected to be told
the worst.

The hundreds of patients passing through an out-patient department,
some for a first visit, some for a check-up, others for routine continuation
care are in an immediate state of apprehension. However, if the patient is
welcomed and accepted as a person, his self-respect is enhanced; if he feels
he is listened to and that his feelings are considered, he becomes less
anxious.

When a patient is in hospital a nurse can be adept at noting his reactions
to a particular situation and how well he seems adjusted to his present
environment and, by personal care, she can diminish the unfamiliar and
orientate the patient to his new surroundings.

A patient may not know of what he is afraid. His fear may be complex—
fear of the unknown, for his future, his family, his job, fear of mutilation,
e.g. colostomy, amputation, fear of cancer. A woman contemplating
hysterectomy may fear the loss of her husband's love. Patients may have
groundless fears that they may not be able to meet with courage what lies
ahead. Most patients are unable to admit or discuss their fears except
occasionally to a comparative stranger, as in the relationship between a
good nurse and a patient. *She creates the listening situation* often at night,
perhaps because it is dark or a patient may think that a night nurse has
more time. The nurse should not think she is called upon to solve a patient's
problems. She is only there to listen, but some of the information she
receives should be passed on to the right channels as part of his medical
history.

The relatives have the same fears as the patient, particularly whether they can be brave in front of him and cope with what may lie ahead. There is often a protective barrier between a patient and his relatives, when it would be more helpful to both if they could face their problems and fears together.

The nurse also is afraid that something will happen she cannot cope with, some crisis she will not know how to deal with and for which she may blame herself needlessly. She may be afraid a patient may die. She is afraid of what a patient, old enough to be her father, may ask of her and yet he hangs on to her for her normality. She derives strength from this dependence on her and behaves with maturity.

The more apprehensive a patient seems to be, the clearer should be the explanation of what is taking place or about to take place in relation to him. This information should include the value of the collaboration he can give. There are always two positive factors which contribute to recovery:

1. The part nature takes in repair.
2. The value of the patient's confidence in his doctors.

The more these points are considered by patients, the greater will be their contentment and sense of security.

There are the psychiatric patients, many of whom are very apprehensive indeed (see note on anxiety by a psychiatric nurse, p. 271); and also the patients with thyrotoxicosis, described on p. 294; those suffering from rectal disorders or disease whose apprehensive state is mentioned by a rectal surgeon, p. 487.

A PATIENT IN DELIRIUM

Delirium may accompany fever, be brought about by toxaemia or arise as the result of the effects of certain drugs. Alcoholic addiction may result in delirium tremens. Delirious patients are restless and confused and this is worse at night. They are disorientated to time and place and subject to illusions and hallucinations.

Nursing measures include protection from injuring himself or others, trying to reduce confusion and disorientation by having the room or ward quiet, restricting any known movement and noise, avoiding all unnecessary conversation. It is wise to use few words but to be concise and repetitive: 'You are in hospital, I am your nurse, other patients sleep, we must not disturb them.' Try and find out if he wants to know the time or wishes to go to the toilet; he might get onto a commode; if offered a urinal its use should be explained. He may be thirsty or hungry and if offered fluid or food may be satisfied. The calmer and quieter a nurse can be in speaking, the better may be the response from the patient. Some can be reassured, others will be more excited if addressed. A delirious patient should be humoured rather than restrained. The nurse will discover the best approach to each; some resent being touched, others relax if gently handled.

An elderly patient admitted to a geriatric unit finds it all so strange; he confusedly realizes that his surroundings are not right. He is used to a lower bed, probably a wider one, and may fall out, which embarrasses him; he is afraid to express his needs and may become incontinent which distresses him very much.

All these factors may result in a patient becoming disorientated even delirious, and project one, who has previously been mentally normal, into a state of senility from which he may or may not return.

SLEEPLESSNESS

It is becoming increasingly common for patients to approach their doctors, complaining that they cannot sleep. The treatment for this which may be a difficult psychological problem, can hardly be considered to be within the province of the nurse, although she will often be expected to help.

Nursing measures. A nurse in a general hospital ward will often be faced by the problem of a patient who for some reason or another is unable to go to sleep. It is her duty to attempt to discover the possible cause.

> The patient may be hungry or thirsty, too cold or too hot, or his feet may be cold, his position uncomfortable.
> He may be lying on creases, or on a moist sheet.
> If he is wearing any surgical apparatus this may be uncomfortable, a bandage may be too tight, or a splint may be hurting at some particular point.
> He may be conscious of a lack of movement of air around him.
> He may wish to empty his bladder or bowel. The unaccustomed company, lying in a ward with others, surrounded by new and strange noises, can be very disturbing.

Some of the symptoms of the complaint from which he is suffering may be very irritating and troublesome. He may be in pain or have a headache, his skin may be hot or dry, or he may be perspiring heavily; or again he may have marked restlessness, or be suffering from dyspnoea, palpitation, flatulence or indigestion, or he may be exceedingly uncomfortable if his temperature is raised.

Various little nursing attentions may be carried out in an attempt to relieve discomfort and to obtain the relaxation that is so necessary if the patient is to lie quiet and still, breathing regularly and with his eyes closed —all of which are so important if he is to get to sleep.

These measures include giving the patient a warm, light, nourishing drink, allowing him to empty his bladder, altering his position, rearranging his pillows, so that he is supported and his head is not nodding, straightening his sheets, tightening the undersheet, rearranging the draw-sheet so that he lies on a cool part of it.

It is equally important to see that the patient is not facing or in any way irritated by a light; on the other hand, a patient may be distressed because he is in the dark, and the provision of a suitably shaded night lamp may give the confidence which will render it possible for a patient so worried to relax.

A nurse should be very careful to avoid making a noise. It is essential to move quietly and close doors gently. There must not be any whispering, or clattering of utensils, and she should try to ensure that beds do not creak. However, noise alone does not keep people awake provided they recognize that the noise is of no importance to them. A nurse can help by explaining the source of any unavoidable noise.

When a sedative is ordered for a patient the nurse must take pains to prepare him beforehand for sleep, so that he will be unlikely to ask for a drink or a bedpan minutes after the sedative has been administered. Toilet attention or any other service should have been attended to previously.

Many patients bring medicines, particularly sedatives, they have been taking, into hospital. Often the policy is to remove them all. A patient may need a sedative, but often he is not allowed one of his own, ordered for him by his family doctor whom he trusts, and is given another. He may not sleep simply because of the resistance of mind and body to something strange. At the least this is poor patient-approach. The matter should be fully discussed with the patient, preferably by a doctor.

PAIN

Pain is a very common symptom which often provides the physician with valuable information. It varies much in extent and degree, and is apt to be troublesome, producing not only physical but also mental distress. It is important to investigate its location, distribution and character, whether intermittent or continuous, its frequency and severity. It is useful to know any factors which aggravate the pain and whether it has been found to respond to any treatment.

Pain may be a warning and in some cases a protection. The *character* of pain varies; it may be sharp, dull, aching, burning, knife-like, pulsating, gnawing, a sense of pressure, tingling, pins and needles, intractable.

The reaction of individuals to pain varies. Those with a low pain threshold feel pain most acutely, whilst others with a normal or high pain threshold tolerate pain better. The degree of concentration may intensify the suffering; yet on the other hand, if the mind can be distracted, the pain may be less severely experienced.

The memory of pain is another factor, and the fear of and anticipation of pain cannot be disregarded. A patient who has had a coronary thrombosis or anginal pain is always fearful of any pain in the region of his heart.

The control of pain

A patient's anxiety about his condition can cause pain, generally headache and abdominal pain which may be accompanied by diarrhoea *due entirely to emotional causes* and not to any disease.

In treatment when an analgesic is prescribed to be given when necessary for the relief of pain it is a mistake to wait until a patient is in pain before giving a dose. *It is much easier to keep pain away than to send it away* when it comes. Some analgesics such as sodium salicylate and aspirin are so rapidly excreted that when pain is severe they will probably be ordered every two or three hours. A nurse should be able to help a patient locate and describe his pain so that a lucid account of it can be given.

In the interest of diagnosis and sometimes in the interest of treatment a surgeon or physician may consider it necessary to leave a patient's pain unrelieved by drugs which would mask symptoms and make a probable diagnosis difficult. The nurse in this case should realize that it is the emotional response to pain that matters more than the pain itself and endeavour to relieve a patient's apprehensions and misapprehensions and obtain his co-operation. *For a surgeon's description of pain see p. 481.*

NURSING IN DISORDERS OF RESPIRATION

The breathless patient. Patients with respiratory disorders can be very apprehensive; the thought of what may happen if unable to 'get one's breath' is alarming. The nurse must become expert at recording, estimating and observing the respirations. These patients need compassion, understanding and encouragement. They will breathe more easily if propped up in the sitting position. This is facilitated in hospital by special beds but even then it needs nursing skill to make a patient comfortable in this position; it may take quite a time but is time well spent. The back and head should be fully supported, no hollows permitted between pillows, some support for the arms should be given if this seems desirable, even so this should not restrict the chest movements. There should be a footrest to prevent slipping down the bed and a bedtable on which to rest the elbows. A breathless patient is restless and may need moving frequently.

The temperature of the room should be fairly constant; changes in room temperature make breathing and coughing more distressful. The weight of the bedclothing needs assessing; a type of personal garment with no tightness about the neck or chest should be chosen. Any emotional disturbance due to environmental circumstances ought as far as possible to be avoided.

The **mouth** gets very dry; the patient will appreciate frequent sips of fluid; if a covered drink is left beside him and within reach he will be grateful. A beaker with a handle or a tea-cup is easier to manipulate than a glass. If he is having milky drinks a little water or other clear fluid of his liking will cleanse the mouth and prevent sordes collecting. A lip salve will prevent the lips from cracking. It is most important to keep the nasal passages clear and clean and free from crusts; a bland ointment smeared within the passages and around the margins of the nose, or a salve may be useful.

Cough and sputum. A dry irritating cough which is ineffective should be suppressed by a drink of water, lemonade, or other fruit drink of the patient's choice, or sucking a sweet or pastille may be helpful.

Coughing which results in expectoration should be encouraged, though when accompanied by chest pain a patient tends to suppress it. A nurse might help by support over a painful chest or over an abdominal wound following surgery, while the patient coughs.

A linctus may be ordered as mentioned above or analgesics where necessary; if this is so the nurse should give them when an attack of coughing seems imminent. The physician should be consulted, as some analgesics may further suppress coughing. Steam inhalations help and any other means of moistening the air is of value (see Chapter 9, p. 87). An attack of coughing can be very exhausting, leaving the patient tired and weak.

Sputum should never be swallowed; adult patients usually co-operate well but a nurse will often have to try and get the sputum out of the mouth of a child.

Only paper handkerchiefs should be supplied and a disposable sputum container which should always be within the patient's reach. A patient may not be able to hold the sputum container himself and must be assisted by the nurse who should, if necessary, allow him to rest his forehead on her outstretched hand. The nurse should also help by wiping away shreds of viscid sputum from the patient's lips. The frequency of attacks should be reported to the physician.

A physiotherapist is most helpful to these patients by teaching them breathing exercises and by tipping and chest percussion which all help in loosening and bringing up sputum.

Care in diet. It is wise to discuss with him the food a patient is to have, as he can then say what makes him cough. Usually dry food and any hard particles should be avoided; he will be grateful for frequent, small, easily digested meals. If a patient has to be fed, small portions only should be given, interspersed by rests and sips of water, as swallowing is difficult when breathless.

An early-morning cup of tea gives a sense of well-being, or hot water to sip containing a little saline or sodium bicarbonate may help loosen mucoid secretion.

A breathless patient should be spared muscular activity as far as possible, this includes the effort of talking and visitors should be warned about this. He needs help to get in and out of personal clothing. The physician should be consulted in regard to bowel action, as straining at stool is a great effort. It is better to get a patient out of bed onto a commode or a Sani-chair than to attempt to give a bedpan. Exhausted by the effort he may need help with the anal toilet.

The general toilet also needs consideration, as a patient who is very ill or who has had a bad night with breathlessness and coughing or sweating may be unable to get into a bath even with assistance, but he could probably sit on a chair in the bathroom and be 'bathed' in this way by the nurse. Sponging the face, neck, chest, back, hands, arms and groins can be refreshing. The situation obviously varies from patient to patient and is one demanding skill and discretion on the part of the nurse.

Read also a physician's description of the symptoms common in disorders of respiration, p. 194.

NURSING CONSIDERATIONS IN HEART DISEASE

The therapeutic value of rest on a damaged heart is well recognized. Two nursing problems arise:

> The provision of physical rest.
> Consideration of emotional disturbance.

Physicians alert to a patient's physical needs and temperamental tendencies give encouragement and prescribe treatment. The nurse should be on the watch to allay fear and apprehension, keeping the patient's mind as calm and confident as possible.

Nurses will meet not only young people, but many elderly ones, too, in a cardiac unit, who may be subjected to electrical defibrillation, cardioscopy and external cardiac pacing, who are too terrified to ask questions and need compassion, reasonable explanation and encouragement.

Physical rest

Position. Patients should normally be made comfortable in a semi-recumbent position, provided the systolic blood pressure does not fall below 90 mm. If hypotension is present the recumbent position is used; in severe hypotension the foot of the bed should be raised.

Support should be adequate and no hollows or spaces should be allowed between pillows. Unless a patient is comfortably supported, he may not feel that he is secure enough to rest. In positioning a patient with orthopnoea, for example, there should be a pillow to support his head, a pillow or wedge to support each forearm (a knee pillow should be avoided), and a footrest to prevent slipping down the bed.

Bed rest. A patient with severe heart disease, e.g. acute myocardial infarction or severe heart failure, should be on *absolute rest* and not permitted to make any movement unaided. He should be washed and fed, gently moved and carefully lifted when necessary, his locker should be out of reach and he should be warned against raising his arms above his head. A patient must be informed in advance of any movement about to take place.

Bed rest, however, for patients less dangerously ill needs intelligent application, as the possibility of deep venous thrombosis is present, particularly in those who are overweight and those with varicose veins, therefore the patient should be got up and should move about as soon as possible. He will probably get up for a short period at first, then for a meal, progressing gradually until he is up for two meals and a number of hours, but he must be warned not to wait on other patients and certainly not to act as 'tea boy'.

Effort and exercise. Although patients will be in the care of physiotherapists who will teach and advise them about exercise and effort, nurses should always observe the effect of effort on the patient, noting change of colour and alterations in breathing. The pulse rate is a good indication, and if it is taken before effort and again afterwards and fails to return to its former rate within a reasonable time (5 to 6 minutes) this should be brought to the notice of the physician.

Severe dyspnoea necessitates an upright position and some patients, e.g. with congestive heart disease, are often better nursed in an arm chair with legs and feet elevated for periods of time to prevent swelling. Once respiratory distress is overcome the patient is allowed up for part of the day (see above).

Sleep is necessary as it is the best form of rest, and yet a number of patients with heart disease do not sleep well. Nurses need to exercise great ingenuity in obtaining the best possible conditions for their patients' sleep, particularly with regard to their physical comfort; the correct degree of warmth, the provision of a non-irritating light, the reassurance that someone is within call and will hear the slightest sound, all these points need careful attention. The doctor will usually prescribe a sedative. The nurse takes pains to prepare the patient for sleep so that he will not be disturbed after taking the drug.

General toilet. Mouth care is important as patients with heart disease often sleep with the mouth open. A cup of weak tea on wakening is refreshing as it moistens the mouth and also by stimulating the circulation helps to relieve headache and improve the sense of well-being.

The skin is easily damaged, particularly when stretched by oedema.

Careful drying (the use of an emollient cream when dry), light powdering and gentle handling are essential (see Prevention of Pressure Sores, Chapter 4, p. 50).

The bowels should be regulated to act once or twice a day, producing a soft solid stool and thus avoid straining, for straining at stool means strain on the heart.

Urine. The amount passed should be measured and compared with the intake of fluid; as a rule it is tested daily for albumin.

In patients with oedema it should be realized that quite an amount of fluid is retained in the tissues before any swelling becomes obvious, and diminished urinary output may be the first indication of fluid retention.

VOMITING AND DIARRHOEA

These symptoms may arise independently or together, particularly in the infective types. In both conditions the dehydration due to loss of body fluid and electrolytes must be countered. This is a medical question which is dealt with by the administration of the appropriate fluid, often by intravenous infusion and by drugs, such as anti-emetics in vomiting and codeine phosphate in diarrhoea (see also Chapter 24, p. 239).

Vomiting

The causes of vomiting are numerous, but there are certain observations a nurse will be called upon to make with regard to the manner in which the vomit is expelled and also regarding the character of the vomit. In most cases food, then gastric juice and later bile-stained fluid are brought up. In conditions of *dilatation of the stomach* vomit is copious, at first frothy and offensive and later bile-stained. *In gastro-colic fistula* and sometimes in *intestinal obstruction* the vomit becomes faeculent in odour.

As a rule vomiting implies considerable effort and is associated with nausea except in the following instances:

> In peritonitis and intestinal obstruction it is *effortless and regurgitant* in character.
>
> In pyloric stenosis it is described as *projectile* since the stomach contents are *forcibly ejected.*
>
> Vomiting due to cerebral disease is not directly related to food—it may be projectile in character.

Nursing care. The act of vomiting is preceded by gulping, salivation and often by sweating. Vomiting reflexly stimulates the vagus nerve and so causes the patient to feel dizzy and faint; it may temporarily lower the blood pressure. Moreover, it is a very unpleasant symptom and the patient needs sympathy and attention. The nurse herself may be nauseated as she stands by a patient who is vomiting but she must not show this.

During the act of vomiting the basin should be held for the patient and his head supported by the nurse's hand, his dentures removed; it is essential to provide a suitable receptacle as splashing from vomit travels some distance; a sizable bowl or small plastic pail would be about right. The bedclothes should be protected.

If the patient has an abdominal wound which might be strained it should be supported. After vomiting a patient will like to rinse his mouth or have it cleansed, have his dentures washed and replaced. His general condition should be noted, any distress relieved, he may need a warm covering and would probably like a drink. Sipping tomato juice or slightly fizzy drinks often helps to control vomiting, or sucking ice may help, but these are all short-term measures and in most cases medical help should not be delayed.

There is also the social and emotional side to consider and if a patient has to travel he should be supplied with small paper bags, waxed if possible, plenty of tissues and a receptacle for soiled bags and tissues.

Vomiting in infants

This may be due to an acute or a chronic condition, or it may occur as the result of some deformity or malformation, most commonly that associated with congenital pyloric stenosis.

Acute forms of vomiting occur in acute gastro-intestinal disease as in epidemic diarrhoea and vomiting; and at the onset of acute febrile or infectious diseases such as meningitis. The severe vomiting which characterizes *congenital pyloric stenosis* may also be considered to be acute.

Less acute, or more chronic vomiting is usually due to errors of feeding, which include the swallowing of air, too rapid feeding, during which the infant is not given the rests necessary for him to bring air up, and jumping or jerking the infant about either before or after feeding.

The use of unsuitable foods containing either too much sugar or fat or forming too heavy a curd may also be the cause of vomiting.

A little unaltered food brought up during or soon after a feeding is described as *posseting*.

Nursing care. It is important that the nurse in charge of an infant who may be vomiting should consider whether the cause be attributable to the food given or to the manner of giving it, and note any time factor in relation to food.

In making a report on the vomit she should be careful to state whether it contains curds, and of what type these are; and also to note the presence of blood, bile or mucus.

Ruminating vomiting is a type which occurs in healthy infants; the baby or toddler is seen to make a succession of movements of his jaws and tongue and begin mastication; he gulps and brings fluid, or solid food, in the case of a toddler, into his mouth.

It is thought that the cause may be a psychological factor, and probably the infant wishes to create a disturbance and receive notice.

The *treatment* is to break the habit by giving thickened feedings, in the case of a tiny baby; and limiting the intake of fluid, particularly not to give water between meals, in the case of an older infant.

DIARRHOEA

There are many causes of diarrhoea. If the condition is liable to be infective, spread of infection must be prevented by the precautions described in Chapter 35.

Diarrhoea may be the result of eating unsuitable or contaminated foods (see Food Poisoning, Chapter 36, p. 354). Or the cause may be emotional due to some stress such as an impending examination or interview, or it may be due to some fear, real or imagined.

It is often essential for a patient to be able to get to a toilet quickly.

This point also needs consideration when a patient has to go on a journey. The *frequency, consistency* and the *general appearance of the stools should be noted*; these are the first points to be reported to the doctor. Blood and/ or mucus and occasionally undigested food may be present in the stools.

Cleanliness of the anal area and perineum is imperative and a silicone ointment or spray may occasionally be necessary to prevent maceration of the skin; odour has been mentioned but a patient is often embarrassed by this and thinks it can be detected by those around him, which is not usually so. The use of an aerosol deodorant will give him confidence.

Hand toilet should be meticulously performed and an emollient hand lotion used to prevent chapping. People suffering from diarrhoea should not take any part in the preparation of food, nor if possible should they wash or dry any utensils used for the preparation or delivery of food.

Read also a physician's account of symptoms common in gastro-intestinal disease, p. 238.

FITS AND CONVULSIONS

In all fits or other passing lapses of consciousness, it is important to investigate:

> The age of onset, frequency, usual time of occurrence, any pre-monitory symptoms.
>
> The presence of twitchings or convulsive movements such as tongue biting.
>
> Any irregularity of the pupils or movement of the eyes.
>
> Any incontinence.
>
> The duration of the fit, mode of recovery, and the mental state immediately afterwards.
>
> Any subsequent symptoms.

Fits or convulsions in adults may arise from a number of causes, fairly common ones being uraemia, epilepsy, apoplexy, cerebral tumours, and other organic diseases of the brain. Fits may also arise in cases of tetany, when the calcium balance of the body is disturbed; they also occur in tetanus, and may be met as a complication of pregnancy in eclampsia.

A hysterical fit also may arise as a manifestation of functional nervous derangement (see p. 272).

Care of a patient in a fit

1. See that the airway is not obstructed; provided a clear airway is maintained and the patient is not allowed to roll over on to his face and be suffocated, he is not in real danger.
2. Note whether the teeth are clenched and put a firm article such as a rubber ring or metal spatula between his teeth and keep them apart.
3. He may generally lie where he has fallen provided he is not in danger and that neither his arms nor legs are twisted under him; if moved, have him preferably on one side so that saliva does not trickle into his trachea; the tongue should either lie forward or be held forward.

Convulsions in infants are likely to occur whenever the nervous system is irritated.

In infants and young children convulsions may occur in febrile conditions.

Because the infant is debilitated, particularly when the calcium content of the blood is abnormally low.

At the onset of many diseases such as measles, scarlet fever, broncho-pneumonia and meningitis, or during the course of these diseases; and when an infant is dangerously ill.

Convulsions also occur in infants as a symptom of brain disease, such as cerebral haemorrhage.

A typical fit. The infant becomes rigid and pale, twitches slightly and his eyes become fixed. After a moment or two pallor gives way to cyanosis, and the infant loses consciousness. This usually lasts for a few moments, and then he regains consciousness, but is left weak and falls into a stuporous sleep.

The immediate treatment is to see that breathing is not obstructed, and hold the infant's head over to one side; loosen all clothing; if the teeth are erupted and there is any tendency to bite the tongue, a pad of material or a spatula should be held between them.

In the case of a prolonged convulsion the infant should be kept warm and have a cold-water compress applied to his head. A sedative may be ordered to be given by mouth or alternatively in a suppository.

NURSING THE PARALYSED PATIENT

Traumatic injury of the spinal cord has become more frequent owing to the number of severe industrial and road accidents.

From the time of injury both the paraplegic and quadriplegic face major threats to life. Both types may fail to adapt psychologically and fail to collaborate in preventive self-care; both face the possibility of urinary infection and the formation of deep pressure sores. The quadriplegic faces in addition pulmonary complications owing to involvement of the respiratory muscles and diminished vital capacity of the lung.

Changes and stages. At the outset a state of flaccid paralysis or spinal shock appears, lasting for several weeks. At this stage the patient does not react to his injury or understand its severity.

Emotional reactions follow. Though a patient may appear to accept his diagnosis, his behaviour belies this; he may decline to take the amount of fluid needed to keep the urinary output adequate or he may become anxious, depressed and withdrawn. At this stage the nurse should refrain from persuading him to accept his symptoms as this would only accelerate his non-acceptance. She should concentrate on providing for his physical needs and thus demonstrate the care he needs.

The patient will gradually begin to accept his limitations and turn towards adapting himself to the life which lies before him. During this stage the nurse can begin to teach self-care; above all she must show how confident she is in his ability to reach a point where he can approach normal living.

For the paraplegic, this will include exercises to strengthen the muscles of arms, shoulders and trunk. Proper diet and nutrition must be maintained and weight control is necessary to decrease the possibility of complications. Encouragement must be given to increase fluid intake to ensure a minimum urinary output of 3,000 ml per day, and proper care of the urinary tract must be followed. An in-dwelling urinary catheter maintains drainage and avoids distension; the nurse must be on the watch for distension and bring this to the notice of the doctor. Careful catheter technique is essential, with bathing of the urinary meatus and perineum. Strict aseptic technique is equally essential in bladder irrigation and/or continuous drainage (see p. 254). Careful watch must be kept for reflux due to kinking of the tube, and the position of any drainage bag attached to the patient, whether lying, sitting or standing, should be lower than the pelvis.

There is a variety of equipment for male bladder drainage (women are less fortunate); in this aspect self-care should begin from the outset, in order to avoid embarrassment and maintain the patient's independence. Down's male pubic pressure urinal may be used but as there are several sizes it should be fitted by the maker. The patient will soon learn to adjust it for himself; the bag attached to the leg will need emptying several times a day. At night a Paul's tube might be drawn over the penis to drain into a Urisac; alternatively a urinal might be placed in position. It is essential to remember that accidents may happen as patients with spinal cord injury have no sensation of passing urine or stool. The greatest care must be taken to maintain cleanliness of the skin and of any apparatus used.

Scrupulous attention must be paid to all pressure points and the position altered two-hourly. *Friction between the skin and sheet causes abrasions* and so the patient should be lifted when turning (see prevention of pressure sores, p. 49).

Constipation and abdominal distension may be troublesome but nurses and patients become adept at choosing the right suppository or aperient. Only in rare cases should it become necessary to evacuate a loaded bowel by enema or manually.

Quadriplegia (tetraplegia). As already mentioned, these patients have a greater disability, with paralysis of all four limbs, and face even more serious dangers to life than the paraplegic. It is impossible to imagine the emotional reactions and anxieties of a young person with this disability— he sees himself completely dependent on others for the remainder of his life. Good physiotherapy is essential in order to plan how the patient can be moved without injury to the skin. The same nutritional precautions, weight control, skin care, encouragement and urinary tract care as mentioned above in discussing paraplegia are essential.

In most spinal cord injuries at first the paralysis is of a flaccid type, the limbs affected being limp. Later they become spastic or rigid, and in response to reflex irritation become drawn up. This may lead to contractures, and the team-work of nursing and physiotherapy must be patiently and assiduously carried out if these contractures are to be prevented. The mental well-being of the patient is very important and, although progress towards any degree of recovery is usually slow, optimism should characterize his approach. This brings in the whole field of rehabilitation.

When spasticity of muscle ensues many patients assisted by their physiotherapists, nurses and relatives with great perseverance and practice develop trick movements entailed in balancing and using devices, often home-made, to convey food and drink to the mouth, apply cosmetics and so on—the helplessness of one who cannot even blow his own nose is almost unimaginable.

Nevertheless, many of these patients are got out of bed by a hoist into a wheel chair to be moved about, even with their disability. With indomitable courage they often manage shopping and visits.

Hemiplegia, a stroke, usually with paralysis of face, arm and leg on one side of the body, often begins with premonitory symptoms of dizziness and headache. The patient loses consciousness, suddenly or more gradually, which in a favourable case returns in an hour or two. At first the paralysis is of the flaccid type but it soon becomes spastic. There may be difficulty in speaking, *dysphasia*. When the speech area is involved in a right-sided hemiplegia, the inability to express thought by speech, *aphasia*, occurs.

Immediate treatment is as for an unconscious patient—clear the air passages, bring the tongue forward, raise head and shoulders and get a doctor.

Rehabilitation is essential from the outset and the patient's co-operation must be obtained no matter how upset he is at having had a stroke. A *physiotherapist* will teach, guide and encourage but nurse, patient and relatives must follow the aims of treatment and co-operate so that the patient's mind the whole day and every day is directed to educating the muscles affected, correcting positions of trunk and limbs, and preventing contractures. For example, he should have a rolled bandage in the palm of his hand so that the wrist is dorsi-flexed and movements of opposition and relaxation of thumb to fingers frequently made. The joints of his affected limbs should be moved throughout their whole range of movement twice daily.

The patient must not get tired but the tendency to relax in bed should be discouraged. Getting better is slow and though the patient does not act alone, the best results depend upon his own persistent efforts.

A physician's description of the care of a paralysed patient, p. 269, and the notes of an orthopaedic surgeon describing compression injury to the cord following fracture-dislocation of the spine, complications and treatment, p. 556, might usefully be referred to.

NURSING THE UNCONSCIOUS PATIENT

Before considering a few basic nursing points, it is recommended that pp. 411–12 should be read throughout, where the medical aspect and important observations in which the nurse is deeply involved are included in detail.

A nurse thinks and acts for this helpless unconscious patient who is dependent on her for survival and well-being; for example, he should lie in a position that will not embarrass his breathing or restrict the movements of head and abdomen. He must not lie with arms or legs beneath him, as the protective warning signals, pain and cramp, are not felt by him and permanent nerve damage may result. His head should be inclined to the side so that secretions cannot trickle into his trachea. The exaggerated semiprone position suitable for the unconscious patient is shown in

Fig. 8/3, p. 80. A restless patient may roll over and be in danger of asphyxia; his care demands continuous observation.

The causes of unconsciousness are numerous, and a nurse admitting the patient should be prepared to report on the degree of insensibility, be on the look out for injuries to head, back and chest, note the odour of the breath and any odour clinging to the body, observe the state of the mouth, lips and tongue, notice whether the eyes are open or closed, the state of the pupils and the condition of the skin as regards pallor, cyanosis and sweating; any twitchings, fits or convulsive movements should also be recorded.

THE INCONTINENT PATIENT

Incontinence is the involuntary passing of urine or faeces or both, with or without the knowledge of the patient; for example, in lesions of the brain and of the spinal cord as in paraplegia and quadriplegia (see p. 557) the patient has no sensation whatever of his incontinence. It occurs also in extreme weakness, old age, in conditions of prostration and shock, in injuries to the pelvic floor, to the bladder and rectum, including the urethra and anal canal.

In some psychiatric conditions incontinence is normal in early childhood and full continence should not be expected or 'demanded' by the mother too soon.

Incontinence of urine may also occur whenever the urethra or its sphincter has been stretched, as for example after childbirth.

Read also the types of urinary incontinence which may occur as described by a genito-urinary surgeon, on p. 242.

The nurse should look into the possible causes of incontinence, discuss these with the doctor and come to some decision.

(a) As to any measure that can be taken to alleviate the condition.
(b) Care of the patient who has urinary incontinence.
(c) Care of the patient with faecal incontinence.

Observations. Consider whether the incontinence is continuous or tends to occur under stress, excitement, fatigue. The latter might be offset by giving a snack and a nourishing drink, particularly in the elderly when weariness may indicate a low blood-sugar level which needs slight boosting.

In the bedfast person the regular and frequent offering of a bedpan or urinal often prevents incontinence, and similarly the frail ambulant patient should be taken to the lavatory regularly and before need arises. Easy access to a commode or chamber pot at night is important.

Patients are often tempted to drink less than normal, but when they realize that a highly concentrated urine is more irritable to the bladder they will drink reasonably.

Some patients, however clean and careful they are, imagine they smell of urine. This is not usually so and their emotional distress and loss of self-respect can be helped by encouragement. Nevertheless, the regular use of a deodorant (or Air-wick) makes them feel more confident.

For men the equipment available is mentioned on p. 134, where the care of a paralysed patient is considered.

For women specially absorbent cellulose pads which are deodorant and hold from 100 to 150 ml without discomfort are available. These enable women to go shopping, visiting and travelling. Impervious panties are useful on occasions but not recommended for continual use as maceration of the skin occurs.

Cleanliness and great care of the skin is essential, but as all nurses are well versed in this and its care is described on p. 50, it is not dealt with here. The use of an in-dwelling catheter, especially for the female patient may be necessary and although this may give rise to urinary infection, this can be more easily coped with than soreness and maceration of the skin caused by urine incontinence.

Incontinence of faeces is very distressing—it calls for consideration of diet, and an attempt to arrange bowel action to once a day, provided it is adequate, is important. Regular bowel evacuation is important to prevent overloading of the rectum which leads to incontinence. Aperients are best avoided, one does not know when they are going to act, and may lead to loose stools. A suppository or an enema is more controllable. Incontinence pads to protect the bed at night give any incontinent patient some sense of security and save laundry.

Read also the note on urinary and faecal incontinence in the elderly by a geriatrician, p. 340.

HIGH-DEPENDENCY PATIENTS

In a survey conducted in a large general hospital in Greater London, the following categories were observed:

1. *Bedfast, chairfast, totally helpless*, entirely dependent on nursing for all services. *Over 70 per cent of all admissions* fall into this category for an average of 48 hours.
2. *Bedfast, chairfast, partially helpless*, dependent on nursing staff for movement from bed to chair, for assistance with toilet facilities and may require some help with feeding and with all personal services: *68 per cent of the over 70 per cent fell into this category for a further two to three days*. The remainder stayed in category 1 for a much longer time and some died.
3. *Bedfast, chairfast, but not helpless*. Bedfast or dependent on nursing staff from bed to chair and vice versa. Capable of washing (either in bed or taken to a wash basin); feeding self and capable of all personal services. *Fifty per cent of all patients in the hospital at any one time fell into this category*.
4. *Semi-ambulant*. Patients up and moving about part of the day. May need help in getting out of bed, capable of all other services. Only 8 to 10 per cent of patients would fall into this category at any one time.
5. *Totally ambulant*, up and about the ward all day. Approximately 2 per cent of the patients would be in this category at any one time.

A number of patients might be discharged home before reaching category 4.

Most of the patients needing *special nursing care*, mentioned above, would come into one of these first three categories. Any reader could fill in many other conditions requiring special care. For example:

Medical	*Surgical*
Any disease which is progressive	Many cases of carcinoma
Acute disseminated sclerosis	Great number of patients after
Parkinson's disease	major surgery
Rheumatoid arthritis	Ectopic pregnancy
Advanced heart and lung disease	Prostatic enlargement
Ulcerative colitis	Acute urinary retention
Septicaemia	

It is estimated that over 90 per cent of patients are cared for in their own homes or in some form of institution; a number would come into categories 1, 2 or 3 of the highly dependent patient. The function of a nurse has never been adequately defined, but it is fair to say that anyone who contributes to the care, comfort and treatment of a patient, sometimes a very dependent one, is nursing in its widest sense.

A CONCEPT OF INTENSIVE PATIENT THERAPY

Intensive care units are available in many hospitals and there is no set rule or limit to what may be required. Some units admit only one condition as in coronary care, others accept a variety of emergency states. In all, men, women and children may be admitted, each so seriously ill as to be oblivious of the others.

The object is to provide ideal conditions where acutely ill patients *need unremitting medical and nursing care* so that life may be maintained and saved; a service which is very demanding but most rewarding.

Many classes of patients are admitted including those with:

Cardiac arrest.
Respiratory embarrassment.
Cerebro-vascular accident.
Coma.
Acute poisoning.
Multiple injury.
Severe burns.
Those having had major cardio-thoracic surgery, abdominal surgery and neuro-surgery.
Patients with malignant disease who have not responded to medical treatment or radiotherapy.

On average in an acute general hospital the percentage of patients needing intensive care is from 1 to 5 per cent, over a period of 1 to 3 days in the unit. Some passing through crises or developing severe complications may need several weeks intensive care.

A *staff ratio* covering the 24 hours or 3 to 5 nurses per patient is average, depending on the work carried out; this enables each patient to be looked after by one or more nurses at all times. But where a patient needs a special nurse or nurses additional staff must be supplied.

One of the first considerations is the need of adequate permanent staff as observers and therapists with the resourcefulness and stability of temperament required, and the capacity to accept grave responsibilities combined with adaptability to constant change, the ability to get on with others and to learn quickly.

An *experienced doctor and anaesthetist* are present or available within call at all times. An ancillary staff of technicians for servicing equipment, and also physiotherapists and radiographers and adequate domestic staff are needed.

A dated chart which must be comprehensive and accurate is carefully kept, which in addition to the patient's name, address, age, date of birth, occupation, religion, and the address of his nearest relatives, should also record his general condition, the blood pressure, pulse and respiration rate, his temperature and other relevant features.

Following cardiac surgery or myocardial infarction the electro-cardiogram is monitored continuously and arrythmias are reported should they occur. The central venous pressure gives helpful information regarding the circulating blood volume and this is usually monitored.

Reference to pp. 285–6 indicates in some detail how intensive care is applied.

Neurological signs to be observed and recorded in patients recovering from general anaesthesia, in coma, with head injuries, and after neuro-surgery include:

> *Eyes.* Signs and reactions of the pupils—equal or unequal in size—dilated, contracted to pin-point size.
>
> *Responses of the patient* to pain, to commands as to movement of the limbs, to open or close the eyes, to swallowing, and to responses indicating the need for urination or defaecation. Any restlessness.

Nursing measures. *An accurate fluid balance chart* should list *input* by mouth, indwelling gastric tube, intravenous infusion and *output* by urine, vomit, bowels, by gastric and bronchial aspiration, by drainage from indwelling tubes, blood loss and serum loss.

The following points also are noted and recorded:

> Adequacy of all drainage.
> Time, frequency and result of bronchial suction.
> Time and frequency of cuff deflation in intratracheal or trache-ostomy tube.
> Frequency of movement, turning, treatment of pressure area.
> Oral toilet.
> Eye toilet or special eye care as may be needed in coma.
> Frequency of release of indwelling catheter and its time of removal.
> The action of the bowels.

A biochemical analysis of the blood and urine is kept. The nurse records the time any specimen was taken, and the physician or biochemist records the blood and analysis findings, and other details. A chart of the state of the urine, giving reaction, specific gravity, presence of albumin, sugar and ketones is kept.

The nurse will need every item of her professional knowledge from application of the simplest basic nursing procedure to the most complicated nursing skill and management. *By her diligent observation any deterioration in a patient's condition is at once reported to the medical staff so that corrective measures can be taken without delay and by her accurate recordings the medical staff are kept constantly aware of treatments under-taken and drugs given with any reactions noted.* She becomes rapidly aware of her responsibility in maintaining harmony in the life-saving team in which she is deeply involved. She must also have the ability to give clear, concise instructions to junior members of the team.

The nurse must not allow her attention to be diverted from the patient until he is capable of taking responsibility for his own physiological functions.

When a student or pupil nurse is assigned to such a unit there is no cause for apprehension, she will be serving under highly skilled expert nurses who will explain fully any help or procedure asked of her.

Not all nurses are suited for this type of work. They should be able to assess their own limitations. There is a certain degree of self-selection, as only those tend to continue in this work who really like and can accept it.

Read also the treatment of poisoning, p. 283 and nursing in cardiac surgery, p. 610, where intensive therapy is specially important.

THE NURSING OF PATIENTS WITH A COMMUNICABLE DISEASE

In this field the nurse is called upon to consider:

> The nursing care of the sick person.
> The necessity of preventing the spread of infection to others.
> The prevention of infection to herself.

Barrier nursing. The terms barrier isolation and bed isolation mean the same. In certain hospitals wards are set apart, *isolation wards*, in which a variety of communicable diseases are nursed under certain conditions and, when efficiently carried out, cross infection from one patient to another does not occur. *Cubicle nursing* in separate cubicles needs similar precautions.

The principles of this form of isolation are either the separation of all utensils so that each individual patient has his own, or the adequate sterilization of these when used in common. In most instances however certain articles such as the clinical thermometer, and washing and sanitary utensils (unless disposable) are kept separate for each patient.

Two gowns, which may be disposable, are supplied at each bedside, or in each cubicle for the use of doctor and nurse and other gowns should be available for any visitor; disposable masks, caps and gloves may also be supplied: a basin with hot and cold running water with foot or elbow control, a sterilized nail brush in disinfectant, or alternatively chlor-hexidine (Hibitane) cream applied to the hands before washing with the liquid soap. Disposable towels are also provided. The gown should be removed before washing the hands; adequate washing should be employed on each occasion.

Feeding utensils, unless disposable, should preferably be sterilized and should never be washed in the kitchen sink. *All food and drink* left by the patient should be disposed of by means of the sluice which should be adequately disinfected afterwards.

All soiled bed and personal linen should be placed in a disposable waxed container at the bedside and specially treated at the laundry in order to be adequately sterilized before being washed. All dressings, swabs, discharges from the patient should be collected in disposable containers and immediately burnt. Books and papers and toys (only washable ones) tied to the bedside, should be provided. All of these and other personal items and letters, etc., should be disposed of by burning. No articles of any kind should be passed from bed to bed.

Air conditioning is advisable in the prevention of cross infection. When possible swing doors should be used.

Read also Chapters 34 and 35.

Chapter 15

Nursing in Grave Illness. The Needs of a Dying Patient

Many gravely ill patients are nursed in their own homes amongst relatives and friends assisted by the family doctor and district nurses who are so expert in the care of the housebound, bedfast and those with restricted movement. Others go into a home or hostel and some are treated in special hospitals or in the geriatric wards of general hospitals. A few may be in an intensive care unit (see p. 137).

Good nursing is essential. Feeding should be adequate and suitable and patients should use normal utensils for as long as possible. Some nourishment should be given in between meals to avoid hunger, thirst and weariness. Patients need encouragement to eat and dietary restrictions should be avoided when possible. A patient who is used to some alcohol with his meal should not be deprived of it. All patients should be encouraged to do as much as they can for themselves in order to preserve their independence for as long as possible and they should be helped to take an interest in all that is going on around them. A few special nursing points might be mentioned.

Patients should not be allowed to become dehydrated. There are many ways of maintaining an adequate fluid intake so that the tissues are kept moist, including the mouth, lips and tongue, thus enabling the digestive and excretory systems to function comfortably.

Attention to the hygiene of the body means care of the skin, mouth, hair and nails. The prevention of pressure sores is important (for details see Chapter 4, p. 50).

Observation of the state of bladder and rectum. It is important to be on the watch for a distended bladder or loaded rectum as, if neglected, patients become restless and sleepless, and the condition may lead to incontinence.

When analgesics such as aspirin are ordered they should be given before pain sets in (see note on control of pain, p. 126). The doctor will order the use of stronger drugs when necessary to keep a patient free from pain but he should not be demoralized by them and should be able to support the course of his illness and retain his faculties without being mentally confused.

The least sign of change should be noted and reported whether physical or emotional. The latter may include depression and withdrawal; the more dependent the patient becomes so much more may doctors and nurses be involved. *The reaction of the relatives should also be observed* and opportunities made to talk to them, explaining in simple language these changes, which may be temporary, and reassuring them that alterations in mood will vary from day to day. It is essential that the relatives should feel they may telephone at any time if only for a chat about progress to set their minds at rest.

The expression terminal illness has been studiously avoided; it is a depressing term and many grave illnesses and many more chronic illnesses are anything but terminal. But there comes a time when there is a *gradual worsening of the illness, an apparent ebbing away of life* and many more patients than we give them credit for are fully aware of this. It may be accompanied by a final failure of the heart, lungs, kidneys or liver, or a last cerebro-vascular incident or cancer which has defeated surgery and radiotherapy.

An elderly person who is gravely ill feels weak and frail. Physical, mental and moral sufferings take their toll and it is very essential to have time to try to prevent or relieve any distress and to make as good a thing as possible of what may well be a last illness. Nurses should be good listeners, endeavouring to help a patient to express himself when he wishes to do so. *There comes a time when symptomatic relief and good nursing care take precedence over other considerations* with emphasis on consideration and kindness.

Man is a spiritual being and a patient may be glad to receive a visit from a Minister of Religion who can bring him comfort and consolation. Sometimes relatives seem to overlook this need, possibly because they fear the patient may be disturbed and begin to think his illness is more serious; this is not so. A patient knows quite as much, often more, about his condition than they do and this help should not be withheld. Nurses generally realize its value and will suggest a visit, which most patients will be glad to accept.

LONELINESS IN ILLNESS

The loneliness encountered in illness often comes from the knowledge that one is temporarily set apart from others, unable to mix and communicate with them. If in hospital, for example, where the world can only visit occasionally and even then it is quite difficult, often impossible, to feel relaxed and at ease with visitors, the environment is totally different from home.

A patient is both physically and mentally isolated when he is very ill; this loneliness is accompanied by weariness, when a patient may find it impossible to think clearly, read, concentrate and talk, remember what he wants to say or even lie comfortably. He is one mass of discomforts no healthy person could imagine. If he speaks of them he is thought to be exaggerating, which is not so, in reality he is being very brave.

Those who may know, mostly by intuition, that they are probably in their last illness or approaching it are very lonely people who need treating with great consideration when any little attention that seems possible should be given. An observant nurse can enter partly into the sufferings of this patient and try to supply his needs and relieve his loneliness by her presence, her interest, a smile and some friendly words. His knowledge that she will be near enough to hear if he calls can be very reassuring.

Loneliness in serious illness can be the determining cause of death, particularly in infants and elderly people; the nearness of those a patient loves and those who care can help to maintain courage when at a very low ebb. It is vital that nurses should try to understand what he is thinking and feeling and do their best to relieve what may indeed be distress and certainly is great aloneness.

The loneliness of a very sick child following the movements of his mother or nurse with his eyes, dreading lest she should go out of his sight, longing for her nearness, is sad to witness. It is kindness to go often to his side showing some little attention, speaking to him, touching him, stroking his hair, holding his hand and promising to be near and to come back soon and keeping that promise. All this is extremely important.

THE NEEDS OF A DYING PATIENT

Death for mankind is inevitable, it brings to an end our earthly life; there is a deep longing in the heart of all men for immortality.

Sooner or later a nurse will be present at the death of a patient for the first time, and as she closes his eyes or performs other services it is wise to regard this as a continuation of her care of him during life. No one can remain unaffected by a death, for as the poet Donne wrote: 'Any man's death diminishes me, because I am involved in Mankinde.' A sudden un-expected death can be most disturbing, no one need be ashamed at being emotionally distressed but all should endeavour to present a calm exterior.

Death is a time of crisis for the patient, his family and his doctors and nurses. Most conscious patients realize they are dying; they have watched the attitude of their doctors, made an assessment of the various examina-tions and treatments they have undergone and drawn their own con-clusions. A patient may question his nurse as to his condition, or his doctor, who, alive to his responsibilities, must answer. It will depend on circum-stances whether a direct answer can be given, which may often be conveyed by an increased note of sympathy and affection in his bearing rather than by words. *The doctor will continue his regular routine visits to his patient to support him and bring relief from pain and discomforts.* 'Some patients, though conscious that their condition is perilous, recover their health simply through their contentment with the goodness of the physician.'—Hippocrates in The Precepts.

A patient should be aware that his nurses are concerned about him and ready to do all they can to help. They must accept the responsibility of helping to make a good death as they would have helped him, in other circumstances, to make a good recovery. A patient should be allowed to die with dignity and peacefully.

The tendency to belittle or deny death should be discouraged. Patients aware of their state find the false cheerfulness of those around them un-helpful. The dying often long to share their thoughts and feelings with another. A Minister of Religion could help (see note p. 146), or a nurse by finding someone with whom the patient wishes to speak (after warning this person) could bring them together and leave them to chat. Otherwise a dying person deprived of this desire to communicate may, though sur-rounded by relatives and friends, die in isolation and loneliness. Leaving relatives alone with the patient when his condition permits is thoughtful, as this privacy may well be the only opportunity for a last embrace and some final words. Nurses should never intrude.

Death is a reality in nursing and it is natural that a young nurse may feel apprehensive in her first contact with a dying person or in witnessing a death. If uninformed on the points outlined in this chapter nurses may not feel competent to deal with what is a critical situation and will tend either to withdraw or become too emotionally involved. All members of the ward staff can give support to those actually nursing the patient, thus spreading the emotional load. As the result of the spontaneous good comradeship one sees in our wards the sympathy of other patients for the one who is dangerously ill also helps.

The nursing of the dying is extremely demanding. *The grieving relatives need people who understand, with whom they can discuss their feelings of anxiety, depression, a sense of failure or guilt, and will turn to the doctors and nurses who are sharing the situation with them for advice and encouragement.* To let them know, as far as is possible, from day to day, hour to hour what is happening and the help they can give, is very acceptable. For a nurse to notice when the relatives are tired and suggest a change of position, a rest, a cup of tea or some nourishment or a little diversion, is a real kindness.

A patient's condition needs understanding now as never before, for in the last resort death is an individual matter; even when surrounded by the loving care of relatives and friends this 'passing on', as it is so often called, is taken blindfold and alone. The dying must be treated as a person. Don't turn away, speak to the patient, look at him in his helplessness and give what help you can. Your presence lets him see he is cared for. *Care is the operative word.* Try not to hide behind a cloak of professionalism, let your human feelings show so that a patient, if conscious, and his relatives always can see that you care.

When conscious of what is taking place about him a dying person is very lonely. If his relatives are present they should be encouraged to hold his hand, caress him, place a hand on his forehead, thus manifesting their presence. His sense of vision may have gone (for this often goes before feeling), but feeling and other forms of perception may still be present.

A few considerations might be mentioned. Conversation the dying person is not meant to hear should not take place at his bedside, for even apparently unconscious patients may have quite an acute sense of hearing. Incapable of movements or speech, unable to express his needs, he will be grateful when discomforts are relieved such as wiping the sweat from his brow, taking the hair back out of his eyes, giving him a drink or a sip from a teaspoon, and when unable to swallow moistening his tongue and lips frequently, every 15 minutes to be effective, sponging his face and hands, altering his position in the bed, raising his head and shoulders to relieve his breathing. *All general nursing measures should continue to be meticulously carried out, slowly and gently.*

CONSIDERATION OF A PATIENT'S FEARS

The process of dying is generally feared more than death itself. A patient fears he may not be able to accept what is involved: suffering, anxiety and increasing dependence on others; if he is confident that he will not be allowed to suffer pain and that he will not be left alone he will be comforted. The following authentic article shows this clearly.

Death in the First Person

Anonymous

I am a student nurse. I am dying. I write this to you who are, and will become, nurses in the hope that by sharing my feelings with you, you may someday be better able to help those who share my experience.

I'm out of the hospital now—perhaps for a month, for six months, perhaps for a year . . . but no one likes to talk about such things. In fact, no one likes to talk about much at all. Nursing must be advancing, but I wish it would hurry. We're taught not to be overly cheery now, to omit the 'Everything's fine' routine, and we have done pretty well. But now one is left in a lonely silent void. With the protective 'fine, fine' gone, the staff is left with only their own vulnerability and fear. The dying patient is not yet seen as a person and thus cannot be communicated with as such. He is a symbol of what every human fears and what we each know, at least academically, that we too must someday face. What did they say in psychiatric nursing about meeting pathology with pathology to the detriment of both patient and nurse? And there was a lot about knowing one's own feelings before you could help another with his. How true.

But for me, fear is today and dying is now. You slip in and out of my room, give me medications and check my blood pressure. Is it because I am a student nurse, myself, or just a human being, that I sense your fright? And your fear enhances mine. Why are you afraid? I am the one who is dying!

I know, you feel insecure, don't know what to say, don't know what to do. But please believe me, if you care, you can't go wrong. Just admit that you care. That is really for what we search. We may ask for why's and wherefores, but we don't really expect answers. Don't run away . . . wait . . . all I want to know is that there will be someone to hold my hand when I need it. I am afraid. Death may get to be a routine to you, but it is new to me. You may not see me as unique, but I've never died before. To me, once is pretty unique!

You whisper about my youth, but when one is dying, is he really so young anymore? I have lots I wish we could talk about. It really would not take much more of your time because you are in here quite a bit anyway.

If only we could be honest, both admit of our fears, touch one another. If you really care, would you lose so much of your valuable professionalism if you even cried with me? Just person to person? Then, it might not be so hard to die . . . in a hospital . . . with friends close by.

THE MINISTER OF RELIGION

Far more often than we think, dying people think of God and are grateful that a minister of the religion to which the patient belongs should visit him. Religion matters: it is concerned with man's relationship with God and with man's destiny. In this country the frequent presence of ministers in our hospital wards makes it easy and acceptable for one to be asked to go to the bedside of a patient. No matter what the beliefs of a nurse may be (and they are numerous in this multi-racial society) she must respect those of others and obtain for a dying patient whatever she may judge that he or his relatives would wish for him. A nurse acting thus is simply performing an act of great kindness and a worthy professional service for the mental comfort of her patient.

She should send without delay, day or night, when a patient is seriously ill and may die. It is an error to wait until death is imminent, as a patient's co-operation is of value.

Information to give. A minister may have left instructions. Some like to know whether the patient is conscious, if he can swallow or is vomiting, so that the minister may judge whether to bring Holy Communion. If a patient regains consciousness a minister may wish to visit again whilst he is in possession of his faculties. Even if a patient has died the minister should be notified as soon as possible.

As life draws to a close and the relatives, the nurse, and perhaps the doctor if he is a family friend, stand round the bed it can truly be said: 'They also serve who only stand and wait.'

Cardinal Newman wrote in his *Dream of Gerontius*:

Pray for me, O my friends; a visitant
  Is knocking his dire summons at my door,
The like of which to scare me and to daunt,
  Has never, never come to me before:
'Tis death O loving friends, your prayers! 'Tis he!
  As though my very being had given way,
As though I were no more a substance now,
  And could fall back on nought to be my stay,
(Help, loving Lord! Thou my sole refuge, Thou)
.   .   .   .
So pray for me, my friends, who have not strength to pray.

WHEN A DEATH OCCURS IN HOSPITAL

The *time of death* is entered on a patient's case notes which are then sent to the Medical Records office.

The *relatives* are generally left alone at the bedside for a short period to recover and regain equilibrium: they are then taken to a room where they can be alone, a side ward or waiting room, and given tea or coffee. Before they leave the head nurse will discuss with them the procedure for collecting the death certificate and the patient's property and she may arrange for them to see a member of the medical staff.

The patient. The bed is kept screened. The patient is laid flat with the hands resting at his sides. The eyes are closed gently and damp cotton wool swabs are placed on the lids. Dentures are replaced. Any jewellery being worn should be removed and put in safe keeping. It is essential to ask whether a wedding ring is to remain or be removed. If necessary the mouth is kept closed by means of a small pillow or a pad placed beneath the chin.

Apparatus and equipment which has been in use is removed. Drainage tubes should be left in position, the tubings attached are removed and the area covered lightly with cotton wool.

The top sheet is now drawn up over the patient's face, the blankets and counterpane are removed. All equipment, other than the patient's personal property is removed from the bedside or from the room. The body is left for approximately one hour when the *last offices* are carried out according to the custom of the hospital and preferably by two nurses. An identity tape is attached to one wrist or ankle and one mortuary card attached to the front of the shroud, a second one is handed to the porter who takes the body to the mortuary, varying with the custom of the hospital. He is accompanied by a senior nurse.

A director of funerals will arrange, if wished, to collect a body from any house or building and transfer it to his establishment where the last offices can be carried out. The dead person will then be laid in a chapel or viewing room where relatives and friends may visit, bringing flowers, etc. This provides a very valuable service to the community.

Certain groups object to Christians touching their dead: when known their wishes should be respected. The Jews are one group and a Rabbi attached to one large London general hospital issues these instructions:

> Close the patient's eyes.
> Remove any equipment attached to the body.
> Lay the body flat with arms by the sides.
> Wrap in a sheet for transfer to the mortuary.

The immediate post-mortem Jewish Rites will then be carried out by specially appointed persons of their religion.

Section 2

Chapter 16

Understanding Nutrition

by W. T. C. BERRY

> *Introduction—nature and prevalence of nutritional deficiency in Great Britain—energy considerations—practical points—nutrition in developing countries*

INTRODUCTION

Good food like good air is essential to health. Yet we eat the one, breathe the other and get on very well, often without giving a thought to the ways in which these function. When, however, something goes wrong with either, we find that in order to understand it properly, complex physiological and other concepts may have to be mastered. Nurses do not have to master all the complexities of nutrition, but they should have sufficient theoretical knowledge to speak with reasonable authority on the sorts of problems about which they are likely to be consulted (see p. 153).

The food we eat and its relation to our nutrition

Foods are often classed as body builders, protective foods and fillers (energy suppliers), but no common food except sugar falls entirely into one category. Meat is a 'body builder' because of its protein but it also supplies energy and vitamins. Bread is classed as an energy supplier because of its starch, but provides useful amounts of protein, minerals and vitamins. **Energy** throughout this chapter refers to the electrical energy which is liberated from food and measured in calories or preferably joules.

Through the National Food Survey and other nutrition surveys in Britain, it is consistently found that *on average* the diet contains enough of nearly all the nutrients for which the experts have formulated Recommended Allowances. The typical national diet is an adequate one and what need to be sought are departures from this. Moreover, these usually have to be gross because man has an instinct or desire for variety in his diet. Thus, where there is not much meat, he may 'liven it up' with cheese, fish or eggs and so get the necessary protein and other body-building nutrients. *A nutritionally adequate diet is a varied one*, and the reverse is also true.

Therefore be on the watch for monotonous diets. A rule of thumb measure is that if a diet contains at least one daily helping of meat, fish or cheese and one of green vegetables or fresh or canned citrus fruits or tomatoes, the rest can consist of foods which are not usually highlighted by nutritionists, such as bread, potatoes, butter or margarine, even sugar in moderation, and so on, and still be adequate for an adult. An additional important safeguard is milk, which plays a substantial part in our national diet and is rich in most nutrients essential for life.

Children, particularly early in life when growth is most rapid, need a higher proportion of body-building foods than adults. They also need more of some vitamins which are usually regarded as protective but which are also needed to build the body. *So do pregnant women*, for similar reasons, and *lactating women because they are secreting the milk required to construct their babies' bodies*. Therefore, pregnant women and children up to the age of five (or their mothers if the children are breast fed) are entitled, where the family is large or needy, to receive free of charge one pint of milk daily or its equivalent in dried milk powder under the Welfare Milk Scheme. They are also entitled to free preparations of vitamins A, C, and D. Such preparations are also available at cost for smaller and more prosperous families.

Schoolchildren are growing, and a third of a pint of milk is provided free at infant school. But active children expend calories and eat increased amounts of food in order to restore this energy to their bodies. A child who needs and gets a large amount of food is more likely to eat a sufficiency of protein and other nutrients than one who needs and takes little food. The large amounts of food thus consumed need to be of a nutritious sort and the school lunch is designed to be both nutritious and cheap, or free in cases of hardship. (There are children who need little food because they lead inactive lives but who eat too much and become obese.)

THE NATURE AND PREVALENCE OF NUTRITIONAL DEFICIENCY IN BRITAIN

Besides the National Food Survey and other nutrition surveys, we have another source of information about the prevalence of malnutrition from the reports of clinicians and biochemists (some of whom devote much time to nutritional inquiries) when they encounter cases of overt deficiency disease. The two sets of data should tie up. The smaller the margin, over the Recommended Allowances (see p. 156), shown on the average figures of the National Food Survey (N.F.S.), the more often the clinician ought to see cases of malnutrition.

The value of vitamins in nutrition

Deficiencies of vitamin A, calcium and protein are seldom seen in adults, and the N.F.S. indicates a satisfactory margin. This is of interest because formerly it was thought that 'protein foods' were of special importance for all groups, whereas now it is realized that their contribution of other nutrients such as riboflavin (see p. 151) is often as important as their contribution of protein or more so. Deficiency due to thiamine (B_1) or niacin (nicotinic acid, nicotinamide, the *pellagra-preventing fraction of the vitamin B complex*) is rare even though the margin of safety is no more impressive than in the case of other nutrients, but one reason for this is that these nutrients are added by law to flour, and bread is still the staff of life for the worst paid. As a result beri beri and pellagra are rarely seen except among alcoholics and others on peculiar diets.

Riboflavin is a part of the B complex of vitamins present in almost all protein-rich foods. From the N.F.S. averages the margin above Recommended Allowances seems small, but in two tests on schoolchildren and youths no improvement followed the administration of this vitamin. A useful source of riboflavin is milk and it is worth asking how much milk is drunk when angular stomatitis and cheilosis (cracks at the angles of the mouth and sore lips) are encountered. A test on old people showed that though most of such lesions were due to other causes, some of them were associated with deficiences of riboflavin or of pyridoxine (another part of the vitamin B complex).

Vitamin C. Though the position seems from N.F.S. data to be secure, this is a vitamin which is present in useful amounts only in certain foods like vegetables and fruit, which some people rarely eat, and is liable to be reduced by overcooking. *Scurvy or near-scurvy is the only proven manifestation of vitamin C deficiency* and this can in most people (not necessarily all) be prevented by the limited amounts present, after cooking, in green vegetables. *All vitamin C can be destroyed in potatoes* if they are peeled the night before and left to soak, and then mashed well before need so that they have to be kept hot. Despite much teaching to the contrary some cooks responsible for the feeding of large numbers of people still do these things, but they are not characteristic of ordinary households. It is in institutions and places of communal feeding that scurvy has to be feared; otherwise it is a disease of the very young, where mothers fail to give preparations of vitamin C, and the very old at the stage where they can or will no longer feed properly.

Vitamin D. The average supply recorded in the N.F.S. includes the amounts eaten by adults with virtually no need for any vitamin D in their diet, as well as children, some of whom need a great deal. In a sense, *vitamin D preparations should be regarded as concentrated sunlight* rather than as a nutrient, because much of what we require is formed by sunlight falling on the skin; the children of sunny lands who run about naked do not develop rickets. Much of our sunlight comes through window panes which check the ultraviolet rays which form vitamin D in the skin, and when we are in the open much of the sunlight which might fall on us is blocked by tall buildings and the smoke of cities. Nevertheless, rickets is rare in this country because dried and evaporated milks are fortified with vitamin D. *Theoretically children need a medicinal preparation of vitamin D up to the fifth year of life.*

Though *the iron supply in the diet* seems adequate, iron-deficiency anaemia is common in women, but research has shown that this is more closely related to the large amounts of blood some lose in their menses than to defects in their diet. *Deficiency of folic acid* (which is not analysed in the N.F.S. because the amounts in many foods have not yet been determined) appears as anaemia in some pregnant women, particularly multiparae, because of certain demands of pregnancy, and many doctors when in doubt prescribe tablets during pregnancy; research is in progress as to whether there is any deficiency of this nutrient in old people.

ENERGY CONSIDERATIONS

When energy is mentioned in this section kilocalories and their equivalents in joules are understood, e.g.:

1 kilocalorie equals 4·186 joules.
1,000 kilocalories equal 4·186 megajoules.

There exists a superbly accurate instinctive mechanism, sometimes called the *appestat*, which ensures that most of us eat a sufficiency of calories. How it operates we do not know; probably a variety of impulses, from an empty stomach, from a brain not receiving enough glucose in the bloodstream, and so on, tell us to eat more; distension, restoration of glucose levels, and other less obvious mechanisms limit our consumption, and some of these operate quite slowly; there is often an interval of some days before appetite rises or falls to match the alterations in energy requirements which follow changes in the amount of exercise that we take. The accuracy of this mechanism which controls the appetite may be judged by assessing the weight gain which, all else being equal, can be expected to follow the addition to or subtraction from the diet of one pat of butter daily. After a month or so, the body will come into a new equilibrium with a weight gain (if an *extra* pat of butter has been eaten) of about 1 kg.

OBESITY

Obesity can result from greed. Yet many obese people eat less food than the average, and many, who loathe their obesity, go to great lengths to be rid of it, yet all too often they relapse. Therefore, it is obviously something more than greed and it is unhelpful, however true, to say that obesity results from a calorie intake that is higher than the energy expenditure. There are explanations of the failure of the obese to slim which do not involve either greed or lack of willpower, and the obese deserve and need our sympathy in their struggles to get slimmer. The earlier and milder the degree of overweight the better the chances of cure before the biochemical pattern becomes geared to deal with a state of chronic overnutrition. School nurses, health visitors and others working in the field have a better chance than anyone else of catching overweight at the preventive stage, where little is usually needed but a friendly warning and advice which will be respected because it comes from them, particularly if it is simple and does not involve great hardship. This is not to say that success must necessarily result.

Obesity can begin at as early an age as six months. Usually this is because the milk formula is over-concentrated or an excess of other foods is given. Sometimes the child is thirsty but is given milk and becomes more thirsty. Ideally babies should be breast fed. If not, careful attention must be paid to the directions for mixing formulae. There is no need to be in a hurry to introduce mixed feeding.

In the case of *toddlers*, mothers need to understand that overweight is undesirable. *Among older children*, however, overweight and obesity have a multiple origin. Consumption of sweets and sweet dishes contribute, but lack of opportunity for exercise can be important where playing fields are restricted; so can a positive inducement towards a sedentary habit such as television, as well as in some instances too much homework. At low levels of activity and caloric expenditure, the mechanisms that keep us in equilibrium, yet slim, are liable to be less efficient; it was found in one study that summer camps, with intensive training programmes, brought the body fat of obese children closer to values of the normal child despite temporary deterioration during the school year. Finally, *some children and adults too, feel more secure while they are actually eating*, and periods of stress or overwork are palliated thus.

The obese school child is in some measure a victim of our way of life, and unless that can be radically changed the chances of recovery depend upon the extent to which the child really wants to avoid getting fat. The co-operation of the mother is essential, because even moderate overweight can need a strong will to overcome, *but the motivation of the child is the critical factor*. Girls may 'slim' successfully in order to become attractive; but all too often by the time a boy reaches the stage of loathing his fatness, so long and so grim a struggle awaits him that it is wiser to refer him at once to his doctor.

Much of what has been said above about exercise applies also to adults. The housewife, when her children are out in the world, has less housework to do and may be able to afford more labour-saving devices. Her husband with increasing responsibility becomes more deskbound. *The former athlete is particularly prone to fat*. Depending on the amount of overweight, the adult faces an unpleasant period of 'reducing' and though it is easy to lose half a stone, larger losses than this are in the province of the doctor (see weight-reducing diet, p. 159). Depending on the duration of the overweight it means a period of self-discipline—sometimes lifelong—in which the subject has to rise somewhat unsatisfied from every meal. But an intelligent adult often comes to terms with his body; his brain takes over the functions of his appestat mechanism, and if he can find ways of taking daily physical exercise so much the safer for him.

PRACTICAL POINTS

A nurse should, if possible, not be seen to know less than her patient even when the latter has been reading an article on diet in some glossy magazine. She needs a reference book such as the *Manual of Nutrition* published by H.M. Stationery Office. The most frequent question asked is whether such and such a food is fattening. Since this depends on a number of things, such as how much bulk (roughage) there is, there is no sure guide. Nurses must use their common sense. Fatty, sugary and starchy foods without much bulk are all fattening. There is no such thing as a true slimming food. The most that can be said is that some may make the process of dietary restriction a little less unpleasant. They include:

> *Bulky foods* designed to produce a feeling of distension without providing calories. Green vegetables do the same.
> *Starch-reduced foods*. These operate on the assumption that a bread

which contains less starch is less fattening. The flaw is that if it contains less starch it must contain more of something else, usually protein. The argument then is that diets high in protein and low in starch are less fattening. It would be as sound to replace some of the bread we eat with lean meat or Cheddar cheese.

Aerated, fluffy foods aim to delude the subject into eating less solid with each portion then he otherwise would.

Some 'complete' (in all nutrients) foods, available in amounts of which the energy content is known, are sometimes useful to bring weight down (the patient cannot cheat in the way that he can with slices of bread, helpings of food, etc.). In the long run none of these foods is a satisfactory substitute for simple reduction in the amounts of foods eaten. Alcohol is fattening.

Breakfast is a vexed topic. Should a child have a 'cooked breakfast'? Need he even have any breakfast at all? The answer probably is that at no age is it essential for a child to have more than milk plus cereal and bread and butter for breakfast, but up to the age of five it is as well to provide an egg or some other small cooked dish in addition. Some older children can go without breakfast (particularly obese ones); others cannot.

Every child should be allowed at least one fad. Even a dislike of milk can be got round by including it in cooked dishes, and by providing substitutes (such as cheese). In an inquiry into the health and growth of school-children who, because of dislike, ate either no meat, or no liquid milk, or no eggs, or no fish, or no vegetables, no difference was observed compared with others who had none of these fads. Their diet was sufficiently varied in other ways. The hazard arises where there are several fads, and sugary foods and sweets bulk large in the diet, for sugar provides joules and nothing else. If 20 per cent of the joules are provided from sweets and sugar (quite a common figure, amounting to about $2\frac{1}{2}$ oz. daily for the average child) then the *nutrients* which the child needs must be got from the remaining 80 per cent of the diet. This is achieved in practice, but when the figure rises much above this and when in addition much fat (also a conveyor of 'near-empty' joules) is eaten, then the margin gets tighter.

NUTRITION IN DEVELOPING COUNTRIES

The commonest nutritional problem is to wring from the soil an adequate energy supply. To grow crops such as beans, and to include animals in the system of husbandry, may be not merely desirable for good nutrition but necessary in order to maintain the fertility of the soil, but these, viewed purely as producers of energy, are wasteful compared with cereal and starchy root crops.

In the diet of the poor, starches predominate to such an extent that the nature of the common nutritional deficiencies can often be predicted simply from a knowledge of the staple crop grown. *In maize-growing areas* the deficiency to be expected is pellagra (niacin deficiency or deficiency of tryptophane, a constituent of protein which is utilized as niacin and which is deficient in maize protein). *In sorghum areas* it is angular stomatitis and cheilosis (lack usually of riboflavin, see p. 151). *In cassava and dioscorea* *yam-eating areas protein deficiency* is to be expected to a degree much greater than where cereals are grown, because the latter contain 8 to 10 per cent of a protein which though not as valuable to man as is, for example, meat, nevertheless do help to prevent deficiency, whereas roots contain proportionately less protein. Cassava has leaves which are usually eaten and supply *carotene from which vitamin A is formed in the body*.

The adult male in a family is at least nutritional risk but usually gets the best food. This paradox stems from days of war and danger, but it still has its justification in that if the man becomes too malnourished to do the heaviest work in the fields a vicious circle begins for his whole family The other individual not at risk is the adequately breast-fed child and in rural areas particularly breast feeding should be encouraged for as long as possible. By the middle of the second year breast milk may be scanty and thin, particularly in times of hunger, but what there is of it is usually a better source of essential nutrients than the other foods in the weanling's diet. Much damage has in the past been done by nurses who advised weaning from the breast in conformity with European practice without ascertaining whether supplies of cow's milk were available or whether there was money to buy them.

Next to the weaned infant and growing child, the member of the family at greatest nutritional risk is the mother. She bears the burden of pregnancy and lactation and when times are lean she will deprive herself to feed her family.

Kwashiorkor

This is the result of a protein-deficient diet after weaning. *Marasmus* results from inadequate supply or assimilation of energy due to food which is either too little or too ill digested. Every gradation between marasmus and true kwashiorkor may be encountered, and added to them may be the patina of other nutritional deficiencies due to the shortcomings of the staple food; diarrhoea, malaria and other parasitic and infective diseases may be superimposed. In short, all the afflictions of tropical rural poverty seem to converge upon the child at once.

The *protein deficiency* which is the essential element of true kwashiorkor results in obvious malaise and misery, retarded growth and oedema, which on treatment may reveal a grossly wasted child. There is impairment of all tissues, particularly organs that are the seat of much chemical activity such as the liver, and of rapid cellular reduplication such as the hair which becomes sparse and without pigment, spring or curl.

Severe cases should be treated in hospital with food rich in the missing nutrients; skimmed-milk powder is essential. *Prevention* is a matter of securing a proper balance of nutrients and energy supply in children's diets. It is difficult to make adults realize that what is good enough for them may not suffice for their children with added requirements for growth. All children save the last-born are apt to be forgotten and may be expected to stay their hunger with a corncob or a root of sweet cassava, or with leftovers from the last night's cooking, and this in areas where climate favours the multiplication of infective and protozoal parasites. *The problem is only one of many which wait for their solution upon a general improvement of conditions in developing countries.* In many areas protein-rich foods have been introduced with locally produced proteins of vegetable origin. Ideally, all children should have these in kwashiorkor areas. In practice,

Excerpts from 'Recommended Daily Intakes of Energy and Nutrients for the U.K.' from the Report on Public Health and Medical Subjects, No. 120

Age range	Occupational category	Body weight kg	Energy requirements Large calories	Protein g	Ascorbic acid mg	Calcium mg	Iron mg
Boys and girls							
0–1 year		7·3	800	20	15	600	6
1–2 years		11·4	1200	30	20	500	7
3–5 years		16·5	1600	40	20	500	8
Boys							
9–12 years		31·9	2500	63	25	700	13
15–18 years		61·0	3000	75	30	600	15
Girls							
9–12 years		33·0	2300	58	25	700	13
15–18 years		56·1	2300	58	30	600	15
Men							
18–35 years	Sedentary	65	2700	68	30	500	10
	Moderately active		3000	75	30	500	10
	Very active		3600	90	30	500	10
35–65 years	Sedentary	65	2600	65	30	500	10
	Moderately active		2900	73	30	500	10
	Very active		3600	90	30	500	10
65–75 years	Assuming a sedentary life	63	2350	59	30	500	10
75 years and over		63	2100	53	30	500	10
Women							
18–55 years	Most occupations	55	2200	55	30	500	12
	Very active		2500	63	30	500	12
55–75 years	Assuming sedentary life	53	2050	51	30	500	10
75 years and over		53	1900	48	30	500	10
Pregnancy 2nd and 3rd trimester			2400	60	60	1200	15
Lactation			2700	68	60	1200	15

1. Figures for iron and calcium under 1 year apply to those who are *not* breast fed. Infants entirely breast fed get smaller quantities; these are adequate since absorption from breast milk is higher.
2. Note the necessary increase in energy requirements, protein, ascorbic acid, calcium and iron recommended in pregnancy and during lactation.
3. In the age group for men 18–35, the average taken is 25 years. In the age group for women 18–55, the average taken is 35 years.
4. There is a new issue of Recommended Intakes, Report No. 120 to which is added: Megajoules (10⁶ joules), calculated from the relation 1 kilocalorie equals 4·186 kilojoules and rounded to one decimal place.

it may be necessary to limit them on the one hand to the children of intelligent and prosperous mothers, and on the other to children who are brought for treatment of other conditions superimposed on early kwashiorkor. It is as well to remember that kwashiorkor can occur in older children, though as a rule the element of undernutrition becomes the more obvious.

Chapter 17

Samples of Normal and Therapeutic Diets

by MARJORIE McLAUGHLIN

> *Examples of a normal diet for a moderately active woman and examples of simple menus for use in conditions of obesity, diabetes mellitus, coronary, hepatic and renal diseases and abnormal conditions of the alimentary tract—tube feeding—dietary adaptations in special circumstances*

A normal diet has different connotations for different people but some attention to the composition of the diet must be paid if the recommended intakes (summarized on p. 156) are to be met. Foods containing protein, iron and calcium always contain other nutrients: if there is a sufficiency of these items together with a daily intake of ascorbic acid (vitamin C) then the total adequacy of the diet is assured. On p. 159 is an example of a good diet which meets the recommended intakes for a moderately active woman.

Some interesting deductions about the incidence of different nutrients can be drawn from these figures.

Protein. Ample servings of animal protein (eggs, meat, milk) are necessary to meet the recommendations, but bread and potatoes, if eaten in larger quantities than above, add significant amounts to the diet.

Ascorbic acid (vitamin C). One citrus fruit (e.g. grapefruit) will nearly meet the recommendation. Since this vitamin is not stored there is a daily need for it.

Calcium. Milk (or cheese) is the best source.

Iron. Meat and eggs are the best sources but cocoa (or chocolate) provides an appreciable amount.

Additions of calcium and iron are made, by law, to flour in the U.K. and may provide a large part of the intake if sufficient bread and cakes are eaten.

Calories. Sugar, marmalade and butter provide relatively large numbers of calories (energy) without giving good value in nourishment. For good health, foods which provide both energy and nourishment must be eaten.

In the treatment of certain diseases an adjustment of some of the constituents of food is as necessary as drugs or surgery. The following pages give directions for achieving this. Unless otherwise stated all diets meet the recommended nutrient intakes summarized on p. 156.

	Calories	Protein (g)	Ascorbic acid (mg)	Calcium (mg)	Iron (mg)
Breakfast					
½ grapefruit	20	—	25	10	0·2
1 slice toast	70	2	—	25	0·5
1 boiled egg	90	6	—	30	1·4
Butter, sugar, marmalade, etc.	300	—	—	30	—
Mid-morning					
Coffee with sugar	50	—	—	—	—
Bar of chocolate	160	2	—	25	1·3
Lunch					
1 ham roll	250	7	—	45	1·3
Coffee with sugar	50	—	—	—	—
Tea					
Tea with sugar	50	—	—	—	—
1 currant bun	150	2	—	40	1·0
Supper					
1 large chop	450	20	—	5	2·0
Potatoes	150	3	—	7	0·8
Cabbage	10	—	7	35	0·3
Tinned fruit	100	—	5	15	0·8
Jelly	100	2	—	10	0·6
Bedtime					
Cocoa with sugar	100	2	—	5	2·0
Daily intake of milk—½ pint	190	9	3	340	0·2
Totals	2290	55	40	622	12·4

Example of a good diet for a moderately active woman.

WEIGHT-REDUCING DIET

Low-calorie diet for patients who are overweight or whose obesity has caused or aggravated a condition such as hernia, joint or back pain, diabetes mellitus, coronary incompetence or high blood pressure.

The *calorie content* is approximately 1,000, the *carbohydrate content* 80 g.

Breakfast   Tea or coffee with a little milk.
1 egg or 1 rasher of grilled bacon or 1 slice of ham or a kipper or piece of smoked fish or 1 oz. cheese.
Tomatoes, mushrooms and ½ grapefruit if desired.
30 g (1 oz.) bread in any form and thinly buttered.

Mid-morning, Tea or coffee with a little milk or Bovril, Oxo, Marmite
Tea-time and or lemon juice and water.
Bedtime

Lunch and   An average helping of meat, offal, poultry, game, fish,
Evening meal eggs or cheese.
Cooked vegetables or salad as desired.
Either 30 g (1 oz.) bread and butter or 1 small potato
or 1 tablespoonful of rice.
1 portion of fruit. This may occasionally be varied by
the substitution of a small helping of egg custard or
junket, a plain yoghurt or 2 cream crackers with the
cheese.

No sugar or sweet foods of any kind should be taken. Artificial sweet-
eners (not sorbitol) should be used throughout. With the exception of
squash, diabetic foods must not be taken. No fried food, cream, oil or
pastry is allowed. Alcohol of all kinds is forbidden.

DIABETIC DIET

Diets in the treatment of diabetes are ordered where a restriction of
carbohydrate is necessary. Diabetes may be due to failure of the pancreas
to secrete sufficient insulin or, more rarely, to the action of steroid drugs
such as cortisone. In the first instance the diet must be followed for life. In
the second the necessity for the diet ceases when the drug is stopped.

Overweight patients, usually over 35 years of age and not receiving
insulin, may safely use the low-calorie diet found on p. 159. If oral hypoglycaemic drugs are prescribed the carbohydrate content of the diet should
be fairly evenly spread throughout the day.

Diabetics on insulin are usually allowed more carbohydrate, the intake
of which should roughly coincide with the peak action of the insulin. The
physician should be consulted if hypoglycaemic attacks intervene. Two
lumps of sugar or two teaspoonfuls of glucose, dissolved in a little water if
necessary, should be given in the event of a hypoglycaemic attack or
insulin reaction. This may be repeated in five minutes if recovery is not
immediate.

A diabetic diet containing 180 g of carbohydrate is evenly distributed
throughout the day; the calorie content of this diet is approximately 2,000.

Breakfast   15 g ($\frac{1}{2}$ oz.) cornflakes.
A little milk, for tea or coffee and cereal.
Egg, bacon, fish or cheese.
Tomatoes, mushrooms, $\frac{1}{2}$ grapefruit if desired.
60 g (2 oz.) bread and butter.

Mid-morning Tea or coffee with a little milk (1 oz.).
Tea-time   1 Marie or Osborne biscuit.

Lunch   An average helping of meat, offal, poultry, game, fish,
cheese or egg dish. ·
Cooked vegetables or salad as desired.
Either 90 g (3 oz.) bread with butter or 240 g (8ʹ oz.),
4 small potatoes or 6 dessertspoonfuls cooked rice.
1 portion of fruit or 1 brickette ice cream or 1 plain
yoghurt or 2 cream crackers and cheese.
Tea or coffee with a little milk (1 oz.).

Evening meal	Meat, fish, eggs or cheese. Cooked vegetables or salad. 60 g (2 oz.) bread or 180 g (6 oz.) potato or 4½ dessert-spoonfuls rice. Fruit, etc., as at lunch.
Bedtime	1 tumbler of milk (7 oz.). 1 Marie or Osborne biscuit.

Sugar, sweet foods, jams should not normally be taken. Foods such as diabetic chocolate and sorbitol should only be included with the knowledge of the physician. Spirits and dry wines may occasionally be taken (providing there is no weight problem, since all alcohol adds to the calorie content) but the carbohydrate content of beers and cider must be calculated into the diet.

LOW-SODIUM DIETS

Low-sodium diets are for use whenever oedema is present or threatened. The causes may be renal or hepatic failure, coronary incompetence, hypertension or the administration of steroid drugs such as cortisone.

The following diet contains approximately sodium 0·5 g. No salt should be added to food either at the table or in cooking.

Breakfast	Tea or coffee with milk from the day's allowance (see below). Shredded or Puffed Wheat with milk from the day's allowance. 1 egg, a fresh herring or a portion of white fish. Unsalted bread, salt-free Ryvita or Motza. Unsalted butter or Kosher margarine. Fruit, sugar, marmalade, honey.
Mid-morning, Tea-time and Bedtime	Fruit or fruit juice, tea or coffee with milk from allowance, homemade lemonade (not synthetic) or unsalted Marmite. 1 plain sweet biscuit.
Lunch and Evening meal	An average helping of meat, fish or egg dish. Potatoes, rice, pasta or unsalted bread. Fresh or frozen vegetables. Fruit, fruit pie, crumble or fritters, jam tart, pancakes, jelly. An occasional ice cream or a small milk pudding. Sugar, jam, nuts, double cream as appropriate.

A daily allowance of 300 ml (½ pint) of milk is allowed which will be sufficient for tea and coffee.

Foods which must never be included in any low-sodium diet:

Bacon, ham, tinned meat, salt beef, sausages, cheese.
Smoked or tinned fish, kippers, salt cod.
Commercially prepared sauces, mayonnaise, ketchup, pickles.
Tinned vegetables.
Bovril, Oxo, Marmite, meat and fish pastes, celery or garlic salt.

DIETS LOW AND HIGH IN PROTEIN

Low-protein diets are used in renal and hepatic disorders. All low-protein diets must provide adequate calories for energy requirements, otherwise there will be a breakdown of body protein leading to wasting of tissue and increased work for the kidney. *Sugar or glucose* added to the appropriate foods will provide most of the calories.

Minimal-protein diets (5 g) should be used for a few days only. A choice from the following foods may be made for all meals:

> Porridge, arrowroot, cornflour, rice or other cereals cooked in water or fruit juice and sweetened with sugar, glucose or honey.
> Salad, boiled, fried, curried or pickled vegetables.
> Potatoes or rice.
> Fruit, fruit juice, squash, jam, boiled sweets, black coffee and Russian tea.

Fat is sometimes disallowed or not tolerated, as in hepatic conditions. If it can be used it is an excellent source of calories and will enliven the diet.

30 g protein diet

Breakfast	Cereal or porridge with milk from allowance, fruit and sugar. 1 slice of bread with plenty of butter, honey or marmalade. Tea or coffee with milk from allowance.
Lunch and Evening meal	A small helping of meat or fish or 1 egg or 30 g (1 oz.) cheese. Salad, cooked vegetables, potatoes, rice or pasta. Fruit, fruit pie, fritters, crumble, jelly.
Tea-time	Tea with milk from allowance. 1 slice of bread with plenty of butter and jam or a small piece of cake or biscuit.

A daily allowance of 300 ml ($\frac{1}{2}$ pint) of milk is allowed and all foods on the minimal protein diet (see above) should be included.

Giovannetti diet (12 g animal protein plus 6 g from vegetable sources). This diet is used for conditions of chronic renal failure. The animal protein replaces endogenous protein losses; the vegetable protein is an unavoidable addition.

Breakfast	Fruit or juice and sugar. Fried bacon *fat* with tomatoes, apple rings and fried protein-free bread. Protein-free bread, butter, marmalade, honey.
Lunch and Evening meal	Fried, curried or boiled vegetables or salad. 1 medium potato or 2 tablespoonfuls of rice. Fruit or any fruit pie, pastry or crumble made with non-protein flour.

Mid-morning,   Tea or coffee with milk from the day's allowance (see
Tea-time and   below) or fruit juice.
Bedtime   Non-protein biscuits or bread with butter and jam.

Daily allowances (very important)—1 egg cooked in any way, and 195
            ml (6½ oz.) milk.

This diet will be deficient in methionine, vitamins, iron and calcium.
Methionine 0·5 g must be given daily.

The following substances are high in protein and must not be given in
any low-protein diet:

> Complan, Casilan, Ovaltine, Horlicks and other milk powders.
> Peas, broad or soya beans, lentils.
> Energen rolls.

Low-potassium diets, in conjunction with low-protein diets, are used in
conditions of chronic renal disease where excretion of potassium by the
kidney is insufficient to maintain the normal physiological balance. Since
potassium is contained in all foods except refined sugar and fats it is
impossible to lower the intake by much more than half. Protein restriction
automatically results in a reduced potassium intake: in addition the
following foods should not be given:

> Chocolate, cocoa.
> Instant coffee, Coca-cola, beer, cider, wine.
> Marmite, Bovril or other meat or vegetable extracts.
> Dried fruit (including dates), dried vegetables.
> Rhubarb, citrus fruits, fruit juices.
> Spinach, fried mushrooms, vegetable juices, including tomato juice,
>   potato crisps.
> Nuts, peanut butter.
> Treacle, golden syrup, brown sugar.
> Salt substitutes, Carrageen moss.

Curry powder, ginger and mustard should be used infrequently and in
small amounts. Large quantities of fruit and vegetables, including potato,
should not be given.

As a concurrent restriction of protein, and possibly sodium, is likely it is
obvious that the low-potassium diet may be inadequate in calories and
tasteless. Great care must therefore be taken to cook and present the food
attractively and to increase the caloric intake by the use of the following
protein-, potassium- and sodium-free foods:

> White sugar, unsalted butter and margarine, oil, fried foods.
> Commercial foods specially prepared for this condition such as
>   Hycal, Caloreen.
> Spirits if allowed by the physician.

High-protein diets, containing up to 130 g daily, may be used in conditions of malabsorption, malnutrition, proteinuria and in chronic hepatic
disease, and are also used wherever new tissue is required as in burns or
surgery and wherever there is a heavy exudate such as in ulcerative colitis.
It is useless giving a high-protein diet unless the total calories are adequate.
Samples of protein foods are eggs, meat, fish, cheese, milk, Complan (a
total food) and Casilan.

FAT-RESTRICTED DIETS

A low-fat diet is used in cases of gall-bladder and hepatic disease. It is also ordered where there is a failure to absorb fat (steatorrhoea).

The diet should be a normal one with a high carbohydrate content to compensate for the calories lost through the fat restriction. Protein should be of average content. The following foods should be omitted:

> Fried food, cream, oil (a small quantity of butter or margarine may be taken).
> Fatty meat, including goose and duck.
> Herrings, salmon, sardines, trout.
> Suet, lard, pastry, rich cakes, nuts, marzipan.

Ordinary milk may be used if the cream is decanted and, unless there is a protein or calorie restriction, two pints may be taken daily. Skimmed milk is necessary only when the patient is very nauseated or if he is jaundiced. It is easily obtainable in powder form.

Egg yolk contains fat. Patients suffering from gall-bladder disease may tolerate up to one egg daily but eggs may have to be omitted altogether in severe liver disease. Similarly, small amounts of butter or margarine are tolerated by the less severe cases but may have to be omitted.

Low animal-fat or *low cholesterol* diets may be ordered by physicians who believe that restriction of foods containing either or both these substances may result in lowered blood cholesterol. A high level of cholesterol is part of the chain of events leading to coronary disease.

In a low animal-fat diet the following foods should be omitted:

> Butter, cheese, cream, suet, lard, dripping, fatty meat.
> Eggs should be used sparingly.
> Margarine or vegetable oils may be used for any purpose.

In a low-cholesterol diet, sweetbreads, roes and brains should be omitted and liver, kidney and butter only taken sparingly. Egg yolks are extremely high in cholesterol and their use should be restricted to two a week.

DIETS FOR DISORDERS OF THE ALIMENTARY TRACT

Peptic ulcers

It is now known that diet plays no part in the cause of this condition. There is one golden rule in the dietary treatment of peptic-ulcer pain—meals must be small and frequent. No more than a few hours should elapse between meals or snacks. A number of patients find that their pain is often worse after fried, curried, spiced or pickled foods which they should therefore avoid.

Coeliac disease in children and adults

Sensitivity to the wheat protein, *gluten*, results in childhood and adult coeliac disease (Chapter 24, p. 236). The most important part of the treatment of this condition is therefore the exclusion of gluten from the diet. Wheat and rye should be excluded from the diet in every case. Oats and barley also need to be avoided by some coeliac patients.

The essence of a gluten-free diet is to omit entirely all forms of flour. Meat, fish, eggs, cheese, milk, fruit and vegetables may be eaten so long as their preparation does not include flour (usually incorporated as gravy, sauce, batter or breadcrumbs). Fats, sugar, jams and boiled sweets are also permissible. The difficulty in the diet lies in the fact that ordinary bread, bread substitutes such as Ryvita, oatcakes, Energen rolls, cake and biscuits and many manufactured products may not be taken. Gluten-free bread or rusks or cakes made from gluten-free flour must be substituted. These may be obtained commercially but some patients prefer to bake their own.

A low-lactose diet

This is prescribed when lactase, the intestinal enzyme responsible for splitting the milk sugar, lactose, is deficient. This diet involves the omission of all foods containing milk, milk powders such as Complan, Ovaltine, Horlicks and Bournvita and many commercially prepared foods some of which (for example certain sausages) may appear to be unlikely vehicles for milk. As butter and cheese contain no significant amounts of lactose there is no ban on these foods.

LIQUID FEEDING BY MOUTH OR TUBE FEEDING

All diets, whether liquid or solid, must meet the recommended intakes for principal nutrients (see p. 156).

1. By mouth

This may be simply a means of supplementing solid food in a seriously ill patient or it may be the total intake for patients suffering from oesophageal obstruction or having surgery to the mouth, jaw or oesophagus. Variety of taste may be important but blandness may outweigh this where ulceration or soreness is present.

Unless contra-indicated the diet should consist basically of milk, eggs, fine cereals such as cornflour or groats and sugar; cream, fruit juices or purées may be added to produce egg flips, milk shakes, porridge, milk puddings and other foods; the thickness can be determined by the addition of plain or evaporated milk. Soups, cheese sauce and some commercial products, listed below, will also be useful: A liquidizer is of great value in preparing such a diet.

As a very rough guide 2 pints of milk, 3 eggs and 60 g (2 oz.) of Complan powder, together with half a teacupful of Ribena and any of the items listed above would supply at least, 1,700 kilocalories (or the equivalent in megajoules), 75 g of protein and adequate minerals and vitamins.

Useful commercial products
  Complan—a milk powder containing protein, carbohydrate, fat, vitamins and minerals.
  Carnation Instant Breakfast food—a flavoured milk powder.
  Lucozade and Hycal—supply calories from their carbohydrate content only.

2. Tube feeding

Patients suffering from a severe obstruction in the upper gastro-intestinal tract may need tube feeding. It may also be used where patients are unable to take food in sufficient quantities to meet their nutritional requirements. This particularly applies to cases of severe burns, malignant disease, prolonged fever or infection. Certain points need to be considered:

(i) The protein, calcium and vitamin D intakes should not *exceed* the recommended intakes (see p. 156) if no increased need for them exists. It is possible to cause kidney damage or calcium deposition if these nutrients are given in excess.

(ii) Sufficient water is taken to ensure that waste products are excreted.

(iii) The osmolarity of the feed is such that it does not draw water and electrolytes into the intestine from the surrounding tissues. Milk powders mixed in milk can cause diarrhoea if insufficient attention is paid to this.

The following recipe provides a tube (or oral) feed which satisfies these requirements particularly in regard to osmolarity.

Masterton feed, which supplies 70 g of protein and contains 3,000 kilocalories (or 12·558 megajoules).

1 litre of milk
270 ml Prosparol (a proprietary fat emulsion)
250 g glucose } all mixed together.
35 g Casilan (a proprietary protein powder)
1,700 ml water

Iron and vitamin supplements should also be given.

SOME DIETARY ADAPTATIONS IN SPECIAL CASES

Some foods may be unacceptable because of ethnic or religious prohibitions or customs. The following notes may be useful. Fuller information can be obtained from religious group leaders, embassies, consulates and race-relation officers.

Buddhists vary in their observances but generally follow a vegetarian regime, including eggs, cheese and milk in their diet. They avoid food such as meat which has involved the taking of life.

Hindus. The various sects differ in their food observancy. Gujurati and Punjabi Hindus, and some Sikhs are mostly vegetarians, and those of the Hindus and Sikhs who do eat meat avoid beef and veal. In some sects this prohibition is extended to milk, butter and cheese.

Jews vary from the orthodox to the liberal. The orthodox will not eat shellfish, or meat which has been killed or prepared by non-Jews. Liberal Jews will eat any food except pork, bacon, ham, sausages and lard. Some prefer Motza and Kosher margarine to bread and butter; for many milk should never be included in a meat meal.

Moslems do not eat pork, and pork products such as bacon, ham or sausage. Lard and fish are seldom eaten.

Vegetarians omit meat and fish from their diets but will eat cheese, eggs and milk.

Vegans are strict vegetarians who eat no animal food. Thus cheese, eggs and milk (as well as meat and fish) are precluded.

Chapter 18

The Feeding of Infants up to Two Years

by B. E. CHADNEY

> *Types of feeding and feeds—preparation of feeds—precautions—
> weaning*

The following chapter is designed to help those nurses who have little or no knowledge of infants and infant feeding and who during the course of paediatric experience may need some guidance in normal feeding procedures.

One of the most important factors necessary for the maintenance of good health and normal growth and development of the infant is the provision of an adequate well-balanced and nutritious diet. The nurse should know the composition of milk and have some basic principles to which she may refer, as an aid to memory.

Approximate percentage composition of milk (g per 100 ml)

Human milk (transitional)			*Cow's milk*		
Protein 2	Caseinogen 0·6		Protein 3·4	Caseinogen 2·8	
	Lactalbumin 1·4			Lactalbumin 0·6	
Fat	3·7		Fat	3·7	
Sugar	6·9		Sugar	4·8	
Mineral salts 0·25			Mineral salts 0·75		

Vitamins
Water
to 100 in each case

68 Calories   *66 Calories*

It should be remembered that boiling cow's milk destroys vitamin C.

During the prenatal period the advantages of breast feeding should be fully discussed with the expectant mother, and though she must not be made to feel guilty if she does not wish to breast feed, it is well known that breast-fed infants are happier, more resistant to infection, particularly gastro-intestinal, and are more secure in their emotional development than artificially fed ones. Even a short period of breast feeding is worth while, since this establishes a closer relationship between the infant and the mother.

To encourage lactation the breasts need to be stimulated and it is important that the newborn infant is put to the breast at regular intervals either three- or four-hourly according to weight. Smaller infants require feeding more frequently. Alternatively 'on demand' regime may be practised. This means putting the infant to the breast when he appears hungry and not keeping to regular times, though after the first few weeks these will tend to be about every four hours.

During the first few days colostrum, a high-protein fluid, is excreted by the breast; this is gradually replaced about the third day by breast milk.

There are, however, some contra-indications to breast feeding, but rarely to breast milk. The infant may not be able to feed from the breast either because he is too ill or too feeble; some mothers may have retracted nipples, be averse to breast feeding or have insufficient milk, or may be unable to breast feed for social reasons as in the case of the unmarried mother who has to earn her living. In these circumstances artificial feeding has to be considered.

Artificial feeding

These feeds can be readily adjusted to suit the infant's requirements. It is usual practice to select from one of the following:

1. Liquid cow's milk
2. Evaporated milk
3. Dried milk—roller or sprayed
   (This is a product which does not readily support bacteriological growth and in powder form can be kept for some time in opened tins. For this reason it is particularly useful in the absence of refrigeration, and in countries where refrigeration facilities are limited it is the milk of choice.)

But infants on these feeds will require added vitamin C in the form of rose-hip syrup or orange juice, and vitamins A and D in the form of a cod liver oil preparation or one of the concentrated preparations containing vitamins A and D if these have not been added to the milk formula by the manufacturer.

Infant feeding in the first few weeks of life

Caloric requirements approximately 115 Calories (kilocalories) per kg per day.

Protein 2·5 g per kg per day.

Fluid 150–200 ml per kg per day.

But there are great individual variations in requirements and in rate of weight gain.

Type of milk	Ca mg	P mg	K mEq	Na mEq	kcal	Carbo-hydrate g	Protein g	Fat g
Cow and Gate (full cream) water to 100 ml	105	80	3·0	2·3	68	7·5*	3·0	3·1
Cow and Gate (half cream) water to 100 ml	84	70	2·6	2·0	55	7·1*	2·5	2·0
For comparison: Cow's milk (100 ml)	120	95	4·1	2·2	66	4·8*	3·4	3·7
Human milk (transitional) (100 ml)	25	16	1·8	2·1	68	6·9*	2·0	3·7

* sucrose-free

On the first day of life one-seventh of the daily fluid requirement, on the second day two-sevenths and so continue to increase until on the seventh day of life the infant is receiving the full fluid requirement.

To work out expected body weight there can be no hard and fast rules, but an infant usually loses weight in the first week of life, regains the birth weight at the end of the tenth to fourteenth day of life and should then continue to gain weight.

Naturally as the infant gets older the fluid and nutritional requirements based on weight become less and at one year total calories required are 1,000.

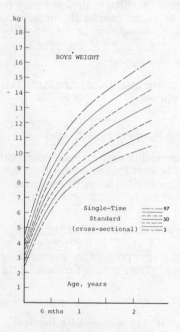 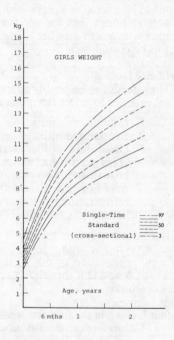

Preparation of feeds

Feeds should be prepared in a milk room away from the wards by someone who is not nursing the infant. Great care must be taken that no infection is introduced. The room and all equipment must be scrupulously clean. The nurse or milk room technician should change into a clean overall, cover her hair and wash her hands and then lay out everything she may require.

> Feed order book, or card.
> Dried-milk tin with lid off.
> Funnel.
> Sugar.
> Feeding bottles that have been sterilized.
> Kettle of boiling water.
> Jug or bottle of cooled boiled water.
> Mixing bowl and fork or electric mixer (of a make which can be sterilized).

Metric scales.
Cow's milk.
Any special feed.

Before preparation of the feed the hands should again be washed.

The milk powder is measured into the mixing bowl or machine with the scoop which is supplied with the tin, or weighed in the scales. It is important not to touch the inside of the tin with the hands. Sugar is added and both are mixed to a smooth paste with the boiling water. The remainder of the water is then added. Vigorous stirring is necessary to prevent lumps forming. It is usual in hospitals for the feeds to be made up each day for the whole 24 hours.

The mixture is then poured into a measure held at eye level for accuracy, and the feeding bottles are filled with the help of a funnel.

Every baby should have his own teat. This may be put onto the feeding bottle and a teat cap or seal placed over it. Each feed should have the infant's name, a brief description of the feed formula and the time it should be given to the infant.

Bottles are then placed in crates and 'terminal heat sterilized' in an autoclave or pressure cooker, or pasteurized by heating to a temperature of 82·2 °C (180 °F) for one minute. The upright bottle is now used almost exclusively.

Feeds may be given at room temperature, but some babies prefer them to be warmed to a temperature of 37 °C (98·6 °F). This is done by standing the bottle in a jug of hot water for approximately 10 minutes. Whenever the feed is left standing the teat cap must be replaced.

The bottle and teat should be rinsed in cold water immediately after use. Later the bottle will need to be thoroughly cleaned with a bottle brush or electric rotating brush, and the teat with salt. Both should then, with equipment used in making up the feed, be either autoclaved or kept in a solution of Milton according to the method adopted by the nursery or paediatric unit.

A number of new methods of making up feeds are now available.

1. *The Axifeed dispensing unit*
   This unit contains the necessary sterile ingredients, i.e. milk, water, sugar with a disposable bottle and teat—for any choice of feed.
2. *The Ostermilk mixer-dispenser*
   10,000 ml of feeds can be made up in a matter of minutes and put into any type of feed bottle.
3. *Cow and Gate mixer*

Pre-packed feeds
1. Cow and Gate sterilized prepared feeds, see Fig. 18/1 (full cream and half cream).
2. S.M.A. (Scientific Milk Adaption) ready-to-feed system.
3. Ostermilk ready-to-feed system.

Instructions for using pre-packed feeds, after the correct feed has been selected:
1. Warm bottle or alternatively give feed at room temperature.
2. Shake bottle—remove cap.

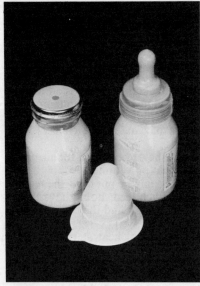

Fig. 18/1 Pre-packed baby feed commercially prepared and presented.

3. Check vacuum seal.
4. Screw teat unit into position through plastic cap—do not touch the actual teat.
5. When teat unit is firmly secured, remove plastic cap.
6. Check temperature, if feed has been heated, by shaking a few drops onto wrist.

Note: Bottles are graduated and at a glance the amount of feed the baby has taken can easily be noted. After the feed the bottle and teat and any remaining feed can be discarded. The teat unit is intended for use once only, but it can be re-used if cleaned and sterilized.

A great deal of time is saved when pre-packed feeds are used and the infant is given a feed which is prepared under ideal conditions. It is estimated that at least 60 per cent of infants in hospital could be given these feeds of varying amounts but the rest may need 'special' feeding because of various pathological conditions.

Position of infant for feeding

The infant should be changed before feeding so that he is comfortable and can enjoy his feed. After carefully washing her hands the nurse should, if his condition allows, lift him out of the cot or pram and hold him in the same position as for breast feeding. The bottle must be tilted so that feed is against the neck of the bottle otherwise air will be sucked. The hole in the teat should be a size according to the condition of the infant and its strength for sucking.

At least once during the feed and at the end the infant must bring up wind. This is done by sitting him upright, with one hand on his abdomen and one hand supporting his head and back. Until the wind is brought up the infant will not be comfortable. If necessary he must be changed at the end of the feed.

After feeding, time should be taken by the nurse to talk and play with the infant. Physical contact and the sound of her voice are important, particularly when he is temporarily separated from his mother.

To increase the caloric value of feeds

This can be done in several ways without increasing the bulk or fluid content of the feed by:

1. Adding sugar
2. Adding a dried milk which has a high protein content, e.g. Prosol (Trufood)
3. Adding a baby cereal
4. Giving pre-digested milk, e.g. Bengers 4 g to 100 ml of reconstituted feed

Thickened feeds

This can be done by adding a thickening agent, e.g. arrowroot or one derived from carob seed, e.g. Nestargel (Nestlé) or Carobel (Cow and Gate). Thickening a feed may be necessary for some special purpose, e.g. the infant with an oesophageal reflux or persistent regurgitation, as in hiatus hernia (see Chapter 24, p. 224), when placed in the recumbent position. These infants if they are kept in an upright position and have feeds which are thick and therefore difficult to vomit, generally do very well.

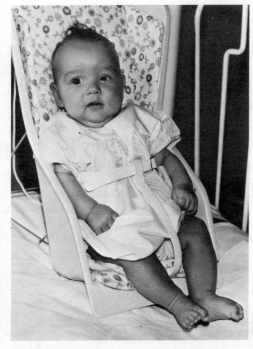

Fig. 18/2 A baby-sitter chair as used in the prevention of oesophageal reflux as in hiatus hernia.

PRECAUTIONS
Vomiting
If the infant vomits, this should be reported. It may not be serious but the cause should always be investigated. A small regurgitation may be normal, but it may mean the feed is too large, being given too quickly or too frequently, or due to underfeeding and air swallowing. Persistent vomiting is frequently a sign of a disturbed mother-infant relationship. There may, however, be other reasons of a more serious nature requiring medical or surgical intervention.

Condition of stools
The newborn infant will pass meconium during the first two to three days. This greeny-black, tarry substance will, between the third and sixth days, change to yellow. These stools are odourless. After mixed feeding is introduced the stool will become brown in colour, formed and with a slight odour. Any abnormality in the stools, curds, bulky stools, undigested food, blood or failure to pass meconium within 24 hours should be reported to the doctor.

Intravenous feeding
If for some reason the infant is unable to feed orally, the administration of intravenous fluid may be required. A special regime will be ordered by the doctor which will give the required fluid, salts and calories until such time as normal feeding can be recommenced. It is possible to give complete nutrition by the intravenous route if this is required.

Tube feeding (by naso-oesophageal tube)
Seriously ill infants are often tube fed. This method requires no effort on the part of the infant and there is the minimum of handling. The nurse should remember, however, that it is still necessary for the infant to bring up wind.

Premature infants who are too weak to suck will be fed in this manner.

Gastrostomy tube feeds may be given in the same way as oral tube feeds. Special feeds may also be given in those renal conditions in which low protein or low sodium intake is indicated, or for infants who cannot digest lactose (milk sugar) or sucrose (cane sugar), and other rare diseases.

Weaning
Weaning means teaching the infant to accept food other than from the breast or bottle. It should start when the child needs additional iron or when very hungry. Usually this will be at the age of about four months.

Principles to be followed
1. Start with one food at a meal—broth or fruit purée.
2. Give a small quantity at first, of a thin consistency. Gradually increase amount and thicken consistency.
3. Introduce new foods one at a time—savoury then sweet.
4. Introduce second meal after one to two weeks, third meal after second is established, including protein and iron-containing food—e.g. egg yolk, minced meat and vegetables.
5. Gradually introduce additional tastes.
6. Avoid foods containing pips or other indigestible matter.

7. Decrease milk feeds as solids are introduced and substitute these with
   water.

Food should be offered in purée form until the child has learned to
masticate. By the age of five months, he should be having three meals a
day and diet should include egg, meat, vegetables, stewed fruit and milk
puddings. A rusk or crust can be given when he starts teething.

As food is increased fluid should gradually be decreased. At the age of
one year approximately 600 ml of fresh cow's milk, water and fruit juices
should be given. As he gets older, bacon, ham, fish, mashed or soft fruit,
apples, bananas, prunes, toast, marmalade, jam and sponge cake can all be
given, so that by the time he is two years old he should have a diet similar to
that of an adult, varying only in size. When the infant changes to cow's
milk, vitamin A and D drops should be given and this should continue
until the child is five years of age.

A toddler may, however, derive considerable comfort from a bottle
before settling to sleep and it is particularly important that this should be
continued if he comes into hospital. At all times the nurse must be understanding and flexible in her attitude. Each infant or child should be treated
as an individual.

Section 3

Pharmaceutical Preparations

Chapter 19

The Administration of Drugs

by G. BRYAN

Introduction—the laws which control drugs—the Pharmacy and Poisons Act 1933—the Misuse of Drugs Act 1971—the Therapeutic Substances Act—safe custody of drugs—containers and their labels—newer systems of prescribing and recording—routes of administration of drugs

Introduction

It cannot be too strongly emphasized that every drug should be regarded as being a possible source of danger to a patient in addition to its being of potential benefit and therefore should be handled with great care. It is perhaps unfortunate that in the past the name 'drug' has been given to particularly potent or dangerous substances with special properties, and the less sinister sounding term 'medicine' to less dangerous or even supposedly harmless substances. It is true that the law differentiates between poisons and non-poisons and it further subdivides poisons into a number of classes. The narcotic drugs of addiction are regarded by the law as requiring more careful control than any other class of drug or poison. But, this is solely because of their addictive properties and it is unfortunate that for many years they have been known in this country as 'Dangerous Drugs', because the implication is that other drugs are not dangerous, whereas it is possible that morphine or pethidine when properly used may be a good deal less dangerous to a patient than, say phenylbutazone, which can cause agranulocytosis and peptic ulceration, or even aspirin, which may cause gastric erosion and a lowered prothrombin level.

Thus, although we have to recognize and observe the legal status of some drugs and the resulting controls imposed upon their use, *the purpose of this introduction is to warn the nurse against complacency and the mistaken view that less care is needed in the handling of some drugs than others.*

THE LAWS WHICH CONTROL DRUGS

The laws which control the handling of drugs and poisons were designed by the Home Office primarily to affect the situation outside the hospital service because it was felt unnecessary to place rigid controls on hospitals which were capable of devising their own control systems according to local circumstances. After the introduction of the National Health Service, however, it became clear that a uniform system of control was desirable and the Minister of Health accepted the Report of a Joint Sub-Committee on the Control of Dangerous Drugs and Poisons in Hospitals published in 1958, containing a number of recommendations which ought now to be practised throughout the hospital service.

THE PHARMACY AND POISONS ACT 1933

This Act and its Regulations restrict the supply, labelling and use of poisons. The Act provides a number of schedules into which various poisons are classified and which provide for specific restrictions or exemptions. Thus, poisons listed in Schedule 1 are the more potent substances which can only be purchased under certain circumstances, whereas poisons listed in Schedules 4A and 4B may only be obtained by members of the public in the form of dispensed medicines on properly written prescriptions by medical, dental or veterinary practitioners. Schedule 4 drugs include those such as barbiturates, sulphonamides, tranquillizers, hormones and central nervous system stimulants.

In hospitals the law states that poisons may only be supplied to out-patients by, or on and in accordance with a prescription of a qualified medical or dental practitioner. Where the substance supplied is a *First Schedule poison*, a record of the transaction must be kept on the premises for two years from the date of supply and the container of the medicine supplied must be labelled with a designation and address sufficient to identify the hospital from which it was supplied.

For in-patient use all medicines containing poisons may only be supplied by the pharmacist provided he has a written signed order from a doctor, dentist or sister or nurse in charge of a ward, theatre or department. First Schedule poisons are required to be labelled with words describing them and the container must bear a label or mark from which it is clear that the poison must be stored in a cupboard reserved solely for poisons and other dangerous substances.

THE MISUSE OF DRUGS ACT 1971

This Act and its Regulations, which supersede the Dangerous Drugs Act and Regulations, control the possession and supply of certain habit-forming narcotic drugs and some other drugs which produce profound effects on the central nervous system. These include morphine, diamorphine, pethidine, methadone and cocaine from the former group and amphetamine, methaqualone, methylphenidate, mescaline and LSD from the latter group. All drugs which are subject to the provisions of this Act and its Regulations are known as Controlled Drugs. Detailed records must be kept by pharmacists with regard to the purchase and sale of all such drugs.

In hospitals, Controlled Drugs may only be supplied to patients on the written and signed instructions of a qualified medical or dental practitioner, who must also specify the total amount of drug to be supplied or administered. The pharmacist must keep records of all such drugs obtained and supplied by him.

For in-patient treatment, the drug may be given from a ward stock supply which the sister, or acting sister for the time being, in charge of the ward or department is authorized to possess. Of all the persons who are authorized by law to possess Controlled Drugs, ward sisters are almost alone in not being required to keep a register of drugs obtained and issued although in most hospitals a record of drugs administered has been kept. It was because this led to different degrees of care in the handling of such drugs that the Joint Sub-Committee referred to on p. 177 was asked to recommend a uniform code of practice which could be applied to all hospitals throughout the country.

THE THERAPEUTIC SUBSTANCES ACT

This Act and Regulations provide for safeguards of adequate biological testing of substances whose potency and purity cannot be adequately determined by chemical means and they control the sale to the public of those substances capable of causing danger to health if used without proper safeguards. Nearly all the antibiotics and their preparations are covered by Part 2 of this Act, as are the corticosteroids such as prednisone, prednisolone and hydrocortisone.

SAFE CUSTODY OF DRUGS AND THEIR ADMINISTRATION

In most hospitals a system is used whereby those drugs which are in constant use are held as ward stocks and those which are used only from time to time are dispensed by the pharmacist for individual patients as they are needed. *The ordering of Controlled Drugs and Schedule 1 Poisons for stock is a responsible and important task and whenever possible it should be done by the sister herself.* There is no standard requisition form for drugs other than Controlled Drugs and each hospital has its own code of practice. The system for Controlled Drugs recommended by the Joint Sub-Committee which is now in use in most hospitals makes use of standard requisition and ward record books. It involves a balancing of receipts against outgoings in respect of each drug so that any loss is automatically brought to notice and it lays the ward record open to scrutiny.

Storage of drugs

Each ward or department should have a minimum of five cupboards for the storage of pharmaceutical preparations and they should all be kept locked. They should consist of:

A Controlled Drugs cupboard which should be within the Schedule 1 Poisons cupboard.
A medicine cupboard.
A cupboard for external preparations, disinfectants, etc.
A cupboard for reagents.

The keys of the Controlled Drugs and Schedule 1 Poisons cupboards should always be carried on the person of the sister or nurse in charge of the ward. Drugs and medicines should be locked away in their appropriate cupboards immediately they are received from the pharmacy and no unauthorized person must be given access to any of these cupboards. A doctor may sometimes ask for the key to one of the ward cupboards where drugs are stored for the purpose of getting a drug for a patient. This request must always be resisted because the custody of drugs in the Controlled Drugs and Schedule 1 Poisons cupboards is the legal responsibility of the ward sister or her deputy.

Some drugs require cool storage in order that their potency is maintained. When a drug is included in the Schedule 1 list but requires cool storage, the latter requirement takes precedence. A refrigerator which is set to be maintained at a temperature of about 4 °C (39 °F) is necessary for these drugs, examples of which are all vaccines, some antibiotics, insulin and suxamethonium chloride injection.

CONTAINERS AND THEIR LABELS

In every hospital where a pharmacist is employed he has legal responsibility for his dispensing activities. *For this reason a nurse should never transfer the contents of one bottle to another, nor should she ever alter the label on a dispensed medicine.* In some hospitals the members of the resident medical staff have access to the pharmacy at night or at weekends in order to obtain drugs for patients newly admitted. Their choice of containers and labels does not always conform to standard pharmaceutical practice, and it should be a rule that the nursing staff should return to the pharmacy any unused portions of drugs so dispensed at the earliest opportunity so that they may be adequately labelled by the pharmacist.

NEWER SYSTEMS OF PRESCRIBING AND RECORDING

In recent years various workers in this country and elsewhere have investigated what they describe as 'errors of administration of drugs in hospitals following complex prescribing'. These errors are found to occur more frequently when patients are prescribed several drugs to be taken concurrently and particularly when one of them has to be administered four or more times a day. It must be remembered that an error has occurred when the administration of a prescribed drug is omitted and there are occasions when such an omission is quite as important as would be the case if the wrong drug had been given. There are many reasons for these errors but some workers believe that the design of the drug treatment sheet and its careful use by the prescriber could be the most important single contribution to reducing errors. Some of these newly designed treatment sheets are combined with a drug recording sheet which is filled in by the nurse each time a drug is administered. Much work remains to be done in this field before the ideal solution is found but the aim should always be the complete elimination of errors whether they are errors of commission or of omission.

ROUTES OF ADMINISTRATION OF DRUGS

This section should be read in conjunction with that part of Chapter 20 which describes the forms in which drugs are presented for use.

Oral administration

This is the most widely used method of administering drugs which are required to produce a systemic effect. From the patient's point of view it is the easiest and most convenient method and unless there is some over-riding reason why another route should be used it should always be regarded as the method of choice.

Liquid medicines are used less now than formerly, particularly since the art and skill of the tablet maker is fully recognized (for administration see Chapter 9, p. 83).

Tablets, capsules and cachets are the most frequently used dose forms for oral administration. Some drugs are not absorbed from the alimentary tract after passing through the oesophagus but are well absorbed through the oral mucous membrane. Glyceryl trinitrate is an example, and tablets containing this drug are made in such a way that they dissolve when placed under the tongue, thus releasing the active medicament for absorption through the mucous membrane of the mouth.

Rectal administration

Enemas and suppositories have long been used as a means of evacuating the colon (see p. 91) or for their astringent action on the rectum, but, in recent years suppositories have been found to be a useful way of introducing drugs into the body to produce a systemic effect. In this way patients who cannot tolerate oral therapy, perhaps because of gastric irritation by the drug, may be adequately treated with suppositories containing the drug. Phenylbutazone, aspirin, aminophylline and some anti-emetic agents are examples of drugs which are administered in this way in doses not significantly larger than when given orally (see Chapter 10, p. 94 for methods of administration).

Parenteral administration

This term implies administration by means of injection into the body. The main routes of injection are intradermal, subcutaneous, intramuscular, intravenous, intrathecal and intra-articular.

Administration by injection

Intradermal injections are used for diagnostic purposes.

Subcutaneous injections are used for small-volume injections of 1 or 2 ml. which are not irritant to superficial tissues. Insulin is usually given subcutaneously and patients are taught to administer injections themselves. The enzyme hyaluronidase is sometimes used in conjunction with subcutaneous injections to increase the rate at which solutions are carried from the site of injection and thereby increase the speed of absorption into the systemic circulation. (For method of administration, see Chapter 9, p. 84.)

Intramuscular injections are used when quicker absorption is required than is obtained from the subcutaneous route or when the drug would be irritant to superficial tissues. Most injections are made isotonic with blood serum if this is possible, but when this would result in a greatly increased volume the intramuscular use of a hypertonic solution is permissible.

Intravenous injections are used when a very rapid action is needed or when the volume to be given is so large as to preclude the use of any other route or when the preparation is so irritant to the tissues that it would be dangerous to use other routes. (See Chapter 9, p. 86, and for intravenous infusion, Chapter 49.) Thus insulin would be injected intravenously in a patient in diabetic coma to obtain an immediate response. Large volumes of dextrose and electrolyte solutions are given by intravenous infusion, and there are times when this is the only way of maintaining a patient's fluid and electrolyte balance in addition to supplying essential calories. Mustine hydrochloride, a cytotoxic drug, must be given intravenously in dilute solution because it would cause necrotic damage to tissues if given outside a vein.

Precautions. Great care is needed in the handling of large-volume intravenous injections, and if the entire contents of a bottle are not used the remaining portion must be discarded. Even though a bottle appears to be full, if the seal is broken it should not be used. This is because large-volume injections in single-dose containers contain no antibacterial agent, and growth of micro-organisms can take place in opened containers.

Intrathecal injections are used when a drug is needed in the cerebrospinal fluid. Great care is needed in the preparation of such injections which can have no added bacteriostatic substance, and an equally good aseptic technique is needed in handling such injections at the time of administration. Drugs such as penicillin and streptomycin may be given by this route in the treatment of meningitis.

Intra-articular injections are used in the treatment of inflamed joints. Hydrocortisone acetate suspensions are used in this way and again great care is needed in the handling of such injections. Because chemical bacteriostats may be irritant to the tissues, such injections should be free from these added substances and this precludes the use of multi-dose, rubber-capped containers.

Chapter 20

Drugs and Their Presentation for Use

by G. BRYAN

> *Definition of terms used in consideration of drugs and medicines—classification of drugs—dosage—the metric system—forms in which drugs are presented for use—some abbreviations used in prescriptions*

A drug is a substance used to treat or relieve the symptoms of disease or is a prophylactic agent used to prevent disease. The term Materia Medica is an old one which has been misused in the past and means simply 'medicinal substances'. In years past it has embraced much wider meanings and has included the study of pharmacy, pharmacognosy and pharmacology. Because these are themselves precise terms no purpose is served by perpetuating the use of the out-dated term Materia Medica.

Pharmacy is the science and art of preparing drugs, standardizing them and formulating them into preparations for use in the treatment or prevention of disease.

Pharmacognosy is the study of the structural, physical, chemical and sensory characters of crude drugs of vegetable and animal origin.

Pharmacology is the study of the mode of action of drugs and **Therapeutics** is the application of this study in the treatment of disease.

The British Pharmacopoeia (*B.P.*) is an authoritative book produced by the Pharmacopoeia Commission and published at the direction of the Medicines Commission, which describes and provides standards for many drugs in common use. It is under constant revision and Addenda are produced at intervals during the five-year life of each edition. The Pharmacopoeia Commission is also responsible for devising Approved Names for drugs. These names become the Pharmacopoeial names of drugs when they are given official status by being included in the *B.P.*

The British Pharmaceutical Codex (*B.P.C.*) is a book produced and published by the Pharmaceutical Society to supplement the information contained in the *B.P.* It includes standards for drugs which are not referred to in the current *B.P.* and for surgical dressings and sutures. It also contains a number of formulae for preparations of drugs in regular use.

The British National Formulary (*B.N.F.*) is a book produced by the Joint Formulary Committee composed of representatives of the medical and pharmaceutical professions and it lists a selection of drugs and preparations which should serve the needs of most prescribers. In addition, it contains a section devoted to notes for prescribers on the actions and uses of drugs.

Proprietary drugs and preparations are those which are protected by patent or other means against competition in respect of name, composition or process of manufacture. It is necessary to use proprietary names with care since it would be an infringement of the law to use one in describing a drug or preparation manufactured by a company other than the company in whose name the proprietary name is registered. For example, there is only one manufacturer entitled to use the name 'Dindevan' to describe his brand of phenindione tablets B.P. although there are several manufacturers of phenindione tablets B.P. It is good practice to use ·Approved Names for drugs whenever possible.

CLASSIFICATION OF DRUGS

There are two methods of classifying drugs—either by grouping them according to their sources of origin or by arranging them into groups based on their pharmacological action.

Source classification

There are four main groups when defined by the first method—vegetable, inorganic or mineral compounds, animal products and synthetic drugs.

Vegetable drugs are less used now than formerly, but some potent drugs are still derived from vegetable sources such as morphine from the opium poppy, atropine from belladonna and digoxin from the foxglove.

Mineral salts account for a number of important drugs which are used in medicine. Ferrous sulphate, calcium chloride and sodium chloride are examples of this group.

Animal products are relatively few in number but of tremendous importance. Insulin, for example, is obtained from the pancreas of the ox or pig and many of the immunological products are obtained from the blood serum of specially treated horses.

Synthetic compounds account for the largest number of drugs used today. These are chemicals which are made in the laboratory by organic chemists. Sometimes they are exact copies of compounds which occur in nature such as benzoic acid or camphor but which can be produced more cheaply by synthesis. More often they are unrelated to natural products and include groups such as sulphonamides, thiazide diuretics, tranquillizers and barbiturates.

Pharmacological classification

The pharmacological classification groups together those drugs which have similar actions or those which have a common site of action. For example, antibiotics are grouped together, as are analgesics or antacids or immunological preparations.

DOSAGE OF DRUGS

In practice, the dosage of many drugs—and this applies particularly to the older ones—is determined solely by experience, provided they have been accurately standardized either chemically or biologically, with little or no regard to the age or size of the patient. With newer drugs it is often necessary to determine the dose with great care to meet the needs of a particular patient and sometimes the presence of unwanted effects will determine the safe upper limit of dosage. Thus, the dose of a powerful anti-hypertensive drug needs to be carefully adjusted in order that postural hypotension is not produced in a given patient.

The formulation or presentation of a drug can have a profound effect upon its dosage. For example, it is no longer possible to assume that equal doses of a pure chemically standardized drug will always produce the same response in the same patient. With many of the new synthetic drugs which have low solubilities in water, the particle size of the drug within a tablet can have a marked bearing on the patient's response to it. When the makers of spironolactone tablets ('Aldactone') first marketed their product, it was in tablets containing 100 mg of active drug. An average dose was 400 mg daily in divided doses. It was discovered that if the drug was powdered much more finely before it was incorporated into tablets it was possible to reduce the dosage by 75 per cent, and the tablets marketed today contain only 25 mg of the finely powdered drug.

Another factor which affects the dosage of a drug is the possibility that a second drug which a patient is taking concurrently may potentiate its action. For example, aspirin potentiates the anticoagulant action of phenindione, and sodium bicarbonate by delaying its excretion by the kidneys produces an enhanced effect when a standard dose of amphetamine is administered. Chlorpromazine enhances the response to some analgesics and sedatives and use is made of this to achieve a given response to morphine without increasing the dose.

Sometimes the size of a patient is used as a guide to correct dosage of a drug. Size has been interpreted as weight in the past, and the dose of a drug such as nitrofurantoin, for example, has been stated as 5 to 8 mg per kg body-weight daily in divided doses. More recently it has been suggested that surface area of the patient is a better criterion than body-weight in assessing the size of a patient.

Infants and children pose a special problem and a number of formulae have been devised as aids to the calculation of doses for children. Young's formula has served as a rough guide for many years:

$$\text{Dose} = \frac{\text{age of child}}{\text{age of child} + 12} \times \text{adult dose}$$

An alternative to Young's formula is given in the *British National Formulary* which is no doubt more reliable though less easy to memorize. Provided the child is of average weight for his age the dose for most drugs can be expressed as a percentage of the adult dose as follows:

Age 12 years = 75 per cent
Age 7 years = 50 per cent
Age 3 years = 33 per cent
Age 1 year = 25 per cent

For infants below one year the dose is based on body-weight and is 2·5 per cent of the adult dose per kg body-weight of the infant.

Idiosyncrasy. This term implies an inherent grossly abnormal reaction to a normal dose of a drug and is probably due to a genetic abnormality. This is different from hypersensitivity which is due to an antibody-antigen reaction, and a patient who is hypersensitive to penicillin, for example, must have been exposed to the antibiotic on a previous occasion without ill-effect.

Cumulation. Drugs should only be administered at the rate at which they will be metabolized or excreted. This explains why some drugs may need to be given four times a day whereas others which are slowly eliminated are only given once a day. If a drug which is slowly excreted is given too frequently, a toxic level is built up and a cumulative effect is produced. This applies to drugs such as the digitalis glycosides.

Tolerance is said to have developed when a patient requires increased doses of a drug to obtain an effect which was previously obtained with smaller doses. This is very liable to happen with the opium alkaloids such as morphine. Tolerance may lead to dependence which can be either physical, which means that the patient is physically ill if the drug is withheld, or psychological. This state is very liable to occur in the case of central nervous system stimulants or depressant drugs and powerful analgesics which produce euphoria.

It will be seen from this examination of the subject that there are many criteria which govern the choice of the correct dosage of any drug for a given patient.

THE METRIC SYSTEM

For many years, as new drugs have been introduced, their doses have been expressed in metric terms, but the older drugs have been prescribed in the Imperial system of weights and measures. Since March, 1969, it has been illegal for any drug or pharmaceutical preparation to be dispensed in any other than the metric system and all preparations in the *B.P.*, *B.P.C.* and *B.N.F.* have been formulated in metric units since that date. The linctuses, elixirs and paediatric mixtures have a unit dose of 5 ml and the adult mixtures a unit dose of 10 ml. The single-dose forms of medication—tablets, capsules and injections—have all been formulated in the metric system since 1963 so that now all prescribing and dispensing should be carried out using metric measurements only. (For metric measurements and milli-equivalents, see Appendix i, p. 754.)

FORMS IN WHICH DRUGS ARE PRESENTED FOR USE

Applications. These are liquid preparations for external application and often contain antiparasitic compounds. Benzyl benzoate application for the treatment of scabies is an example.

Cachets. These are small circular shells made of rice paper which are used to enclose powdered drugs which are given in fairly high dosage. The cachets are softened in water and then swallowed whole. This enables unpleasant tasting powders to be taken with reasonable ease. Sodium aminosalicylate and Isoniazid cachets are frequently used in the treatment of tuberculosis.

Capsules. There are two kinds of capsule—soft gelatin capsules which are used to contain liquid drugs and hard gelatin capsules to enclose powders. Halibut liver oil or oil-soluble vitamins are frequently presented in soft gelatin capsules which are spherical or ovoid in shape. Many bitter tasting drugs are available in hard capsules which are cylindrical in shape. Examples are ampicillin, chlordiazepoxide and amylobarbitone sodium.

Collodions. Flexible collodion contains pyroxylin, colophony, castor oil, industrial methylated spirit and solvent ether. Because of its volatility it should always be kept in a well-closed container. When applied it quickly dries to form a flexible artificial 'skin'. It is sometimes used as a vehicle for an active drug such as salicylic acid which may be used as a corn paint.

Creams. Creams are semi-solid preparations containing water which are used as vehicles for active ingredients to be used in treating diseases of the skin (see Chapter 31). Sometimes the water content of creams is as high as 70 per cent. Because of this, great care must be taken to prevent bacterial contamination of creams. It is for this reason that they are usually packed in collapsible metal or plastic tubes or in screw-capped jars. Creams are of two varieties:

1. Water-in-oil creams which are greasy and not miscible with water—e.g. zinc cream.
2. Oil-in-water creams which are not greasy and are readily removable by washing with water and which vanish when rubbed into the skin. Many of the corticosteroids are incorporated into this type of cream base—e.g. betamethasone valerate cream.

Draughts. There is now only one draught included in the *British National Formulary* (*B.N.F.*) and this type of preparation is rarely used today. It is a large-volume, single-dose, liquid preparation usually of 50 ml. Male fern extract draught which is an emulsion of a vegetable drug used for the eradication of tape-worm infestation is an example (see Chapter 24, p. 238).

Dusting powders are used to carry to the skin an active ingredient or may be used solely for their lubricant properties. Talc and starch are commonly used as the base in dusting powders. Caution should be exercised in applying dusting powders to raw and weeping surfaces because of the possibility of absorption of toxic substances used as ingredients.

Ear drops are solutions or suspensions of drugs in an aqueous vehicle or other organic solvent. For example, phenol ear drops are always made in glycerin because of the caustic properties of aqueous solutions of phenol.

Elixirs are clear, pleasantly flavoured preparations of potent or nauseous drugs. The vehicle may contain a high proportion of alcohol or other solvent such as glycerin. Sugars or other sweetening agents are frequently present. Ephedrine elixir is a typical example.

Emulsions. An emulsion consists of two normally immiscible liquids, one of which is finely subdivided and dispersed in the other, the system being stabilized by the presence of an emulsifying agent. Thus, liquid paraffin which is immiscible with water can be formed into a stable emulsion by the inclusion of methylcellulose. Because such emulsions are usually thick creamy products the term is frequently wrongly applied to any white viscous preparation. In pharmaceutical practice the term 'emulsion' should be restricted to oil-in-water preparations for internal use.

Enemas are aqueous or oily solutions or suspensions intended for rectal administration. Any solid substances or oils contained need to be uniformly dispersed (for examples and modes of administration see p. 91).

Eye drops are sterile, aqueous or oily solutions or suspensions of drugs for instillation into the eye. They usually contain medicaments with antiseptic, anaesthetic, anti-inflammatory, mydriatic or miotic properties, but some eye drops contain substances which are used for diagnostic purposes. All aqueous eye drops contain a substance which is bactericidal and fungicidal in order that their sterility is maintained during use. It is necessary to limit the 'life' of eye drops once the container has been opened and the *B.P.C.* specifies that not more than 10 ml should be supplied in one container which should be discarded 14 days after opening by a domiciliary patient, after 7 days for a ward patient and after being used once in an operating theatre.

Eye lotions are sterile aqueous solutions used undiluted for bathing the eyes. They should be discarded 24 hours after being opened.

Eye ointments are sterile preparations for application to the conjunctival sac or lid margin and are usually made in a greasy base. They contain the same type of active drugs as are contained in eye drops and are presented in small collapsible tubes with very fine nozzles. Great care should be exercised in the handling of eye ointments so as to prevent bacterial contamination during use. A separate tube should be used for each patient.

Gargles are aqueous solutions in concentrated form intended to be diluted with warm water before use. They are used as a prophylactic or for the treatment of an affection of the throat.

Implants are sterile cylinders prepared by fusion or heavy compression of a drug for subcutaneous implantation in order to produce slow absorption and prolonged action over several weeks or months. Hormones such as testosterone are administered in this way.

Inhalations. There are now two types of preparation which are used by inhalation. The older one is a liquid preparation composed of or containing volatile ingredients which when vaporized in a suitable manner can be brought into contact with the lining of the respiratory tract. This is done by adding hot, not boiling, water and inhaling the vapour. The newer type of inhalation consists of a very fine suspension of an active drug in an inert propellant in a pressurized aerosol (see p. 90). On pressing the release button a measured dose of the drug is released which is inhaled by the patient. Isoprenaline is administered in this way. (For details of administration see Chapter 9, p. 87.)

Injections are sterile solutions or suspensions intended for parenteral administration by the subcutaneous, intramuscular, intravenous or intrathecal routes (see Chapter 9, pp. 84–6). They are used to administer drugs which may be inactivated or not tolerated when given by mouth. Drugs given by injection usually produce a more rapid response than is the case when they are given by mouth.

Linctuses. These are viscous, liquid preparations usually containing sugar and possessing soothing, expectorant or sedative properties. They are usually given to relieve cough and are administered in 5 ml doses which should be sipped and swallowed slowly without the addition of water.

Liniments are liquid preparations intended for external application to the skin and may contain substances which possess analgesic, rubefacient, soothing or stimulant properties.
Liniments are usually applied with friction by massaging with the hand. They should not be applied to broken skin.

Lotions are liquid preparations which are applied to the skin without friction. They usually contain ingredients which are anti-inflammatory or soothing.

Lozenges are solid preparations prepared by moulding or compression, consisting of medicaments incorporated in a flavoured basis, and are intended to dissolve slowly in the mouth. They usually contain anti-bacterial drugs or anaesthetic drugs such as chlorhexidine or amethocaine.

Mixtures are liquid preparations for oral administration and consist of one or more drugs suspended or dissolved usually in an aqueous vehicle. The normal dose for an adult is 10 ml and for a child is 5 ml.

Mouth washes are aqueous solutions in concentrated form intended to be diluted before use and usually contain antiseptic or astringent substances.

Nasal drops. These are liquid preparations for instillation into the nostrils by means of a dropper. They may be aqueous or oily but the prolonged use of oily nasal drops is not to be recommended since it may cause lipoid pneumonia. Nasal drops may contain drugs which have antiseptic, local analgesic or vasoconstrictor properties.

Ointments. These are semi-solid preparations containing one or more medicaments dissolved or dispersed in a suitable base, and are intended to be applied externally. The base usually contains fatty substances and is often anhydrous. Soft paraffin and lanolin are frequently used, but the newer bases although having a greasy appearance are capable of emulsifying water and can therefore be readily removed from the skin. Emulsifying Ointment B.P. is an example of this type of base.

Paints are liquid preparations for application to the skin or mucous surfaces. They are usually medicated with a substance possessing antiseptic, astringent, caustic or analgesic properties. The base often contains a volatile ingredient such as spirit when rapid drying on the skin is required.

Pastes are semi-solid preparations for external use and they usually contain a high proportion of finely powdered medicaments in soft paraffin. Zinc paste, for example, contains a very high proportion of zinc oxide and starch. They are principally used as protective soothing dressings and are applied thickly on lint.

Pastilles are used for the same purpose as lozenges but are made with a glycerin and gelatin base.

Pessaries are solid bodies suitably shaped for vaginal administration and containing drugs to act locally. The base is sometimes cocoa butter or glycerin and gelatin, but many pessaries today are made by compression in the way that tablets are produced. It is important, however, that whatever base is used, the pessary will either melt or dissolve at body temperature and so release the active drug at its site of action. (See Insertion of Medicated Pessaries, p. 750.)

Pills are spherical masses containing one or more active ingredients. They are prepared by being massed with a moistening agent or exipient, cut and then rolled to their familiar shape. It will be seen from this description that a pill is quite different from a tablet. Pills are now almost obsolete for two main reasons: they are difficult to mass produce and they do not have reliable disintegrating properties.

Poultices are viscous, pasty preparations for external use, usually employed with the object of reducing inflammation or relieving pain. Kaolin poultice is one of the few remaining poultices in current practice (see p. 103).

Powders are usually mixtures of active constituents in dry form for oral administration. Many are used for the treatment of gastric disorders and are taken by measurement using the 5 ml medicine spoon and mixed with a little water.

Solutions are liquids containing one or more active ingredients usually in water. They may be for internal or external use or for instillation into body cavities, when they must be sterile.

Sprays are preparations of drugs in aqueous, alcoholic or glycerin-containing media intended to be applied to the nose or throat by means of an atomizer. Those which are intended for the treatment of asthma and similar conditions of the respiratory tract should be used with a nebulizer capable of producing a 'dry mist'. Oily sprays which were formerly used should be abandoned because drops of oil may enter the trachea and cause lipoid pneumonia.

Suppositories are solid conical or torpedo-shaped bodies for rectal administration. The base is usually a suitable solid vegetable oil such as cocoa butter or a hydrogenated vegetable oil derivative with a melting point of about 37 °C (98 °F), i.e. just below body temperature. A wide range of drugs may be administered in the form of suppositories and whereas until fairly recently they were used for the treatment of haemorrhoids and proctitis alone, when they contained astringent substances and local anaesthetic drugs, they are now widely used as a means of introducing drugs into the bloodstream. Suppositories can be used to administer drugs to patients who are unable to take them by mouth and for whom injections would be tiresome.

Tablets. Compressed tablets are usually circular in shape with flat or convex faces. They are made by compressing a granulated preparation of a drug or mixture of drugs by means of punches in suitable dies. Tablets may be coated to improve their appearance and stability, to mask an unpleasant taste or to protect the drug from the action of the acid juices of the stomach. The preparation of tablets is a skilled process and the *British Pharmacopoeia* lays down stringent tests which must be applied to ensure that all tablets in a batch are of a uniform weight and that they will disintegrate under prescribed conditions within a specified time. Some tablets are formulated in such a way that they do not disintegrate until they have passed through the stomach. This may be desirable if the drug is liable to cause gastric irritation, e.g. prednisolone, or it may be necessary to protect the drug from the acid contents of the stomach, e.g. erythromycin. This type of coating is known as enteric coating. Other tablets are prepared in such a way as to provide a slow release of a drug over a period of several hours. This is done to achieve a longer duration of action and therefore results in less frequent administration. Some tablets are taken by allowing them to dissolve under the tongue and the drug is absorbed through the mucous membrane of the mouth, e.g. glyceryl trinitrate.

Vitrellae are thin-walled glass capsules containing a volatile medicament. They are protected by a wrapping of fabric and are used by crushing the capsule and inhaling the vapour which spills out onto the absorptive and protective fabric. Amyl nitrite is used in this way in the treatment of angina.

Vaccines and antisera (formerly known as antitoxins) are preparations used in the treatment of diseases due to specific micro-organisms or for the prophylaxis of patients exposed to such diseases. Antisera only provide temporary protection, but vaccines which contain antigenic substances are administered with the object of inducing in the recipient a specific active immunity (see also Chapter 42, p. 399).

SOME ABBREVIATIONS USED IN PRESCRIPTIONS

The use of Latin in the writing of prescriptions is discouraged in most English medical schools, but a custom which has become established over a period of centuries will take a long time to disappear. It is because of this that a list of commonly used Latin abbreviations is appended in order that the nurse may be able to interpret a doctor's intentions when he uses this mode of expression.

Abbreviation	Latin	English translation
a.c.	ante cibum	before food
aq.	aqua	water
aq. ad.	aquam ad	water up to
aq. dest.	aqua destillata	distilled water
b.	bis	twice
b.i.d.	bis in die	twice a day
c.	cum	with
d.	die	day
ex aq.	ex aqua	in water
garg.	gargarisma	a gargle
gutt.	gutta	a drop
G. or gm.	gramma	a gram
m.	mane	in the morning
m. et n.	mane et nocte	morning and night
mist.	mistura	a mixture
n.	nocte	by night or at night
p.c.	post cibum	after food
q.d. *or* q.i.d.	{ quater die { quater in die	four times a day during the 24 hours
q.q.h.	quaque quarta hora	every four hours
q.s.	quantum sufficit	as much as is required
stat.	statim	immediately
t.	ter	three times
t.i.d.	ter in die	three times a day
t.d.s.	ter die sumendum	to be taken three times a day
ung.	unguentum	ointment

Section 4

Medical Conditions, Treatment and Care

INTRODUCTION

Medicine, even in the restricted sense of the word—the province of physicians as distinct from surgeons, gynaecologists, pathologists, etc.—is a wide field and classification is difficult. One method of classifying medical diseases is by the system of the body predominantly affected: thus, diseases of the digestive system, of the nervous system, of the respiratory system, and so on. However, this method leaves it difficult to define the place of certain diseases that affect more than one system. The chief examples of such multi-system diseases are the *infectious diseases*, which are best classified according to the causative micro-organism.

The present section covers the diseases of single systems, the next (Section 5) covers infectious diseases. There is bound to be some overlap between these sections: for example, tuberculosis is described under infectious diseases because it may affect all systems of the body, but it may predominantly attack the respiratory system and is therefore also mentioned in the chapter on diseases of the chest. The subdivision into these two sections is thus largely a matter of convenience and does not imply a rigid differentiation between the diseases described in the two sections.

Chapter 21

Disorders of Respiration

by P. E. BALDRY

> *Applied physiology—symptoms of respiratory disease—diseases of the airways: acute and chronic laryngitis, acute and chronic bronchitis, asthma, bronchiectasis, bronchial carcinoma—diseases of the lungs: the pneumonias, pulmonary infarction, the pneumoconioses—diseases of the pleura: pleural effusion, spontaneous pneumothorax—pulmonary tuberculosis*

APPLIED PHYSIOLOGY

Efficient lung function depends on (1) the airways (trachea and bronchi) being free from obstruction; (2) good inspiratory and expiratory movements; any interference with the movement of the thoracic cage such as occurs with paralysis of the chest-wall muscles or from the splinting effect of obesity, will affect inspiration, whereas expiration is impaired when there is loss of elasticity of the lung tissue itself such as occurs in emphysema; (3) the absence of any pathological process in and around the air sacs interfering with the exchange of gases. The air sacs, or alveoli, are surrounded by thin-walled capillaries (the alveolo-capillary membrane). The close proximity of these structures allows oxygen to diffuse readily into the blood from the atmospheric air, and carbon dioxide to pass in the reverse direction. In certain diseases such as pneumonia or heart failure, the outpouring of fluid into the air sacs seriously interferes with this gaseous exchange and in an attempt to compensate for this the rate of respiration is increased.

The control of respiration

Respiration is partly under voluntary control, but in addition the rate and depth of breathing are automatically adjusted in accordance with the changing requirements of the body by a control unit in the medulla of the brain (the respiratory centre) which responds to changes in the arterial carbon dioxide pressure and hydrogen ion concentration. A rise in carbon dioxide pressure, such as occurs with exercise or with obstruction of the airways or in certain diseases affecting the lungs, stimulates the respiratory centre to effect a compensatory increase in the rate and depth of respiration. Similarly, any increase in the blood hydrogen ion concentration as occurs in uraemia and in diabetic coma results in very deep sighing respiration (Kussmaul's breathing).

The action of the respiratory centre is depressed by excessive amounts of narcotic drugs such as morphine or barbiturates in the circulation: for this reason, in certain cases of self-induced drug poisoning, breathing has to be maintained artificially by a respirator.

The respiratory centre is responsive normally to slight variations in blood chemistry; at times it loses this degree of sensitivity and only stimulates respiration when the carbon dioxide pressure has risen considerably. This results in a type of breathing known as Cheyne-Stokes breathing which is seen in left ventricular failure and in certain cases where there is a raised intracranial pressure. In such cases the amplitude of respiration deepens progressively until a maximum is reached (*hyperpnoea*) and then diminishes progressively until finally there is a period when breathing ceases (*apnoea*). During this phase of apnoea the carbon dioxide in the blood rises to a level sufficiently high to stimulate the respiratory centre to restart breathing (see Fig. 21/1).

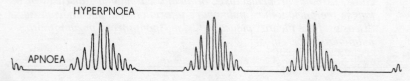

Fig. 21/1 Cheyne-Stokes breathing showing periods of hyperpnoea and apnoea (see text).

Lack of oxygen has little direct influence on the respiratory centre but affects mainly nerve endings in the walls of the carotid artery and aorta which in turn relay impulses to the control centre in the brain.

SYMPTOMS OF RESPIRATORY DISEASE

Careful history taking with the skilful evaluation of symptoms is of the greatest importance in the diagnosis of disease. Certain symptoms associated with disorders of respiration will therefore be discussed in detail.

Dyspnoea. In health breathing is carried out automatically and without conscious effort. An early symptom of disturbed lung function is an uncomfortable awareness of respiration with shortness of breath known as dyspnoea. This symptom is not confined to diseases of the lungs and bronchi; it occurs in heart failure and in severe anaemia, and in addition may be present in anxiety states. Patients with emotional disturbances often feel that they cannot get sufficient air into their lungs and consequently take deep gasps with much sighing. Some hysterics breathe very deeply (hyperventilate) with the liberation of excessive amounts of carbon dioxide from the body; this disturbs the body chemistry with the production of severe cramp in the hands and feet (tetany).

Cough. A cough may be dry, irritant and unproductive or it may result in the expectoration of sputum. An irritant dry cough may result from the inhalation of a foreign body or from virus infections of the respiratory tract. In children it is often caused by enlarged infected tonsils or from secretions dripping down the back of the throat from infected adenoids.

Sputum. The walls of the bronchi contain a large number of glands which secrete sufficient mucus to form a protective layer over the epithelium. In disease this mucus is produced in excessive amounts and when expectorated is known as sputum. The mucoid type of sputum is a colourless, sticky jelly. In the presence of bacterial infection it becomes mixed with pus cells and this purulent type of sputum has a yellow or green colour with at times an offensive smell. On occasions sputum is bloodstained or there may be a large amount of almost pure blood expectorated which is then known as a *haemoptysis*. The common causes of haemoptysis are: carcinoma of the bronchus, pulmonary tuberculosis, bronchiectasis, pulmonary infarction, and mitral stenosis. A haemoptysis is always frightening to a patient so those in attendance should behave in a calm and reassuring manner. It is better to encourage expectoration of the blood rather than to allow it to be retained in the lungs where it may obstruct the airways. The patient may require sedation. Blood transfusion is rarely necessary although occasionally a haemoptysis may be massive and even fatal.

Wheezing. Narrowing of the air tubes from spasm of the muscle in the bronchial wall or because of partial obstruction from retained sputum leads to the production of a wheezing noise often audible to the patient and those nearby.

Pain. The character of this symptom depends on whether it arises from disease affecting the muscles, ribs, nerve roots, or pleura. Disease confined to the lung alone does not cause pain. Pain in the muscles of the chest wall due to *fibrositis* is common; it gives rise to an intermittent stabbing sensation or a continuous dull ache, often shifting from one place to another. Severe pain is experienced when the ribs are damaged; even when they are only bruised there is discomfort for many weeks, but when they are fractured or eroded by neoplasm the pain is agonizing and further aggravated by coughing or sneezing. Girdle pains radiating around the chest wall occur when nerve roots are affected by disease. Inflammation of the pleura (pleurisy) causes a severe knife-like pain, made worse by taking a deep breath.

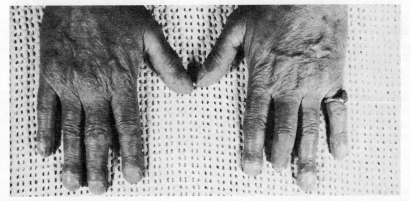

Fig. 21/2 Clubbing in the fingers of a 40-year-old man with long-standing bilateral bronchiectasis.

Clubbing of the fingers. The changes in the appearance of the fingers known as clubbing are of much diagnostic significance (see Fig. 21/2). It may be considered a symptom when complained of by the patient, but more frequently the patient is unaware of the changes and it is the doctor or nurse, who, as trained observers, first recognize clubbing as a physical sign of underlying pulmonary or cardiac disorders including bronchial carcinoma, bronchiectasis, lung abscess, bacterial endocarditis and cyanotic types of congenital heart disease.

DISEASES OF THE AIRWAYS

Acute tracheitis, laryngitis and bronchitis often occur together as a complication of the common cold or one of the childhood fevers such as measles. The symptoms include a sore throat, hoarse voice, dry painful cough and wheezing. In addition, in small children, whose airways are normally narrow, inflammation may lead to dangerous obstruction with the production of a harsh, strident, inspiratory noise known as a *stridor*.

Chronic laryngitis which causes persistent hoarseness of the voice for days or weeks may result from excessive use of the voice (speaker's throat), but if it persists for more than three weeks the larynx should be examined to exclude either a carcinoma arising at that site or paralysis of the vocal cords from interference with the nerve supply to the larynx by a growth in the lungs.

Chronic bronchitis is an extremely common disease in the British Isles, also a very serious one as it may be associated with crippling, and at times fatal, complications. Its course may be divided into four stages:

1. Enlargement and overactivity of the mucus-secreting glands in the walls of the bronchi
2. Bacterial infection of the mucus
3. The development of emphysema
4. Cardiac and respiratory failure

Stage 1. The reason for the sudden production of excessive amounts of thick tenacious mucus is not known. It usually occurs in men over the age of 40, often seeming to follow an acute virus infection of the respiratory tract, and once the condition is established it is aggravated by many factors. Bronchitis is always worse in cold damp winter weather. The irritant effect of fog and industrial smog is particularly harmful but the prevalence of this has been reduced since the creation of smokeless zones following the passing of the Clean Air Act by Parliament in 1956. The disease is also made worse by exposure to dust, fumes or sudden changes of temperature. *In particular the dangerous irritant effect of cigarette smoking cannot be overemphasized.* As soon as the diagnosis is made the patient must stop cigarette smoking and avoid all forms of bronchial irritation even if this means changing his job. Mucoid sputum is sticky and difficult to expectorate but this is often made easier by increasing its water content, either by inhalations of steam or by the use of a humidifier. The suppression of an irritant cough at night by a linctus containing codeine is helpful.

Stage 2. Intermittent acute episodes of infection are common. The patient feels toxic, is febrile, the wheezing and shortness of breath become more marked and in addition the sputum increases in amount and changes to a yellow or green colour. The bacteria usually responsible for this type of infection are the *Haemophilus influenzae* and pneumococci. The antibiotics tetracycline and ampicillin (Penbritin) are equally effective against these organisms. Sometimes a combination of penicillin and streptomycin (Crystamycin Forte) is administered by intramuscular injection.

Stage 3. Repeated episodes of bronchitis associated with severe bouts of coughing put a great strain on the tissues of the lungs resulting in the development of *emphysema*. In this condition the walls of many of the alveoli rupture with the formation of large balloons or bullae while at the same time many of the surrounding capillaries are destroyed; in addition the lung tissue loses its elasticity with resultant difficulty in expelling air from the lungs. After a time the lungs remain in a constantly distended state with the chest assuming the shape of a barrel. These structural changes result in a serious reduction in the amount of oxygen entering the blood and an accumulation of carbon dioxide in the tissues.

Stage 4. When lungs already severely damaged by chronic bronchitis and emphysema are subjected to the added strain of an acute respiratory infection, *respiratory failure may develop* with a further marked lowering of the oxygen pressure and sharp rise in the carbon dioxide pressure in the blood. The amount of carbon dioxide retained in the blood is so excessive that it has an action similar to a powerful narcotic drug (carbon dioxide narcosis) with drowsiness, disturbance of behaviour with agitation at times amounting to violence, rambling delirium, coarse flapping tremor of the hands similar to that seen in liver failure, and marked depression of respiration. This severe disturbance of the blood gases also adversely affects the heart and blood vessels with the development of cardiac failure. Cardiac failure when it arises as a complication of disordered lung function is sometimes referred to as *cor pulmonale*.

Treatment includes the use of diuretics and the administration of oxygen. It must, however, be clearly understood that as carbon dioxide narcosis has a severe depressive effect on the respiratory centre in the brain the only stimulus to breathing is oxygen lack. If this stimulus is removed by the administration of pure oxygen the patient becomes increasingly drowsy and comatose until finally breathing ceases altogether. In view of this paradox a compromise has to be reached whereby the patient is given a mixture of oxygen and air using a Venti-mask (see Chapter 47, Fig. 47/1, p. 450) which is specially designed to deliver a 30 per cent mixture of oxygen with air. When respiration is markedly depressed the respiratory centre can sometimes be artificially stimulated by the use of drugs such as amiphenazole (Daptazole) or nikethamide (Coramine). Occasionally a tracheostomy has to be performed and breathing maintained by a respirator.

Bronchial asthma is characterized by episodes of severe spasm of the muscle in the walls of the bronchi. The attacks usually begin in childhood or adolescence but in some people the onset is later. When the disease begins in childhood there is often a history of other members of the family suffering from either hay fever, urticaria, infantile eczema or a combination of these. The constriction of the bronchi is produced by an abnormal hypersensitivity or allergic reaction to proteins in the environment. This is called *extrinsic asthma*. The proteins include ones which are inhaled, such as pollens, moulds, house dust, animal hair, face powder and dandruff: also, but less commonly, proteins in food such as eggs, milk, fish or chocolate. In addition, the bronchi in an allergic subject may go into spasm in response to emotional stress. When the disease starts in middle age there is often no evidence of allergy to external proteins and it is assumed that such a patient must be allergic to his own internal body protein. This is called *intrinsic asthma*.

An attack of asthma starts suddenly with intense constriction of the bronchi so that within minutes the patient is wheezing loudly and gasping for breath. Cough and sputum do not appear until the attack has been present for some time. There is a wide variation in the frequency and duration of attacks from patient to patient. In between, an asthmatic may often appear to be in good health but frequent severe episodes lead to the development of emphysema, and in children result in loss of weight, stunted growth and deformities of the chest wall.

In asthma, as in other allergic disorders, there is a considerable increase in the number of eosinophil cells in the blood; in addition the sputum often contains solid plugs in which eosinophil cells may be found.

Status asthmaticus is a severe, prolonged, life-threatening attack of asthma requiring prompt, skilled and energetic treatment. Such an attack may be controlled by an intravenous injection of aminophylline but often the violent allergic reaction in the bronchi has to be suppressed by the injection of corticosteroids using either hydrocortisone, intravenously, or intramuscular injections of corticotrophin.

Formerly the routine treatment of asthma included sucking a tablet of isoprenaline sulphate or the subcutaneous injection of a 1 in 1,000 solution of adrenaline, but these methods have been superseded since the introduction of *bronchodilator aerosols* containing either isoprenaline or adrenaline or orciprenaline (Alupent) or salbutamol (Ventolin) which are easy to use, readily portable and very efficient as they deliver a measured dose of the substance directly into the respiratory tract. Persistent incapacitating asthma requires the use of oral steroids such as prednisone or the twice or thrice weekly injections of corticotrophin (ACTH).

It is essential to try to prevent future attacks. The recent introduction of disodium cromoglycate (Intal), a substance which when regularly inhaled suppresses bronchial allergy in a large proportion of people affected, is already proving useful in reducing the frequency of attacks. In addition it is sometimes helpful to ascertain which proteins are particularly harmful by taking an accurate history, paying special attention to the circumstances in which the attacks usually occur. Such information may be supplemented by that gained from skin testing. Occasionally, when the patient is found to be allergic only to one protein, it is possible to undertake desensitization, which involves giving injections of a very dilute solution of the protein once a week and gradually increasing the strength until finally a large amount can be injected without ill effect. This procedure is of particular value in those who suffer from hay fever and grass pollen asthma.

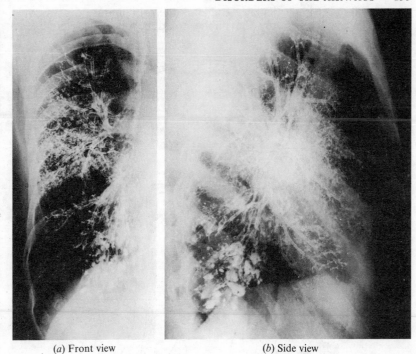

(a) Front view   (b) Side view

Fig. 21/3 Bronchogram showing bronchiectasis of the right lower lobe.

Bronchiectasis. In this disease the bronchi are abnormally widened, the bronchial mucus collects in large pools where it readily becomes infected, and this leads to the expectoration of large quantities of purulent, foul-smelling sputum which for some unknown reason is associated with the development of gross clubbing of the fingers.

The widening of the bronchi may be the result of a developmental error or may arise from disease acquired after birth. This occurs when the airways become weakened by acute bronchopneumonia (either primary or secondary to whooping cough or measles) in infancy; also, when pressure from an enlarged tuberculous lymph gland against a main bronchus or a foreign body impacted within one, leads to collapse of part of a lung with distension of the smaller bronchi contained within it. These dilated air tubes may be demonstrated on an X-ray after filling them with a radio-opaque iodized vegetable oil (see Fig. 21/3).

Treatment includes regular emptying of the damaged bronchi by postural tipping: the combating of infection by antibiotics; and in cases where the disease is localized, the surgical removal of the affected part.

Carcinoma of the bronchus (lung cancer). During recent years deaths from lung cancer have increased far more than from any other malignant disease. It attacks ten times as many men as women and mostly affects people in middle life. At the present time there are about 30,000 deaths a year in England and Wales from this disease, in a population of approximately

50,000,000. This is particularly tragic as these premature deaths could mostly be avoided if only the public could be persuaded to give up cigarette smoking.

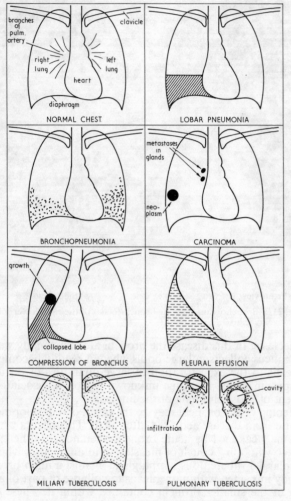

Fig. 21/4 Drawings of chest radiographs. In routine X-rays of the chest, normal air-containing lung appears black whereas solid structures such as the heart, blood vessels and areas of diseased lung cast white shadows. (a) Normal chest. (b) Solidified lobe of lung in pneumonia. (c) Bronchopneumonia with foci of infection around terminal bronchi. (d) Bronchial carcinoma with metastases at the root of the lung (e) Compression of bronchus by a growth, resulting in a collapsed lobe. (f) Pleural effusion. Note that the heart and the trachea are displaced to the opposite side. (g) Miliary tuberculosis, showing widespread seeding of the lungs with foci of infection around arterioles. (h) Pulmonary tuberculosis, showing cavity formation on each side with infiltration of the lungs surrounding the cavities.

Cancer of the lung is caused by malignant changes in the epithelial cells lining the wall of a bronchus. A tumour growing in a main bronchus eventually blocks it, cutting off the air supply to the area of the lung beyond, which therefore collapses (Fig. 21/4e). Stagnant secretions in the collapsed area of lung may then become secondarily infected with the development of an acute pneumonia (see p. 202). A tumour arising in the periphery of the lung (Fig. 21/4d) may invade the pleura with the production of a pleural effusion which is often bloodstained. In addition central and peripheral tumours may extend into neighbouring structures with the enlargement of lymph glands, erosion of ribs and vertebrae, irritation of nerve roots, compression of the superior vena cava with the development of obstructive swelling of the face and neck and, most important of all, invasion of the pulmonary veins with spread to other parts of the body including the brain, the bones and the liver.

Carcinoma of the bronchus may present in a variety of ways. Persistent cough and sputum in an otherwise fit middle-aged person or increase in the cough and sputum of a chronic bronchitic, should rouse suspicion. The sputum may be bloodstained or there may be a frank haemoptysis. The possibility of a growth has to be considered when a pneumonia recurs or takes a protracted course. Not infrequently the presenting symptoms are from metastases outside the lung, before the tumour in the lung is recognized. The onset of a neurological disorder or the development of severe pain in a bone are common examples.

Investigation and treatment of bronchial carcinoma. In any suspicious case a chest X-ray is essential. This may show either a rounded opacity or collapse of part or of the whole of a lung with or without evidence of secondary infection, or there may be the appearance of a pleural effusion. Bronchoscopy is a very important investigation as the tumour arising in a main bronchus may readily be seen and a small piece removed for histological examination. The sputum and any pleural fluid should be examined for neoplastic cells; if there is an enlarged lymph gland in the neck this should be removed for histological examination.

When the growth is confined to the lung without evidence of metastases in other parts of the body it is removed, together with surrounding healthy lung and neighbouring lymph nodes. Unfortunately, approximately three out of four patients are unsuitable for surgery when first seen, either because the growth in the lung has extended too far up the main bronchus or because of the presence of metastases in other organs or because the patient is too short of breath. Of the minority of patients who are fit for surgery only about 25 per cent survive for five years. Deep X-ray therapy (see Chapter 64, p. 680) is useful in the relief of symptoms, particularly those associated with superior vena caval obstruction and for the relief of pain arising from bone erosion.

DISEASES OF THE LUNGS

The pneumonias. The term pneumonia is used to describe any inflammation of the lung. There are several different types including:

    Lobar pneumonia.
    Bronchopneumonia.

Virus pneumonia.
Inhalation pneumonia.
Aspiration pneumonia.
Pneumonia secondary to bronchial obstruction.

The term *pneumonitis* has also been introduced in connection with inflammation of the lung other than that associated with lobar pneumonia and bronchopneumonia but there is little to recommend this.

Lobar pneumonia. The inflammation involves the whole of one or more lobes, causing the affected tissue to be airless and solid. The area of consolidation shows on an X-ray as a large dense opacity (Fig. 21/4b). The illness has a sudden onset, usually affecting fit young adults. The patient quickly becomes ill with fever, rigors, rapid breathing, pain in the chest, cough and purulent sputum which may be bloodstained. Before the introduction of antibiotics this disease was frequently fatal but if the patient survived for eight days the temperature suddenly subsided and from then on recovery was usually uneventful. This dramatic course is no longer seen because although the infective organism is a virulent strain of pneumococcus it is readily killed by penicillin.

Bronchopneumonia. Localized patches of consolidation form around the ends of the bronchi usually in the lower part of both lungs. On an X-ray these patches appear as diffusely scattered small opacities (Fig. 21/4c). The clinical picture is similar to that seen in lobar pneumonia except that bronchopneumonia occurs in those whose resistance to infection is poor so that the very young, the elderly and those whose health is undermined by chronic disease are particularly prone. Also it is liable to affect anyone whose respiration is depressed when in coma from a cerebral haemorrhage or drug poisoning, or whose chest movements are restricted because of pain following a surgical operation, or whose lungs are oedematous from cardiac or renal failure. Finally it may complicate an acute exacerbation of chronic bronchitis.

The causative organisms are those usually found in the nose and upper air passages of healthy people and include streptococci, *Haemophilus influenzae* and non-virulent strains of pneumococci which, when the body's resistance becomes lowered, spread down the airways to infect the lungs. Antibiotics used to combat these organisms include a combination of intramuscular penicillin and streptomycin or the oral administration of tetracycline or ampicillin.

Inhalation pneumonia. An area of pneumonia may be caused by the inhalation of food material into the respiratory tract; this may occur when an anaesthetized patient inhales vomit or when an obstructive lesion in the oesophagus, such as a carcinoma, results in food material spilling over into the lungs when the patient is asleep.

Aspiration pneumonia. A segment of a lobe may become infected when pus is aspirated into a bronchus from a site of infection in the upper respiratory tract. It may therefore be a complication of acute sinusitis or occur after the removal of infected teeth.

Complications of pneumonia

When the infective organisms causing a pneumonia are especially virulent there is destruction of lung tissue with the formation of an *abscess cavity* containing a large quantity of pus. The patient becomes extremely ill with high fever, marked constitutional disturbances and clubbing of the fingers. After some days the abscess may burst into the bronchus with the expectoration of large amounts of foul-smelling purulent sputum. The patient requires energetic postural drainage skilfully applied by a qualified physiotherapist, in addition to antibiotics.

An *empyema* is a collection of pus in the pleural cavity: its treatment is described on p.582.

Pulmonary infarction. The death or necrosis of an area of lung, caused by the sudden arrest of its arterial blood supply, usually occurs when a clot of blood (thrombus) in a peripheral vein undergoes fragmentation and a part of the clot (embolus) is carried in the circulation until eventually it plugs a terminal pulmonary arteriole. These conditions and their management are described on p. 469.

The Pneumoconioses are a group of lung diseases caused by the inhalation of dust during the course of work. One of the best known is widespread fibrosis of the lungs occurring in coal miners exposed to a mixture of silica and coal dust. More recently the danger of exposure to asbestos has been recognized. Mined in Canada, Italy and South Africa, it is widely used as an insulating material and for the lagging of pipes and boilers. Not only may it cause widespread fibrosis of the lungs but it is also associated with the development of a highly malignant type of growth known as a mesothelioma.

DISEASES OF THE PLEURA

Pleural effusion. Disease of the pleura may lead to the outpouring of fluid into the pleural cavity. This may complicate pneumonia, pulmonary infarction, bronchial carcinoma and tuberculosis. Also fluid in the pleural cavity may arise during the course of cardiac failure (Fig. 21/4f).

Spontaneous pneumothorax. Rupture of the lung wall with escape of air into the pleural cavity may occur in otherwise fit people. Sometimes there is an obvious cyst on the lung surface which ruptures, but often there is only a minute hole arising at the site of a localized area of developmental weakness in the wall. Rarely it is a complication of some underlying disease in the lung such as tuberculosis. (See also Chapter 58.)

PULMONARY TUBERCULOSIS

Tuberculous infection of the lungs is of two types:

primary and
post-primary reinfection, or adult type.

Primary infection. Tubercle bacilli on first entering the lungs set up a localized reaction usually no larger than a small coin (*Ghon focus*). From there the organisms are carried by the lymphatics to the neighbouring lymph glands at the hilum or root of the lung causing them to undergo considerable enlargement. Usually the infection in the lung and the regional lymph glands, known collectively as the *primary complex*, heals spontaneously without the development of any symptoms, but occasionally the infection in the lymph glands leads to complications which cause the person concerned to become ill.

The course of the infection depends largely on the age at which it is first acquired. The resistance of infants to the disease is very poor so that infection occurring in the first year of life is always dangerous, but natural immunity gradually improves so that from the age of 5 to 12 any infection usually passes unnoticed. Once adolescence is reached, however, resistance once again diminishes so that infection at this time may be accompanied by ill-health.

It must be emphasized that primary infection in childhood is usually a symptomless self-healing disease but occasionally the enlarged hilar lymph glands compress a bronchus, causing collapse of part of the lung, or worse still erode the wall of the bronchus, discharging infected material into the air tubes which then becomes widely disseminated throughout the lungs with the production of a tuberculous bronchopneumonia. Even more serious is when the glands erode the pulmonary veins, causing infected material to be carried in the blood and disseminated throughout the body. When a large number of virulent tubercle bacilli are released into the circulation, multiple small foci of infection appear around the terminal arterioles in every organ of the body, producing what is known as *miliary tuberculosis* (Fig. 21/4g). This term is derived from the appearance of these small foci of infection, which are considered to resemble millet seeds. Before effective chemotherapy was discovered miliary tuberculosis was invariably fatal, but this type of infection can now readily be brought under control. When the number of tubercle bacilli released into the circulation is smaller infection may be confined to an individual organ such as the brain, causing *meningitis*, or a joint with resultant *arthritis*, or the kidney with the production of a *pyelonephritis*.

Tuberculin tests

A person suffering from a tuberculous infection or who has had the disease in the past reacts strongly to tuberculin (a protein derived from tubercle bacilli) when it is injected into the skin. The test devised by the French physician Charles Mantoux entails injecting various dilutions of tuberculin (1 in 10,000, 1 in 1,000, and 1 in 100) into the skin. The skin is examined 48 to 72 hours later and a positive reaction consists of an area of oedema 5 mm or more in diameter with surrounding erythema.

Another test now widely used was devised by Professor Frederick Heaf: an instrument known as a Heaf gun is pressed against a drop of concentrated tuberculin placed on the skin; the gun is then fired releasing six needles which penetrate the skin, driving the tuberculin into it. This test is also read about 72 hours later when a positive reaction consists of an area of oedema around four or more of the needle marks (grade I) or the coalescence of the oedematous areas to form an elevated ring (grade II) or the replacement of the whole area by a plaque of oedema (grade III). More extensive induration with central blistering is known as grade IV.

Until some years after the Second World War pulmonary tuberculosis was so widespread in Great Britain that by the time adolescence was reached most people had a positive tuberculin skin test, denoting that at some time in their childhood they had had a tuberculous infection. In recent years not more than about 5 to 10 per cent of school leavers are found to have a positive test. The majority, therefore, are in danger that if they should become infected for the first time during early adult life it is at a time when their natural resistance is diminished.

In 1911 two Frenchmen, Calmette and Guérin, grew a particularly weak strain of tubercle bacilli known as B.C.G. vaccine, which when injected into the human body produces only a localized reaction but which at the same time promotes the development of acquired resistance against any future infection with virulent tubercle bacilli. The vaccine is usually given into the skin in the outer part of the upper arm where it produces a raised papule 7 to 10 mm in diameter, together with, particularly in babies, some enlargement of the neighbouring lymph glands. At the present time in this country B.C.G. vaccine is given to all babies exposed to infection, also to tuberculin-negative school leavers and in addition to people whose work brings them into contact with the disease.

Adult post-primary or re-infection type of tuberculosis. Tuberculosis in the adult differs from that of childhood insomuch that instead of the lymph glands being mainly affected the disease is confined to the lungs. It starts with a localized area of inflammatory change, usually in the upper part of one lung, from where it spreads to adjacent lung tissue and by way of the bronchi to other parts of the lung. On an X-ray, inflammatory changes appear as fluffy cotton wool areas of infiltration with cavities in places where the inflammation has destroyed the lung tissue (Fig. 21/4h).

Adult type tuberculosis may be relatively advanced and yet remain symptomless: it is because of this that until recently large groups of apparently fit people in offices, factories and the armed services, have had periodic examinations by *mobile mass miniature radiography units.* When this method of detection was first introduced during the Second World War large numbers of apparently symptomless but in fact infectious cases of tuberculosis were discovered, but as in recent years the number of cases found by this method has become progressively less the mobile X-ray service is being curtailed.

Most large hospitals have static miniature X-ray units, and general practitioners are encouraged to refer to them anyone who has a persistent dry cough or cough with sputum, particularly if it is bloodstained, and in addition anyone complaining of undue tiredness, loss of weight or fever. Hoarseness of voice may occur in advanced cases from spread of infection from the lung into the larynx. Pain, however, is not a symptom of pulmonary tuberculosis unless the infection is involving the pleura.

Tuberculosis may be extensive and still not produce any physical signs on clinical examination of the chest, so that radiological investigation is essential for its diagnosis. At the same time sputum should be stained and examined under the microscope for tubercle bacilli. This type of direct examination, however, will only reveal tubercle bacilli when present in large numbers. If there are only a few it is first necessary to encourage their growth by culturing the sputum in an incubator for up to six weeks, after which time the characteristic colonies of tubercle bacilli may be seen.

Treatment. At one time the only treatment available was bed rest, good food, fresh air, with, in addition, methods of immobilizing a lung either temporarily or permanently. Temporary procedures included injecting air into the pleural cavity, *pneumothorax*, or into the peritoneal cavity, *pneumoperitoneum*, so that the lung might be rested by restricting its movements. There were also several methods of permanently collapsing part of a lung. The most effective but deforming procedure was a *thoracoplasty*, an operation involving the removal of several ribs (see p. 588).

Treatment underwent a radical change following the discovery of streptomycin by Selman Waksman in 1944, a bacteriologist working in America. He showed that this substance inhibits the growth of tubercle bacilli in the laboratory and when the drug was first given to tuberculous patients the effect was remarkable, with almost immediate control of fever, reduction in the volume of sputum and improvement in the disease as shown by the clearing of radiological shadows. The benefit, however, proved to be short lived, for after about three months' treatment it was found that the bacteria had become resistant to the effects of the drug. This was the first time that *the phenomenon of drug resistance* had been encountered although since then it has been observed with several other organisms. In the same year another drug, para-amino-salicylic acid (PAS), was discovered, which also had an adverse effect on the growth of tubercle bacilli in the laboratory, but when it was first given by itself to tuberculous patients its action proved to be very disappointing.

This observation that antituberculous drugs can be given effectively for long periods was a major advance in the battle against tuberculosis, because experience has shown that these drugs may have to be given for up to eighteen months to two years, in order to be certain that infection has been completely eradicated. In 1951 another powerful antituberculous drug known as isonicotinic acid hydrazide or Isoniazid (INAH) was introduced and this, together with streptomycin and PAS have been the drugs of first choice for many years. Recently two other drugs, rifampicin and ethambutol, have also proved to be extremely useful in the treatment of this disease.

When tuberculosis is first diagnosed it is essential to show, by laboratory tests, that the tubercle bacilli in the sputum are not resistant to any of these drugs. These tests take three months to complete, during which time, as a precautionary measure, three drugs are administered. Once the result of the tests is known, two drugs of proven efficacy are continued for several more months.

It is important that a nurse should be familiar with the various side-effects that may arise from the use of these drugs. Streptomycin may produce an allergic or hypersensitive reaction with fever and/or rashes. In addition it sometimes has a toxic effect on the vestibular apparatus with resultant giddiness; a symptom which is especially likely to occur in those over the age of 40, causing the patient to stagger, particularly in the dark. The condition is reversible provided there is no appreciable delay in stopping the drug. A further disadvantage is that the drug has to be administered intramuscularly whereas the other drugs are given by mouth. PAS may also produce allergic reactions with fever, rashes, enlargement of lymph glands and sometimes jaundice. Also it commonly has an irritant effect on the gastro-intestinal tract with the development of diarrhoea and vomiting; for this reason, since drugs with less tendency to side-effects became available, its use has declined considerably. Isoniazid has no side-effects in the dosage usually employed, neither has rifampicin, providing it is not used in the presence of pre-existing liver disease. Ethambutol may occasionally cause disturbances of vision but these are reversible providing the drug is promptly discontinued. Since the introduction of effective chemotherapy the indications for surgery have become remarkably few. Occasionally resection of a damaged lobe or lung becomes necessary when the causative organisms are resistant to the principal drugs, or when there is severe secondary infection not readily controllable by antibiotics.

The general management of a case of pulmonary tuberculosis depends on the circumstances of each individual. Certain cases of non-infectious tuberculosis may be given chemotherapy while continuing at work; most patients, however, require to stop work for two to three months. Some people, particularly the elderly, can have all their treatment at home, but it is usually wise to admit a recently diagnosed case to hospital for six to eight weeks so that the initial stages of chemotherapy can be supervised and the patient instructed in taking the drugs strictly as prescribed. Bed rest is not required unless the patient is toxic or febrile.

On discharge from hospital another month should be spent at home and then, provided sputum tests and X-rays show that satisfactory progress has been made, a return to work should be encouraged while chemotherapy is continued, to complete a two-year course. Patients who take their chemotherapy conscientiously and for the required period of time, may confidently be reassured that recovery is always complete without any fear of relapse.

Chapter 22

Disorders of the Heart and Circulation

by T. M. CHALMERS

> *General considerations: disturbances of heart rate and rhythm—heart failure—atherosclerosis—ischaemic heart disease—hypertension—rheumatic heart disease—infective endocarditis—venous thrombosis and pulmonary embolism—drugs used in heart disease (for nursing considerations see Chapter 14)*

DISTURBANCES OF HEART RATE AND RHYTHM
(see also pp. 34–6)

Tachycardia, or a rapid heart rate, is found in anxiety, shock, haemorrhage, fever, hyperthyroidism and many other conditions.

Bradycardia, or a slow heart rate (less than 60 per minute), is not unusual in athletes. A slow heart rate may be associated with jaundice and increased intracranial pressure. The rate accelerates with exercise unless it is due to heart block. Bradycardia is common after myocardial infarction.

Extrasystoles, or premature beats, are due to abnormal stimuli arising in various parts of the heart, particularly the ventricles. They are common in organic heart disease, but more frequently no other cardiac signs are detected. They are sometimes due to overdosage with digitalis when *coupled rhythm* may appear, the heart beats being grouped in pairs followed by a pause.

Atrial fibrillation is an irregularity in which there is an absence of co-ordinated atrial contraction, tumultuous rapid twitching of atrial muscle fibres and total irregularity of the ventricular beats. Apart from extrasystoles, atrial fibrillation is the most common disturbance of rhythm. It is usually associated with organic heart disease, and may occur transiently in acute rheumatic fever, pneumonia, myocardial infarction and pulmonary embolism. It is common in chronic rheumatic heart disease, especially mitral stenosis, and in hyperthyroidism. The pulse is rapid and totally irregular in rate and volume. Simultaneous auscultation and palpation of the pulse usually reveals a *pulse deficit*. Digitalis slows the ventricular rate and reduces the deficit by allowing more time for diastolic filling. Patients may carry on satisfactorily for years when the rate is controlled. However, sluggishness of blood flow in the atrial appendages plus lack of co-ordinated contractions promotes *formation of clots* and their dispersal in the bloodstream.

Infarction of brain, spleen and kidneys, and occlusion of peripheral arteries may occur. Pulmonary infarcts result from thrombi from the right atrium. To prevent these complications younger patients with chronic fibrillation are often maintained on an anticoagulant drug. When fibrillation is not associated with severe heart disease normal rhythm may be restored by electrical treatment, *cardioversion*.

Heart block, or atrioventricular block, occurs when stimuli arising in the atria are delayed or obstructed in their passage down the atrioventricular bundle. Block may be partial or complete. In complete heart block the ventricle beats regularly at 10 to 50 beats per minute and the patient often complains of syncopal attacks. Heart failure may result. Exercise does not increase the rate. Electrical pacemakers or isoprenaline may be used to increase the heart rate. Heart block complicating myocardial infarction may respond to atropine.

In **ventricular tachycardia** there is a fairly regular rhythm with a rapid rate caused by stimuli arising from an irritable focus in one of the ventricles. It may follow myocardial infarction or may be a toxic effect of digitalis. Ventricular tachycardia and frequent ventricular extrasystoles may herald the appearance of *ventricular fibrillation*, a common cause of cardiac arrest and sudden death, especially in coronary patients. Ventricular arrhythmias may be prevented by intravenous lignocaine or oral procainamide or in some cases by atropine. The management of cardiac arrest is discussed on p. 448.

HEART FAILURE

Heart failure exists when the amount of blood pumped out by the heart is insufficient for the needs of the tissues. Although the heart may fail as a whole it is helpful to consider failure of the left and right sides of the heart separately.

Left ventricular failure is usually due to hypertension, coronary artery disease or aortic valve disease. The patient complains of weakness from decreased blood supply to the tissues and shortness of breath, *dyspnoea*, due to pulmonary congestion. At first dyspnoea occurs only on exertion. Later, as failure progresses, the patient becomes breathless at rest and may be unable to lie flat because of breathlessness, *orthopnoea*. He is subject to severe attacks of breathlessness, particularly at night, *paroxysmal nocturnal dyspnoea*, in which he wakes up gasping for breath and may cough up watery, bloodstained sputum. Severe attacks can usually be cut short by intravenous injections of morphine, aminophylline and frusemide (a rapidly acting diuretic): mild attacks subside in 20 to 30 minutes if untreated.

Right ventricular failure (congestive failure) is most often secondary to preceding left ventricular failure. It can also be caused by lung diseases, such as severe chronic bronchitis, or by congenital heart defects. The main features of right heart failure are (1) *increased central venous pressure* leading to distension of the neck veins and enlargement of the liver; and (2) *oedema*. The oedema is found in the dependent parts of the body, that is, in the feet and ankles if the subject is up and about and in the sacral region if he is confined to bed. Fluid may also collect in serous cavities to form a pleural effusion or ascites. Right-sided failure is treated by rest, digitalis to increase cardiac output and diuretics to promote the excretion of sodium and water.

ATHEROSCLEROSIS

Atherosclerosis is an extremely common form of arterial disease in which narrowing due to deposits of fatty material beneath the inner lining of the vessels leads to diminution or failure of blood supply to various tissues. When the blood supply is sufficiently reduced symptoms and signs appear. The organs most commonly affected are the heart, brain and kidneys. Atherosclerosis of limb vessels also produces typical clinical syndromes.

There is a great deal of clinical and experimental evidence that athero-sclerosis is intimately related to lipid metabolism. It is aggravated by diabetes, hypertension, obesity and cigarette smoking. It is uncommon in women before the menopause.

The most important clinical manifestations of atherosclerosis are undoubtedly cerebro-vascular disorders (p. 259) and ischaemic heart disease.

ISCHAEMIC HEART DISEASE

Narrowing or blockage of the coronary arteries impairs the function of the myocardium due to an insufficient supply of blood (ischaemia). The classic symptoms and signs are those of angina pectoris and myocardial infarction.

Angina pectoris is a syndrome consisting in paroxysmal substernal or precordial pain or discomfort of short duration, frequently radiating to the shoulders and inner aspects of the arms, usually precipitated by exertion, emotion or other states in which the work of the heart is increased, and relieved by rest or trinitrin. Exertion is the usual precipitating factor. Attacks are more readily induced after meals and also in cold weather by chilling or walking against the wind. The patient is usually forced to stop and rest and the pain then passes off within a few minutes. Trinitrin helps to relieve the pain and may prevent it if taken before exertion. In obese patients weight reduction may greatly reduce the frequency of attacks. Elimination of smoking is also beneficial. Adrenergic nerve blockade with drugs such as propranolol can be extremely helpful.

Acute myocardial infarction (coronary thrombosis) is characterized by prolonged substernal oppression or pain, progressive electrocardiographic changes, fever, leucocytosis, increased sedimentation rate and aspartate transferase (AST). It affects men about six times as often as women and is commonest after the age of 50. However, it is by no means rare in the thirties and forties and may even occur in the twenties. The mortality from the acute attack may be as high as 60 per cent. By far the commonest cause of death is *ventricular fibrillation* leading to cardiac arrest. The treatment is immediate electrical defibrillation. Where this can be carried out promptly, as in coronary care units, the prognosis is very good. External cardiac massage (p. 448) and mouth-to-mouth breathing followed by defibrillation within 5 to 15 minutes can also save lives. Unfortunately, most coronary deaths occur in the first two hours, before the patient can reach hospital.

One of the causes of ventricular fibrillation is believed to be the *intense vagal discharge* which follows infarction: the resultant sinus bradycardia or heart block increases ventricular irritability. Therefore if the heart rate is found to be less than 60 when the patient is first seen he should receive immediate treatment with intravenous atropine to block the vagus and increase the heart rate. An irregular heart rate in the absence of bradycardia may be an indication for the administration of lignocaine intravenously and intramuscularly to reduce ventricular irritability. Morphine 10 mg or diamorphine 5 mg may be given intravenously to relieve pain.

As soon as possible the patient is admitted to hospital, preferably to a coronary care unit.* It is desirable that the electrocardiogram should be continuously monitored for 48 to 72 hours so that cardiac arrest or pre-monitory irregularities can be immediately recognized and treated. To prevent venous thrombosis and pulmonary embolism an anticoagulant drug such as Warfarin is given for as long as the patient remains in bed (usually two to three weeks). Treatment with atropine or lignocaine may be needed as indicated above. Heart failure is treated with digitalis and diuretics. Cardiogenic shock, characterized by severe hypotension and collapse, may respond to atropine if bradycardia is present. Usually it is associated with very severe myocardial damage: treatment is ineffective and the prognosis is grave.

For the first few days strict rest is needed. The patient should not wash nor feed himself but may be allowed to use a bedside commode. He should not smoke. Pain and anxiety must be relieved. Gradual mobilization is usually possible after 10 to 20 days. Return to normal activity can be expected within about three months in most cases.

HYPERTENSION

Hypertension is present when the blood pressure exceeds 140/90 mm of mercury. Primary (essential) hypertension, of unknown aetiology, constitutes about 85 to 90 per cent of all cases. The remainder include various disorders in which there is a known underlying pathological process giving rise to secondary hypertension, such as acute and chronic glomerulone-phritis or an adrenal tumour.

Patients with *primary hypertension* are often symptomless and may survive for many years. Morning headaches may be present, disappearing when the blood pressure is lowered with drugs. There is a gradual hypertrophy of the left ventricle and eventually left ventricular failure may appear. Secondary to atherosclerotic changes in the coronary and cerebral arteries, angina pectoris, myocardial infarction and cerebro-vascular disorders are common. About 10 per cent of patients sustain a cerebral thrombosis or die from a cerebral haemorrhage. In the *accelerated (malignant) form*, diastolic pressure usually exceeds 130 and papill-

---

* The value of hospital admission has recently been questioned. A large-scale controlled trial of home versus hospital care is in progress in Britain.

oedema is present. Renal damage is progressive and death occurs within two years if the hypertension is untreated.

Management. Obesity should be corrected and smoking discouraged. Salt should not be added to food at meals. An antihypertensive drug such as methyldopa is prescribed in all but the mildest cases and may be combined with a diuretic such as bendrofluazide. Careful search is made for possible causes of secondary hypertension and where possible they are removed.

RHEUMATIC HEART DISEASE

Whereas hypertension and coronary artery disease are the commonest causes of heart disease in the middle aged and elderly, rheumatic fever is by far the commonest cause in childhood, adolescence and early adult life. Rheumatic heart disease includes inflammation of the endocardium, myocardium and pericardium occurring in the course of acute rheumatic fever; also those sequelae which persist after the acute process has subsided.

Rheumatic fever is a febrile disease which occurs as a delayed sequel of infections with group A haemolytic streptococci. It is primarily a disease of childhood with a peak incidence between the ages of 5 and 15 years. It is characterized by fever and migratory joint pains coming on typically one to four weeks after a streptococcal throat infection. Cardiac involvement is present to some degree in all cases although clinical evidence may be slight. Tachycardia, cardiac enlargement, various murmurs, electrocardiographic changes, pericarditis and heart failure may occur. The illness may last only a few weeks or continue for many months. Recurrences are common.

Treatment consists of bed rest together with salicylates or corticosteroids to suppress the inflammatory response. The prevention of recurrence depends on the prevention of streptococcal infections, and every rheumatic patient should receive continuous *prophylactic therapy* with penicillin through the school age and for at least five years following the last attack of the disease. Penicillin may be given orally twice a day or by long-acting injections at monthly intervals.

Most **chronic valvular heart disease** is of rheumatic origin. The diseased valve becomes stenosed (narrowed) or incompetent or both. Stenosis of a valve increases the work of the chamber behind the obstruction, while incompetence tends to increase the work both of the chamber in front of the incompetent valve and the one behind it.

Mitral disease is the commonest form of chronic valvular heart disease. In mitral *stenosis* there is interference with the flow of blood from the left atrium into the left ventricle during diastole. The increased pressure in the left atrium is transmitted backwards to the lungs causing exertional dyspnoea and sometimes haemoptysis. Later pulmonary arterial pressure rises and eventually right ventricular failure develops. Atrial fibrillation is common. *Arterial embolism is not infrequent*, most commonly affecting the brain, spleen, kidneys or extremities. Pulmonary infarction may also occur. Where disability from mitral stenosis is significant, and contraindications, such as long-standing right heart failure, are absent, mitral valvotomy (see p. 603) can offer the prospect of considerable benefit at reasonably low risk. *Mitral incompetence* causes left ventricular hypertrophy as well as producing a rise in left atrial pressure, etc. When it is severe an artificial valve is sometimes inserted. Stenosis and incompetence may occur together.

Aortic valvular disease is less common than mitral disease, with which it is frequently associated. *Aortic stenosis* is chiefly a disease of older men. The diseased valve often becomes calcified. Stenosis tends to develop slowly and there is time for considerable left ventricular hypertrophy to occur. Anginal pain is frequent and often severe. Some patients may develop symptoms of deficient cerebral blood flow with faintness and dizziness. Sudden death is common. The classic signs of aortic stenosis include a small, slowly rising pulse. Surgery may benefit certain patients. *Aortic incompetence* develops more rapidly than stenosis and is likely to produce left ventricular failure at an earlier age. If incompetence is of significant degree it is accompanied by peripheral signs of a widened pulse pressure, such as a collapsing pulse and arterial pulsation in the neck, see p. 36 (Corrigan's sign). Valve replacement is carried out in suitable cases.

INFECTIVE ENDOCARDITIS

Infective (subacute bacterial) endocarditis is a serious and often insidious complication of chronic valvular heart disease and congenital heart lesions. Repeated blood cultures are indicated in any patient who develops fever or malaise lasting more than a day or two. Clinical evidence of infective endocarditis includes changing murmurs, microscopic haematuria, splenomegaly and tender nodules in the fingers (Osler's nodes). Emboli may occur in any part of the arterial system: thus the presenting feature may be a stroke or sudden blockage of a limb artery.

The commonest infecting organism is *Streptococcus viridans* which is present in the mouth: it may enter the bloodstream during dental fillings or extractions. Patients at risk for infective endocarditis should always be protected with penicillin during dental treatment.

Treatment consists in the prolonged administration of a bactericidal antibiotic, e.g. penicillin for six weeks. This usually eradicates the infection. Valve replacement is required where damage has been severe.

VENOUS THROMBOSIS AND PULMONARY EMBOLISM

Clotting of blood within the veins is an extremely common and serious condition. Predisposing factors are prolonged bed rest or external pressure, local injury to the vein wall and increased coagulability of the blood following childbirth, surgical trauma or myocardial infarction. *Thrombosis* usually begins in the deep veins of the calf. It may be accompanied by pain, swelling and tenderness in the limb. The most serious complication is *pulmonary embolism* which follows dislodgement of a thrombus shortly after it has formed and before organization has fixed it firmly in the vein of origin. Forty per cent of pulmonary emboli occur postoperatively, 30 per cent in cardiac patients and 30 per cent in non-cardiac medical patients. Emboli may occur singly but are more often multiple.

The commonest symptoms of pulmonary embolism are sudden chest pain, sometimes pleuritic, moderate fever, cough and bloodstained sputum. With larger emboli or repeated small ones cyanosis, dyspnoea and right-sided heart failure may occur. Massive pulmonary embolism is associated with profound shock, acute right-sided failure and not infrequently sudden death. Pulmonary embolism and infarction should be suspected in chest pain without known causes, in atypical pleural effusion or pneumonitis and in any lingering low-grade unexplained fever, especially after operation. Clinical evidence of peripheral venous thrombosis, such as a swollen leg, is frequently absent.

Preventive measures include early ambulation, leg exercises and frequent turning in patients confined to bed, and the use of anticoagulant drugs. With an established pulmonary embolus or deep venous thrombosis anticoagulant therapy with heparin and Warfarin should be started immediately. Heparin may be stopped after the first few days but Warfarin should be continued for several months. In severe pulmonary embolism it may be necessary to remove the clot surgically or by infusion of streptokinase.

DRUGS USED IN HEART DISEASE

Digitalis and aminophylline

Digitalis, originally derived from the foxglove, is usually given in the form of *digoxin*. It slows and strengthens the heart beat. *Slowing of the heart* is most striking when atrial fibrillation is present, the effect being due to interference with the transmission of impulses from the atria to the ventricles. Slowing of the ventricular rate allows more time for diastolic filling and pumping becomes more efficient. The second important action of the drug is to *increase the force of contraction* of the failing ventricular muscle.

Enough of the drug must be given in the first 24 to 48 hours to produce full 'digitalization'—this usually requires 1·5 to 3 mg of digoxin in divided doses. Thereafter a maintenance dose varying from 0·05 to 0·5 mg daily is given. *Symptoms and signs of overdosage are common and include anorexia, nausea, vomiting, bradycardia and frequent extrasystoles.* If they occur the drug is withheld for one to two days until toxic manifestations disappear and then continued in a reduced dose. Serious intoxication with digitalis can induce arrhythmias and sudden death. Toxic effects are more likely in the presence of potassium depletion which frequently complicates diuretic therapy unless potassium supplements are given.

Aminophylline increases cardiac output and is of value in acute left ventricular failure. It is given by slow intravenous injection.

Diuretics

Diuretics act on the renal tubules to decrease the reabsorption of sodium from the glomerular filtrate. As a result more sodium and water are excreted in the urine. Oedema diminishes and venous pressure is reduced.

Thiazides (e.g. chlorothiazide, bendrofluazide) are effective by mouth in a single morning dose. Initially, daily treatment may be required but subsequently the frequency of administration should be reduced as much as the condition of the patient permits. If a thiazide diuretic is required on more than two days a week supplementary *potassium chloride* should be given.

Frusemide and *ethacrynic acid* have a more rapid and powerful action than thiazide derivatives. They should be reserved for emergency use and for cases with resistant oedema.

Anti-arrhythmic drugs

Atropine blocks transmission at cholinergic (parasympathetic) nerve endings. It is used in the emergency treatment of sinus bradycardia and heart block following myocardial infarction. The dose is 0·6 mg intravenously repeated at two-minute intervals until the heart rate reaches 90 (the total dose should not exceed 3 mg).

Lignocaine and *procainamide* reduce ventricular excitability and are used to prevent serious ventricular arrhythmias after myocardial infarction. Since it is rapidly inactivated, lignocaine is usually given in hospital by intravenous infusion. (If required before admission to hospital 200 mg intramuscularly will maintain an effective blood level for two hours.) When intravenous lignocaine is no longer required procainamide may be given by mouth.

Practolol and other agents which block β-adrenergic receptors are used in the treatment of supraventricular arrhythmias, especially those induced by digitalis.

Isoprenaline increases the ventricular rate. A long-acting oral preparation (Saventrine) may be of value in chronic heart block.

Antihypertensives

Methyldopa reduces the vasoconstricting effects of sympathetic impulses on arteries and can bring about large falls in blood pressure. Usually the drug produces a fall in pressure both when the patient is lying and standing, but postural hypotension occurs and the patient should be warned of the danger of fainting on standing; the blood pressure should always be checked in both postures when adjusting the dosage. The usual starting dose is 250 mg twice daily; the maximum dose is 3 g daily. The effect is potentiated by diuretics. Side-effects may include stuffy nose, dry mouth, drowsiness, depression and gastro-intestinal upsets.

Guanethidine reduces sympathetic tone and causes a fall in blood pressure because it blocks the transmission of impulses in the sympathetic nerves. It is slowly excreted and can therefore be given in a single daily dose. Hypotension and faintness on standing up or after exertion are common. Weakness and diarrhoea and failure of ejaculation of semen are also troublesome side-effects.

Propranolol blocks β-adrenergic receptors. It reduces cardiac output and lowers blood pressure gradually. Postural hypotension does not occur because the vasoconstrictor pathway is intact. The drug is contra-indicated in patients with incipient heart failure, heart block and asthma.

Thiazide diuretics have an important role in the treatment of hypertension, usually in combination with another agent. Their action is due mainly to a reduction in plasma volume.

Drugs used in angina pectoris

Nitrites cause vasodilatation by a direct action on smooth muscle in the walls of blood vessels. Glyceryl trinitrate, *trinitrin*, tablets are used in anginal attacks to increase coronary blood flow. The tablet should be crunched up in the mouth so that the drug can be rapidly absorbed through the oral mucous membranes. Trinitrin is also useful as a prophylactic measure before a patient undertakes an activity which may produce anginal pain.

Propranolol protects the heart against inappropriate sympathetic stimulation. It is useful in the management of angina. The usual dose is 20 to 80 mg four times daily (see p. 215).

Chapter 23

Diseases of the Blood and Lymphatic System

by A. J. E. BRAFIELD

*Introduction—conditions involving the red cells—the white cells—
the platelets—the plasma constituents—diseases of the lymphatic
system*

Blood is composed of cells and plasma and either may be involved in
disease. Most of the cells are derived from the bone marrow, and it is for
this reason that a *marrow puncture* is performed in many blood diseases,
since an examination of the young cells to be found there may give a clue
to the diagnosis.

An increase in the number of leucocytes is termed *leucocytosis*; a decrease,
leucopenia. *Thrombocytopenia* is a decrease in the number of platelets.
An increase in all types of cells is termed *polycythaemia*, while a decrease
in the red cells or haemoglobin is *anaemia*.

Haemoglobin is a red substance which is carried inside red cells. It has
a very complicated chemical structure, of which iron forms an important
part. Its function is to carry oxygen from the lungs to the rest of the body.

CONDITIONS INVOLVING THE RED CELLS

Anaemia is by far the commonest condition to be found in hospital
patients; probably more than 50 per cent have some degree of anaemia.
Certain *symptoms* are common to all anaemias whatever the cause; these
are due to the diminished oxygen-carrying capacity of the blood, and
include *fatigue, breathlessness, palpitation, headache* and *loss of appetite*.

The anaemias may be grouped as follows, according to their cause.

(*a*) Deficiency anaemias.
(*b*) Haemolytic anaemias.
(*c*) Aplastic anaemias.
(*d*) Haemoglobinopathies.

In the **deficiency anaemias** there is a lack of the materials necessary to
build red cells and haemoglobin, such as *iron, protein, vitamin B_{12}* and *folic
acid*. This occurs when the patient takes an inadequate diet. Pregnant
women and growing children need more iron than a healthy adult male,
and unless they are provided with extra iron in their diet they will develop
an *iron deficiency anaemia*. The same will occur if the body is depleted of
iron by chronic haemorrhage as happens in menorrhagia or bleeding

peptic ulcer. The anaemia is described as *hypochromic* because the red cells are poorly coloured due to a low content of haemoglobin.

When vitamin B_{12} is deficient the anaemia is characterized by red cells which are very large (*macrocytic*). This vitamin is found in meat, eggs and milk, but can only be absorbed after combination with a substance known as the '*intrinsic factor*' which is secreted by the stomach. Surgical removal of the stomach will be followed by *macrocytic anaemia*.

In *pernicious anaemia* the stomach is unable to secrete the intrinsic factor and so the patient cannot absorb vitamin B_{12}. In addition to the usual symptoms of anaemia (see p. 217), these patients are often prematurely grey, while the tongue is often smooth and very sore, and the skin has a lemon-yellow tint. Diarrhoea is sometimes troublesome. Paralysis occasionally results from degeneration of the spinal cord.

An almost identical anaemia results from a *diet deficient in folic acid* (found in green vegetables), especially when the need of the patient is increased, as happens particularly in pregnancy.

To *treat a deficiency anaemia* it is necessary to provide that which the patient lacks. *Iron* is usually given in tablet form, e.g. as ferrous sulphate or gluconate, or by intramuscular or intravenous injection, over a period of weeks or months. Sometimes the total deficiency is calculated and given as a single intravenous infusion. This method of *total dose infusion* (T.D.I.) has the advantage that the patient requires no further treatment, but it is not without risk and requires very careful supervision. *Vitamin B_{12}* is administered by injection. *Folic acid* is prescribed in tablet form. A liberal well-balanced diet is prescribed in all cases.

The haemolytic anaemias. Anaemia may also result from the premature destruction of red cells within the circulation. Such haemolytic anaemias are of two kinds. There may, for instance, be an *antibody* present in the plasma which destroys the red cells. A report from the laboratory of a positive Coombs' test indicates that such an antibody has been discovered. Alternatively the red cells may themselves be abnormal and consequently unable to live for more than two or three weeks. (The normal life of a red cell is four months.) The commonest anaemia of this second group is *congenital spherocytosis* in which the cells tend to be spherical in shape instead of flattened and disc-shaped.

All these patients exhibit the usual symptoms of anaemia, but in addition they are jaundiced. This is a direct consequence of the large amount of haemoglobin which is being destroyed.

Treatment is not always satisfactory. Steroids are of value if an antibody is present. If the cells are abnormal, the spleen (whose normal function is to remove abnormal cells) may be removed with some benefit to the patient.

Aplastic anaemias. Occasionally anaemia is caused by the marrow being damaged and unable to produce cells. Such aplastic anaemias may follow the use of drugs, such as chloramphenicol. More often no cause is discernible. Red cells, white cells and platelets are all reduced in number, so that in addition to anaemia the patient may suffer from severe infections and from haemorrhage.

Treatment. Steroids are sometimes helpful and repeated transfusions are necessary to sustain life. The long course of treatment and frequent transfusions are demoralizing and the patient requires consideration and reassurance. Infection must be combated by antibiotics.

Haemoglobinopathies. These form a group of cases in which the patients are unable to synthesize normal haemoglobin. Adult haemoglobin is designated by the letter A—haemoglobin A. The fetus has a different haemoglobin—haemoglobin F, which changes to A as the fetus matures. These two are normal haemoglobins, but amongst some peoples, notably Africans, are to be found many with *abnormal haemoglobins* which are designated by the letters C, D, E, etc. The majority do not give rise to symptoms, but one is of major importance—haemoglobin S. This is the cause of *sickle cell anaemia*, in which condition the red cells assume the shape of a sickle when the patient is starved of oxygen such as might occur at a high altitude. The distorted cells block small blood vessels and cause a variety of symptoms. Leg ulcers, haematuria and abdominal crises are common. The patient is often markedly anaemic.

In *thalassaemia* the patient has difficulty in producing normal haemoglobin A, but does not substitute an abnormal haemoglobin as far as we know. In consequence he suffers a *hypochromic anaemia* (see page 218) which may be very severe, but which does not respond to iron. The condition is found amongst the peoples of South-east Europe and those living on the borders of the Mediterranean.

Both sickle cell anaemia and thalassaemia are ultimately fatal if the patient has inherited the disease from both parents. There is no cure for either condition. Sickle cell cases should be protected from conditions of low oxygen tension as occurs, for example, in high flying aircraft and during general anaesthesia. Pneumonia is a serious hazard to these patients.

Polycythaemia is a condition in which there is an excess of all cells, but the red cell increase predominates. Sometimes this merely indicates that the body is suffering from a shortage of oxygen, as in bronchitis, and the extra cells represent an attempt by the body to compensate. At other times the cause for the marrow activity remains a mystery. Patients with polycythaemia are recognizable by their florid complexions.

Treatment consists of removing the cause, if known. The second variety is treated by radiation and by regular blood letting.

CONDITIONS INVOLVING THE WHITE CELLS

There are three kinds of white cell in the blood.

1. Polymorphs (also referred to as 'granulocytes').
2. Lymphocytes.
3. Monocytes.

Their number varies between 5 and 10 thousand per cubic millimetre of blood. Their function is mainly to combat infection.

Leukaemia is a malignant condition of the blood. The disease may be acute or chronic. *In the acute disease* death usually occurs within six months, while chronic cases may live for years even without treatment. The condition may be *lymphatic, monocytic* or *granulocytic* (myeloid) according to the type of cell involved. Blood leucocyte counts range from below normal to half a million per cubic millimetre. There are a host of drugs which may be used in treatment, particularly of acute leukaemia, but results are disappointing. Frequent blood transfusions may be required because of the profound anaemia which occurs in all cases. The patients are susceptible to infections and may require antibiotics. *In chronic leukaemia* life may be prolonged for months or years with suitable treatment.

Agranulocytosis is a serious condition marked by the disappearance of granulocytes (polymorphs) from the circulation. The usual cause is damage to the marrow by drugs such as the sulphonamides. With the removal of the protective effect of the polymorphs, micro-organisms act unhindered and necrotic ulceration of the mucous membranes occurs, particularly of the mouth and throat. *Treatment* is with antibiotics in an attempt to control the infection until the marrow has had time to recover.

CONDITIONS INVOLVING THE PLATELETS

Platelets are tiny cells whose function is to prevent bleeding. A healthy person has between 200,000 and 500,000 platelets per cubic millimetre of blood.

Purpuras are a group of conditions in which a decrease in the number of platelets is manifested as minute haemorrhages into the skin, *petechiae*, and sometimes as haemorrhage from mucous membranes such as found in the gut, bladder or uterus. The cause of the platelet decrease may be allergy, or infection (as in acute fevers) or drugs. In the commonest variety the cause is unknown. *Treatment* is with steroids. Platelet transfusions are given in serious cases.

CONDITIONS INVOLVING THE PLASMA CONSTITUENTS

The plasma becomes altered in many diseases. Most striking are the changes which account for the congenital bleeding disorders, of which haemophilia is the best known. In these patients there is a lack of one or more of the so-called 'factors'—there are thirteen of them—which are necessary for normal clotting of the blood. In **haemophilia** the missing substance is factor VIII. The disease occurs in males, but is transmitted only by females, who do not themselves suffer any of the unpleasant consequences of the illness. *Christmas Disease* is clinically identical with haemophilia, but laboratory studies show that in these patients it is factor IX which is missing, not factor VIII. The condition derives its name from the first patient in whom it was described.

The simplest method of *treating* these patients is to give an infusion of *fresh frozen plasma* which contains all the necessary factors.

DISEASES OF THE LYMPHATIC SYSTEM

The lymphatic system is part of the circulatory system, behaving, as it were, as the middleman, working between the tissues and the blood, and acting as a filter which tries to prevent disease organisms or other poisonous products from reaching the blood from the tissues. Occasionally the lymphatics become blocked with dangerous waste matter, setting up local inflammation (lymphangitis).

Lymphangitis or inflammation of the lymphatic vessels is characterized by the presence of red lines under the skin; these are the inflamed vessels and can be traced to the nearest gland, which may also be affected (see also adenitis, below). The area around the inflamed lymphatics is tender and swollen, and signs of general constitutional disorder will accompany the condition when severe.

Adenitis is inflammation of the lymphatic glands, one gland or more being affected. As in lymphangitis, when due to the presence of a septic focus, the glands which drain the area will be infected. In the *upper limb* the first lymphatic gland is on the inner aspect of the elbow; very important large groups of glands lie in the axilla and below the clavicle. In the *lower limb* the first groups are the popliteal glands, then come large groups of inguinal glands in the groin. Several groups of glands lie in *the neck*, and these drain the mouth, nose and throat, so are often affected by septic inflammatory conditions.

Adenitis may be *simple* when the gland is inflamed, enlarged, tender, red and hot, but does not suppurate. *Suppurative adenitis* occurs when the inflammatory lesion forms pus. Adenitis may also be *tuberculous*, or *carcinomatous*.

The *treatment of simple adenitis* is by the administration of sulphonamides or antibiotics; *suppurative adenitis* necessitates incision and drainage of the infected gland.

When adenitis is severe it will be accompanied by a rise of temperature and the symptoms which are associated with this, and it will demand the ordinary nursing care applicable to such a condition.

Tuberculous adenitis is a chronic condition and does not cause the discomfort of an acute adenitis. The glands enlarge and may soften and require to be aspirated, but apart from this, modern treatment is strictly conservative, using only the appropriate antituberculous drugs.

Tumours of the lymph nodes are known as *lymphomas*. They may be benign, in which case simple surgical removal may be all that is required. *Lymphosarcoma* and *Hodgkin's disease* are malignant tumours which are very similar in their presentation and treatment. Both sexes and all ages are affected, though Hodgkin's disease tends to occur in a slightly younger age group (20 to 40 years). Lymphosarcoma tends to be more malignant than Hodgkin's disease, in which condition the patient may survive for many years. One or more groups of lymph nodes may be affected, and the tumours may reach considerable size. When the nodes within the chest or abdomen are affected there may be no external evidence of disease. Pressure internally may produce cardiac, respiratory, gastric, or renal symptoms. Variable fever may be a feature, and anaemia is common. The *diagnosis* is established by surgical removal and examination of a gland.

Treatment. General measures are most important. The patient should have a good diet well served, for he may have a poor appetite. Infections should be treated early and effectively. Anaemia may require blood transfusion. *Radiotherapy* is very successful in the early stages with large tumours melting away in a few days. In the later stages *chemotherapy* is usually necessary (see p. 681).

Chapter 24

Diseases of the Digestive System

by JAMES S. STEWART

> *The mouth—achalasia—hiatus hernia and reflux oesophagitis—carcinoma of the oesophagus—the stomach—peptic ulcer—carcinoma of the stomach—gastritis—regional enteritis—liver and biliary tract—pancreas—malabsorption—diseases of the colon—dysentery—worms—symptoms of gastro-intestinal disease*

Many patients with gastro-intestinal disorders are best managed by the closest co-operation between the medical and surgical teams of doctors and nurses or even on joint units. Where surgical treatment is mentioned in this chapter the reader is referred to p. 470 for operations on the stomach and biliary tract and to p. 487 for the large bowel. Food poisoning is dealt with in the Section on Communicable Diseases, p. 354.

Diagnosis, on which specific and curative treatment depends, relies first and foremost on an accurate analysis of the patient's symptoms. Inevitably, most patients give their medical histories by describing how their symptoms affect their everyday lives. While both nurses and doctors must always remain sympathetic, they must also draw out sufficient information to enable them, often together, to define a recognizable symptom pattern. You will be able to recognize a diagnostic pattern only when you are familiar with the group of symptoms which tends to be characteristic of one particular condition. Therefore, this chapter describes first the common disorders of the alimentary system which bring patients on to a 'medical' ward and then, in retrospect, the symptoms which most often take these patients to their doctors.

THE MOUTH

While the food is being chewed it is moistened by saliva which helps both tasting and swallowing. The saliva contains ptyalin which starts the digestion of starch. Ptyalin is an enzyme, a substance produced by the cells of the body which promotes and controls chemical reactions without being changed itself. Enzymes, also present in trace amounts in pancreatic juice and elsewhere, play an important part in digesting food and, later, making it available for use by the tissues.

The chewing, or mastication, of the food by the teeth is an important preliminary to digestion. Regular visits to the dentist are the best way of ensuring that the teeth remain adequate for this purpose and that, if dentures are necessary, they fit properly and do not cause ulcers on the mucous membranes of the cheeks or tongue. Bacterial infection of the root of a tooth may cause an *apical abscess*, sometimes producing malaise with or without low grade fever and local pain and tenderness. This condition needs dental treatment. Inflammation of the gums, *gingivitis*, is common in people with bad teeth and may proceed to *pyorrhoea*, a septic condition of the gums and underlying bone. The gums are swollen, recede and bleed easily. Pus is produced and swallowed and finally the teeth become loosened. *Although treatment is primarily dental, the nurse can make a good start by giving frequent hydrogen peroxide mouth washes and swabbing with glycerin to keep the mouth moist.* In epileptic patients gingivitis may be caused by phenytoin, an anticonvulsant drug.

Stomatitis, inflammation of the mouth, may be due mainly to poor oral hygiene but is especially liable to develop in association with dental sepsis, during a febrile illness or in seriously ill patients. A severe stomatitis, with ulceration and bleeding, is often seen in acute leukaemia. In most forms of stomatitis the gums and mouth are painful and dry and the mucous membrane is reddened. *Treatment* is by improving oral hygiene, including mouth washes as for pyorrhoea. Sometimes *aphthous ulcers* occur. These are small vesicles on the tongue, gums or inside of the mouth which form painful ulcers. They may be single or multiple, they often occur in healthy people without any other evidence of stomatitis, but they are sometimes found in association with gastro-intestinal or other disease.

Treatment is seldom effective but as the condition is painful the urge to 'do something' is strong and several local forms of treatment are tried, including antiseptics, anaesthetics and steroids.

When stomatitis is caused by infection with the fungus *Candida albicans* it is called *thrush*. Probably the most common predisposing factor to the development of thrush in hospital wards now is treatment with one of the tetracycline group of antibiotics, but oral thrush is also liable to develop in any severely ill patient. White plaques appear, most often on the palate and throat; they join together to form a membrane and peel off to reveal superficial ulceration. The most convenient effective treatment is with amphotericin lozenges sucked after each meal and last thing at night.

Glossitis, inflammation of the tongue, is usually chronic, producing a red, sore tongue made smooth by atrophy of the papillae. It may be associated with any of the above forms of stomatitis or with long-standing deficiency of iron or one of the B group of vitamins, especially folic acid or vitamin B_{12}. The treatment is that of the underlying condition.

ACHALASIA

The gullet, or oesophagus, is a muscular tube lined, like the rest of the alimentary tract, by mucous membrane, and takes the food from the pharynx to the stomach. The muscle in its upper part is striated, 'voluntary' muscle, but in the lower part and right down to the internal anal sphincter the muscle of the gastro-intestinal tract is unstriated, smooth muscle, not under voluntary control. Thus swallowing starts as a voluntary act and then the bolus of food is carried on by involuntary peristalsis, a co-ordinated wave of smooth muscle contraction. Functional sphincters at both ends help to prevent regurgitation.

Achalasia is a condition in which the muscle in the lowest part of the oesophagus fails to relax, so that the swallowed bolus of food cannot pass on into the stomach. The presenting symptom is difficulty in swallowing, *dysphagia*, with a feeling of food sticking in the lower substernal region. This is sometimes painful. The stagnation of food in the oesophagus leads to its regurgitation, so that spill-over may occur into the larynx and bronchi, giving rise to recurrent episodes of aspiration pneumonia. The diagnosis is established by a barium swallow (Chapter 50, p. 473) as described along with the treatment, which is surgical.

HIATUS HERNIA AND OESOPHAGEAL REFLUX

The hole in the diaphragm through which the oesophagus passes from the chest into the abdomen to enter the stomach is called the oesophageal hiatus. A hernia is a bulging out, or protuberance, of part of a body cavity's contents beyond its usual boundaries, and a hiatus hernia is therefore a bulging of the abdominal part of the oesophagus and usually also the upper part of the stomach through the oesophageal hiatus into the chest (see Fig. 24/1). This condition is more common in women than in men, especially with increasing weight and age, although anything that increases intra-abdominal pressure, such as pregnancy, may contribute to its development.

Hiatus hernia is very common and often symptomless, being found incidentally on barium meal examination. The *symptoms are caused* by regurgitation of irritant, acid, peptic juice from the stomach into the gullet, producing a *reflux oesophagitis* because the oesophageal mucosa is not resistant to its acid, peptic, digestive effects. A substernal burning discomfort, known as heartburn, or an aching pain in this region, is the most common presenting symptom, sometimes with regurgitation of acid-tasting fluid into the mouth. *The most readily recognizable feature of this heartburn is its close relationship with posture*, such as bending over forwards, especially to lift something heavy, lying down, or even sitting with the trunk bent slightly forwards, for instance after a large meal. Some patients experience quite severe, substernal pain which may mimic angina pectoris, except that it is not related to exertion in the upright position and is usually relieved by milk or antacids. The oesophagitis may lead to peptic ulceration in the lower oesophagus which may bleed, usually slowly, to produce an iron deficiency anaemia. Occasionally there is haematemesis.

The diagnosis of hiatus hernia is made by barium meal, see p. 691, but reflux oesophagitis may occasionally occur without a hiatus hernia being demonstrable even on the most careful radiological examination unless the patient is well tipped with head down, so as to show a hernia which is present only some of the time. *Treatment* consists of weight reduction on a low-calorie diet if the patient is overweight, avoiding the postures that produce reflux as far as possible and combating its effects with antacids. If symptoms are troublesome at night the head of the bed can be raised on nine-inch blocks, and pillows used to prevent the patient slipping down the bed. Should all these measures fail to relieve symptoms, or if iron

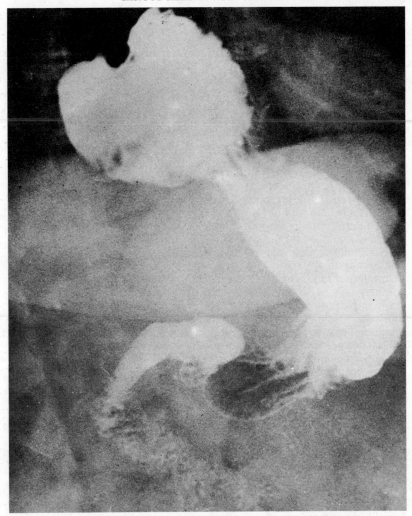

Fig. 24/1 A hiatus hernia shown by barium meal. The patient was tipped head down, supine on the X-ray table, to demonstrate the extent of the hernia above the diaphragm.

deficiency anaemia persistently recurs, or even stricture develops from chronic ulceration, surgical treatment should be considered.

CARCINOMA OF THE OESOPHAGUS

Like achalasia, but unlike hiatus hernia, carcinoma of the oesophagus is relatively uncommon. Also like achalasia it usually presents with dysphagia which may be painful but here the resemblance ends. It chiefly affects men in their sixties and seventies and the dysphagia relentlessly and often rapidly progresses to complete obstruction, when the patient cannot even swallow his saliva. Even in the earlier stages, weight loss is prominent. *Diagnosis is by barium swallow* (Fig. 50/3, p. 473) *and meal or oeso-phagoscopy, and treatment is either by oesophagectomy or radiotherapy or both.* The *prognosis* is almost universally bad but recently surgery of cancers of the lower third of the oesophagus, which is the common site, has given a nearly 50 per cent chance of surviving five years.

THE STOMACH

The upper part of the stomach, that is the fundus and body, acts as a reservoir for the food and secretes gastric juice, containing hydrochloric acid, pepsin, mucus and the intrinsic factor which is essential for the absorption of vitamin B_{12} in the lower ileum. The two vagus nerves and the hormone gastrin, secreted by the pyloric antrum, the lower part of the stomach, control the secretion of gastric juice from the fundus and body of the stomach. The wall of the stomach in the region of the pyloric antrum also contains enough smooth muscle to allow active mixing of the food, which is made semi-fluid and partially digested before being delivered through the pyloric canal to the duodenum.

The output of gastric acid secretion, measured in milli-equivalents of hydrochloric acid (mEq HCl) can be estimated following a maximum stimulus such as histamine or Pentagastrin, a commercially available substance structurally related to gastrin. As Pentagastrin does not have the unpleasant side-effects of histamine and is as effective in stimulating maximum gastric acid secretion it is becoming the method of choice. *The practical procedure is for the patient to fast from midnight. On the morning of the test the nurse passes a soft plastic Ryle's tube into the stomach either through the nose or mouth, whichever is easier for the patient, using a local anaesthetic such as lignocaine.* In most units X-ray screening is used to check the position of the tube. However, recent work has shown that if the patient drinks a small volume of water and this is immediately aspirated, the tube is in a satisfactory position if at least three-quarters of the volume is recovered.

When X-ray screening is used the patient lies on his left side, but it is now doubtful if any one posture makes a real difference to the completeness of collection of gastric juice. The tube is attached to a suction pump and continuous aspiration is started. When the resting juice has been collected a subcutaneous injection of Pentagastrin is given and gastric juice collected by continuous suction for an hour. If no acid is obtained the patient is said to have Pentagastrin-fast achlorhydria (equivalent to augmented histamine-fast achlorhydria). This strongly suggests pernicious anaemia. A low gastric acid output is found with chronic gastritis (see p. 229) and with gastric carcinoma. Patients with chronic gastric ulcer may secrete normal or low amounts but never have complete achlorhydria. Patients with chronic duodenal ulcer may secrete normal or high amounts of acid.

PEPTIC ULCER

A peptic ulcer is an ulcer caused by acid-peptic digestion of the mucosa, usually gastric or duodenal. Occasionally peptic ulceration occurs in the lower oesophagus as already described or, rarely, it is anastomotic, in the small intestine anastomosed to the stomach, for instance, following partial gastrectomy for duodenal ulcer. The cause of peptic ulcer is unknown but the resistance of the mucosa to digestion is probably more important than the concentration and volume of the gastric juice.

There is a tendency for either gastric or duodenal ulcers to run in families. The presenting symptoms of chronic gastric and duodenal ulcers are indistinguishable. Characteristically they both give rise to intermittent epigastric pain which may radiate to the back, and is often worse before meals and briefly relieved by food, to return shortly afterwards. It is also usually, in the early stages at least, relieved by milk and antacids. The severity of pain is hard to assess, but peptic ulcer pain is often bad enough to wake a patient at night, characteristically in the small hours, and it may well cause the loss of many days or weeks off work. Heartburn, nausea, vomiting, which usually relieves the pain, and weight loss are also common. Clinical examination may reveal epigastric tenderness but the

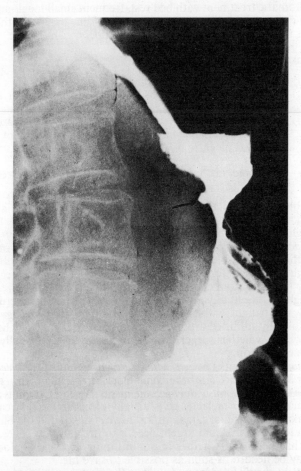

Fig.24/2 A peptic ulcer on the lesser curve of the stomach shown by barium meal. This is a common site for chronic gastric ulcers.

diagnosis is established by barium meal (Fig. 24/2) or by endoscopic examination of the stomach using a flexible fibrescope.

The symptomatic treatment of peptic ulcer consists of the relief of pain by eating 'a little and often', avoiding fried, curried, spiced or pickled foods if this proves helpful; rest when practicable; antacids such as magnesium trisilicate, aluminium hydroxide or calcium carbonate; and anticholinergic drugs to reduce acid secretion. These tend to be more helpful in chronic duodenal ulcer and the dose should be increased to the limit of tolerance. Poldine is probably the most effective, starting at 2 mg four times a day before meals.

In the specific treatment of chronic gastric ulcer three things have been shown to accelerate the rate of healing. These are bed rest in hospital, stopping smoking and the drug carbenoxolone. There is no specific medical treatment for chronic duodenal ulcer which will accelerate healing, but if the pain becomes severe the patient is brought into hospital for full symptomatic treatment with bed rest, frequent small meals and snacks including milky drinks, liberal antacids and poldine pushed to the limit of tolerance, set by blurred vision and dry mouth.

Surgical treatment must be considered:

    (i) when medical treatment has failed

    (ii) for an emergency such as perforation or severe or recurrent haemorrhage

    (iii) for pyloric stenosis, a narrowing of the pyloric canal at the outlet of the stomach due to fibrosis from scarring of a nearby duodenal ulcer, and sometimes associated muscle spasm and oedema

    (iv) for suspicion that an apparently benign gastric ulcer may in fact be a carcinoma.

Slight bleeding from time to time, detected by testing the stools for occult blood, probably occurs in most patients with peptic ulcer. It is often not enough at any one time to cause *melaena, the passage of soft or liquid stools made tarry black by altered blood,* or *haematemesis,* the vomiting of blood (either obvious blood or 'coffee ground' material when blood has been in the stomach for some time). A peptic ulcer may cause iron deficiency anaemia from chronic low grade blood loss.

Although not essentially different, a much more dramatic picture is presented by the patient with *acute gastro-intestinal haemorrhage.* Such a patient is usually admitted to a medical ward because there may be no need for surgery, but whether surgery will be necessary or not usually remains a very open question.

The management of the patient with acute gastro-intestinal bleeding provides an excellent example of the value of close co-operation between the medical and surgical teams of doctors and nurses. When a patient is admitted with haematemesis or melaena he is usually pale, faint and sweating and always anxious. The pulse rate is almost always raised and the blood pressure often low. The first and urgent need is to find out how severe the loss of blood has been and whether it is continuing, because a blood transfusion may be needed as soon as possible to save life.

The patient should be reassured right at the start that this sort of bleeding is a fairly common condition from which he will make a full recovery. He should be nursed in bed and sedated, for instance with full doses of phenobarbitone. The nurse starts to make regular observations of the pulse rate and blood pressure. The frequency of these observations, often hourly, will be determined by the apparent severity of the blood loss and other factors. *A further rise in pulse rate or fall in blood pressure may be the first indication of further bleeding.*

In the meantime the doctor has taken blood for estimation of haemo-globin concentration and for cross matching. The nurse is often asked to pass a Ryle's tube into the patient's stomach for hourly aspiration to see if there is fresh blood. The medical and surgical teams consult from an early stage. The factors in favour of surgical treatment are severe, persistent or recurrent bleeding. These apply especially to older patients with hard arteriosclerotic vessels which are less likely to stop bleeding of their own accord, particularly if hypertension has been present. Medical teams vary in their practice of what to give the patient to eat. On the author's unit a light, nutritious diet according to the patient's taste is given when he feels like starting it.

While this management proceeds, the source and cause of the bleeding are being actively investigated, for instance in an emergency by fibre-optic endoscopy and by X-ray of the stomach and duodenum with Gastrografin. The most common causes of acute gastroduodenal bleeding are chronic peptic ulcer, gastric or duodenal, and acute gastric ulcer, which may be due to aspirin sensitivity or may occur in any severe illness. Occasionally the bleeding may come from a carcinoma of the stomach, gastro-oeso-phageal varices or peptic ulceration in a hiatus hernia (see p. 486).

CARCINOMA OF THE STOMACH

Carcinoma of the stomach may grow for many months or longer with-out producing any symptoms. Anyone over 45 who has unexplained loss of appetite (*anorexia*), loss of weight, or epigastric pain or nausea which does not respond to antacids in a few weeks, or who develops unexplained iron deficiency anaemia, should be investigated for stomach cancer. The cause of this condition is unknown although certain families have several members affected. The *diagnosis* is established by barium meal, although as with other gastro-intestinal cancers, examination of the stool for occult blood can be helpful in first showing the likelihood of organic disease in a clinical situation which is often vague and ill-defined. Sometimes frank haematemesis and melaena occur. *Another diagnostic procedure involving the nurse in the search for suspected cancer of the stomach, or anywhere else, is the erythrocyte sedimentation rate* (E.S.R.). A normal result in the absence of previous information is of no value but a raised E.S.R., like a positive result for occult blood, may be the sole evidence of the likelihood of organic disease. The treatment is surgical but the prognosis is very bad.

GASTRITIS

Gastritis, inflammation of the gastric mucous membrane, may be acute or chronic. *Acute gastritis* can be caused by an acute excess of alcohol or irritant foods, or drugs, or by a severe systemic infection such as influenza. It may be complicated by haematemesis or melaena but improves with the disappearance of the cause. *Chronic gastritis* is different. It is an inflammation which tends to progress very slowly to atrophy of the gastric mucosa. Its cause is unknown and it often produces no symptoms, although some patients with a peptic ulcer type of dyspepsia have chronic gastritis and no evidence of a peptic ulcer.

Diagnosis is by biopsy of the gastric mucosa. The treatment of symptoms is the same as the medical treatment of peptic ulcer (see p. 228). In pernicious anaemia there is a complete atrophy of the gastric mucosa, which fails to secrete the intrinsic factor which is essential for the absorption of vitamin B_{12} in the lower ileum. No one yet understands the relationship between chronic gastritis, as seen in many elderly patients, and the relatively uncommon pernicious anaemia.

REGIONAL ENTERITIS

Crohn's disease, as this condition is also called, is an inflammatory condition usually affecting the small intestine, especially the terminal ileum. It may also affect the colon. Its cause is unknown. The patient, usually a young adult, often presents with recurrent pain in the right iliac fossa and recurrent diarrhoea which is not usually severe and rarely contains blood or mucus. Loss of appetite and weight, occasional nausea and vomiting, low grade fever and mild iron deficiency anaemia are all quite common in Crohn's disease, but any one of these features in a young adult is not very likely to be due to this uncommon condition. There is often tenderness and sometimes a mass in the right iliac fossa.

Diagnosis is established by barium follow-through examination of the small intestine. Treatment is unsatisfactory because the condition has a very strong tendency to relapse. Codeine phosphate is useful for the diarrhoea and may help the pain. Steroids, such as prednisolone, may be helpful in the acute stage. Intestinal obstruction is an indication for surgery but recurrence is common after operation and a *fistula* may develop. This is an abnormal communication between a hollow organ and another, or between a hollow organ and the surface of the body.

THE LIVER AND BILIARY TRACT

The liver is essential to life because it largely controls the metabolism of the proteins, fats, carbohydrates and many of the vitamins brought to it by the portal blood from the absorbing cells of the small intestine. That is, it prepares the absorbed foodstuffs into components suitable for use by the cells of the body. It also inactivates hormones as necessary and detoxicates drugs such as morphine, barbiturates and salicylates. Finally, it produces bile pigment and salts, and excretes them through the biliary tract into the duodenum.

The bile pigment, *bilirubin*, is formed in the liver and spleen from the normal breakdown of red blood cells. In health a small amount is always present in the blood, bound to protein and therefore incapable of being excreted by the kidney into the urine. At this stage, before it is changed within the liver cells, it is known as prehepatic, unconjugated bilirubin. When it enters the liver cells it is split from its binding protein and made soluble in water. Having passed through the liver cells into the bile it is now conjugated, posthepatic bilirubin and, being water soluble, can pass through the kidney into the urine. In the intestine it gives the stools their usual colour. Some is re-absorbed and some of this is excreted as *urobili-nogen* in the urine, which also takes its usual colour from this pigment. The *bile salts*, also formed by the liver and excreted in the bile, help with the digestion of fat.

Jaundice is the yellow colour of the skin and mucous membranes due to increased circulating bilirubin. If mild, it is more easily seen in the day-light and in the sclerae, the whites of the eyes. Jaundice may be due to premature destruction of the circulating red blood cells, *haemolysis,* or to liver cell disease or to obstruction to the outflow of bile, either in the small bile ducts within the liver or in the large ducts outside the liver. Roughly speaking, the causes are prehepatic, hepatic and posthepatic:

1. Haemolysis (uncommon)
    (i) from outside the red cells, e.g. antibodies on their surface
    (ii) from inside the red cells, e.g. congenital spherocytosis
2. Liver cell disease (very common)
    (i) from outside the body, e.g. *virus,* drugs, poisons
    (ii) from inside the body, e.g. cirrhosis (less common)
3. Obstruction (common)
    (i) outside the liver, e.g. gallstone or carcinoma
    (ii) inside the liver, e.g. 'cholestasis', drugs

1. The *haemolytic anaemias* (see p. 218), may be due to antibodies on the outside of the red cells or to abnormalities within the red cells them-selves, as in congenital spherocytosis. This condition is also called *acholuric jaundice* (*achol-* means no bile, *-uric*, in the urine) because the excess circulating bilirubin produced by premature destruction of the red cells, *as in any haemolytic anaemia*, is prehepatic, unconjugated, bound to protein and incapable of passing through the kidney into the urine.

2. *Liver cell disease*, especially virus hepatitis, is the most common cause of jaundice. The causes, symptoms and treatment of the two common forms of virus hepatitis, *infectious hepatitis* and *serum hepatitis*, and also *leptospiral infections*, are described in Chapter 39, p. 383. It is therefore sufficient here to explain that the jaundice in these patients with acute infective liver cell disease is caused by the failure of the liver cells to per-form their function of excreting bilirubin, although they do conjugate it and make it soluble in water. The urine turns very dark about a week after the start of the illness because this posthepatic, conjugated, water-soluble bilirubin accumulates in the blood, produces jaundice, and is excreted by the kidney. Less of it gets into the bowel and so the stools become pale, especially when, a little later in the illness, the small bile ducts within the liver become oedematous so that there is some degree of obstruction to the bile outflow from the liver itself. This type of small duct obstruction is called *cholestasis* and explains why so many of the symptoms of large duct obstruction (see p. 232) may be seen in patients with liver cell disease.

Cirrhosis of the liver is a chronic, diffuse disease of the liver in which some liver cells die and others regenerate, along with fibrous tissue, so that the normal pattern of liver structure is distorted. Its functions tend to become progressively impaired, although the natural history of the disease is very variable over several or many years. The basic causes of cirrhosis seem likely to be related to unusual forms of immune reaction to a number of different factors, including a virus hepatitis which fails to clear, and chronic alcoholism in a person on a poor diet with low protein content. Jaundice may not develop until late. When it does, much of the bilirubin is conjugated and so becomes posthepatic and water soluble and appears in the urine.

Portal hypertension, i.e. a raised pressure in the portal vein and its tributaries, which take blood from the gastro-intestinal tract to the liver, is usually due to partial obstruction to the flow of portal venous blood through the liver (for description and surgical treatment, see p. 520). This complication of cirrhosis arises both from the fibrosis and distorted pattern of liver structure and from transmission of pressure from the arterial system within the distorted network of liver blood vessels. The increased pressure in the portal venous system may lead to recurrent, small bleeds which produce iron deficiency anaemia or to dramatic rupture of dilated gastro-oesophageal veins (varices) with massive *haematemesis*, which can be fatal (for management, see p. 521).

Ascites, i.e. free fluid within the abdominal cavity, may develop in relation to portal hypertension and also because of a fall in the plasma level of albumin (due to reduced production by the liver) with consequent drop in osmotic pressure. Finally, cirrhosis may terminate in liver cell failure with pre-coma, coma and death.

The treatment of cirrhosis can sometimes be remarkably effective if the patient can be persuaded to keep off alcohol (whether there is a history of chronic alcoholism or not) *and stick to the diet prescribed. The nurse can sometimes make all the difference to the patient's acceptance of advice by reinforcing it at times and in ways which she is often best placed to judge.* The diet advised for a particular patient will depend on the results of the investigations but, in general, a high-calorie, high-protein diet with no added salt is helpful, sometimes with supplements of the B group of vitamins. Diuretics, for ascites or oedema, must be given with careful attention to the risk of potassium loss in these patients.

3. *Obstructive jaundice* may be due to a block in the common bile duct outside the liver. This duct is formed by the junction of the common hepatic duct with the cystic duct, which takes bile to the gall bladder to be concentrated, and back again for excretion into the duodenum. This type of extrahepatic, large duct obstruction is usually due to a gallstone or carcinoma of the pancreas.

Partial obstruction of the small bile ducts within the liver substance, from oedema of their walls, produces cholestasis. It may develop during any form of liver cell disease, or it may arise as a direct result of sensitivity to certain drugs such as chlorpromazine (Largactil). Jaundice due to cholestasis has the same sort of features as when it is caused by large duct obstruction, including itching (pruritus), from an increased level of bile salts in the blood. Antihistamines may be helpful in relieving this symptom but it is often resistant to treatment.

Cholecystitis, inflammation of the gall bladder, may be acute or chronic and in both cases almost always develops in relation to *gallstones* (cholelithiasis).

In *acute cholecystitis* a gallstone usually obstructs the cystic duct or neck of the gall bladder, or sometimes the common bile duct, and infection follows the obstruction. The patients are most often women in their forties or fifties who have had several children and they are often overweight. The obstruction causes pain which is usually severe, more constant than inter-mittent, often epigastric, sometimes in the right upper abdomen and sometimes radiating round the right side to the back or further up, to the angles of the scapulae or the right shoulder. Vomiting is common. The patient is often restless, with fever and tachycardia. Bilirubinuria is fre-quently present and jaundice may develop when the common bile duct is obstructed. Medical treatment consists of rest, effective analgesia, anti-biotics and intravenous infusions to maintain electrolyte balance. Surgical treatment by cholecystectomy is usually indicated after the acute stage has passed or if complications develop, such as empyema of the gall bladder or even perforation.

In *chronic cholecystitis* the long-standing inflammation usually leads to thickening and fibrosis of the walls so that the gall bladder shrinks and loses its ability to concentrate the bile. Recurrent biliary obstruction forms the most certain basis for the diagnosis, which may be established by a cholecystogram X-ray of the gall bladder. The most effective treatment is surgical, by cholecystectomy.

THE PANCREAS

The pancreas excretes digestive enzymes into the duodenum. The main pancreatic enzymes are trypsin, for breaking down proteins, lipase, for splitting fats which have been acted on by bile, and amylase for splitting starch, as it also does in the saliva. The pancreas also contains cells, in the islets of Langerhans, which produce an internal secretion direct into the blood, the hormone insulin.

The main diseases of the pancreas in adults are pancreatitis and carci-noma, both largely of unknown cause. *Acute pancreatitis* presents with sudden, severe, persistent abdominal pain due to a spilling of the digestive pancreatic juice into the abdominal cavity because of destruction of the pancreas by its own digestive enzymes. Diagnosis is often difficult but will be revealed by the finding of a very raised level of amylase in the blood. Treatment is by 'drip and suck', i.e. intravenous infusion and gastro-intestinal suction, and also measures to combat the shock and pain. *Chronic pancreatitis* is a slowly progressive condition characterized by recurrent central abdominal pain, sometimes with vomiting and fever and later with malabsorption. Diabetes mellitus and, rarely, obstructive jaundice may develop. The treatment is symptomatic.

Carcinoma of the pancreas occurs more often in men, especially in their fifties and sixties. The symptoms depend largely on the site of the growth. For instance, cancer of the head of the pancreas often produces painless obstructive jaundice and in the body or tail of the gland it may cause epigastric pain boring through to the back, sometimes relieved by sitting hunched over the knees with the legs bent. Diagnosis is often difficult; treatment, which is surgical, is only palliative and the prognosis is very poor.

MALABSORPTION

The gastro-intestinal tract exists to feed the cells of the body by taking proteins, fats, carbohydrates, minerals, vitamins and water from its lumen into the blood which passes through its mucosal lining. This food-enriched blood then travels through the veins of the portal circulation to the liver. The intake, or absorption of these foods occurs mainly in the small intestine, either by diffusion into the epithelial cells lining the mucosal surface or by active transport, a mechanism which depends on the chemical energy of the cell. It follows that the more epithelial cells there are in contact with the food, i.e. the greater the surface area of the mucosa lining the small gut, the greater will be the capacity for absorption. This surface area is greatly increased by mucosal folds and villi (Fig. 24/3), leaving a large absorptive capacity in reserve.

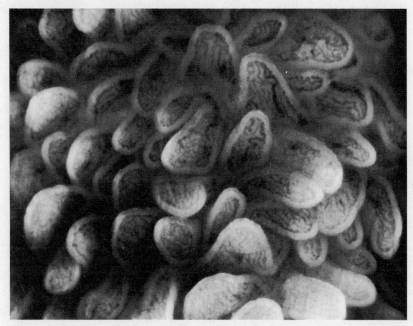

Fig. 24/3 A magnified view (× 70) of the normal mucosal lining of the small intestine obtained by peroral intestinal biopsy, in its natural, unstained state. Note the food-absorbing surface cells which appear in this photograph like a rim around each villus and also the rich network of blood vessels, well placed to start the absorbed food on its journey through the portal venous system to the liver. *Photograph by W. Brackenbury.*

Reduced absorption, i.e. *malabsorption,* may be due to a defect of the function of the stomach, which starts digestion and secretes intrinsic factor; it may be due to a defect of pancreatic juice or bile; or the small intestine itself may be defective in its gross or microscopic structure or in its cell function. Thus the conditions causing malabsorption may be classified in this way:

    1. Defects of gastric function
        (i) postgastrectomy
        (ii) pernicious anaemia
    2. Defects of digestion
        (i) deficiency of pancreatic enzymes
        (ii) deficiency of bile

3. Defects of intestinal absorption
    (i) gross anatomical lesions
    (ii) mucosal (microscopic) lesions
    (iii) apparently normal structure

1. **Gastric function** may be sufficiently defective to cause malabsorption even after partial gastrectomy or a drainage procedure with vagotomy (Chapter 50, p. 476). Organic iron as present in food is liable not to be fully absorbed but this can be overcome by giving inorganic iron such as ferrous sulphate. If there is malabsorption of fat, *steatorrhoea* develops. This is the passage of fatty stools which tend to be pale, bulky, offensive and difficult to flush away from the lavatory pan. Any patient with steatorrhoea, whatever the cause, may malabsorb fat-soluble vitamins such as vitamin D, along with calcium, and so become liable to develop *osteomalacia*, a softening of the bones due to insufficient calcium. Malabsorption of vitamin B_{12} may also develop following gastric surgery. This may be due to removal of intrinsic-factor-secreting gastric mucosa, atrophy of the gastric remnant, or a stagnant loop (see below, 3), for instance the afferent loop of a Polya gastrectomy. Treatment will be dealt with at the end of this section on malabsorption. *Pernicious anaemia* is described in Chapter 23, p. 218.

2. **Pancreatic insufficiency** may be due to chronic pancreatitis or carcinoma of the pancreas. In both these conditions there is defective excretion of pancreatic enzymes into the duodenum. The resulting defect of digestion leads to malabsorption. Thus proteins are lost with the stools because they have not been broken down by trypsin, and the deficiency of lipase leads to steatorrhoea, which may be severe. There may be malabsorption of the fat-soluble vitamin D, producing osteomalacia, but anaemia is not a feature of pancreatic disease unless there is bleeding from a carcinoma. Thus the diagnosis of pancreatic insufficiency may be suspected on the clinical grounds of steatorrhoea without either anaemia or abnormalities in the blood film. It is confirmed by passing a tube into the duodenum and aspirating its contents so that, for instance, the concentration of trypsin can be measured following a fatty meal, as in the Lundh test.
Deficiency of bile, in particular of bile salts, most often results from obstruction to bile outflow by gallstone or carcinoma. As with pancreatic malabsorption, steatorrhoea develops because of defective digestion of fat, in this case from a lack of the emulsifying action of the bile salts.

3. **Intestinal absorption** is liable to be defective when the gross anatomy of the small intestine includes a *stagnant loop*, such as the afferent loop of a Polya gastrectomy, a segment of small bowel proximal to a stricture or adhesion, small fistulae, or diverticula, which produce quite different effects from those in the large bowel. Any stagnant fluid in the body is liable to become infected and the small gut offers no exception. Some of the organisms which may infect a stagnant loop prevent the absorption of vitamin B_{12} and cause steatorrhoea by splitting bile salts abnormally so that they cannot perform their digestive functions properly. *Resection* of sufficient distal ileum, for instance three or four feet for regional enteritis, always causes malabsorption of vitamin B_{12} because this is where it is absorbed, in combination with the intrinsic factor secreted by the stomach.

Coeliac disease is the most common form of malabsorption in this country due to an abnormality of the mucosal lining of the small intestine. A very few people react to the wheat protein, *gluten*, in such a way as to damage their small gut mucosa and reduce their ability to absorb the necessary foodstuffs. 'We call such persons coeliacs'—a direct quotation from the original, second-century, Greek description of the disease. The Greek word means 'suffering in the bowels'. This suffering usually consists of steatorrhoeic diarrhoea and fatigue from anaemia due to malabsorption of folic acid and iron. Many other symptoms may occur, including aphthous ulcers in the mouth, anorexia, weight loss, abdominal distension and flatulence and, less commonly, tetany or osteomalacia from calcium deficiency, or oedema from protein lack, or purpura from malabsorption of fat-soluble vitamin K. Coeliac disease develops soon after weaning on to foods made with flour, which contains gluten. It may present at this time, or later in childhood, or remain latent until any time in adult life.

Diagnosis is by biopsy of the small intestine which shows a bare mucosa without villi (Fig. 24/4). These return following treatment with a *strict* gluten-free diet (Chapter 17, p. 164), always in children and usually in adults. Patients should remain on the diet for life. The *Coeliac Society*, like the *Ileostomy Association*, is run by patients for patients and provides some very useful and practical advice, especially on ways of solving problems caused by the need to remain strictly on the gluten-free diet.

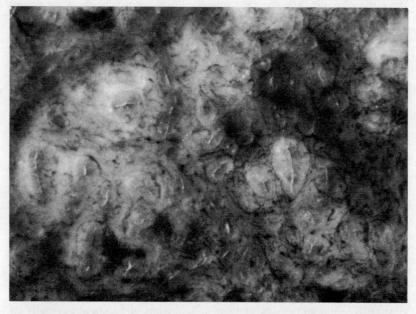

Fig. 24/4 A magnified view ($\times 70$) of the flat mucosal lining of the small intestine obtained by peroral biopsy, in its natural, unstained state, from a patient with untreated adult coeliac disease. Note the complete absence of villi, resulting in a greatly reduced surface area available for absorption. The mouths of the crypts of Lieberkühn can be seen. *Photograph by W. Brackenbury.*

In *alactasia*, apparently normal epithelial cells lining the surface of the villi may be deficient in lactase, the intestinal enzyme responsible for splitting the milk sugar lactose. This deficiency may produce diarrhoea, usually mild, following the ingestion of milk. Everything else in the diet is absorbed normally. Treatment is by a diet low in lactose.

The **investigation of malabsorption** is twofold. *Defects of gastro-intestinal structure* will be revealed by a history of gastric surgery or intestinal resection, by barium meal and follow-through examination of the small intestine, or by biopsy of the intestinal or gastric mucosa. Evidence of pancreatic disease is provided by tests of pancreatic function such as the Lundh test. Second, the extent and severity of *defects of absorptive function* should be investigated so that a full diagnosis may be reached and specific treatment given. *The nurse will be involved in the practical procedures of all these tests, but the details vary from one hospital to another.* Most units use the inert sugar, xylose, as a screening test of intestinal malabsorption. The presence of steatorrhoea is demonstrated by the estimation of excess fat in a stool collection, which must continue for at least three days. The function of the lower ileum or the effect of a gastrectomy or stagnant loop can be assessed by testing the absorption of vitamin B_{12}.

Treatment thus depends on both the cause and the results of the mal-absorption. Antibiotics for a stagnant loop, pancreatic extract for defective pancreatic function, and a gluten-free diet for coeliac disease are specific examples. A low-fat, high-protein diet and codeine phosphate are often helpful symptomatically. Supplements such as iron, folic acid, vitamin B_{12}, calcium and vitamin D may be given according to the specific deficiencies detected by investigation.

DISEASES OF THE COLON

Ulcerative colitis, diverticular disease and *carcinoma of the colon* are fully described in Chapter 51.

The term *irritable bowel syndrome* is now used to describe the condition which used to be known by several different names such as spastic colon, mucous colitis and functional disorder of the colon. The cause lies in the patient's overanxious reaction to stress and there is a tendency for this condition, which is quite common, to run in families. Recurrent episodes of mild or moderate abdominal pain, especially in the left iliac fossa, are often associated with constipation and followed by diarrhoea, sometimes brought on by taking purgatives.

Sigmoidoscopy shows either an entirely normal appearance or an actively contracting colon. *Barium enema* often shows a variably irregular outline. On the X-ray screen the radiologist often sees narrow segments, as if in spasm, but there is no constant deformity of any one part of the bowel as there is, for instance, in the inflamed bowel which may be associated with diverticular disease.

Intelligent reassurance personally suited to the individual patient and his worries is an important part of treatment and one in which nurses can play a most useful role. A sedative such as phenobarbitone may supplement this sort of support and some relief can be provided with methyl cellulose, either as Isogel granules or Celevac tablets, to provide extra bulk for the stool. Failing this, poldine is worth trying as it is probably the most effective of the antispasmodic preparations.

DYSENTERY

Causes, symptoms, preventive measures and treatment are described in the Section on Communicable Diseases, pp. 357–8.

Amoebic dysentery is a tropical disease caused by the protozoon *Entamoeba histolytica*. It is briefly mentioned in a Table, p. 392, under amoebiasis.

WORMS

Threadworm (*Enterobius vermicularis*) is the most common type of worm to cause infection in this country, especially in children, although whole families may be infected. Perianal pruritus, especially at night, when the female worm is laying her eggs in this region, is the chief symptom. Diagnosis is by detecting the eggs (ova) on a Cellophane tape applied to the perianal skin first thing in the morning. Treatment is with piperazine, which is very effective. The main problem is to prevent re-infection. Careful hand washing, especially after bowel actions and before meals, is important and nails should be kept short.

Roundworm (*Ascaris lumbricoides*) is uncommon in Britain. The worm is rather like an earthworm. Infection is by ova being carried to the mouth on the hands. The ova hatch in the duodenum and the larvae pass to the lungs by the lymphatics and blood vessels. They then climb up the bronchi and trachea and are swallowed and mature in the intestine. The diagnosis is by finding ova or an adult worm in the stools and the treatment is with piperazine.

Tapeworm: *Taenia saginata* is the *beef tapeworm*, not uncommon in Britain. Segments are passed in the stools. Treatment is with niclosamide. The bowels should be opened the day before treatment. Two tablets, each containing 500 mg, are taken when fasting and chewed with a little water. One hour later another two tablets are taken in the same way. This treatment rarely fails and there are no side-effects.

The *pork tapeworm* (*Taenia solium*) is rare in Britain. The *dog tapeworm* is *Echinococcus granulosus*, also uncommon in this country. It causes hydatid cysts, usually in the liver, occasionally in the lung or even the brain. If a cyst causes symptoms, it should be removed surgically.

SYMPTOMS OF GASTRO-INTESTINAL DISEASE

Dysphagia, difficulty in swallowing, may be due to obvious local conditions of the mouth or throat like stomatitis, tonsillitis, or quinsy, a tonsillar abscess which is excruciatingly painful. A hemiplegic patient with weakness of the muscles of the soft palate or pharynx will also find swallowing difficult and may need very careful nursing help with feeding. Further down, in the oesophagus, achalasia or peptic ulceration in the lower oesophagus from gastro-oesophageal reflux or, in an older patient, carcinoma of the oesophagus, may be the cause of the trouble, to be shown on barium swallow and meal. Occasionally pressure from outside the oesophagus, from a goitre, carcinoma of the bronchus or glands in the mediastinum may cause obstruction and difficulty in swallowing. Hysterical dysphagia, seen especially in young women, is known as globus hystericus.

Vomiting may be due to a large variety of gastro-enterological or more distant conditions. When the cause of the trouble lies in the gastro-intestinal tract the patient usually feels nauseated first, and often salivates freely. Probably the most common cause of vomiting is so-called gastric 'flu', infectious vomiting and diarrhoea, from which many readers will have suffered themselves. However, among patients in hospital, the common gastro-intestinal conditions causing vomiting are peptic ulcer, especially when complicated by pyloric stenosis, hiatus hernia and acute inflammation further down the alimentary tract like acute cholecystitis, appendicitis or peritonitis from any cause. Apart from anorexia, vomiting is the most common gastro-intestinal symptom to arise from conditions elsewhere in the body. Migraine is the most common everyday example but among hospital patients uraemia or raised intracranial pressure may present in this way. When vomiting is due to direct stimulation of the medulla in the brain stem it often comes suddenly upon the patient without the usual warning signs of nausea and salivation. Vomiting may sometimes be psychogenic, calling for psychiatric diagnosis and treatment (see nursing points, p. 130).

Abdominal pain is probably the most common symptom of disease of the digestive system. It is often due to excessive contraction of smooth (involuntary) muscle, especially in the presence of inflammation, as in peptic ulcer, regional enteritis without obstruction, acute appendicitis, diverticular disease of the colon with inflammation, or ulcerative colitis. In these conditions it usually remains at a relatively constant pitch while it lasts. In contrast, the painful, smooth muscle contraction of acute mechanical obstruction of the small intestine is intermittent, like the severe intermittent pain produced by a stone in the ureter. However, a similar type of obstruction produced by a gallstone in the common bile duct usually gives a constant, though equally severe pain.

Another way in which severe abdominal pain may be produced is by acute inflammation of the peritoneum which covers the outer surfaces of the abdominal organs. Peritonitis may be caused by perforation of a peptic ulcer, an acutely inflamed appendix or, less often, a deep ulcer in ulcerative colitis (see p. 501). It is particularly severe in acute pancreatitis. Abdominal pain may sometimes be related to ischaemia, or to distension of an organ. A dramatic example of both these factors in combination is provided by a strangulated hernia, but a more everyday illustration is offered by the dull ache in the upper abdomen which contributes to the distress of patients in congestive heart failure. This ache, which is usually felt either in the epigastrium or across the right upper abdomen, is due to distension of the liver capsule by venous congestion.

Diarrhoea, the frequent passage of loose stools, is most often due to infection, but if it persists for long enough to bring a patient into a general medical ward it is probably due to disease of the large intestine, trouble in the small bowel or, occasionally, a gastrectomy. The group of closely related conditions ranging from granular proctitis through procto-colitis to full-scale ulcerative colitis is probably the most common cause of persistent severe diarrhoea in a medical ward in this country. Blood and mucus with the stools, a feature of any large bowel diarrhoea, is common.

If the inflammation is confined to the rectum there may still be blood with the stools, but sometimes there may be constipation instead of diarrhoea. This feature of varying bowel habit, between diarrhoea and constipation, is also suggestive of diverticular disease of the colon and carcinoma of the rectum or lower colon. Blood with the stools is more common with carcinoma than with diverticular disease.

If rectal examination, sigmoidoscopy and barium enema show no evidence of large bowel disease, and the patient has not had a gastrectomy, which can cause mild or moderate diarrhoea without significant mal-absorption, then chronic diarrhoea is likely to be due to psychological factors such as chronic anxiety, or to one of the forms of malabsorption discussed earlier. The stool frequency is not usually so great in diarrhoea which originates outside the colon as it is in large bowel disease and there is no blood or mucus with the stool except occasionally in regional enteritis. If there is malabsorption of fat there will be steatorrhoea, with pale, bulky, offensive stools which are difficult to flush away. Psychogenic diarrhoea, whether as part of the irritable bowel syndrome or not, is remarkably common but not usually severe enough to bring the patient into a hospital ward (see nursing points, p. 131).

Constipation, infrequent passing of the stools, often with difficulty, is a relative matter. The normal frequency for one person may be three times a day and for another once every few days. For constipation to be present there must be a significant reduction in the frequency of bowel actions as compared with the previous bowel habit. Probably the most common cause of constipation in a hospital, especially in old people, is the change of habit induced by coming into the ward. However, if constipation was present before admission and before a period of bed rest at home, it could be related to a carcinoma of the rectum or sigmoid, or further up the colon, or to diverticular disease of the colon. In both these conditions constipation may sometimes alternate with diarrhoea. The same is true of the irritable bowel syndrome and, occasionally, granular proctitis.

If dehydration is present for long enough it may cause constipation, as may hypothyroidism. Constipation is no exception to the rule that any symptom of gastro-intestinal disease may in fact be a symptom of the patient's state of mind. The depressed patient is often constipated and may sometimes be very distressed by this symptom, considering it as a sign of being 'inwardly unclean'. Even psychiatrically normal people may some-times be obsessed by the idea of the uncleanliness of constipation and take frequent purgatives. As the colon is the proper place for stools and the normal frequency of evacuation varies widely, this has no factual basis. The nurse can help many such people to rid themselves of their obsession by firm and patient reassurance. Liberal fruit and vegetables and fluids also help to increase stool frequency and are much better for the bowel than purgatives.

Habitual failure to empty the rectum is known as *dyschezia*. This com-monly arises in childhood from poor training or neglecting to act on the sensation of a full rectum. These patients can be helped by training, fruit, vegetables and fluids.

In elderly constipated patients stools may accumulate in the rectum until the faecal mass is large enough to produce partial large bowel obstruction. This is known as *faecal impaction*. As the obstruction is usually only partial it is not uncommon for liquid stool to leak round the hard faecal mass and produce 'spurious diarrhoea' or a form of rectal in-continence which is really a retention with overflow. The treatment is to remove the obstructing faecal mass by manual evacuation, if necessary under anaesthetic.

Chapter 25

Diseases of the Urinary System

by J. E. A. WICKHAM

> *Urological symptomatology—examination—radiological examina-tions—endoscopy—tests of renal function—diseases of the urinary tract: renal failure and anuria, acute tubular necrosis, renal infections, nephritis, acute nephritis, the nephrotic syndrome, chronic nephritis—systemic diseases which involve the kidneys—catheterization—bladder drainage*

The investigation of a patient with urinary disease is designed to elicit a precise diagnosis so that specific treatment may be given. Strict classifica-tion of urology into medical and surgical divisions is to some extent artificial, for the symptomatology, examination and detailed investigation of the patient with urinary disease today does not recognize these boun-daries. Only in terms of treatment is dichotomy to some extent justified.

UROLOGICAL SYMPTOMATOLOGY

Patients with urinary disease may complain of some or all of the following:

Frequency is due to irritation of the bladder lining or bladder wall either from inflammation or inability to empty completely the bladder due to outflow obstruction. Conditions producing *polyuria* may cause frequency.

Difficulty. Straining and inability to void easily signifies outflow obstruc-tion as from prostatic hypertrophy or urethral stricture.

Incontinence. When *passive* the patient leaks urine continuously due to derangements of the bladder sphincter mechanism either from direct damage or denervation, commonly seen after severe spinal cord trauma.

Stress incontinence is due to weakness of the bladder sphincter mecha-nism occasioned by stretching of the pelvic floor during childbirth. Urine is lost intermittently during coughing or sneezing, but normally the patient remains dry.

Urge incontinence. In severe inflammatory conditions of the bladder the desire to void is so urgent that the patient leaks urine before reaching the toilet. This usually resolves rapidly after treatment of the infection.

Enuresis is seen in children and adolescents who fail to establish a complete control of micturition especially at night. The bladder mechanisms are normal and the fundamental cause of this trouble is not always clear but a large number of these patients appear to sleep very deeply and do not wake to the normal stimulus of a full bladder. *Administration of the drug Tofranil 25 mg at night* has aided these patients dramatically during the last few years, probably by making them more aware of the neurological stimuli to void produced by a full bladder.

Haematuria. Blood passed with the urine is usually of serious significance and commonly indicates the presence of a tumour in the lining epithelium of the urinary tract. Less frequently haematuria is seen in inflammatory disorders such as tuberculosis.

Pain. Renal pain is characteristically a dull aching pain in the loin below the last rib and is caused by inflammation or obstruction of the kidney.

Ureteric colic. This is an intermittent severe pain referred to the line of the ureter and implies ureteric obstruction by stone or blood clot.

Bladder pain and dysuria is associated with inflammation and produces a suprapubic dull aching pain when the bladder is full. On voiding, the pain is intensified and accompanied by a burning discomfort in the urethra. The whole symptom complex is then known as *dysuria* and if severe as *strangury*.

Perineal pain is a continuous dull ache in the perineum associated with prostatic inflammation or cancer.

Testicular pain is a constant burning ache in the scrotum associated with inflammation or trauma of the epididymus and testis.

EXAMINATION

A *general* examination should be made to reveal evidence of any other systemic diseases which can contribute to urological symptomatology. For instance the patient may be found to be in heart failure or suffering from severe conditions such as hypertension which may require primary treatment.

Abdominal. The presence of a renal mass suggestive of renal tumour, or a distended bladder confirmatory of outflow obstruction may be revealed. Tenderness may be elicited over the inflamed kidneys, ureters or bladder.

Genital examination on a male patient may reveal the presence of scrotal masses or inflammation or anatomical abnormalities of the penis such as phimosis or hypospadias.

A rectal examination will provide information as to the size and consistency of the prostate gland and confirm the presence of benign hypertrophy or malignant enlargement.

A neurological examination may well reveal evidence of primary neurological disease which may secondarily cause defects in bladder function.

Special investigations

Urine tests. Ward tests are carried out for reaction, protein and sugar. *A midstream specimen* (for method of collection see Chapter 5, p. 64) is needed for laboratory tests which may reveal the presence of casts indicative of glomerulonephritis, excess red cells which may indicate neoplasm or bacterial infection. The urine is then cultured bacteriologically to identify specific infecting organisms and the sensitivity of these organisms to various antibiotics is also tested.

RADIOLOGICAL EXAMINATIONS

These investigations are probably the most important in the elucidation of urological disease.

Intravenous excretion pyelogram (see Chapter 66, p. 694). The patient is given an intravenous injection of an iodine-containing compound. The dye is concentrated and *excreted* by the kidneys to outline the urinary collecting system. X-ray films are taken at intervals after the injection and the progress of the dye observed. In this way non-function or partial function of the kidneys may be seen. Tumours may be outlined and distortions of the renal collecting system recognized. Delay in bladder evacuation may be seen and bladder outlet obstruction observed.

Cystogram. To study bladder function alone it is often sufficient to instil a radio-opaque medium into the bladder by way of a catheter; this is removed and the process of bladder evacuation may then be observed under the X-ray screen as the patient voids. Ciné films may also be taken during micturition.

Retrograde pyelogram. When kidney function is depressed it may not be possible to obtain an excretion pyelogram, and to gain information about the urinary collecting system it may be necessary to pass a small ureteric catheter in a retrograde manner into the kidney by way of an operating cystoscope (see p. 695). Radio-opaque dye can then be injected directly into the kidney and ureter to produce a high-contrast pyelogram.

Urethrogram. The urethral canal is outlined by a radio-opaque jelly injected retrogradely into the *urethra*, and X-ray films are taken to demonstrate the presence of narrowing or stricture of the lumen.

Arteriography. A small catheter is passed into the femoral artery and upwards by way of the aorta into the renal artery. Radio-opaque dye may then be injected directly into the renal circulation to outline abnormal tumour circulations or to reveal blockage in the main renal vessels.

Radioactive renogram. The way in which the kidneys take up a substance from the bloodstream, and then pass it down the ureters to the bladder, can be studied by injecting the substance labelled with a radioactive isotope. The rise and fall of radioactivity in the kidneys is measured externally by counters sensitive to radioactivity, placed over the renal areas.

ENDOSCOPY

Endoscopy. The inside of the bladder can be examined directly by the passage of a small illuminated telescope along the urethra. The outer sheath of the instrument provides a water channel which allows the bladder to be distended with water or other irrigant fluid, and the bladder wall and ureteric orifices are viewed through this fluid medium with a telescope passed into the sheath. There are various modifications to the simple viewing cystoscope known as *operating cystoscopes* which permit the introduction of fine catheters into the ureters, or the treatment of bladder tumour by means of small diathermy electrodes passed alongside the cystoscope. With a *resectoscope*, which carries a small cutting diathermy loop,

it is also possible to cut away intruding and obstructing prostatic tissue—
the so-called *transurethral prostatic resection*.

TESTS OF RENAL FUNCTION

Specific gravity. The main function of the kidney is to concentrate the
urine. When renal substance is lost by disease the ability to produce a
concentrated urine is much diminished and a simple test is to estimate the
patient's ability to produce a concentrated urine while fluid is restricted for
12 hours. At the end of this time the urine specific gravity should have
risen to at least 1·022. Lesser figures imply impairment of renal function
and concentrating ability.

Blood urea or serum creatinine. Both these substances are produced as
end-products of protein metabolism and are excreted in the urine. An
impairment of renal excretory capability will cause the quantity of these
substances in the peripheral blood to increase above their normal levels
of about 30 to 40 mg per 100 ml for urea and 0·5 to 1·2 mg per 100 ml for
creatinine, which provides a rough guide to *any impairment of renal function*.

The creatinine clearance test. Creatinine, like urea, is an end-product of
metabolism that is continually excreted in the urine. By measuring the
concentration of the creatinine in the blood plasma and the concentration
of creatinine in a known volume of urine secreted *in a known time*, it is
possible to derive a simple expression, the *creatinine clearance*, which
accurately reflects the excretory ability of the kidney. The normal value in
the adult is 120 ml per min. With failing renal function this value gradually
falls and at a level of 7 to 8 ml per min. treatment by dialysis becomes
necessary to maintain life.

It cannot be over-emphasized that careful ward collections of all 24-hour
urine specimens are essential for this test.

DISEASES OF THE URINARY TRACT

A number of these disorders have become the province of the renal
physician or nephrologist and are considered in this chapter. Others,
because of the nature of the treatment required, come under the care of the
urological surgeon and are described in Chapter 54, p. 529. Many conditions, however, require the combined expertise of both specialists.

Renal failure and uraemia

Many diseases of the kidneys destroy the renal tissue, giving rise to the
condition of renal failure or uraemia. The patient suffers from general
malaise. He is anorexic and vomits frequently. There is headache, breathlessness and insomnia. If unrelieved the patient deteriorates into cardiac
failure, coma and death. This sequence of events is due to two principal
causes:

Failure to excrete the end-products of protein metabolism. Forty g of
protein is broken down in the body every 24 hours and the end-products of
this metabolism are excreted in the urine. The principal substances released are urea, potassium and acid radicals such as sulphate and chloride.
In renal failure these substances are not excreted and accumulate within
the body to toxic levels.

Failure of water excretion. If a patient with complete renal failure continues to drink water in normal quantities, it is obvious that a rapid accumulation of excess fluid within the body will occur. The patient will become waterlogged, causing cardiac-circulatory failure and death from water intoxication.

The treatment of renal failure whether acute or chronic is designed to avoid these two major complications and may be conservative, by dialysis or by means of transplantation.

Conservative treatment is used for the management of acute renal failure which is normally a fully recoverable disease. The treatment consists of fluid restriction to 500 ml in 24 hours to avoid water overload, and the restriction of diet to carbohydrates *only* to minimize urea and acid production from ingested protein. With this regime patients may be maintained in water balance with reasonable levels of urea and potassium for periods of two to three weeks while recovery of renal function ensues.

In the pre-terminal phases of *chronic renal failure*, although a little urine is passed there tends to be a degree of sodium retention which leads to hypertension and cardiac failure. In these patients conservative treatment includes the restriction of sodium and protein intake (Giovannetti diet, see p. 162).

Treatment by dialysis

This is used for cases of acute renal failure associated with much tissue destruction as after a major accident. Here protein is rapidly broken down and end-products released in amounts too great to be managed conservatively. Dialysis is also used in chronic renal failure when kidney function has been reduced to negligible levels and death would otherwise occur.

Treatment by dialysis depends upon the fact that if two solutions of different concentration are separated by a semi-permeable membrane then solutes in high concentration will diffuse across the membrane to an area of lower concentration until both solutions become identical. If, therefore, blood of a patient suffering from renal failure and containing a high concentration of urea is passed through an exteriorized tube made of semi-permeable material lying in a bath of fluid from which urea is absent, urea will diffuse from the blood into the bath fluid. In the course of time excess urea will be removed from the vascular system of the patient and the body urea content lowered to normal levels. Similar considerations apply to other unwanted or toxic metabolic end-products. *There are two methods of dialysis*:

Haemodialysis is carried out with the *'artificial kidney'*. This consists essentially of a Cellophane tube, permeable to water and solutes but not to blood cells or protein molecules, lying in a bath of saline. Blood from the patient is conveyed from an artery or vein through the tube and back to a second vessel. The dialysis is continued until the correct composition of the blood is restored.

In *acute renal failure* this treatment is carried out every few days until renal recovery occurs. In *chronic renal failure* the patient must be dialysed twice a week in order to maintain reasonable health. In this latter group to obviate the necessity for repeated vascular cannulations it is now standard practice to insert a small tube of Silastic rubber with a Teflon tip into an adjacent small artery and vein at wrist or ankle. The Silastic tubes are exteriorized and connected together with a further small Teflon tube to make an artificial external arterio-venous fistula, through which blood flows continuously from artery to vein. When haemodialysis is performed the shunt is disconnected and the vessels attached directly to the artificial kidney.

Peritoneal dialysis. The same principle of solute diffusion applies but in this technique the peritoneum of the patient constitutes the semi-permeable membrane. The equivalent of the saline bath fluid of the artificial kidney is run by gravity into the peritoneal cavity of the patient through a small plastic catheter inserted into the lower abdominal wall. Fluid is instilled in 1·0 litre quantities and is allowed to remain in the peritoneal cavity for about 15 minutes while solute diffusion takes place. The fluid is then siphoned by gravity into a receiver at the bedside and the same cycle repeated as many times as is required to return the patient's blood constituents to normal: usually a period of 12 hours is necessary. Contrary to expectation, infection of the peritoneum is exceedingly rare.

Renal transplantation. The successful transplantation of organs between closely related animals was first performed over 30 years ago, but it was Murray in 1961 who demonstrated that such a procedure was possible in man when he grafted the kidney of one of a pair of identical twins into a second twin who was dying of renal failure. The graft worked successfully but unfortunately the further step to transplantation of kidneys between entirely unrelated persons has not been so simple, for these kidneys are treated as foreign protein by the host and are immunologically rejected (see Chapter 44, p. 419).

Considerable effort has been devoted to methods for overcoming this rejection reaction and in the last few years appropriate suppressive drugs such as Imuran have been developed which selectively suppress the immunological reactions of the recipient and allow graft survival. With such a regime it has been possible to achieve transplantation of kidneys from both related and unrelated cadaver donors to large numbers of prepared recipients and the technique has now reached a degree of success sufficient to warrant its adoption as a routine treatment of chronic renal failure.

SPECIFIC RENAL DISEASES

Acute tubular necrosis gives rise to the state of *acute renal failure* described on p. 245. It is most commonly seen in situations where the patient has been exposed to severe circulatory depression and shock as in massive haemorrhage after operation or childbirth, bacteraemic shock or severe crushing injuries. During these insults the kidney blood supply becomes impaired with ultimate death of renal tubular cells. Occasionally poisonous substances such as mercury or carbon tetrachloride cause direct destruction of the renal tubules to produce a similar acute cessation of renal function. The immediate picture is usually that of the precipitating condition, but once this has been corrected, for example by re-transfusion after massive haemorrhage, it is noted that the patient passes only a very small quantity of urine (*oliguria*) or none at all (*anuria*). Once this fact is recognized the patient must be immediately treated by the conservative regime for renal failure outlined on page 246. Careful watch is kept of the blood urea and serum potassium level and should these rise above the levels of 400 mg per cent and 6·0 mEq per litre respectively dialysis is normally undertaken.

The natural history of acute tubular necrosis is divided into three phases:

The *oliguric phase* which may last for up to three weeks when little or no urine is passed. The tubular cells are regenerating during this period.

The *diuretic phase* of about 10 days when large quantities of dilute urine begin to be passed by tubules which are healed but cannot concentrate urine.

The *late diuretic phase* with gradual return to near normal renal function in approximately two to three weeks.

In the majority of patients the condition is fully reversible with ultimate recovery.

Renal infections

Acute and chronic pyelonephritis account for nearly half of all cases of renal disease. The brunt of the disease falls on the kidney tubules. The *bacteria* normally giving rise to acute renal infections are of the Coliform group. Urine is an ideal culture medium for bacteria, and once organisms are introduced into the urinary tract multiplication may rapidly occur, particularly if there is any interference with the free drainage of urine. Most bacteria are introduced into the lower urinary tract by the urethral route. The frequency with which women suffer from urinary infections supports this suggestion. Bacteria once established in the urine may ascend to the kidney.

Acute pyelonephritis. The initial symptoms are frequency and dysuria followed a little later by loin pain and malaise. The patient is febrile, with tenderness over the renal area. The urine may be offensive and occasionally contains blood; it must be cultured to identify the appropriate organism.

Treatment. A high urine output should be induced to wash bacteria out of the kidney mechanically, and the appropriate antibiotic administered. Symptoms usually settle within three days and the urine should be subsequently examined to make sure that all organisms have been eradicated. Any patients with recurrent infections must be fully investigated in case an anatomical abnormality in the urinary tract predisposes to infection and might be amenable to surgical correction (see Chapter 54, p. 532).

Chronic pyelonephritis is the end stage of recurrent attacks of acute pyelonephritis. Both kidneys are affected, with destruction of many renal tubules and much scarring and shrinkage of the renal substance. Other renal insults, for example, excess phenacetin intake, gout and lead poisoning, may, however, produce a picture similar to that described above. A large number of patients may sustain major renal damage from untreated childhood urinary infections.

Symptoms vary: some patients present with recurrent dysuria and frequency, whilst others present with the symptoms and signs of chronic renal failure discussed above.

The intravenous pyelogram reveals evidence of loss of renal tissue with shrinkage and scarring. Renal function tests reveal diminution in concentrating ability and urinary culture may reveal evidence of persisting infection.

Treatment. When infection is found this must be treated by appropriate antibiotics. With the onset of renal failure the treatment outlined on p. 246 is instituted. Almost half of all patients coming to dialysis and transplantation suffer from this condition.

Nephritis

This refers to a group of conditions that primarily affect the glomeruli rather than the tubules. Strictly, the word is inaccurate because it implies inflammation of the kidney and nowadays very few of the conditions labelled nephritis are thought to be primarily inflammatory in nature. The *clinical picture* produced falls into three main types:

> *Acute nephritis,* which leads to the presence of red blood cells and protein in the urine.
> *The nephrotic syndrome,* in which the protein loss in the urine is much greater and the patient becomes oedematous.
> *Chronic nephritis,* in which the gradual destruction of the *nephrons* (the functioning unit of each glomerulus with its tubule) and their replacement by fibrous scar tissue results in an increasing failure of renal excretory function and a raised blood pressure.

The fact that there are three typical syndromes must not be allowed to obscure two important considerations. First, each syndrome has a wide variety of causes. Secondly, the idea that an acute nephritis may progress through the nephrotic syndrome to chronic nephritis is only occasionally accurate; in most cases of the latter two syndromes, no evidence of a previous acute nephritis can be found.

Acute nephritis. The commonest condition producing this picture is *acute glomerulonephritis.* Other causes are *Henoch-Schönlein purpura,* collagen diseases such as *polyarteritis nodosa* and *radiation nephritis* due to damage by X-rays, but they will not be considered further here.

Acute glomerulonephritis is a specific disease in which acute glomerular damage occurs following distant infections, particularly with certain streptococci. It usually affects children and young adults. The *clinical picture* is commonly one of a dramatic onset of *oedema* or *haematuria,* and the patient may complain of malaise, pain in the loins, and a reduction in urine output. In most patients there is a history of a recent sore throat, and streptococci may be grown from the throat swab. There is usually a moderate increase in blood pressure. *Investigations* reveal red cells, tubular casts and protein in the urine, and the blood urea rises moderately.

The *pathology* appears to be an allergic reaction induced in the glomeruli by distant streptococcal infection. The basement membrane of the glomerulus through which the plasma is filtered becomes disorganized and allows protein and blood to leak from the circulation into the urine, but the total volume of the liquid filtered is reduced. The normal response of the tubules to this reduction in the volume of the glomerular filtrate is to increase their extraction of water and sodium from the filtrate, and the resultant expansion of the extracellular fluid is responsible for oedema.

There is no known *specific treatment.* Any streptococcal infection is treated, but the principal management is that of the secondary renal failure. The patient is put to bed and fluid intake is restricted to 500 ml per 24 hours plus the volume of any urine passed. Sodium intake is reduced to control the oedema, but protein is not usually restricted unless there is severe oliguria. Blood pressure if grossly elevated is treated with antihypertensive agents or by venesection. After a few days a diuresis usually ensues with loss of oedema and a gradual return of the blood pressure to normal, but bed rest is usually maintained for three weeks. If oliguria persists the resulting uraemia very occasionally may need to be treated by dialysis.

The *prognosis* is good, complete recovery occurring in most patients. If the patient continues to pass red cells and protein in the urine for several months, the chances of the condition merging into the nephrotic syndrome or chronic nephritis increase.

The nephrotic syndrome

Among the many causes of this clinical picture are some in which the kidney damage is *secondary* to a more widespread general disease; important examples of these are given later (p. 251). The *primary renal diseases* producing the nephrotic syndrome include the common so-called 'minimal change' glomerular lesion and those few cases of acute glomerulonephritis which gradually pass into the nephrotic state.

Clinical features are largely common to all cases, whatever the cause of the syndrome, although the nature of the underlying disease affects the likelihood of the development of renal failure and hypertension, and also the prognosis. Patients may be any age, but the condition is twice as common in children as in adults. In children the syndrome is nearly always due to primary renal disease—usually the 'minimal change lesion'—but in adults 20 per cent of cases are due to secondary renal involvement from other generalized diseases.

The patient presents with oedema which may become very severe, affecting the face as well as the legs and sacral area, and is due to a reduction in plasma protein concentration following the leakage of proteins into the urine. The plasma volume shrinks, and this may produce hypovolaemic shock. The patient is weak and ill and is liable to infections. Frank haematuria is rare, but microscopic examination may reveal red cells in the urine, and the blood urea may rise a little because of the interference with excretion produced by the state of shock. *Renal biopsy* by needle puncture is an important investigation since it may reveal the underlying cause as well as giving evidence about the progress of the disease.

In patients with the 'minimal change lesion', 40 per cent recover spontaneously or with treatment. The remainder usually have one or more relapses, and the chance of permanent renal damage with a terminal chronic nephritis is correspondingly greater.

Treatment. When the condition is secondary, the underlying cause is treated if possible. *The control of oedema is most important* with rigid restriction of sodium in the diet (but a high protein intake), diuretics such as chlorothiazide, and drainage of oedema from the subcutaneous tissues by multiple punctures. Corticosteroids such as prednisone may induce remissions or cure, particularly in the 'minimal change group'.

Chronic nephritis is the end-result of chronic damage to the kidneys from a wide variety of causes, and there may not have been any preceding acute glomerulonephritis or nephrotic syndrome. The clinical picture is proteinuria for some years, gradually progressing to renal failure with hypertension and uraemia (see p. 245). Renal biopsy may help in the diagnosis of the cause, and in giving a prognosis. Treatment is of the cause, and of the renal failure when this supervenes.

SYSTEMIC DISEASES WHICH INVOLVE THE KIDNEY

There are a number of generalized systemic disorders which give rise to secondary renal damage and are worth noting.

Diabetes. Patients suffering from diabetes are frequently subject to recurrent attacks of urinary infection leading to chronic pyelonephritis and finally renal failure. Renal failure may also arise from diabetic vascular involvement of the glomerulus leading to a diabetic type of chronic glomerulonephritis and renal failure. *Treatment* is directed to the primary treatment of the diabetes and to the specific type of renal failure produced (see p. 302).

Gout. The hyperuricaemia of gout can result in deposition of crystals of uric acid around the kidney tubules leading to cellular destruction and fibrosis. Renal failure may follow. *Treatment* is that of the hyperuricaemia (see p. 309) with secondary attention to the renal failure.

Hypercalcaemia from hyperparathyroidism may result in interstitial renal calcification, overt renal stone formation and ultimately renal failure. *Treatment* is correction of the parathyroid abnormality and surgical treatment of any renal calculi.

Amyloid disease arising from chronic infection anywhere in the body may result in the deposition of amyloid material in other organs. In the kidney deposition occurs in glomeruli and tubules leading to ultimate renal failure. *Treatment* is of the infective focus and may result in improvement or resolution of the amyloid deposition with reversal of the renal failure.

Drug nephropathy. More and more evidence is being obtained of the deleterious effects of various drugs upon the kidney. More especially drugs of the mild analgesic group have been implicated, phenacetin being the most potently nephrotoxic in this respect. Some antibiotics have been shown to be nephrotoxic as have some of the barbiturates, and the damaging effects are mostly on the renal tubules. *Treatment* is the avoidance of the specific drug and treatment of any renal failure induced by exposure to the damaging agent.

Hypertension is not only a *result* of chronic nephritis: it may be the *cause* of chronic renal damage. In late cases it may be difficult to decide which condition came first.

CATHETERIZATION

Catheterization is the passage of a fine tube into the male or female bladder by way of the urethra to drain the urine. It may be either *intermittent* when the tube is passed at specified intervals, or *indwelling* when the tube is allowed to remain permanently in the urethra for long-term urinary drainage.

Types of catheter. *Those introduced via the urethra* are non-retaining or self-retaining. For types see Fig. 25/1.

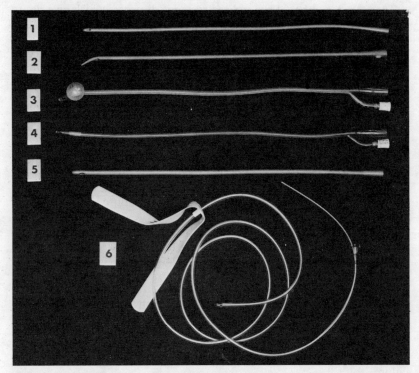

Fig. 25/1 Standard catheters. 1. Jacques' catheter. 2. Tiemann's catheter. 3. Foley catheter with balloon inflated. 4. Foley catheter with balloon collapsed. 5. Harris 'whistle tip' catheter. 6. Gibbon catheter.

The non-retaining for intermittent catheterization are simple tubes about 12 inches long and about a quarter of an inch in diameter. The last half inch of the catheter is often angulated at about 30 degrees to enable the catheter to negotiate the prostatic urethra in the male and the tip may be rounded or pointed. The one most commonly used for intermittent catheterization is the *Tiemann catheter*.

The self-retaining catheter is modified from the simple tube by the addition of a bulbous device at the bladder end which is larger than the internal urethral diameter. The commonest catheter of this type is the

Foley balloon catheter. The retaining device is a small Latex balloon near the catheter tip which may be inflated or deflated by fluid or air introduced from the external end of the catheter along a fine side tube welded to the catheter. The catheter is passed with the balloon collapsed until the tip lies within the bladder. The balloon is then filled rendering withdrawal of the catheter impossible. The balloon is deflated prior to removal. Another type of self-retaining catheter is the *Gibbon catheter.* This is essentially a fine plastic tube which is passed into the bladder and retained by means of two plastic flanges cemented to the tube 12 inches from the tip. The flanges are strapped to the penis or labia with Elastoplast strapping to prevent extrusion of the catheter.

There are several designs of catheters which are only *introduced into the bladder by the surgeon at operation* and are not intended for ward use. The common catheter of this type is the *Harris 'whistle tip' catheter* which is put into the bladder during prostatectomy and retained by a nylon stitch passed through the abdominal wall and tied over a small metal bar or clamped with a Harris button. These catheters are retained during the immediate postoperative period only and are removed by the surgeon.

Catheter sizes. Catheter sizes are graduated on the Charrière or French scale, the number being the circumference of the catheter in millimetres. A size 18 French catheter is the one most generally used. Female catheters are normally half the length of the full-sized male catheter and are about 6 inches long.

Technique of catheterization. It is essential to appreciate that the passage of a catheter into the bladder can cause considerable urinary contamination with bacteria if the utmost care is not taken by the operator. First the genitalia must be cleansed as far as possible, and secondly, handling of the parts of the catheter that will actually be within the bladder must be avoided and contact made only by sterile forceps or sterile rubber gloves.

For female catheterization see p. 748.

Male catheterization

Articles required. These are the same as those required for female catheterization except for the addition of a tube of sterile urethral local anaesthetic (2 per cent Xylocaine) in a small tube with sterile nozzle adaptor and a penile clamp.

Procedure. The patient lies on his back with the legs abducted and the bedclothes removed from the operating area. The hands are scrubbed and sterile rubber gloves put on. The penis is held in the fingers of the left hand and the prepuce retracted fully. The glans and the external meatus are carefully cleansed with Hibitane 1 : 5000 or Savlon. Sterile towels are then placed over the abdomen and over the scrotum and between the legs to leave only the penis available. The sterile nozzle is attached to the tube of local anaesthetic and the nozzle introduced into the external meatus. The contents of the tube are squeezed into the urethra and massaged into the prostatic portion, and then a penile clamp is applied behind the glans for five minutes. A receiver is placed between the legs. The clamp is then removed and the catheter picked up with the dissecting forceps and the tip introduced into the urethra. The catheter is then advanced until urine begins to flow from the lumen of the catheter into the receiver.

It cannot be overemphasized that if the catheter meets with obstruction or if bleeding or pain should be experienced, the procedure should be abandoned and the advice of an experienced urologist be sought.

When the bladder has been emptied, the catheter is either removed or the self-retaining balloon inflated and the catheter connected to the drainage apparatus. Finally, the prepuce is reduced to prevent paraphimosis.

BLADDER DRAINAGE

If the catheter is to be retained then some form of drainage apparatus to collect the urine is required. Two principal methods are available:

1. Simple continuous closed drainage
2. Drainage with irrigating facility

In simple continuous closed drainage the lumen of the catheter is connected directly to the connecting tube of a pre-sterilized plastic drainage bag of one or two litres capacity which is suspended from the bed frame by a metal hanger. When the bag is full the drainage tube is disconnected and a fresh bag substituted. Details of some bag systems vary slightly but the essential point to be appreciated by the nurse is that on each occasion that the bag or tubing is disconnected from the catheter there is a considerable hazard of organisms being introduced by way of the catheter lumen into the bladder with the consequence of serious morbidity for the patient.

It should be routine when such disconnection is necessary that the end of the catheter must always be laid on a sterile towel and swabbed with a disinfectant prior to re-connection to the new drainage tube. Also the nurse should scrub the hands thoroughly at the start of the procedure and keep the fingers well away from the junctional area while manipulating the tubes. Generally this procedure need only be carried out once in 24 hours if two-litre bags are utilized.

Drainage with an irrigating facility. When a patient has been subjected to an operation where blood or blood clot is expected to drain by way of the catheter, for example after prostatectomy, the drainage system may be modified as follows.

The catheter instead of being connected to a urine bag is connected to a sterile plastic 'Y' piece. One limb of the 'Y' piece is attached to a sterile drip-set through which standard bottles of intravenous fluids may be administered. The other limb of the 'Y' piece is attached directly to a Urisac by its connecting tube. Both limb tubes are fitted with occlusive gate clips. When it is desired to flush blood clot from the bladder or to irrigate the bladder, the clip on the drainage limb is closed and that on the infusion limb opened. About 200 ml of irrigant, water or saline, is run into the bladder and the clip closed. The drainage tube clip is then released, allowing the irrigant plus debris to flush into the drainage bag. Occasionally to dislodge troublesome clots a Higginson syringe without its valve is introduced into the drainage limb tubing. Gentle squeezing of the bulb when the bladder has been filled with irrigant then permits dislodgement of clot from the catheter and connecting tubing. If much irrigation is required the plastic drainage bag is substituted by a large volume sterile glass jar containing a few millilitres of Hibitane as disinfectant.

Care of the catheter. It must again be emphasized that the greatest care must be taken to avoid accidental disconnection of these drainage systems

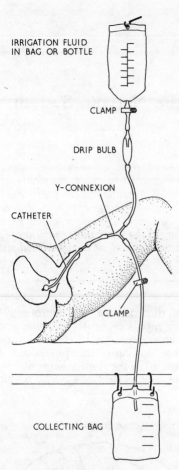

IRRIGATION FLUID
IN BAG OR BOTTLE

CLAMP

DRIP BULB

Y-CONNEXION

CATHETER

CLAMP

COLLECTING BAG

Fig. 25/2 System for closed
drainage and bladder irrigation after prostatectomy.

during other ward procedures such as bed making. If the system has to be
broken for bag changing, etc., then precautions already noted must be
carefully observed. Care must also be taken that the connecting tube of the
indwelling catheter is not pulled upon and dislodged. It is a good idea to
pin the drainage tube to the lower sheet, leaving some slack to allow for
movement while the patient is in bed.

When an indwelling catheter is used a sticky secretion forms around the
external meatus in both men and women. This should be cleansed away
each day with a dilute solution of Hibitane 1 : 5000 using a pledget of sterile
cotton wool held in dissecting forceps.

Chapter 26

Disorders of the Nervous System

by J.C.MEADOWS

Introduction—neurological examination—upper and lower motor neurone lesions—cerebro-vascular accidents—paraplegia—multiple sclerosis—epilepsy—presenile dementia—Parkinson's disease—chorea and athetosis—subacute combined degeneration of the spinal cord—migraine—infective disorders of the nervous system—neuro-syphilis—disorders of the lower motor neurone—peripheral neuritis—disorders of muscle—nursing of the paralysed patient

An understanding of disorders of the nervous system requires some familiarity with the essentials of neuro-anatomy and neuro-physiology. Fig. 26/1 recalls the gross anatomy of the brain and Fig. 26/2 shows a diagrammatic transverse section of the spinal cord. The neurones which supply muscles are situated in the *ventral horns* within the whole length of the spinal cord, and in special collections, *nuclei*, within the brainstem. The

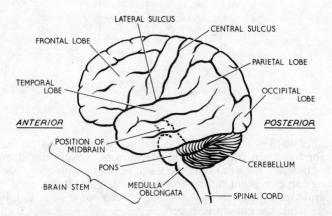

Fig. 26/1 The brain and brainstem. The position of the four lobes (frontal, parietal, occipital, temporal) which arbitrarily divide each cerebral hemisphere are shown. The component parts of the brainstem—mid-brain, pons and medulla—are also shown with the cerebellum lying behind.

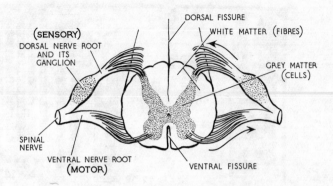

Fig. 26/2 Transverse section of the spinal cord. The grey matter is shown stippled, the ventral horn of grey matter giving rise to the ventral root in front, and the dorsal horn of grey matter giving rise to the dorsal nerve root behind. The arrows indicate direction of flow of impulses.

ventral horn cells (and the corresponding neurones in the brainstem) are known as *lower motor neurones*. They have long axons which pass out into the spinal (or cranial) nerves, eventually to reach the muscles.

Voluntary acts are initiated by the upper motor neurones whose cell bodies are situated in that part of the cerebral hemispheres known as the *motor cortex*, a narrow strip of brain lying immediately in front of the central sulcus (Fig. 26/1). The long axons of these upper motor neurones pass down to the lower motor neurones at all levels of the brainstem and spinal cord and it is always through these lower motor neurones that the voluntary act is finally carried out. Thus damage to any part of the upper or lower motor neurones will cause weakness in the muscles supplied.

NEUROLOGICAL EXAMINATION

Fig. 26/3 shows a typical setting of the equipment for a full neurological examination.

UPPER AND LOWER MOTOR NEURONE LESIONS

Damage to the upper motor neurones produces weakness associated with increased tone (resistance to passive movement of the limb) and brisk tendon reflexes; wasting is typically absent. Babinski's sign is present, the big toe moving upwards (towards the face) when the sole of the foot is stroked. In a lesion of the lower motor neurones, tone is decreased, reflexes are reduced or absent and wasting pronounced.

Examples of upper motor neurone lesions are strokes, brain tumours, cervical spondylosis and disseminated sclerosis, while causes of *lower motor neurone lesions* include Bell's palsy, poliomyelitis, carpal tunnel syndrome and peripheral neuritis.

Upper motor neurone lesions. The long axons (which pass down in the *pyramidal tracts*) cross over in the medulla and a lesion in one cerebral hemisphere will therefore cause weakness of the *other* side of the body.

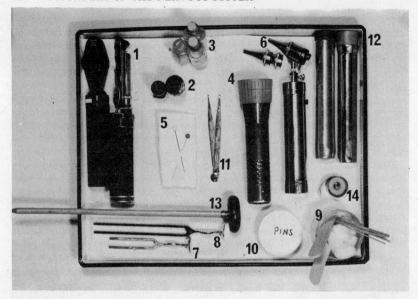

Fig. 26/3 Tray for neurological examination. 1. Two common types of ophthalmoscope. 2. Homatropine and eserine eyedrops. 3. Bottles containing different substances to test the sense of smell (e.g. oil of cloves, peppermint). 4. A torch for examining the throat and pupillary reactions. 5. Red- and white-headed hat pins, or some similar alternative, for testing the visual fields. 6. Auriscope. 7. Small tuning fork for bone and air conduction tests. 8. Large tuning fork for testing vibration sense. 9. Supply of wooden spatulae, 'orange sticks' and cotton wool. 10. Pins for testing sensation. 11. Calipers for testing two-point discrimination. 12. Two metal or glass tubes which can be filled with hot or cold water for thermal testing. 13. Hammer for tendon reflexes.* 14. Tape measure. See also Chapter 61, p. 637 for Snellen's types for testing visual acuity.

* Tendon reflexes are produced by tapping the tendons of certain muscles to produce a momentary stretch in the muscles. This stimulates tiny structures within the muscle known as muscle spindles, resulting in impulses being sent to the spinal cord to activate the lower motor neurones supplying the muscle. Thus a brief jerk of the muscle results. Tendon reflexes are reduced or absent if either the motor or sensory nerve fibre is damaged, and are increased in disorders of the upper motor neurones.

Various clinical patterns may occur:

> *Hemiplegia*, paralysis of one side (face, arm, leg).
> *Monoplegia*, paralysis of one limb.
> *Paraplegia*, paralysis of the lower part of the body on both sides.
> *Quadriplegia*, paralysis of all four limbs.

A *hemiplegia* is usually caused by a lesion in one cerebral hemisphere. Commonly the onset is abrupt, and a vascular cause is then responsible ('*stroke*' or '*cerebro-vascular accident*'). Less commonly, the condition develops slowly over a few weeks and a tumour may then be present. In either case, other functions are often affected, *impairment of intellect*, *sensory symptoms* (numbness or tingling in the weak limbs) or *defective speech*. Speech is controlled by the left cerebral hemisphere and is thus usually only affected with right hemiplegias: the patient is unable to think of, or use words correctly (*dysphasia*) and may be unable to understand the speech of others. *Dysarthria* is another form of speech disorder—a disorder of articulation, the words being chosen correctly but pronounced incorrectly—occurring in brainstem and cerebellar disorders, and in bilateral cerebral disease.

CEREBRO-VASCULAR ACCIDENTS (Strokes)

Cerebro-vascular accidents are of three main types, though clinically they are sometimes difficult to distinguish.

Cerebral haemorrhage.
Cerebral thrombosis.
Cerebral embolism.

Cerebral haemorrhage results from rupture of a cerebral artery or aneurysm, and is commonest in patients with high blood pressure. Apart from cutting off the blood supply to the relevant part of the brain, the leaking collection of blood forms a space-occupying lesion within the brain, pressing on adjacent areas and causing *raised intracranial pressure*. The clinical picture is often more severe and of more abrupt onset than cerebral thrombosis or embolism and the patient may lapse into coma and die quickly.

Typically the onset is with headache, mental confusion and hemiplegia, the patient often losing consciousness almost immediately. In many cases, death follows rapidly, but when the haemorrhage is smaller, the course is correspondingly less rapid. Occasionally it is possible to evacuate a clot surgically, but otherwise there is no treatment.

Cerebral thrombosis is due to clotting of blood in a cerebral artery usually as a result of arteriosclerosis (*atheroma*). The *clinical picture* depends upon the size and importance of the occluded vessel and may vary between a trivial and transient weakness of a single limb to profound weakness of one side of the body, followed by coma. There is no effective treatment, unless the thrombosis is extending, when anticoagulants may sometimes be given.

Cerebral embolism is due to obstruction of a cerebral artery by an embolus. The latter is usually a clot, which has formed either in the heart (in mitral stenosis, atrial fibrillation, or after myocardial infarction), or on an atheromatous patch in one carotid artery. *The clinical picture* is often the same as that causing cerebral thrombosis (see above) and the diagnosis is usually made by finding the embolic source. It is no use removing the embolus because brain tissue is dead within a few minutes of losing its blood supply. *Treatment* is therefore aimed at preventing further episodes; anticoagulants, and possible surgical attack on the embolic source.

Prognosis of strokes. Many patients with cerebral haemorrhage quickly die but most patients with cerebral thrombosis or embolism survive. In such cases the paralysed limbs are often flaccid at first but before long the tone increases to produce the typical picture of an upper motor neurone lesion. The disability is at its greatest in the first few days; thereafter improvement occurs slowly, but what disability remains in several months is usually permanent, depending upon the size of the initial stroke and the age of the patient.

Treatment. Apart from the specific medical measures already mentioned, management depends largely upon the conscious level of the patient and whether or not his condition is deteriorating. In severe cases, the patient may be comatose on admission and management is then as for the unconscious patient (see Chapter 14, p. 135) both as regards nursing care and regular observations to detect a possible intracerebral haemorrhage (haematoma) which might be surgically evacuated.

In milder cases, the patient's conscious level may be little affected and attention should then be directed to his comfort. Until it is certain that deterioration has ceased, four-hourly records of pulse and blood pressure should be made. If there is obvious deterioration and coma seems imminent, this is increased to half-hourly observations with regular assessment of pupil size. Under these circumstances it is important to keep the attendant doctor informed of the patient's condition.

If deterioration does not occur during the first 24 to 48 hours the patient should be mobilized with the help of physiotherapy. Some patients are immediately ambulant but in others progress may be painstakingly slow. The patient may need help in dressing, feeding and performing toilet functions but constant encouragement to use the affected muscles is essential. Communication may be difficult if dysphasia is present and an understanding attitude on behalf of the nursing staff is required.

Those in whom quick mobilization is not achieved are frequently elderly; the position should be changed every two hours to prevent pulmonary congestion and pressure sores. Care of the bowels and bladder is important; constipation is common and retention of urine occasionally develops. Oral hygiene should be maintained if the patient is severely paralysed or his consciousness clouded.

PARAPLEGIA

Paraplegia is paralysis of the lower part of the body due to damage to the spinal cord, where, because of the compactness, both pyramidal tracts are liable to be affected. Typical causes include spinal fractures, prolapsed intervertebral discs (called cervical spondylosis when the neck is involved), and disseminated sclerosis. When the lesion is high in the spinal cord (e.g. in the neck) or in the brainstem all four limbs may be affected (*quadriplegia*). Sensory loss often accompanies the weakness, and nervous pathways to the bladder and bowel may also be interrupted, leading to retention or incontinence of urine and constipation.

If the lesion *severely* damages the spinal cord at one level, paralysis and sensory loss below this level may be complete. If the onset is sudden as in trauma, the muscles may be quite flaccid initially but in some weeks increased tone appears and involuntary movements may develop; in particular, the legs may develop flexor spasms which are especially prone to occur if the patient is disturbed or the legs touched. This is a reflex mechanism and the patient has no control over it.

The most important *nursing points* are to prevent pressure sores or infection of the bladder and to avoid contractures by regular passive movements through a full range at all joints at least once a day.

DISSEMINATED SCLEROSIS (Multiple Sclerosis)

This is one of the commonest neurological diseases, affecting both sexes, with onset usually between the ages of 20 and 40. It is characterized by scattered patches of degeneration in the brain and spinal cord. These come on at different times so that the progress of the condition is typically episodic. They may be separated by months or years and in the early stages each episode often makes a complete recovery. In later episodes recovery may occur but commonly some permanent deficit remains. The outcome varies; at one extreme there may be little or no disability after 20 or 30 years while at the other there may be complete paralysis within two or three years and death may follow from respiratory or urinary infection.

Early symptoms may include transient dragging of a leg, clumsiness of an arm, blurring of vision in one eye, double vision or retention or urgency of micturition. In advanced cases, examination may reveal quadriplegia of variable degree, together with features of cerebellar and ocular dysfunction. Sometimes there is *euphoria* (inappropriate cheerfulness), or intellectual deficit.

Treatment. There is at present no specific treatment although ACTH or steroids are sometimes given in acute episodes. *It is important that patients should remain ambulant for as long as possible.* Physiotherapy plays an important part in management and patients should be encouraged to do things for themselves. In advanced cases the nursing problems may be similar to those encountered in any severely paralysed patient (see Chapter 14, p. 133).

EPILEPSY

Epilepsy is caused by an abnormal electrical discharge within the brain. Various forms can be recognized, not all of which result in loss of consciousness. Some, such as *petit mal* and many cases of *grand mal* (see below) occur in otherwise normal people and there may be a family history of epilepsy. Other cases of grand mal (particularly when first occurring in adult life) and *focal epilepsy* result from organic disease of the brain, e.g. tumour, scarring, encephalitis. Grand mal may also occur in metabolic disturbances such as uraemia or hypoglycaemia.

Petit mal occurs in children and commonly disappears before adult life is reached. The attacks consist of impairment of consciousness lasting a few seconds during which the child appears 'blank' but does not fall.

Grand mal (major epilepsy) is the typical convulsion. Sometimes the patient has an *aura* (some type of preliminary sensation, the content of which varies from case to case, e.g. a strange smell or an odd feeling in a limb) before losing consciousness. More commonly this stage is omitted and there is sudden loss of consciousness, associated with 'tonic' (maintained) contraction of all the muscles which causes the body to become rigid. Respiration stops during the spasm. Sometimes there is a cry at the onset due to air being forced past the narrowed vocal cords, whose muscles are in spasm. After a variable period, usually less than half a minute, the tonic phase is replaced by a *clonic phase* during which the muscles jerk regularly, usually for about 30 to 60 seconds although this duration is variable. When the movements stop the patient is usually *deeply unconscious*. This stage sometimes merges with a state of *deep sleep* sometimes lasting several hours from which the patient eventually wakes, tired and often with headache. Commonly there is incontinence of urine or sometimes faeces during an attack, and the patient may bite his tongue or lip during the clonic phase because of convulsive movements of the jaws.

Focal epilepsy. Convulsions may affect predominantly one side of the body; the abnormal electrical focus responsible for the attack is then on the opposite side of the brain. When an aura occurs in grand mal and is referable to a particular part of the body, e.g. twitching or numbness of an arm, this too should be strictly regarded as focal epilepsy for it indicates that a particular part of the brain is primarily at fault. There are two other well-recognized forms of focal epilepsy.

Jacksonian epilepsy. This consists of twitching that starts in one place, typically a finger, a toe or the corner of the mouth, and then spreads slowly to all parts of that side of the body. The whole process may take many minutes and may culminate in loss of consciousness. It is caused by an abnormality, often a tumour, in the opposite motor cortex.

Temporal lobe epilepsy. With abnormalities in the temporal lobe, a curious form of epilepsy may occur which may result in episodes of alteration of consciousness, temporary mood changes (e.g. fear, depression), automatic behaviour of which the patient subsequently has no recollection (e.g. he might make a journey, or go to bed), hallucinations of special senses (particularly hearing and smell) and memory disturbances (such as a vivid revival of past memories, or a feeling that whatever he is doing, he has done before—'*déjà vu*').

Treatment of epilepsy. When epilepsy first develops in adult life it may be due to a tumour, so appropriate investigations should be done. If no underlying cause is found, the treatment is medical. Phenobarbitone and phenytoin (Epanutin) are the two most effective drugs for grand mal and focal epilepsy. Primidone (Mysoline) may also be used, particularly in temporal lobe epilepsy, and there are other drugs available in difficult cases. These three drugs cause sleepiness in large doses but phenytoin is the least likely to do so; rarely they may cause megaloblastic anaemia responsive to folic acid, and phenytoin may also cause swelling of the gums. Unsteadiness is common with large doses.

Ethosuximide (Zarontin) may be given for *petit mal*, but if the attacks are infrequent treatment may be unnecessary. Petit mal commonly diminishes with age but is sometimes replaced by grand mal.

Management during a grand mal seizure is directed at preventing the patient from injuring himself. A padded spatula (or any convenient object if this is not at hand) must be manipulated between the jaws on one side to prevent the patient biting his tongue. Care should be taken not to obstruct respiration. In addition, the head and limbs should be protected from injury since they may be undergoing quite violent movements. For nursing observations and care during a convulsion, see p. 132.

Status epilepticus. Occasionally, a patient may have repeated convulsions every few minutes without recovering consciousness between attacks.

It is a serious condition and untreated may be fatal from exhaustion. Fortunately, the attacks can usually be terminated by intravenous paraldehyde or diazepam (Valium) which leaves the patient in a state of deep sleep for several hours.

PRESENILE DEMENTIA

Dementia (intellectual deterioration) is normal in old age, but sometimes occurs in younger people (under 70) when it is known as presenile dementia. Usually the patient is middle-aged. He or she may have few complaints and it may be relatives who are responsible for his referral to hospital. The commonest cause is Alzheimer's disease, a degenerative disease of unknown cause. There are other rarer degenerative diseases but these too are not treatable. However, occasionally a treatable cause is found and most patients with presenile dementia should therefore be investigated in hospital. Amongst these treatable causes are cerebral tumours, 'general paralysis of the insane' (G.P.I.—a form of neurosyphilis), and vitamin B_{12} deficiency.

PARKINSON'S DISEASE (paralysis agitans)

Parkinson's disease is one of the commonest chronic diseases of the nervous system. It is a *disorder of the basal ganglia*, large groups of nerve cells deep in the substance of the brain that are necessary for the control of movement. The exact cause is unknown but some cases develop after encephalitis lethargica. Both sexes are affected and the onset is usually in middle life. It is a slowly progressive disorder of the motor system and is characterized by slowness of voluntary movement, rigidity of the muscles and tremor at rest which usually disappears on movement. One of the most characteristic features is the immobile 'mask-like' face. There is also a disturbance of balance so that the patient may tend to topple backwards, forwards or sideways at the slightest provocation.

Treatment is initially medical. Benzhexol (Artane) is usually the drug of choice but there are several alternatives, e.g. orphenadrine (Disipal), all of which act in a similar way and all of which have the side-effect of causing dryness of the mouth and blurring of vision. A new substance, L-Dopa, which acts in a totally different way has recently become available and in some patients results in dramatic improvement. However, none of these drugs is curative and in selected cases stereotactic surgery has a special place in management (see p. 664).

Encephalitis Lethargica. This disease is probably caused by a virus. It occurred in epidemic form between about 1915 and 1930 but is now rare. The features of an acute encephalitis were usually present but certain other features occurred—in particular a reversal of the normal sleep rhythm leading to wakefulness by night and drowsiness by day. Manifestations of Parkinson's disease sometimes developed in the early stages but in other patients these have developed months or years after the original illness.

CHOREA AND ATHETOSIS

These are also disorders of the basal ganglia. The salient feature in both is involuntary movement. In *chorea*, these resemble fragments of inappropriate voluntary movements and in mild cases may appear simply as undue restlessness. In more severe cases, the movements may be pronounced, usually affecting the arms more severely than the legs, and the hands may be held together in an attempt to control the movements. When an arm escapes his control, the patient may try to hide the movement, for example, by pretending to straighten his hair. There may be grimaces of the face and the tongue may be seen moving in the cheeks or may be protruded involuntarily at intervals.

In *athetosis* the movements are slower and more writhing but the two conditions sometimes merge and the term *choreathetosis* is then used. Athetosis is usually congenital.

Chorea is seen in two main forms: *Sydenham's (rheumatic) chorea*, now uncommon, is a post-infective phenomenon that may follow streptococcal sore throats. It occurs in childhood, rather more commonly in girls. In common with most other forms of involuntary movement it is made temporarily worse by emotional stress. Therapy is usually aimed at avoiding such stresses by keeping the child in a quiet but happy environment. In the uncommon event of movement being so severe as to injure the child, padded cot sides and other preventative measures may be necessary.

Huntington's chorea. This is an inherited condition that develops in middle life and is characterized by progressive chorea and dementia, with a chronic and ultimately fatal course.

SUBACUTE COMBINED DEGENERATION OF THE SPINAL CORD

This condition is caused by deficiency of vitamin B_{12} which results in damage to the spinal cord (particularly the dorsal and lateral columns) and peripheral nerves. The symptoms consist of numbness and pins and needles in the extremities and a progressive difficulty in walking. In most cases, pernicious anaemia is present. *Treatment* is with regular injections of vitamin B_{12} (cyanocobalamin) which initially must be given every few days; subsequently a monthly injection is usually adequate but this has to be continued for the remainder of the patient's life. Substantial improvement usually occurs although some permanent deficit may remain.

MIGRAINE

While not a serious condition, migraine is a common cause of absenteeism. The onset is usually in adolescence or early adult life and a family history is frequently present. In the typical attack, visual symptoms appear first—usually flashing lights or zigzags on one side of the visual field of both eyes. As this subsides, it is replaced by headache that is typically one-sided and usually lasts for the remainder of the day. Nausea and vomiting often occur. Photophobia, a dislike of bright light, is usual, and classically the patient goes to lie down in a room with the curtains drawn.

However, not all attacks are of this type. Visual symptoms may sometimes occur without headache or vice versa, or headache may be generalized rather than one-sided. Occasionally the visual symptoms may be replaced by sensory symptoms or transient weakness of one limb or one side of the body, or even a transient disorder of speech (dysphasia).

The symptoms of migraine result from changes in calibre of the arteries supplying the scalp and brain. The cause is not certain but there is some evidence of a disturbance in metabolism of serotonin, a substance normally occurring in the body.

Treatment is mainly with ergotamine preparations (e.g. Migril, Cafergot) which are taken at the beginning of an attack orally or by injection or occasionally by suppository or inhaler.

INFECTIVE DISORDERS OF THE NERVOUS SYSTEM

These include *meningitis, encephalitis* and *syphilis* (see below), *poliomyelitis* (see p. 376), and *cerebral abscess* (see p. 660).

Acute meningitis may be produced by bacteria (meningococcus, streptococcus, staphylococcus, pneumococcus, *Haemophilus influenzae*) or viruses. Bacterial meningitis is severe and usually fatal within a few days if untreated, but viral meningitis (benign lymphocytic choriomeningitis) is milder and subsides spontaneously. The patient develops severe headache with fever, neck stiffness, photophobia and irritability (he often resents being examined). In the case of meningococcal meningitis, blood infection (septicaemia) may be prominent and may cause petechial haemorrhages in the skin.

Diagnosis is by lumbar puncture (see p. 120) which reveals many leucocytes and bacteria in the cerebrospinal fluid. Some fluid should be sent for culture to identify the organism and its antibiotic sensitivity.

Treatment is urgent in bacterial meningitis. Antibiotics usually result in rapid improvement. They may have to be given by injection as vomiting frequently occurs. No specific treatment is available in viral meningitis but recovery is the rule; analgesics should be given if necessary for headache.

Nursing care is important in meningitis. The patient is usually curled up and resents disturbance. Excessive interference should therefore be avoided and routine nursing procedures should be carried out gently. Encouragement to drink may be necessary since the patient may be dehydrated from vomiting and sweating. If the patient has lapsed into coma, or is vomiting profusely, tube feeding or intravenous fluids may be necessary.

Tuberculous meningitis is a chronic form. The symptoms are similar to those of acute meningitis but of much more insidious onset. In other cases, the patient may appear very ill, with malaise, loss of appetite, fever and headache, and the diagnosis of meningitis may not be immediately obvious. In general, however, the features which suggest meningitis— neck stiffness and rigidity, photophobia and cerebral irritability— eventually develop. Untreated, the patient lapses into coma which may end fatally but in contrast to acute meningitis this may take many weeks.

Diagnosis is again by lumbar puncture. Treatment is with standard antituberculous therapy (streptomycin, PAS and isoniazid; see p. 206). Steroids are sometimes given in addition, as these may prevent fibrous adhesions developing around the brain.

Nursing attention depends upon the clinical state and is essentially as for acute bacterial meningitis (see above).

ENCEPHALITIS

This is a diffuse inflammation of the brain and in nearly all cases is caused by a virus. It may develop after common viral infections (e.g. measles, chickenpox, rubella) or even after vaccination. The damage may then be due to an allergic reaction against viruses which have reached the brain. In other cases (e.g. herpes encephalitis) damage may be due to multiplication of the virus itself. *The symptoms of encephalitis* are headache, fits, delirium and deterioration in level of consciousness. There may also be signs suggesting meningitis (neck rigidity, etc.) but these are mild in relation to the severe cerebral symptoms. Specific treatment is limited but steroids may be of value to counteract inflammation and brain swelling, and in the case of herpes encephalitis an antiviral substance, idoxuridine, is now used.

SYPHILIS OF THE NERVOUS SYSTEM (Neurosyphilis)

In a small proportion of cases an acute meningitis may develop within weeks of primary syphilitic infection. Apart from this, neurosyphilis is a late manifestation occurring years after primary infection. There are several forms:

Meningovascular syphilis—a chronic inflammation of the meninges and of the arteries which pass through the meninges to reach the brain and spinal cord. Occlusion of these vessels may cause strokes, and when these occur in a younger man, meningovascular syphilis should always be borne in mind as a possible cause.

General paralysis of the insane (G.P.I.)—an old-fashioned and now inappropriate title since it is usually diagnosed and treated before the classical syndrome has had time to develop. It is a syphilitic infection of the brain itself. The initial symptoms are impairment of memory and concentration. Dementia supervenes, sometimes accompanied by 'delusions of grandeur', fits, and eventually paralysis of the limbs due to bilateral upper motor neurone involvement.

Tabes dorsalis. In this condition the dorsal nerve roots and dorsal root ganglia are involved. The sensory nerves entering the spinal cord are therefore affected. Stabbing pains ('lightning pains') and paraesthesiae (pins and needles) may occur in the legs. Voluntary movements may be poorly controlled (ataxia) because of lack of sensory information telling the patient the position of his limbs in space. There may also be a disturbance of bladder function due to lack of awareness of a full bladder. Examination reveals absent tendon reflexes and sensory loss, together with an abnormality of the pupils (Argyll-Robertson pupil) that often accompanies other forms of neurosyphilis.

Syphilitic optic atrophy: a degeneration of the optic nerves which leads to failure of vision. It may accompany tabes dorsalis.

Treatment of all forms of syphilis is by penicillin once the diagnosis has been established by serological tests (Wassermann reaction and treponemal immobilization tests). Sometimes this is so effective that during the first few days of treatment, the toxic products from the dead organisms cause a temporary aggravation of symptoms (Herxheimer reaction).

DISORDERS OF THE LOWER MOTOR NEURONES

Good examples of this are seen in the following conditions: Bell's palsy (see below), poliomyelitis (see p. 376), motor neurone disease, peripheral neuritis, carpal tunnel syndrome (see p. 268).

Bell's palsy. This is a lower motor neurone paralysis of the seventh cranial nerve (supplying the muscles of facial expression) which develops over a few hours, often with some discomfort behind the ear, and usually recovers within a few weeks or months. Its cause is unknown. Occasionally it is permanent. The whole of one side of the face is limp and expressionless, but sensation and the muscles of chewing are unaffected as these are supplied by the fifth cranial nerve. On smiling or talking, the mouth is drawn over to the normal side because the muscles on that side are unopposed in their action. Blinking and eye closure may be incomplete on the affected side and this results in exposure of the eye, with, occasionally, the development of corneal ulceration.

Treatment. Some physicians give steroids or ACTH in the early stages, to counteract the nerve swelling that is thought to be responsible for the paralysis. If corneal damage occurs, it may be necessary to stitch the eyelids together temporarily (tarsorrhaphy—see Chapter 61, p. 647). In the small proportion who do not recover, plastic surgery may be carried out, using fascial slings beneath the skin to lift that side of the face, or another nerve (e.g. the hypoglossal) may be transferred in the hope that it will re-innervate the face. These manoeuvres are not very effective.

MOTOR NEURONE DISEASE

This is a progressive disorder of lower and upper motor neurones, usually affecting both together, but sometimes one may be affected more severely. The onset is typically in middle life and the condition is usually fatal within two to three years. Its cause is unknown and there is therefore no specific treatment. In most cases the patient eventually becomes completely paralysed, and death results from respiratory failure, either because the respiratory muscles fail, or because the swallowing muscles are defective and allow food and liquid to spill over into the trachea. In either case there is usually a terminal pneumonia.

Nursing attention is as for the paralysed patient (see p. 133). In particular, extreme care must be taken during feeding to prevent choking. Indeed, feeding may become so hazardous that tube feeding must be considered; unfortunately, there is no cure for this condition and such procedures may only be delaying a very unpleasant end.

PERIPHERAL NEURITIS (polyneuritis, polyneuropathy)

This is an inflammation or degeneration of the peripheral nerves and there are many possible causes. It may follow infections (e.g. upper respiratory tract infections), drugs (e.g. isoniazid, nitrofurantoin), ingestion of chemicals, or dietary deficiency (particularly thiamine deficiency as in alcoholics). Both sensory and motor nerve fibres are affected and the longest nerves are most involved. Thus the peripheral parts of the legs and arms are affected by weakness, numbness and paraesthesiae and tendon reflexes are reduced or absent.

Treatment is directed against the causative agent. Those cases following infections usually recover spontaneously, but occasionally paralysis may become so widespread that even the muscles of respiration and swallowing are affected. If this occurs, all measures are taken to save the patient—including tracheostomy and positive pressure respiration if necessary—because if this difficult period can be overcome, complete recovery occurs after some weeks or months.

Nursing care depends upon the severity of the condition. If weakness is widespread, appropriate measures must be taken, as for the paralysed patient.

CARPAL TUNNEL SYNDROME

This is very common, but not serious. The median nerve at the wrist passes through a narrow tunnel and is liable to compression. Typically the patient is a middle-aged woman. Pain and paraesthesiae are experienced in the thumb and adjacent two and a half fingers, particularly at night. In severe cases the small muscles of the thumb may also become weak due to damage to the motor nerve fibres.

Treatment. Wrist splints that cock the wrist back relieve the pressure in the canal and may be worn at night. Hydrocortisone injections into the canal also relieve the symptoms but usually only for a month or two. Permanent cure is obtained by opening up the canal surgically.

DISORDERS OF MUSCLE

Myopathy is the name given to disorders of the muscle fibres. There are several forms of inherited myopathy which are known as *the muscular dystrophies.* Those developing in adolescence or adult life are usually mild but the type with onset in early childhood, *Duchenne dystrophy* or *pseudo-hypertrophic muscular dystrophy*, is much more severe, leading to progressive paralysis which eventually involves the respiratory muscles; such patients do not usually reach adult life.

Other myopathies. Generalized weakness due to myopathy may occasionally occur in other conditions, for example carcinoma and endocrine disturbances (hyperthyroidism, Cushing's syndrome, steroid administration). In these cases, treatment is directed at the primary disorder.

Polymyositis is an inflammatory disease that may resemble a myopathy.

Myasthenia gravis. This is not a disorder of the muscle fibres themselves, but of the 'neuromuscular junction', where the nerve fibre activates the muscle fibre in contraction. This activation is normally produced by acetylcholine which is liberated from the termination of the nerve fibre.

Myasthenia can begin at any age, but most commonly does so in early adult life, affecting females more commonly than males. The symptoms of myasthenia consist of an abnormal fatiguability of muscle. Sometimes this is generalized, but in other cases it may predominate in either muscles around the eye, causing double vision and drooping eyelids, *ptosis*, or the muscles of speech and swallowing. Whatever the distribution of weakness, the characteristic feature is that use of the muscles rapidly causes their strength to decline, although this will recover within a few minutes on resting. For a similar reason, symptoms are usually least on rising, and worst at the end of the day.

Treatment is by drugs (neostigmine and pyridostigmine), which prevent the breakdown of acetylcholine and therefore improve the function of the neuromuscular junction. Sometimes steroids are used. Although the cause of myasthenia is not known, there is sometimes an associated tumour of the thymus gland, and even when there is no such tumour removal of the thymus (thymectomy) may benefit selected cases.

Carcinomatous myasthenia. Occasionally a distant carcinoma (e.g. of the bronchus) may produce a condition mimicking myasthenia gravis but this can be distinguished by special electrical tests. If the tumour is removed the condition may disappear.

CARE OF THE PARALYSED PATIENT

The paralysed limbs of the *recently hemiplegic patient* are usually flaccid and should be arranged and supported with pillows or sandbags. The arms should be in a comfortable position, usually slightly flexed and the legs should be straight with sandbags or pillows separating the pressure points at knee and ankle. The foot is kept dorsiflexed by means of sandbags, or splints, to prevent the development of foot drop. Contractures must be avoided by regular passive movements through a full range at all joints at least once a day.

The problem in the paraplegic patient is usually more complex as the disturbance is bilateral and is often accompanied by loss of cutaneous sensation (predisposing to pressure sores), and urinary retention or incontinence (predisposing to urinary infection).

In the *quadriplegic* (or *tetraplegic*) *patient*, the same problems apply, but the patient is unable to feed or wash himself and requires correspondingly more attention (see Nursing the Paralysed Patient, Chapter 14, p. 133). Because the intercostal muscles are paralysed, coughing may be inadequate and in high cervical lesions there is the added danger that the phrenic nerve (arising from the third to fifth cervical nerves) may be damaged, leading to diaphragmatic paralysis. The rate and depth of respiration should therefore be carefully observed; in severe or acute cases, tracheostomy and positive pressure respiration may be necessary. Even when respiration is adequately maintained for everyday needs, its shallow nature coupled with the paralysed state of the patient may favour the development of pneumonia. Antibiotics may also be necessary. Preventive measures include regular physiotherapy to the chest.

Care of the patient with muscular dystrophy is similar although sensory involvement and bladder dysfunction are not present. However, as in other types of paralysis, the patient should be encouraged to use the affected parts for as long as possible, as disuse may lead to further deterioration.

Chapter 27

An Introduction to Psychiatric Conditions, Treatment and Nursing Care

by JOHN GREENE

> *Introduction—the neuroses—the psychoses—addiction, alcoholic, drug—disorders of intelligence, behaviour, personality—general principles of psychiatric treatment, psychological, physical, social—psychiatric nursing—responsibility of the psychiatric nurse*

Psychiatry is the specialized branch of general medicine which deals with the study and treatment of mental disorders. The term mental disorder in its legal sense embraces all forms of mental illness, mental subnormality, and psychopathic states. As psychiatry becomes more closely identified with general medicine the facilities for treating psychiatric illness are increasing. In the past the psychiatric hospital was the focal point of psychiatry. There are now psychiatric units in many general hospitals, more out-patient clinics, day hospitals, specialized treatment centres, and provisions for actual treatment in the patient's own home.

Constitutional, emotional and environmental factors contribute to the causes of psychiatric illness. Prevention and treatment is therefore dependent on using the resources of physical, psychological and social medicine and in seeing the relation between man's body, his mind and the world around him. There are many methods of classifying psychiatric illness using various headings and sub-headings such as:

> The neuroses or psycho-neuroses.
> The psychoses.
> Disorders of intelligence, behaviour and personality.

THE NEUROSES

The common illnesses in the *neuroses* group include: anxiety states, obsessional states, hysteria and some reactive depressions.

Neurotic illness is characterized by the patient's insight into his condition. He recognizes the need for treatment. His symptoms may outwardly appear to be almost entirely of a physical nature and not seriously impair his behaviour and personality. Once physical illness has been eliminated investigation will reveal a history of unresolved conflicts and psychological stress. These may be due to difficulties of adjustment to a new environment or increased responsibilities; family disharmony and problems of interpersonal relationships are frequently elicited.

Anxiety states. The symptoms most commonly mentioned are fear, inability to concentrate and sleeplessness. There may be feelings of panic, phobias about going out, meeting other people, and having to make decisions. These feelings can gradually dominate and produce a disruption of the patient's life. The body reacts to psychological stress by producing symptoms such as excessive sweating, particularly of the palms of the hands, headaches, loss of appetite, gastro-intestinal upsets, tremors of the hands and facial tics. Depression associated with the patient's feelings of misery and despair is also a common feature of anxiety states.

Treatment. Psychological treatment will include individual or group *psychotherapy*. At a superficial level this consists of counselling, reassurance and giving the patient insight into his symptoms. At a deeper level it will mean exploring the emotional factors, analysing the symptoms and leading the patient to an understanding of his illness. A short period away from anxiety-provoking situations may in some cases be all that is necessary in the way of treatment.

Physical treatment will consist of restoring good physical health through diet, exercise, relaxation and sleep.

Drugs in the form of hypnotics, tranquillizers and antidepressants may be used (see pp. 278–9).

Social treatment may involve the removal or at least the reduction of problems in relation to work, finance, housing and other contributing factors. It is important also to improve the patient's capacity to make friends, find fresh interests and live a fuller social life.

Obsessional states. In this neurotic form of illness the patient's behaviour is disturbed by rituals which dominate his thoughts and actions. They tend to occur in people of obsessive personality, who realize these performances are senseless and try hard to resist them. In a simple form they may be no more than repeatedly checking that a light has been switched off or a door properly closed. In severe form they may, for example, actually prevent a housewife from leaving the house in case the cooker is still on, or the telephone rings. Such ideas can be manifest also in ritualistic washing or in fear of touching or being touched by something unpleasant. The effect of these compulsive actions can produce great feelings of anxiety, distress and depression.

Treatment. Obsessional states usually respond to *psychotherapy*. Although the patient can be given insight and guidance into methods of avoiding the situations which worry him, it is unlikely that his obsessional personality will be changed. Treatment is therefore aimed at relieving the distress of the sufferer. *Drugs* of the tranquillizer group help to reduce tension. *Electroplexy* may be necessary to counteract depression. *Leucotomy* may be resorted to if the tension cannot be relieved by other means.

Depressive states. When depression occurs in association with neurotic illness treatment of the primary symptoms may be all that is needed. When the depression persists, *antidepressant drugs* may be used, and in some cases *electroplexy* may be ordered.

Hysteria or *hysterical reaction* is associated with a particular type of self-centred personality. It is said to be more easily recognized than defined, and because so many factors may be involved in the cause, the diagnosis and treatment are extremely complex.

Physical symptoms are abnormalities in function of practically any part of the body supplied with nerves. Many forms of neurological, visceral or skin disease are simulated. *Mental symptoms* can resemble the various types of mental illness. Emotional storms and threats of suicide may follow comparatively minor frustrations and upsets. Amnesia, sleep-walking, or trance-like states are also common. In long-standing cases there is a typical attitude of indifference and cheerful detachment. There is usually a lack of insight and a vehement insistence on a physical basis for the symptoms.

Treatment. Suggestion is useful. Too much sympathy may be harmful and a suitable combination of firmness and sympathetic understanding is what is most needed. Psychotherapy may bring success in the cure of symptoms, and the aim may be to analyse the patient's problems and to re-educate his personality. Subtle adjustment of the environment can relieve stress; drugs may be used to control emotional outbursts and disturbances of behaviour.

The reactive depressions associated with neurosis tend to occur in response to emotional upsets or situational problems in people of unstable personality.

THE PSYCHOSES

The psychoses or psychotic group of illnesses can be described under four main headings. In acute form they produce disturbances of behaviour which usually require treatment in hospital. In a few cases legal formalities for compulsory admission may be necessary when the patient is unable or unwilling to accept that there is a need for treatment.

> Schizophrenia including simple schizophrenia, hebephrenia and catatonic schizophrenia.
> Paranoid states.
> Manic depressive states.
> Organic psychoses.

Schizophrenia is one of the commonest forms of psychiatric illness and a high proportion of beds in psychiatric hospitals are occupied by schizophrenic patients. The condition usually develops in adolescents and young adults and is rarely seen to begin after the age of 40. It is slow in onset and a study of the previous personality usually reveals a history of day-dreaming, undue sensitivity and odd idiosyncrasies.

The *symptoms* associated with schizophrenia include general apathy and loss of interest; shallowness and lack of emotional reaction; withdrawal from contact with other people; loss of initiative in relation to movement and action sometimes leading to stupor; manneristic, ambivalent and impulsive behaviour. Thought disorders, bizarre expressions and feelings of unreality may be present; auditory hallucinations are common and patients frequently have delusions of being affected by rays, or radio waves. Many of the symptoms are found in all forms of schizophrenia and this adds to the difficulty of differentiating between three main types.

In *simple schizophrenia* the main features may be apathy, loss of interest, lack of ambition, unsociability and emotional dullness.

In *hebephrenia* hallucinations of sight and hearing are common. There may be delusions of a bizarre nature with a disturbance in train of thought, incoherence of speech and impulsive activity.

Catatonic schizophrenia is characterized by its sudden onset. A dull stupor may develop from a period of apathy. The patient may become mute and motionless. Bouts of excitement and frenzy may alternate with periods of stupor; in both phases sudden violent attacks may be made on other people or self-destruction attempted. *Hallucinations* and *delusions* are present. The condition of stupor is seen less often as a result of earlier diagnosis and treatment.

Treatment of schizophrenia. The aim of treatment is to relieve the symptoms and prevent deterioration. *Schizophrenia* is now commonly treated with the major tranquillizing drugs of the phenothiazine group see p. 279) in association with a programme of *resocialization* and *rehabilitation. Electroplexy* is effective in relieving the states of excitement and stupor. *Occupational, social* and *recreational* activities combat the tendencies of withdrawal and isolation from normal activities. Continuous persuasive encouragement is needed and may have to be continued for prolonged periods.

Return to normal social habits should be the aim of the rehabilitation process. Schizophrenic patients have a notorious tendency to relapse through not keeping in touch with their doctor and failing to take prescribed drugs. The use of long-lasting tranquillizing drugs such as Modecate and Depixol helps to maintain many of these patients in the community. The inclusion of psychiatric nurses in the after-care team ensures continuity and better supervision of the patients' medication. Unfortunately a proportion of schizophrenic patients require readmission to or continued treatment in hospital. Periodic admission rather than continued hospitalization is considered best in the long term so that the patients do not become institutionalized.

Paranoid states. These are sometimes associated with the schizophrenic group of illnesses. The onset is usually after the age of 40, and the patient generally has a suspicious 'chip on shoulder' personality. Delusions are usually fixed and immovable and persecutory in nature. Intellectual deterioration is rare.

Manic-depressive psychoses. These include the alternating states of *mania* and *depression,* and *involutional depression.* The chief characteristics are extreme mood-swings from elation and excitement to profound despair and feelings of misery. A *cyclothymic personality* and physical *pyknic type* is associated with manic-depressive illness.

Mania can be seen in three forms. The mildest, *hypomania*, presents a picture of sustained elation, overactivity and a marked flight of ideas. To the general public the patient will be seen as a lively, talkative, jolly and generous type. His family may experience this as a passing phase in which he is unusually active, irritating and extravagant with money.

Acute mania. The symptoms mentioned above are more marked. The patient is superior in his attitude and quick to anger if frustrated. Conduct is generally disordered and a period in hospital may be necessary. There will be evidence of fleeting *hallucinations* and *grandiose delusions* with claims to wealth and power. Extreme restlessness may lead to fatigue and exhaustion.

Delirious mania is an extreme state which may follow the hypomanic and acute stages unless they are effectively controlled by drugs.

Treatment. The main consideration is to control the excessive activity and excitement. Heavy sedation may be the first step, followed by the use of tranquillizing drugs over a long period. The atmosphere should be calm and quiet, with external stimuli kept at a minimum. Adequate fluids and solid nourishment are essential as it is difficult to halt the patient's activity long enough for proper meals to be taken. Prolonged *narcosis* may be necessary if the restlessness and excitement persist. *Electroplexy* is also beneficial in controlling excitement.

Depression is in striking contrast to *mania.* Instead of overactivity and elation there is extreme retardation of movement and thought. The patient looks anxious and unhappy and complains of misery and guilt out of all proportion to the circumstances. The most serious symptoms are feelings of guilt and unworthiness which may lead to attempted or actual suicide. The patient also complains of bodily dysfunction, for example an inability to eat and pass food through the body. *Depression,* like *mania,* varies in degree and may be divided into *simple depression* and *acute depression.*

Treatment. Nursing care calls for strict but unobtrusive observation in the acute stage to prevent suicide. Depression quickly responds to electroplexy when given two or three times a week and up to six or eight times in all. *Antidepressant drugs* such as *imipramine* (*Trofranil*) and *amitriptyline* (*Tryptizol*) are used in association with *psychotherapy.*

Involutional depression occurs most commonly in men and women of middle age who have usually had no previous history of psychiatric illness. It can be attributed both to the feeling that the best years of life are over and to the physical aspects of the change of life. The symptoms in general differ little from those of other forms of depression but there may be a greater tendency towards feelings of unreality and hypochondria. Treatment consists of *antidepressant drugs, electroplexy* and *psychotherapy.*

The organic psychoses include a number of conditions in which there is a dysfunction of the brain or central nervous system and an associated disturbance of the mind. Examples are cerebro-vascular disease, alcoholism, cerebral syphilis and after effects of head injuries. Less common conditions such as *Huntington's chorea* also produce dementia in varying degrees.

Senile psychosis. Mental disorder in the elderly may simply consist of depressive, manic or paranoid states, but the disintegration of the personality associated with dementia is much more common. The typical symptoms include loss of memory for recent events, confusion, irritability and restlessness. If the patient lives alone, his self-neglect may lead to a decline in his general state of health and subsequent admission to hospital. There is considerable strain on the family of senile patients if they are wandering around, are incontinent at night, and are in danger of coming to harm if left alone.

Treatment consists of relieving the physical and mental symptoms. The outlook is changing for many of these elderly people as the facilities improve with the development of psychogeriatric services.

The combination of *drug therapy* and attention to diet, combined with a programme of physical and mental rehabilitation can prevent rapid deterioration. It may be possible to discharge the patient, and arrange attendance at a day hospital or care in the patient's own home. Re-admission to hospital for short periods can ensure relief for the family and regular assessment of the patient.

Addiction is included in the organic psychoses when alcohol or drugs cause mental disturbance as a result of damage to the brain or nervous system. *Alcoholic addiction* has always been a social problem. The effects of alcohol may vary from disruption of the patient's own and family life to severe mental disturbance. The habit may be acquired in sociable drinking and become impossible to break, or there may be physiological or psychological need for a feeling of well-being and a means of escape from difficulties and problems.

Treatment. In mild forms the alcoholic can be helped by *psychotherapy* and *social re-education.* Tolerance of the individual's weakness and help from agencies such as Alcoholics Anonymous can do much to assist the patient.

Severe alcoholism will require treatment in hospital or in an alcoholic addiction centre. A gradual or even sudden withdrawal may be prescribed. Sedative or tranquillizing drugs will be used to control excitement and withdrawal symptoms, and the general bodily health will require attention. *Conditioned aversion therapy* through the use of the nauseating and emetic effect of drugs such as apomorphine is sometimes used in association with psychotherapy. *Vitamin B, modified insulin* and modified narcosis therapy are also used as adjunctive treatments.

Drug addiction. The pattern of drug addiction has dramatically changed in recent years despite the legal control of the manufacture, sale and prescribing of drugs like *cocaine, heroin* and *morphine.* A steep increase has occurred in the use of amphetamine as a stimulant, and cannabis and *lysergic acid diethylamide* (L.S.D.) for their psychedelic effects, particularly by young people in the 15 to 25 age groups, which may lead to the more dangerous habits of heroin and cocaine addiction. Drug addiction centres where skilled help is available have been established in many hospitals.

Treatment may take the form of maintenance doses of the drug to prevent withdrawal symptoms. Intensive *psychotherapy* over a long period may be necessary with the aim of getting the patient to give up the drug altogether. Substitute drugs may be ordered in the early stages. *Modified narcosis* using drugs such as *Sodium Amytal, Librium,* or *paraldehyde* may also be prescribed. The combined efforts of the patient, his family, the police, doctors, social workers and nurses may be needed. Permanent recovery is most likely to take place in patients of previous stable personality. The addict may start taking drugs to satisfy a neurotic need but in chronic form addiction can have severe organic repercussions.

Puerperal psychosis is a condition sometimes occurring after childbirth and shown as two main groups of symptoms. A state of *confusion, excitement,* or *delusion* in which restlessness and disturbed perception make it impossible for the mother to nurse her baby may arise. It is attributed to toxaemia, sepsis, pyrexia and exhaustion. Once the underlying cause is cleared up recovery quickly takes place.

Alternatively there may be a *depression* or *schizophrenic* reaction to childbirth. The *depression* develops some days after the birth of the child. It is in this condition that the risk of infanticide may arise through the mother having feelings of general inadequacy, of rejecting the child, and fears of being unable to feed it.

Treatment will include close nursing observation during the acute stage. Some psychiatric hospitals have mother and baby units where the mother can be treated without total separation from her baby. Specific treatment will include *antidepressant drugs, electroplexy* and *psychotherapy.*

In both conditions careful follow-up after discharge from hospital will be necessary so that the patient can be quickly readmitted if there are signs of relapse and consequent danger to the baby.

Childbirth can be the precipitating factor when symptoms of *schizophrenia* occur in mothers who have had no previous history of mental illness.

DISORDERS OF INTELLIGENCE, BEHAVIOUR, PERSONALITY

No introduction to psychiatry and psychiatric nursing would be complete without reference to the disorders of intelligence, behaviour and personality. These include severe subnormality and psychopathic states. Because recent scientific knowledge has thrown new light on the whole subject of mental subnormality the problems of nursing and training have increased. This is partly due to the high survival rate amongst the most seriously handicapped and the consequent standard of institutional care that is required.

Severe subnormality. This grading covers those who are incapable of self-support and vary from the completely helpless to those who are able to perform very simple tasks. An intelligence quotient (I.Q.) of below 50 and a mental age of not more than seven years is another criterion applied. Scientific research has shown that genetic factors and chromosome abnormalities or metabolic disturbance are responsible for conditions such as *mongolism, phenylketonuria, microcephalus, hydrocephalus* and *epiloia.* Other conditions in which severe subnormality may be found are *postencephalitis, postmeningitis, paralysis, epilepsy, spina bifida* and *birth injury.*

The *subnormal* category includes those who have poor mental capacity, an I.Q. of 50 to 69, and a mental age of eight to ten years. The group may also include some cases of *epilepsy, psychosis, autism* or *psychopathic disorder.* One or two out of a hundred in a hospital for the mentally subnormal may be found to have a chromosome or metabolic abnormality.

The *treatment* of subnormal patients is essentially care, education and training. Specific treatment may be aimed at preventing metabolic abnormality. Rehabilitation methods can enable many to live at home, in hostels, or in training centres where the resources of community care are available.

Autism. The word autism which was formerly used to describe a symptom is now associated with a particular form of psychiatric illness in children, also known as *schizophrenic syndrome in childhood*. The condition may fit into the category of subnormality when the overall I.Q. is low. In contrast there may be areas of high intelligence and if selective education and training are available the potential of these patients can be considerably improved.

Psychopathic states, according to the Mental Health (England and Wales) Act 1959, are defined as 'persistent disorders of mind (whether or not accompanied by subnormality of intelligence) which result in abnormally aggressive or seriously irresponsible conduct on the part of the patient, and require or are susceptible to medical treatment.' The main characteristics are emotional instability, psychological immaturity, child-like irresponsibility and an inability to learn from experience. In hospital these patients are demanding, unco-operative, unreliable and often unpredictable in behaviour. They are more likely, however, to respond to tolerant guidance and to sympathetic understanding than to punitive and restrictive handling. Behaviour tends to improve, and after the age of 25 the problems tend to lessen.

GENERAL PRINCIPLES OF PSYCHIATRIC TREATMENT

Once a psychiatric diagnosis has been made treatment will be undertaken in whatever setting is most appropriate. The broad principles of psychiatric treatment can be listed under the three main headings of psychological, physical, and social methods (see below). *Children* can be treated as out-patients at a child guidance clinic or in a children's psychiatric hospital unit. In the case of subnormality it will most likely be in the children's section of a mental subnormality hospital. Occasionally it will be decided to investigate and treat children with psychiatric disorders in a paediatric unit of a general hospital.

Adolescents, like children, have special needs and benefit from treatment in special units where the facilities permit energetic activities. Young people with emotional and behaviour problems require sympathetic understanding. It is therefore important that the staff who work in adolescent units have a good preparation for and an interest in this specialized work.

For *adult patients* treatment may take place at out-patient clinics, in day hospitals, psychiatric units of general hospitals, or in the ordinary psychiatric hospitals. Where it is desirable, some patients will be treated in specialized units such as those for addiction, or in special security hospitals.

The elderly. Ideally all elderly patients should in the first instance be assessed in psychogeriatric centres where the diagnosis, prognosis and the plan of treatment can be determined.

Psychological treatment ranges from simple counselling and reassurance to *deep psychotherapy*. Deep analysis and exploration of the unconscious mind requires the skill of a trained psychotherapist, who is usually a doctor. Individual or group methods may be used. Some nurses are now developing considerable skill in these methods but all nurses can play an important part in psychological treatment by developing the art of listening, counselling and giving psychotherapeutic support to the patient. In short the whole aim of psychological treatment is to give the patient the insight he needs to resolve his problems and lead him towards a healthier way of living. Where the concept of a therapeutic community is accepted every member of the hospital staff and the patients themselves are seen as participants in the process of healing.

The main physical treatments in use at the present time are electroplexy, narcosis, modified insulin and drug therapy.

Electroplexy is a common physical treatment. It is particularly effective in cases of severe depression. The procedure consists of passing a low voltage electrical current between two electrodes, one on each temporal area. The patient is usually anaesthetized with Pentothal, and given a muscle relaxant such as Scoline. A pre-medication of atropine half an hour beforehand is given to reduce salivation. Preparation includes thorough reassurance and explanation of the procedure. During treatment the patient lies on his back on a flat firm surface with the head supported. Support to the lower limbs, hips and shoulders gently and evenly applied to prevent injury when the convulsive action takes place may be necessary. To accelerate the return of normal respiration an airway is inserted and oxygen is usually administered under pressure immediately after the convulsion. The patient is then turned on his side, and kept under observation until consciousness is regained and the period of confusion and restlessness has passed. Complications are rare in physically healthy patients but occasionally fractures, or cardiac and respiratory failures may occur.

Narcosis. Deep and modified narcosis is used in cases of extreme anxiety, manic excitement or in the treatment of drug and alcoholic addiction. Prolonged sleep is induced for as many hours as possible day and night for a period of 10 to 14 days with drugs such as Sodium Amytal and paraldehyde. The treatment calls for skilled nursing attention in a quiet atmosphere where external stimuli can be excluded from the patient. Liberal fluids are needed to counter toxic effects. Blood pressure and temperature should be frequently recorded and a close watch kept for signs of collapse.

Modified insulin therapy. Deep insulin therapy has been almost wholly replaced by drugs in the treatment of schizophrenia. Modified insulin is used mainly as an adjunctive treatment in psychiatry when the physical health is poor and the appetite is in need of stimulation.

Drugs. The drugs most commonly used in psychiatry at the present time can be broadly classified as hypnotics, tranquillizers and antidepressants. The list is constantly changing and it is therefore important that nurses should be aware of the potency of the preparations being used and the need to observe the patient for any possible side-effects of the drug.

Hypnotics: phenobarbitone—Luminal;   quinalbarbitone—Seconal; amylobarbitone—Sodium Amytal; pentobarbitone—Nembutal.

Tranquillizers: chlorpromazine—Largactil;   trifluoperazine—Stelazine;   perphenazine—Fentazin;   promazine—Sparine; thioridazine—Melleril; chlordiazepoxide—Librium; diazepam —Valium; pimozide—Orap; haloperidol—Serenace. In addition long-acting preparations such as fluphenazine—Modecate, and flupenthixol—Depixol, are widely used in psychiatry.

Antidepressants: imipramine—Tofranil;   desipramine—Pertofran;   protriptyline—Concordin;   amitriptyline—Tryptizol; tranylcypromine—Parnate; phenelzine—Nardil.

Social therapy. Under social therapy can be included all activities of an educational and occupational nature designed to improve the patient's capacity to live a full life in the community. The choice of social therapy will usually be decided upon by the doctor in consultation with nurses, social workers and occupational therapists, the aim being to rehabilitate the patient to his optimum capacity. Account will be taken of the patient's age and degree of illness in planning all activities, whether they be of a diversional or occupational nature for short-stay patients or industrial therapy and training programmes which are more suitable for long-stay patients in hospitals for mental illness and mental subnormality. To complete the programme of rehabilitation, after-care on leaving hospital may be necessary. This is where the resources of the hospital and local authority health services can be brought together for effective community care of psychiatric patients.

PSYCHIATRIC NURSING

The role of psychiatric nurses has undergone considerable change in recent years. It was formerly work of a custodial nature when the majority of all psychiatric patients were nursed in locked wards. In this situation it was not easy to establish a satisfactory nurse-patient relationship. The qualities required for a good psychiatric nurse are not easy to define but she should have a stable personality, good intelligence, a friendly disposition and a sympathetic understanding of other people's needs. These are basic qualities but the skills of psychological, physical and social nursing care have to be learned from practical experience and theoretical instruction.

In psychiatric nursing the aim is to treat the whole person and it must never be forgotten that the behaviour of each individual patient is influenced by the action of his mind, body and total environment. The nurse has to learn to know her patients through carefully observing their behaviour, finding out how they feel, and seeing how they react to other people and to the situations in which they find themselves. As interpersonal relationships are so important it is essential that the nurse equally understands her own behaviour because of the way it can influence her attitudes towards her patients.

The psychological content of psychiatric nursing includes counselling and reassuring the anxious, stimulating the depressed and calming the excitable or overwrought. It also includes listening to the patients' outpourings and showing a genuine interest in all that they have to say. Occasionally the nurse will become the target for complaints and verbal abuse; this may be the only way in which a particular patient can express his feelings, and the experienced nurse will accept it as a means of communication. Planned group activities are designed to involve patients in situations where they can discuss their symptoms with one another; they will gain from knowing that other people have problems like their own; they can in a subtle way be encouraged by the nurse to assume responsibility and learn also to put the needs of others before their own. A good deal of the psychological part of nursing consists of doing things *with* patients rather than *for* them so that they do not become dependent on the nurse.

The physical content of psychiatric nursing includes caring for those who are sick or infirm; ensuring that general hygienic habits are encouraged; looking after the general cleanliness, comfort, appearance and physical well-being of the patients.

The social content of psychiatric nursing will include the immediate environment of the patient, such as ensuring that he does not come to harm through avoidable hazards. At times he may need protection from others whose behaviour is disturbed or he himself may threaten injury to others. As a result of his illness he may actually attempt to harm himself deliberately because of *hallucinations* or *delusions*, or he may come to harm simply because he is unable to distinguish what may be harmful to him. If restraint in any form has to be resorted to, it should not be continued for longer than is absolutely necessary.

It must be remembered, too, that all physically sick people undergo some psychological stress during illness and it is therefore an advantage to all nurses to gain some experience in nursing both physically and mentally ill people.

The nurse has responsibilities towards many other people as well as her patients. *She has a duty to keep doctors and her fellow nurses fully informed by accurate verbal and written reports.* She comes into contact with a great many people who have an indirect interest in the patient's welfare, and need accurate information in order to be able to give a patient the most effective help. *The patient's relatives must be given every facility to visit and keep in touch with him.* Their inquiries should be fully answered in so far as it is in the nurse's province to do so, their anxieties anticipated, and they should have reassurance and advice so that they can feel that the patient is receiving the best possible care. A knowledge of the patient's background is also important. The nurse can obtain much of this information from the medical and social histories but her contact with friends and relatives will enable her to get a picture of what the patient was like before his illness, and the kind of situation which he is likely to return to on discharge.

Psychiatric nurses also work as a member of a team with doctors and social workers in community care. Individual patients may be allocated to the nurse if there is still a need for nursing supervision; in cases where it is desirable to continue the relationship that has been built up between the nurse and patient in hospital; or on the principle that the key worker most useful in the situation takes over the task.

As the role of the psychiatric nurse changes, new responsibilities are incurred and fresh opportunities appear. Her influence now extends far beyond the patients and staff of her ward; she meets more of the general public and comes into contact with nurses and health workers in many spheres. In making the most of these opportunities her professional status will be enhanced and her influence as a mental health educator will be of greater benefit not only to her patients but to the entire community.

Chapter 28

Poisoning and its Treatment

by ROY GOULDING

Poisons information service—epidemiology—first aid—accident and emergency treatment—management and nursing care—examples of poisoning

Poisoning occurs when a toxic substance of mineral, animal, vegetable or chemical origin gains access to the body by mouth (orally), via the lungs (inhalation), through the skin (percutaneously), by injection (parenterally), or by any other route. The life or health of the patient is then in jeopardy. To overcome the danger, treatment is imperative, with a rigour commensurate to the degree of poisoning. If, however, the substance taken is not intrinsically toxic, no treatment is called for, only reassurance. Unnecessary treatment can itself be hazardous.

POISONS INFORMATION SERVICE

When poisoning is a likely diagnosis the action to be taken depends very largely on the toxicity of the substance concerned. Carbon monoxide, barbiturates, aspirin, arsenic, strychnine, etc., seldom give cause for doubt. Today a wide variety of substances may be involved and their toxicity is not generally known. For this reason many countries have now established poisons information, or poisons control, centres. In the United Kingdom the National Poisons Information Service has centres in London, Edinburgh, Cardiff and Belfast, while the Republic of Ireland has an associated centre in Dublin.

The position is that a registered medical practitioner dealing with a case of suspected poisoning (but not a member of the general public) may telephone a centre at any hour of the day or night to ascertain the toxicity of any substance or product believed to be contributory, the likely symptoms and a synopsis of the treatment that should be given. Detailed consultant advice cannot be obtained about the clinical management of an individual patient; that remains the responsibility of the doctor directly concerned.

EPIDEMIOLOGY

Poisoning may be *accidental*, or *deliberate*. In children up to about twelve years of age there is seldom any intent to do themselves harm and the highest incidence of accidental poisoning falls in the age group between one and five years. Youngsters in this category are naturally inquisitive and tend to put into their mouths anything within reach. Poisoning will occur if the substance ingested happens to be toxic so, in the interests of prevention, no child should have access to medicines, powerful disinfectants, agricultural chemicals, or any suchlike dangerous products.

Adults too may be the victims of accidental poisoning. A toxic substance may be swallowed by mistake, especially if the container is incorrectly labelled. Or someone may be exposed to a noxious gas or vapour, in the home or at work. These incidents, however, are proportionately few. The majority of adults who take poison do so deliberately, not necessarily with the intention of killing themselves but very often simply as a gesture to attract attention, sympathy and kindness. The term *self-poisoning* is therefore preferable to that of suicide or attempted suicide. (In Britain today, homicide by poisoning is extremely rare, though the possibility should never be overlooked.)

Mortality from poisoning, in most western countries at least, is nowadays attributable mainly to carbon monoxide inhalation (from domestic gas, exhaust fumes, etc.), and increasingly also to overdosage of drugs, principally barbiturates, aspirin and other preparations having an action on the brain. Non-fatal cases of poisoning—the number of which requiring admission to hospital seems to increase yearly—are due largely to drug overdosages, but involve a wider range of substances—various hypnotics, tranquillizers, antidepressants and so on.

FIRST AID

In the treatment of poisoning the use of specific antidotes is the exception, not the rule, but see p. 286 for some examples. There is no point in wasting time trying to ascertain exactly what substance was responsible in order to administer the exact counteractant. Instead, the principles applying to the management of any medical emergency should be followed.

The patient should be removed from a toxic atmosphere, e.g. carbon monoxide or some industrial gas, as soon as possible, taking care not to expose any of the would-be rescuers to danger.

Establish a clear airway. Dentures or other likely obstructions in the mouth or throat should be taken out, the tongue should be drawn forwards and the patient lain on one side to prevent the tongue falling back again. If spontaneous respiration is lacking, artificial ventilation should be instituted (see p. 284).

Remove contaminated clothing and liberally wash with water any skin or mucosal surface similarly contaminated.

Emesis should not be induced as a routine (see Removal of Poison, p. 285).

If *convulsions* appear the patient should be carefully protected from falls or injury (see p. 132).

ACCIDENT AND EMERGENCY TREATMENT

Unless it is certain that the suspected poisoning is not serious the patient should be moved to hospital for care and assessment. It should, however, not be overlooked that certain poisons do not act for some time and then may act rapidly. There the same principles of supportive management are adopted.

Respiration. This is of primary and vital concern. So long as the breathing is natural and unimpeded and the patient is a good colour (but see pp. 286, 287 for exceptions with carbon monoxide and cyanide) no further assistance is immediately required. Otherwise, and especially when coma has supervened, the patient should be lain on one side (see p. 80), the tongue should be drawn forward and the foot of the bed should be raised a little so that the head is lower than the rest of the body. By this means, the risk of bronchial aspiration, notably of vomitus, is reduced. Dentures should be removed and any other possible obstruction to the airway should be overcome. The passing of a cuffed, endotracheal tube, which should then be left in position, may be necessary. (Tracheostomy is seldom demanded at this early stage.)

After these preliminaries have been promptly carried out the respiratory status should again be checked. If spontaneous respiration is still deficient, *artificial ventilation* should be performed by whatever method is at once available and convenient—by the mouth-to-mouth technique, by means of an Ambu bag or, preferably, by means of a mechanical source. Air, or an oxygen mixture, is usually sufficient for this purpose, though with carbon monoxide poisoning it is essential to administer oxygen, or a mixture of oxygen with 5 per cent carbon dioxide.

Constant nursing observation is essential so that immediate intervention can be made if respiratory difficulties should appear.

Cardio-vascular system. Repeated measurements should be taken of the pulse and blood pressure. Any degree of circulatory failure will be treated by routine measures under the direction of the doctor; for example, hypotension can often be corrected simply by further raising the foot of the bed. An intravenous infusion should also be set up and, by this route, a plasma expander such as dextran can be introduced if the blood pressure still remains low. In the same way a drug such as isoprenaline, or nor-adrenaline or metaraminol, can be given in repeated does to afford extra support. Cardiac arrest, of course, demands prompt cardiac massage (see p. 448.

Convulsions. Mere muscular tremors sometimes seen in poisoned patients are seldom of any consequence, but frank convulsions can be disastrous, above all in small children for whom they can be fatally exhaustive in a very short time. Injury to the patient must be prevented; the insertion of a wedge between his teeth will prevent the tongue being bitten. Anticonvulsant drugs, e.g. diazepam, paraldehyde, or sodium phenobarbitone, may be ordered, taking into account that respiration may thereby be further embarrassed.

Hypothermia. Severe overdose with coma may well be accompanied by hypothermia. This possibility should always be borne in mind and the rectal temperature should be checked using a low-temperature recording thermometer. Careful rewarming should be undertaken as necessary, but only in extreme cases of profound hypothermia is actively heating permissible.

Pain. This is rarely a symptom of poisoning, though it may be apparent when, for example, corrosives have been swallowed. A strong analgesic such as morphine or pethidine may then be given under medical direction.

Removal of the poison. Not until the integrity of the vital processes has been ensured by proceeding along the lines already outlined should consideration be given to the removal of ingested poison. Removal should be withheld if:

(i)   The substance or dose swallowed is regarded as insufficiently toxic to cause harm.

(ii) Ingestion took place more than four hours previously—or 12 hours previously for salicylates.

(iii) The material involved is paraffin (kerosene), white spirit, turpentine substitute or products containing ingredients of this kind, e.g. polishes. (With these the complications of bronchial aspiration and bronchopneumonia are likely to outweigh the benefits of gastric lavage.)

(iv) The patient is unconscious—unless a cuffed endotracheal tube has been properly inserted beforehand.

In a child who has swallowed poison and who has an adequate gag reflex, emesis when desirable can be provoked simply by putting a finger down the thoat, or by giving a drink of Syrup of Ipecacuanha 10–15 ml, repeating this dose once if the first is unavailing.

When it has been decided that the stomach should be washed out the procedure adopted should be that described on p. 114.

MANAGEMENT AND NURSING CARE

Severely poisoned patients are best looked after in an intensive care unit. Whatever the ward to which they are assigned the mainstay of successful management is unremitting and skilled nursing care. Experience in numerous hospitals has shown that by adherence to conservative principles alone and without resort to elaborate methods for eliminating the toxin from the body, more than 95 per cent of the patients admitted for severe poisoning survive. *Satisfactory recovery depends more on high-grade nursing care than on any other single factor.*

(i) *Assiduous observation*, notably of the respiratory and cardio-vascular performance, in order that any deterioration of condition is immediately reported and corrective measures are applied without delay.

(ii) *Accurate recording is mandatory* both as regards the general condition of the patient, especially an exact assessment of the depth of coma, and any untoward symptoms developing. Note should always be made of all drugs administered, together, if possible, with any reactions arising therefrom.

(iii) When a urethral catheter is in position and properly functioning so that all urine can be collected and measured an *up-to-date fluid balance chart should be kept.* If a lubricant containing a local anaesthetic, e.g. lignocaine, is used on the urethral catheter, a note to this effect should be made on the request form accompanying any urine sample sent for analysis, otherwise the chemical findings may be confusing. All fluid input, including intravenous infusions and any other artificial means of introducing fluid, and the fluid output should be measured and recorded. Any significant discrepancy should be brought to the notice of the medical staff.

(iv) *Every unconscious patient* should be turned two-hourly, and care given to the pressure areas (see Chapter 4, p. 49). Anyone on a respirator, or who has a defective cough reflex, should be subjected *to repeated bronchial suction carried out under full aseptic technique.*

To combat bronchopneumonia which is a frequent complication from poisoning by drugs that are depressant to the central nervous system, and as a precaution against peripheral venous thrombosis, *physiotherapy to the chest and limbs* should also be carried out every two or three hours.

(v) *A complete, comprehensive and accurate chart should be maintained at the bedside of each patient* so that, as far as possible, every feature of management and treatment, together with every response, both by observation and management, can be seen at a glance.

(vi) Finally, since so many poisoned patients will be in need of, and receiving, psychiatric investigation and help, the nurse is in a virtually unique position to achieve rapport with the individual that she is looking after and to afford invaluable liaison with the psychiatrist responsible.

A few profoundly poisoned patients may be subjected to special techniques designed to accelerate the elimination of the toxin from the body, e.g. forced diuresis, peritoneal dialysis, extra-corporeal dialysis (the artificial kidney). In any such instance the nursing care is no less vital and should be carried out in the same way and just as conscientiously as for the conservative regime.

One cardinal dictum should always be borne in mind; today in clinical toxicology there is practically no valid argument at all for using so-called analeptics—bemegride, picrotoxin, lobeline, leptazol, nikethamide (Coramine), etc. Their alleged advantages are usually illusory and in themselves they may prove harmful.

EXAMPLES OF POISONING

For overdosages with *barbiturates, non-barbiturate hypnotics* and *sedatives, tranquillizers, antidepressants* and most of the other so-called *psychotropic drugs* the care of the patient should follow the recognized conservative principles, and forced diuresis, peritoneal dialysis and use of the artificial kidney will be reserved for a few very severe and selected cases. In *aspirin poisoning* emphasis is placed on forced alkaline diuresis, again not neglecting the usual supportive measures.

Carbon monoxide over-exposure demands prompt attention to the respiratory function and the administration of oxygen. Cerebral oedema can prove a complication and this may be relieved by the intravenous administration of mannitol, or by giving corticosteroids or by administering a diuretic, e.g. frusemide. Physiologically, hyperbaric oxygen is the treatment of choice, but the transference of a patient to a hyperbaric unit should never be allowed to interfere with, or delay, the immediate giving of oxygen at atmospheric pressure and its continuous provision until arrangements can be made for removal to a suitable unit. Carbon monoxide sometimes causes brain damage and recovery from this may be delayed over weeks, or it may even prove permanent. (Nothing special can be done to overcome this, only general rehabilitation.)

Corrosives and *caustics*, such as strong mineral acids, sodium hydroxide, phenolic disinfectants, e.g. lysol, or formic acid (a common ingredient of kettle-descaler), are now infrequently taken. Supportive management is again imperative, with particular attention to the alimentary tract and to the possibility of gastric and intestinal perforation, for which surgical intervention is urgently required. *Demulcents*, such as milk, egg white or olive oil can be given by mouth, both to soothe and counteract the mucosal damage, while pain may be relieved by injected analgesics, e.g. morphine.

In the healing process, cicatricial narrowing of the alimentary tract, usually at the upper level, may become manifest. This may be prevented to some extent by the prophylactic administration of corticosteroids; otherwise, surgical dilatation must be performed.

Iron in the metallic form is virtually non-toxic but the various pharmaceutical preparations of iron, like ferrous sulphate, ferrous gluconate, ferrous succinate, etc., designed for the treatment of anaemia, can be disastrously toxic in overdose, especially in children. Once again the patient must be given general support and, in addition and urgently, the specific antidote, which is desferrioxamine (Desferal), will be ordered. After vomiting and/or gastric lavage, 5 g desferrioxamine in 50–100 ml water are left in the stomach and further doses of this preparation are given by injection at the rate of 15 mg per kg body-weight per hour, up to a total of 80 mg per kg in 24 hours.

Patients who have taken *morphine* and other *opiates* in excess should be looked after in the same way as those who have taken barbiturates, and the respiratory depression treated by a specific antagonist, e.g. naloxone, nalorphine or levallorphan repeatedly by injection.

Cyanides can prove fatal in a matter of minutes, or even seconds. In works, laboratories and similar places where cyanide exposure is likely to occur the specific antidote must be kept immediately to hand. Either amyl nitrate is given by inhalation, followed by 10 ml sodium nitrite injection (3 per cent) intravenously and then by 25 ml sodium thiosulphate solution (50 per cent) slowly by the same route, or more simply, when available, cobalt edetate solution is the specific antidote, and to be effective it should be given intravenously over the course of about a minute.

Arsenic is not often taken as an acute poison but it can be deadly, especially as the inorganic arsenical, and the possibility should always be borne in mind. The vomiting, diarrhoea and collapse must be overcome by the customary supportive regime and the specific antidote, dimercaprol (BAL) must be given to neutralize the action of arsenic in the tissues and to promote its excretion via the kidneys.

Chapter 29

Diseases and Disorders of the Endocrine Glands

by QUENTIN J. G. HOBSON

> *Introduction—the hypothalamus—the anterior pituitary—the posterior pituitary—the thyroid gland—the parathyroid glands—the adrenal glands—the male gonads—diabetes mellitus—insulin.*

INTRODUCTION

The maintenance of normal health and the repair of tissues when diseased or injured depends on the regulated function of the endocrine glands.

In contrast to the exocrine glands, which secrete their contents to the outside of the body, the endocrine glands have no ducts and their secretions (hormones) pass into the circulation and body fluids.

Many of the endocrine glands are themselves controlled by hormones secreted by the anterior pituitary, the pituitary secretion itself being controlled by chemical substances released by the brain cells in the hypothalamus.

The endocrine glands may be destroyed by disease, or be subject to malignant changes and benign tumours, or hyperplasia of the gland may cause excessive hormone secretion. These diseases, except for diabetes mellitus, are not common, but the changes caused by altered hormone secretion are often characteristic.

The importance of these hormones extends far beyond the few patients with diseases of these glands. These very active substances can be extracted or artificially produced and used to influence disease processes to the benefit of the patient.

Many patients receiving hormone treatment are critically dependent on accurate dosage and regular treatment to avoid serious and sometimes even fatal side-effects. The nurse must be well informed about the often complicated effects of hormone treatment (see Appendix ii, p. 756 for untoward side-effects of some endocrinological products).

THE HYPOTHALAMUS

In the small area below the thalamus and in the walls of the third ventricle extending into the pituitary stalk are the nuclei of the hypothalamus. These nuclei, though very small in size are the command centres controlling many bodily functions through the nervous system and the endocrine glands. These centres have direct nervous connections with the autonomic nervous system—the sympathetic and parasympathetic pathways. Some of the nerve cells are also 'neuro-secretory' cells secreting the hormones *vasopressin* and *oxytocin* which pass down with the nerve fibres to the posterior pituitary where these hormones are stored before release.

In other hypothalamic centres the neural cells secrete at least seven different chemical substances—of uncertain structure—which are 'hypophysiotrophic', passing by the vessels to the anterior pituitary.

There are no nerve fibres from the hypothalamus to the anterior pituitary but these chemical substances secreted by the hypothalamus pass to the nearby anterior pituitary stimulating the release of one of the hormones of the anterior pituitary into the general body circulation.

The hypothalamic centres control many bodily functions. In this area are centres controlling appetite and body weight; the onset of puberty and reproductive cycles. The body temperature is controlled through the autonomic system and the control of thyroid activity; and the body's water balance through the action of vasopressin from the posterior pituitary. The normal daily 'diurnal' rhythm of hormone changes and of waking and sleeping depend on the normal function of these centres.

The hypothalamus is concerned with the 'feedback' control of pituitary hormone release. If the level of thyroxine in the body falls, this is appreciated by the appropriate centre. The neural cells secrete the thyrotrophin releasing factor which passes to the anterior pituitary releasing thyroid stimulating hormone into the circulation to act on the thyroid gland. The presence of excessive thyroxine will shut down this action of the hypothalamus. Similar mechanisms control the secretion of ACTH and sex hormones.

The hypothalamus is only rarely affected by disease. Injury or tumours may damage the centres causing complex effects on growth, sexual development, sleep or endocrine function. There may in addition be damage to the adjacent optic nerves or to the anterior and posterior pituitary glands.

THE ANTERIOR PITUITARY

The anterior pituitary gland has no nervous connection with the hypothalamus but is closely controlled by the chemical hypophysiotrophic hormones secreted by the hypothalamic nuclei. These substances pass through vascular channels to the pituitary.

The hypothalamus and the pituitary itself are sensitive to changes in the level of hormones in the blood, the 'feed-back' mechanism stimulating the production of thyroid, adrenal and sex gland hormones if one of these is deficient in the circulation.

The anterior pituitary secretes at least six different hormones:

Anterior pituitary hormone	Effects
Growth hormone	Growth of all tissues
Prolactin	Lactation
ACTH	Control of adrenal cortex
TSH	Control of thyroid secretion
Gonadotrophins	Control of sex glands
(a) FSH	Follicle-stimulating hormone
(b) LH	Luteinizing hormone

The cells of the anterior pituitary control these functions individually, and although in disease a single hormone may be deficient the secretion of several hormones is usually affected.

Hypopituitarism. The anterior pituitary may be destroyed by injury, cysts or tumours (often a chromophobe adenoma). The gland is vulnerable to infarction when postpartum haemorrhage causes shock in a woman at childbirth (Sheehan's syndrome). In some patients with breast or other cancer the tumour growth may be limited by deliberate destruction of the anterior pituitary, by surgery or irradiation.

In the child hypopituitarism causes dwarfing (from lack of the growth hormone) and sexual development may fail to occur, and thyroid and adrenal deficiency may be found.

In the adult hypopituitarism may cause loss of gonadotrophins (sexual function); of TSH (myxoedema); of ACTH (adrenal insufficiency) and of prolactin (preventing lactation in the puerperal woman).

The symptoms are usually insidious in onset with amenorrhoea, impotence, fatigue, sensitivity to the cold. Mental changes and even psychotic symptoms may occur. Occasionally the onset of symptoms may be sudden, the patient developing stupor or coma.

Treatment. Pituitary extracts are not suitable for treatment, but treatment with cortisol for adrenal insufficiency, and thyroxine for thyroid deficiency are effective; and fertility may sometimes be restored by treatment with human gonadotrophins. If the cause is an enlarging tumour surgical removal may be required to relieve pressure on the optic pathways.

Hyperpituitarism (*gigantism and acromegaly*). Tumours of the anterior pituitary may secrete excessive growth hormone. In the child this causes excessive growth in size and height—gigantism. In the adult further growth of bone is not possible but the soft tissues grow. The appearance of the patient may be characteristic, the hands, feet and face enlarging and outgrowing the patient's normal size of rings, shoes or dentures.

Amenorrhoea, impotence, diabetes and arthritis may occur, and a big tumour may affect the optic pathways.

Treatment. The function of the tumour may be destroyed by implantation of radioactive seeds. Large tumours require surgical removal to relieve pressure on the optic nerves.

Cushing's syndrome. In a few patients with this syndrome, the primary cause is an ACTH-producing tumour of the pituitary. The excessive ACTH secretion causes bilateral adrenal cortical hyperplasia, and in some patients pigmentation, similar to that of Addison's disease, may occur.

THE POSTERIOR PITUITARY

Some nerve fibres from the hypothalamus descend through the pituitary stalk to the posterior pituitary gland and conduct two hormones secreted by the neuro-secretory cells of the hypothalamus to the gland where they are stored.

Vasopressin, or antidiuretic hormone (ADH). The main action of this hormone is on the distal tubule in the kidney, ensuring that water is re-absorbed to prevent excessive loss in the urine. Vasopressin also causes contraction of smooth muscle in blood vessels and the gut.

The osmolarity (the total concentration of all particles dissolved in body fluid) normally controls the rate of release of vasopressin. When the release is absent due to disease of the hypothalamus or posterior pituitary, excessive urine is passed—a rare condition, *diabetes insipidus*. This may follow injury or tumours in the region of the hypothalamus. The affected patient has severe thirst and polyuria. Five to fifteen litres of urine are passed each day, disturbing sleep and threatening dehydration.

The hormone, vasopressin, can be given as a nasal spray, or Pitressin Tannate as an injection in oil to correct the deficiency.

Oxytocin. A hormone very similar in structure to vasopressin is secreted. The hormone has little effect on the kidney but acts on muscle in ducts in the breast ejecting milk in the lactating woman, and stimulates the uterus to contract at the end of pregnancy. It may play a part in initiating the normal onset of labour, and is used in obstetric practice to induce parturition.

THE THYROID GLAND

The thyroid gland secretes hormones affecting growth and metabolism. Two very similar substances are secreted having the same qualitative actions but differing slightly in structure and iodine content. They are:

Thyroxine.
Tri-iodothyronine.

In practice we can consider these as one substance, thyroxine. A third hormone, calcitonin, is secreted by some thyroid cells. Calcitonin lowers the serum calcium but the part it plays in health and disease is not yet known.

The activity of the thyroid gland is controlled by the thyroid stimulating hormone (TSH) released by the anterior pituitary gland.

Thyroxine secretion may alter in response to changes of environment and pregnancy and there is normally a close interaction between the thyroid activity and the pituitary. If the level of thyroxine falls the release of TSH is increased.

Thyroid cells are unique in their ability to concentrate iodine from the blood, linking this to tyrosine and to protein to form thyroglobulin which is stored in the thyroid follicles. When stimulated the protein is broken down and thyroxine is released into the circulation. Thyroxine is essential for normal growth of body and brain and is a major factor in controlling the rate of metabolism of all tissues.

Clinical tests of thyroid function. *The measurement of the basal metabolic rate* (B.M.R.) is an indirect measure of thyroid activity. The consumption of oxygen by the patient is measured with the patient in a basal state, at rest and without food. The normal value lies between $+15$ to -15 per cent, but as other factors may influence the metabolic rate it is less used today than in the past.

Thyroxine is unique in its large content of iodine, and the chemical measurement of protein-bound iodine (PBI) in the plasma can be used to assess the circulating level of thyroxine. New methods for estimating the concentration of thyroxine itself are becoming available.

The uptake of iodine by the thyroid and the manufacture of thyroxine can be tested by giving the patient iodine with very small quantities of radio-active iodine. Subsequent measurement of radioactivity in blood and urine traces the passage of the normal iodine in the body. Iodine-containing drugs or treatment may confuse this test. Furthermore *the local function of the thyroid tissue* may be studied by 'scanning' the neck for radioactivity with an 'external counter'. The gland can be identified, and altered function within the gland can be demonstrated which may assist the diagnosis of malignant or other thyroid diseases.

Hypothyroidism (see below) is occasionally the secondary consequence of abnormal pituitary function, and in such patients the response to a diagnostic injection of TSH may indicate that there is no primary disorder of the thyroid gland itself.

Goitre. Goitre *describes visible enlargement of the thyroid gland* in the neck.

Simple goitre. The thyroid may be diffusely enlarged with normal secretion of thyroxine. When there is iodine deficiency due to inadequate iodine in the diet the pituitary stimulates the thyroid to work harder to produce its normal secretion. This deficiency causes goitre particularly in adolescent girls and in some families and races. This 'simple' or iodine-deficiency goitre may be 'endemic' in mountain communities where the diet is often iodine-deficient, in contrast to those eating fish and other iodine-containing foods commonly found in sea or fresh water.

Increasing the iodine intake by providing iodized table salt avoids this condition. When simple goitre is found in young people iodine treatment or treatment with thyroid or thyroxine tablets will cause the goitre to diminish. If untreated the goitre may become with time large and nodular.

Non-toxic nodular goitre. The smooth goitre of iodine deficiency may become lumpy and ugly and even massive in size, pressing on the trachea, but still without over- or under-secretion of thyroxine.

Medical treatment is usually ineffective and surgical removal of the gland may be required.

Hypothyroidism (cretinism, myxoedema). The infant may be born without thyroid tissue or have at birth a goitre, the thyroid being enlarged but incapable of normal thyroxine formation.

In infancy thyroid deficiency is called 'cretinism', which if untreated leads to retardation of mental development and defect of growth (dwarfism) in addition to the other changes seen also in thyroid deficiency in adult life. In the adult when the deficiency is marked the skin and other tissues are swollen by 'mucous oedema' and this is given the name myxoedema.

Hypothyroidism is usually due to primary atrophy of the gland, which is probably the result of autoimmune thyroiditis. The thyroid may be destroyed by surgery or radioactive iodine treatment. It may follow in-advertent administration of antithyroid drugs, and occasionally thyroid failure is secondary to anterior pituitary failure.

Hypothyroidism is commonest in women and in middle life. *The onset of symptoms is insidious*: the changes may be attributed to age by those nearest to the patient, though the true diagnosis may strike the nurse or doctor on first acquaintance. *The patient has increasing fatigue, dryness of the skin, absent sweating, sensitivity to the cold, aches, cramps and paraesthesiae in the limbs. The voice may be hoarse, constipation and weight gain are usual, the skin is cold and dry with puffiness about the eyes, the movement and thinking are slow. The pulse is slow, the reflexes are sluggish.* Mental changes may be marked, thinking and reactions are slow, while paranoia and delusional states may occur. Occasionally the slowing of metabolism may lead to mental confusion and coma, often associated with hypothermia (see p. 342).

The *diagnosis* is confirmed by demonstrating low thyroid function with radioactive iodine tests and the low value of the PBI. Only when tests are inconclusive is a trial of treatment with thyroxine given, for it is important to have a firm diagnosis before starting lifelong treatment.

Treatment. Thyroxine can completely replace the deficiency and return the patient to normal. Thyroxine is a pure chemical and replaces the less certain action of the dried thyroid extracts used previously.

The starting dose is small, especially in the elderly, when a too sudden increase in metabolism may affect the heart. The initial dose is 0·05 mg sodium thyroxine daily, increased gradually in four to eight weeks to a maintenance dose of 0·3 mg daily.

Thyroxine takes some days to have any effect and acts for some weeks. The dose may be given once daily, and patients should know that symptoms of deficiency will not reappear until some weeks have passed if treatment is stopped. Tri-iodothyronine, 40 micrograms (μg) twice daily, has a quicker action and occasionally its use is preferred to thyroxine.

Maintenance treatment must be continued for life in the patient with myxoedema. Unnecessary treatment with thyroid is sometimes given in error to fat patients; although this dose has no immediate adverse effects on the normal person it suppresses thyroid function and may lead to thyroid atrophy.

Hyperthyroidism. The excessive secretion of thyroid hormone, or the administration of excessive thyroxine, produces hyperthyroidism.

The symptoms are the result of increased tissue metabolism, and increased sensitivity to the circulating adrenaline-like substance (catecholamines). Many of these symptoms can be suppressed by adrenaline-blocking drugs such as propranolol, which may have some place in treatment. The primary cause of hyperthyroidism in patients with exophthalmic goitre (Graves' disease) is probably the secretion of long-acting thyroid stimulating substance (LATS) secreted outside the normal endocrine mechanism but stimulating on the one hand the development of prominence of the eyes and also thyroid activity with the consequent metabolic changes. Sometimes the eye changes are very marked and the thyroid overaction trivial (ophthalmic form of Graves' disease). Hyperthyroidism may appear in several forms:

> *Toxic adenoma.* The rare form in which a single benign tumour of the thyroid secretes excessive hormone.
> *Toxic nodular goitre.* The patient may have had a nodular goitre without symptoms for many years, but in later life the lumpy goitre secretes excessive hormone.

Exophthalmic goitres, Graves' disease. Some outside factor causes hyperthyroidism with diffuse enlargement of the thyroid and also proptosis of the eyes, which does not occur with toxic adenoma, toxic nodular goitre or overdosage with thyroid hormone.

The symptoms and signs of hyperthyroidism are indicative of increased metabolism and exaggeration of the normal action of adrenaline-like hormones. *The onset is usually insidious and occasionally exophthalmic goitre appears precipitated by psychological stress. The appetite is increased but weight is lost, sweating is prominent, the skin flushed and circulation overactive, and the patient may feel the heat unduly. The pulse is fast, the sleeping pulse rate raised, palpitations and shortness of breath are common, the pulse may be irregular (atrial fibrillation) and congestive heart failure may occur, see p. 209. The muscles may be wasted and weak, the hands and fingers may have a tremor. The reflexes are brisk; nervousness, irritability and anxiety are usual, and rarely psychotic mental symptoms occur, see p. 272. Occasionally, all these symptoms appear in hours with dramatic suddenness, thyroid crisis (for treatment see below).*

The physical changes usually, but not always, include evident goitre or thyroid enlargement. The eyes may stare due to retraction of the lids, and in Graves' disease true protrusion of the eyeball occurs which, if severe, may cause double vision, paralysis of eye movement, swelling of the conjunctivae and even ulceration of the eyes through failure to close the eyelids.

Diagnosis is confirmed by the tests described. Before modern times some patients recovered spontaneously without treatment after years of illness. Nowadays when the diagnosis is made treatment is initiated to control symptoms promptly and obtain permanent relief from hyperthyroidism.

Treatment. *In nursing management the patient's anxiety and irritability must be appreciated and allayed.* When symptoms require prompt control, as in a thyroid crisis, propranolol may be given, 40 mg three times daily, but this does not alter thyroid hypersecretion which can be controlled in three main ways by:

Medical treatment. Thyroid secretion can be blocked by drugs which if continued for some 18 months may allow normal thyroid function to be resumed. In some patients, however, hypersecretion returns when treatment is withdrawn. The drugs used are carbimazole (initially 30 mg a day, 5 to 15 mg a day maintenance); potassium perchlorate 600 mg a day. Tablets must be taken regularly. Some patients are sensitive and skin rashes, fever, and potentially fatal agranulocytosis may appear and must be watched for, especially in the first six weeks of treatment. Iodine can be used but its effect is short-lived and can only be used as preparation for surgical treatment.

Surgical treatment (see p. 523). Partial thyroidectomy when the hyperthyroidism has been controlled with medical treatment is usually chosen for patients with large or nodular goitres.

Radioactive iodine treatment. A large calculated dose of radioactive iodine is given. No immediate symptoms occur, but local concentration of radioactivity in thyroid tissue destroys the gland over some weeks. This treatment is usually reserved for patients over 45 years of age because radioactivity can after many years produce cancer. Excessive destruction of thyroid with consequent myxoedema in later life may occur.

Thyroiditis due to infection is very rare but thyroiditis due to 'autoimmune' processes is more common, as in Hashimoto's disease, and the same process may be the common cause of thyroid-atrophy producing myxoedema.

The thyroid may be diffusely enlarged, the normal thyroid working increasingly hard until overtaken by the destructive changes of thyroiditis which lead in the end to atrophy. The patient's blood contains 'autoantibodies' to thyroid tissue.

Treatment. The symptoms of hypothyroidism and the thyroid enlargement usually respond to maintenance treatment with thyroxine. Surgery is occasionally needed to confirm the diagnosis or remove a large goitre.

Thyroid tumours. *Benign tumours* of the thyroid may occur as a solitary nodule in the gland. These are not usually associated with hypersecretion, and have to be distinguished from malignant tumours, a distinction which may only be possible by surgical removal.

Malignant cancer of the thyroid is rare and not associated with hyperthyroidism. There is often invasion of the glands and tissues of the neck, but occasionally the thyroid swelling is small and secondary tumours may be found in the lung or bones. *Treatment* with a combination of surgical removal and radioiodine therapy may be required.

PARATHYROID GLANDS

There are usually four small parathyroid glands, two glands on each side closely applied to the lateral lobes of the thyroid gland. The glands may vary in size, which may complicate the identification and removal of a suspected parathyroid tumour.

The secretion of parathormone by the glands is controlled by the level of ionized calcium in the blood acting on the parathyroid cells which are independent of pituitary or other control.

The effect of parathormone is to regulate the level of serum calcium. Parathormone releases calcium from the bones, and increases the absorption of calcium from the bowel, increasing the loss of phosphate and calcium passed in the urine by the kidneys.

Disease of the parathyroid glands is uncommon. The destruction of function incidental to operation on the adjacent thyroid gland is perhaps the commonest.

Hypoparathyroidism. When this occurs it has usually complicated thyroid surgery and very rarely it occurs without an obvious cause. The symptoms the patient suffers are due to the fall in serum calcium which increases neuro-muscular irritability. The symptoms of cramp, muscle stiffness and paraesthesiae, odd sensations such as pins and needles in the hands and feet, may pass unrecognized until the patient shows spasms of tetany.

Tetany may result from hypocalcaemia, reduction of the total calcium concentration in the plasma from any cause, or may be due to a fall in the ionized fraction of the total calcium as may happen in alkalosis. The facial nerve when tapped may show spasm of the face, Chvostek's sign, the small muscles of the hand may become stiff from spasm, Trousseau's sign. *In children particularly spasm may cause flexion at the wrist and ankle* (carpo-pedal spasm) *and the laryngeal muscles may be in spasm causing laryngeal stridor.*

Prolonged unrecognized hypocalcaemia may also lead to cataract formation in the lenses and to epilepsy.

Treatment. The hormone parathormone cannot be used satisfactorily for increasing the serum calcium.

Tetany is treated by intravenous injection of calcium gluconate (10 to 20 ml of a 10 per cent solution). With less urgent symptoms, hypocalcaemia is treated by giving added calcium in the diet (calcium effervescent tablets, calcium gluconogalactogluconate, 1 tablet three times a day) and by increasing calcium absorption from the gut by giving vitamin D 50,000 to 100,000 units a day or the similar dihydrotachysterol (AT10). The treatment has to be followed by repeated serum calcium estimates to ensure that a normal serum level is maintained.

Hyperparathyroidism may be due to:

1. A primary tumour of a parathyroid gland
2. Hypertrophy of parathyroid glands developed in response to loss of calcium, as may happen in chronic renal disease and some bowel disorders
3. Very rarely this hormone is produced 'ectopically' in malignant tumours quite apart from the normal parathyroid.

The symptoms of parathormone excess are of insidious onset and are the consequence of the raised serum calcium level, the resorption of bone, and the excessive urinary excretion of calcium.

In hypercalcaemia symptoms and changes include:

Weakness, fatigue, nausea, vomiting, loss of weight, mental change.
Renal changes—kidney stones, polyuria.
Bone pain and pathological 'bone fractures'.

All patients with calcium-containing renal stones are investigated for hypercalcaemia, for stones may appear many years before other symptoms. The diagnosis is confirmed by finding high serum calcium values and often characteristic X-ray changes in bone.

The *treatment* is the surgical removal of the parathyroid tumour. The serum calcium falls to normal and bone pain is relieved and further renal stone formation prevented.

THE ADRENAL GLANDS

The adrenal (suprarenal) glands lie above the kidneys. The outer adrenal cortex develops to surround the adrenal medulla which has a separate origin from sympathetic nervous tissue.

The *adrenal cortex* secretes three main groups of steroid hormones:

Glucocorticoids (cortisol).
Mineralocorticoids (aldosterone).
Androgens, masculinizing hormones.

Adrenal cortical deficiency. The clinical effects of adrenal cortical deficiency are associated with the name of Thomas Addison who first described them.

The adrenal cortex may be destroyed by 'adrenalitis', of uncertain mechanism (similar to Hashimoto's disease found in the thyroid, see p. 295). Tuberculosis occasionally spreads to destroy both adrenals. In some patients with cancer deliberate surgical removal of the adrenal cortices may benefit the patient. *The symptoms of adrenal cortical deficiency* may appear as:

> Chronic adrenal deficiency.
> Acute insufficiency (Addisonian crisis).

Chronic adrenal insufficiency. The progressive destruction of the adrenal cortex is associated with the insidious onset of symptoms, unaccompanied initially by physical changes and often mistakenly thought to be psychogenic in origin. As adrenal function fails symptoms and signs of disease are more evident, and the patient is exposed to the hazard of sudden adrenal failure.

The common symptoms are *tiredness and fatigue, gastro-intestinal upsets, vomiting and diarrhoea, pigmentation of the skin, faintness due to hypotension, loss of weight, and of body hair, hypoglycaemic symptoms and psychotic changes.* These symptoms follow the fall in secretion of cortisol, aldosterone and androgenic steroids.

The *diagnosis* may be confirmed by estimating the level of cortisol in the serum and demonstrating the absence of the response to stimulation by ACTH.

The patient is rapidly improved by treatment with cortisol (hydrocortisone), 20 mg in the morning, 10 mg at night, or cortisone acetate 25 mg in the morning and 12·5 mg at night. In many patients additional salt-retaining hormone is required, for example alpha-fluorohydrocortisone (Fludrocort) 0·05 to 0·2 mg each day. If tuberculosis is present routine antituberculous treatment will be given.

The nurse must ensure that the patient knows that continued treatment is vital and the patient must carry a steroid treatment card detailing his daily dose (see p. 83). In the event of illness, injury, or operation the dose should be increased under medical supervision. In some patients mental symptoms may appear unless the individual's dose is accurately assessed, and normal health can only be maintained by strict and regular daily treatment.

Acute adrenal insufficiency (Addisonian crisis). *This medical emergency may arise in a patient with unrecognized chronic deficiency, often precipitated by incidental infection or operation.* In children especially, the adrenals may be suddenly destroyed by haemorrhage or infection. Symptoms of acute adrenal crisis may occur in patients on long-term treatment with steroid drugs who suddenly stop their treatment. Such patients may also respond poorly to stress or show signs of acute deficiency for some months after steroid treatment is stopped, because this treatment suppresses the normal pituitary-adrenal axis.

Adrenal deficiency may play a part in patients who are shocked or collapsed due to other causes, such as severe infection or hypothermia.

Symptoms may be of very sudden onset. Weakness, collapse, vomiting, diarrhoea are associated with hypotension, confusion progressing to coma, and death within hours.

Treatment requires an immediate intensive therapy regime in hospital, and may be started even before laboratory tests to confirm the diagnosis can be completed. *Intensive nursing care will include frequent observation of temperature, blood pressure, state of consciousness, fluid balance and urinary output.* The first hours of treatment are critical. Special measures include:

> Intravenous hydrocortisone, 300 mg followed by four-hourly doses.
> Intravenous infusion of fluid and electrolytes.
> Treatment with antibiotics may be required and in some patients hypoglycaemia may need treatment.

With prompt steroid treatment and supporting measures recovery should proceed, the patient's steroid dose being reduced to a maintenance level in a few days.

Adrenal cortical hypersecretion (Cushing's syndrome). The excessive production of adrenal cortical hormones produces striking changes. This may follow large doses of steroids given as treatment to patients and similar appearances may accompany the development of tumours or hyperplasia of the adrenal cortex. *Cushing's syndrome* may be due to:

> A single tumour in the adrenal cortex.
> Release of excessive ACTH from the pituitary with bilateral hyperplasia of the adrenal cortices.
> Occasionally cancer cells arising in tissues outside the adrenals may make ACTH causing adrenal hyperplasia.

The *physical changes* are the result of excessive cortisol levels and in some patients with tumours there may be masculinizing changes from increased androgen secretion.

The patient feels unwell with increasing obesity, puffiness and 'mooning' of the face and often oedema. Increasing growth of hair and amenorrhoea occur in women. The deficiency of protein metabolism may lead to thinning of the skin with 'striae', and thinning of the bones, osteoporosis. Hypertension and diabetes mellitus are common and resistance to infection is lowered.

The *diagnosis* may be confirmed by finding greatly raised levels of cortisol in the blood, and with radiological and other investigations the primary cause of the Cushing's syndrome can be located. *Treatment* may require removal of the greater part of both adrenal cortices, or of the single tumour if this is the cause. In many patients treatment of the anterior pituitary by irradiation will be needed. The physical changes regress with treatment.

The adrenal medulla. The sympathetic nervous system stimulates the cells of the adrenal medulla to secrete the catecholamines, adrenaline and noradrenaline. These hormones, which are also secreted by the sympathetic nerves, play a part in the control of metabolism, and of the circulation, the pulse and blood pressure. The adrenal medulla may be destroyed without causing symptoms, its function being taken over by nervous tissues.

Phaeochromocytoma. This tumour of the adrenal medulla may cause excessive catecholamine secretion. This results in some patients in a continued hypertension, and in other patients in intermittent bouts of hypertension which may be sufficiently characteristic to suggest this diagnosis. The attacks may last minutes or hours, causing headaches, vomiting and abdominal pain, with distress and anxiety, and sometimes heart failure, raised blood sugar and increased metabolism.

The diagnosis may be confirmed by finding an excessive excretion of the products of catecholamines in the urine. Special X-rays may reveal the tumour. This rare cause of hypertension has to be distinguished from the commoner causes (see Chapter 22, p. 211).

Treatment. The effects of the catecholamines can be reduced by propranolol and phenoxybenzamine, drugs which block the action of these hormones. These drugs control the blood pressure and enable surgical removal of the tumour to be completed.

THE MALE GONADS (Testes)

The *testes* develop from primitive germ-cells in the abdomen and descend during development through the inguinal canal to lie in the scrotum. In some infant boys the testes may not have descended. This may be due to defect of the testis itself or to mechanical interruption of its descent. The testes will only develop normal spermatozoa if they lie in the scrotum, and if retained in the abdomen sterility results.

The boy with undescended testes may be treated before puberty with injections of chorionic gonadotrophin to try to stimulate descent, and if this fails, by surgical correction. At puberty the testes increase rapidly in size due to the action of pituitary gonadotrophins.

The testis contains two types of tissue:

Seminiferous tubules form the major part in which spermatozoa are developed, passing through the epididymis and vas deferens to the seminal vesicles.

The interstitial cells secrete male hormone, which is responsible for masculinizing changes, growth of muscle, genital development, hairiness on the face, limbs and pubic region, libido, and baldness.

When gonadotrophic hormones are absent the stimulus of male hormone is lacking and the testes are small and the patient has a 'eunuchoid' physique. Similar changes occur if the testicles are destroyed, the affected male being termed a 'eunuch'.

An inherited defect with absent spermatozoa and varying degrees of eunuchoidism is common. This condition, *Klinefelter's syndrome* (or seminiferous tubule dysgenesis), is usually associated with readily detectable chromosome abnormality, the male patient having the chromosomes XXY and not the normal XY complement.

The physical changes of male hormone deficiency can be readily corrected by treatment with male hormone. Oral tablets are relatively ineffective and regular injections of testosterone or implantations of tablets are preferred.

Fertility. Infertility in the male may be due to absent or defective spermatozoa of unknown cause. This may be an unexpected (and often untreatable) finding in a male with normal sexual habits and physique.

Sometimes infertility may follow infections obstructing the ejaculatory ducts, and rarely from bilateral disease of the testes as may happen with mumps orchitis. Fertility may be reduced when a varicocele (dilatation of veins accompanying the vas deferens in the spermatic cord) is present.

Vasectomy. Division of both vasa deferentia makes the man infertile without affecting sexual function and this is an increasingly popular method of sterilization.

Impotence. The normal act of intercourse may fail if penile erection does not occur or cannot be sustained or if ejaculation is premature.

It is exceptional for physical changes to be found in this complaint though such causes must be excluded by examination. In most patients psychogenic causes predominate; these may be trivial and transient, or continued and often resistant to psychoanalytic or other methods of treatment.

Gynaecomastia. The male breast may appear of female outline due to fat, but when due to the presence of true breast tissue the condition is called a gynaecomastia.

Some change of this type is common at puberty or during recovery from severe or wasting illness. It may be due to administered female hormone, and occasionally unexpectedly to other drugs, e.g. chlorpromazine, spironolactone.

Gynaecomastia may accompany Klinefelter's syndrome. Rarely it is evidence of malignant tumours of the testes or of other tissues that secrete sex hormones. The appearance often distresses the patient, and if no special cause can be identified cosmetic surgical removal may be justified.

DIABETES MELLITUS

Diabetes mellitus is a disorder of metabolism in which the most evident change is an increase of the level of blood sugar which causes excretion of sugar in the urine (glycosuria). There are other less recognized changes in protein and fat metabolism. These changes appear initially to cause a functional disturbance of blood chemistry, but when long continued, physical changes in the blood vessels and tissues appear, these complications being probably the consequence of the abnormal chemistry.

The diabetic state is commonly the result of deficient insulin production, though in some patients insulin may be present but functionally inadequate. In the pancreas the microscopic 'Islets of Langerhans' contain β (beta) cells which secrete insulin (also a (alpha) cells which secrete glucagon).

In the great majority of diabetic patients there is no gross disease of the pancreas, though in some patients the pancreas may be seen to be damaged by pancreatitis, tumour or haemochromatosis. In some patients diabetes is associated with other endocrine diseases such as acromegaly, Cushing's syndrome, thyrotoxicosis or phaeochromocytoma. The chemical changes of diabetes may also be precipitated by drugs such as thiazide diuretics, steroids, 'the Pill', and, rarely, other chemicals.

The incidence of diabetes. Diabetes is common in most peoples. Six in every thousand are known to be diabetic and examination of people without symptoms would reveal a further six. In the United States some 4,000,000 people are diabetics.

Diabetes is especially common in those who become obese; it is commoner in later life, and in some families. It may occur at any age but usually comes on between 50 and 60 years of age.

The abnormality of sugar typical of diabetes can be defined but there are many patients with abnormal tests of 'glucose tolerance' which though not diabetic are not normal, and it is supposed that such persons are liable to develop diabetes in the future. The obese and women who give birth to large babies (over 4·5 kg) are especially prone to diabetes in later life.

Clinical symptoms. In many patients there are no symptoms, but glycosuria is discovered at a routine medical or insurance examination. The majority develop symptoms over a period of some weeks and occasionally the patient is seen first confused or in coma.

Common symptoms are, *thirst, polyuria, fatigue, weight loss* and in women *pruritus vulvae*—skin infection, boils, furunculosis are often found. The first symptoms may be those of diabetic complications or associated diseases such as peripheral vascular disease, ischaemic heart disease, poor vision due to retinopathy or cataracts, neuritis, or nephropathy.

Diagnosis. Glycosuria may be caused by low renal threshold or for other reasons but the presence of diabetes must be confirmed by a formal glucose tolerance test. The blood is examined each half-hour after the patient has drunk 50 to 100 g of glucose, the level being followed for $2\frac{1}{2}$ to 3 hours.

The complications of diabetes include *diabetic ketosis, coma* and *hypoglycaemia* (the consequence of treatment with insulin or oral drugs).

Diabetic ketosis and coma. This results from inadequate insulin activity. The blood sugar rises, the glycosuria is marked with polyuria causing dehydration, the combustion of fats leads to excessive ketone bodies in the blood and urine, acidosis, overbreathing, vomiting, later stupor and coma. These changes cause severe biochemical cell change with the loss of sodium and potassium and water from the tissues.

The diagnosis is confirmed by blood chemistry. The blood sugar is raised, ketone bodies are present, and the alkali reserve lowered, the pH is lowered (acid), the serum potassium may be low, the concentration of the plasma (the osmolarity) is increased.

Treatment. Immediate treatment with detailed nursing as in intensive care units will be needed for severe cases. The pulse, blood pressure, urine output are watched, the stomach contents are aspirated, intravenous infusion is started immediately. Many patients are deficient of 7 litres of body fluid and the contained electrolytes; 2 litres of fluid may be needed in the first hour of treatment with normal saline with added alkali (sodium bicarbonate) and potassium. Insulin in a dose of 100 to 200 units is given, at least half the dose being given intravenously. The blood sugar, ketone level, potassium are followed if possible each two hours and further treatment planned. When improvement is achieved, urine testing may serve for control and the patient is able to take fluids and food by mouth.

Acute Complications. *Hypoglycaemia.* The patient on insulin and on some oral drugs may have symptoms due to abnormally low blood sugar. These symptoms are of sudden onset, unlike diabetic ketosis; altered vision, paraesthesiae, may be followed by objective evidence of mental confusion, aggression, 'drunkenness', finally stupor and coma.

The onset is sudden, the patient usually sweating and not dehydrated. He may be known to be a diabetic on insulin who may have missed his normal meal. Where there is doubt an immediate test of a drop of blood will confirm the low blood sugar (Dextrostix). The treatment is to give 10 to 20 g of glucose if the patient will swallow; if he won't glucagon 2 to 5 mg intramuscularly. If the patient has not roused in 10 to 20 minutes intravenous glucose 20 ml of 50 per cent solution is given. If recovery has not taken place within the hour admission to hospital is desirable. *Prolonged hypoglycaemia may cause permanent brain damage.*

The chronic complications of diabetes. The majority of persons who have had diabetes for 15 years show some physical changes on detailed examination. These changes may be the first symptoms noted, and they seem most evident in patients whose diabetes has been inadequately controlled.

Diabetic retinopathy results in damage and scarring of the retina which is a common cause of blindness in later life. *Diabetic neuropathy* causes neuritis involving often the voluntary muscles and sensory fibres as well as the autonomic system, causing impotence, diarrhoea, absent sweating, hypotension. *Diabetic nephropathy* damages the renal glomeruli with albuminuria, oedema, and finally, often in association with renal infections, uraemia. Vascular disease is common in diabetics, causing ischaemia of the legs and feet, and an increased incidence of *coronary disease in diabetic women.*

Treatment. The treatment of the diabetic state requires assessment of the severity of symptoms, the age, weight, sex and intelligence of the patient.

The aim of treatment is for the patient to achieve a normal weight and to lead a normal and active life without diabetic complications. There are four main aspects of treatment:

> Diet.
> Oral drugs.
> Insulin.
> Education of the patient.

Diet. All diabetic patients must attend to their diet. The diet should aim to achieve normal weight. In the obese, weight reduction on a standard low calorie diet (800 to 1,000 calories a day) is mandatory. In most patients some attention to carbohydrate intake and restriction of this is needed. Normal weight will be maintained on a diet adjusted for the patient's sex, age and activity in the range of 1,500 to 3,500 calories a day, the carbohydrate content being limited to 150 to 300 g a day. In a few patients weighing the diet may be of value. The protein and fat content are not prescribed in detail, but in pregnancy adequate protein intake must be ensured. Details of a diabetic diet are given on p. 160.

In the event of illness the normal carbohydrate intake is taken in liquid form, and if vomiting occurs in a patient on insulin, admission to hospital and intravenous infusion may be needed. In patients on insulin, or oral drugs, the daily routine of meals must be ensured and the relation to injections or tablets maintained.

Oral hypoglycaemic drugs. Two main types of drug can be given by mouth to lower the blood sugar: the sulphonyl ureas which stimulate the release of insulin, and the biguanidines which increase the uptake of sugar by muscle (see Table below).

These drugs are not used when the diabetes is severe, or in children, but when diabetes is not controlled by diet alone.

The patient is observed and the dose increased to the maximum, then if control has not resulted, combined therapy with a drug of the different group is given. A change to another drug in the same group is not usually effective. In some unstable persons on insulin these drugs may be added with advantage.

Complications of treatment. The largest doses may cause gastro-intestinal side-effects—nausea and diarrhoea—which may prevent their use. Skin and other sensitivities are rare. In the elderly, especially when uncertain about their meals, and with renal impairment, hypoglycaemia must be watched for when the sulphonyl urea drugs are being given.

Oral Diabetic Drugs

S.U. (Sulphonyl urea)	*Tablet*
Tolbutamide	500 mg
Chlorpropamide	100 mg
	250 mg
Glibenclamide	5 mg
Tolazamide	100 mg
	250 mg
Acetohexamide	500 mg
Glymidine	500 mg
BiG (Biguanidines)	
Metformin	500 mg
	850 mg
Phenformin	25 mg
	(50 mg slow release capsules)

INSULIN

Insulin is a protein which is digested in the gut and must be given by hypodermic injection. The precise structure of insulin is known but all the material used in clinical practice is extracted from animal sources. There are small variations in structure between animal species. The trivial differences raise the possibility of antibody reactions to insulin, which is largely obtained from beef and pigs killed for human consumption. Pig insulin resembles the human insulin more closely than beef insulin.

Very many types of insulin are available, coming from either the pig or from beef, and chemically modified so that they may be quickly or slowly absorbed (see list below).

Treatment is usually initiated with soluble insulin given twice daily, followed by a major meal. The dose required cannot be precisely predicted and the initial dose is adjusted by testing the blood sugar and urine sugar in the individual being treated.

In many patients a routine of treatment with one dose of long-acting insulin given, usually, before breakfast can be achieved.

The complications of treatment are few if the patient masters the snags of hypodermic injection, in particular intravenous injection must be avoided as this produces an extremely rapid response whatever the type of insulin used. Sensitivity to insulin is very rare. The commonest problem is ensuring that the dose given is suitable and that excessive lowering of the blood sugar is avoided by balancing the dose given against the intake of food, so that symptoms of hypoglycaemia are avoided.

Insulins available as either 40 or 80 units per ml.

'Quick acting'	*Total action*
Soluble insulin	6–12 hours
Neutral insulin	
'Semi-quick acting'	
ISOphane insulin	12–24 hours
Globin insulin	
Semi-lente insulin	
'Long acting'	
Protamine insulin	24–30 hours
Ultralente insulin	
'Mixed quick and slow acting'	
Insulin zinc suspension (Lente)	24–30 hours
Biphasic insulin (Rapitard)	

THE EDUCATION OF THE PATIENT

The diabetic must be encouraged to lead a normal life while keeping a watch on his weight and diet. In a few patients weighing the diet initially may be instructive, but this need not be continued. Knowledge about diet and other matters of care can be derived from diabetic associations, such as the British Diabetic Association (3 Alfred Place, London), which will assist its members.

The diabetic on insulin should carry a card stating his dose to assist in his management if he is taken ill. When driving or travelling special care is required to avoid hypoglycaemia.

The control of hyperglycaemia can be roughly assessed by the patient testing his own urine (collected usually before meals), and all patients should know that occasional tests of the blood sugar as well are essential to ensure that control is adequate and so try to avoid the development of diabetic complications.

Chapter 30

The Chronic Rheumatic Diseases

by A. C. BOYLE

> *Rheumatoid arthritis—osteoarthritis—ankylosing spondylitis—less common forms of arthritis—soft tissue rheumatism—gout*

The chronic rheumatic diseases are a group of conditions which affect the musculo-skeletal system, giving rise to pain and loss of function. Affection of the joints (arthritis) is usually serious, since it may lead to deformity and crippling; affection of the soft tissues (e.g. fibrositis, tendinitis, bursitis), although often painful, is usually short-lived, and complete and rapid recovery is usual.

RHEUMATOID ARTHRITIS

This is an inflammatory disease, mainly affecting the peripheral joints, and of unknown cause. A great deal of research over the years has failed to establish its nature—indeed, in the present state of our knowledge we cannot even be certain into which category of disease it falls—i.e. infective, endocrine, etc. Currently, it is considered by many to fall within the group of disorders in which an abnormality of the immune mechanisms of the body plays a part—the so-called *autoimmune diseases*.

Rheumatoid arthritis is a common condition. Estimates of its frequency in the population of this country vary between 1·6 and 5 per cent. It is three times more common in women than in men, and may occur at any age, although the usual age of onset is in the mid-forties in both sexes. Since it is so common and often disabling, it contributes substantially to the 25 million or so working days lost each year in this country because of the rheumatic diseases.

As the course of the disease is often protracted, no single clinical description can cover it adequately. In the early stages there may be no more than one or two mildly swollen and painful joints, without any disturbance of general health; *the more acute* case may present a pitiful picture with multiple swollen and intensely painful joints, making the patient fearful of movement, while the associated feeling of ill-health and depression contributes to the patient's misery. *In the later stages of the disease* one or more joints may be so deformed that the patient is reduced to complete dependence on others.

The basic pathology starts with a low grade inflammation of the synovial membrane; at this stage in the disease the joints will be found to be warm, swollen and tender. If the disease progresses, the inflamed synovial membrane may gradually spread over the articular cartilage and erode it, so that the joint may now be painful and limited in movement. Finally, the bone ends themselves may be eroded by the same process, so that the architecture of the joint is gradually destroyed (Fig. 30/1). The end result may be fibrous or bony ankylosis, leaving permanent deformity and stiffness.

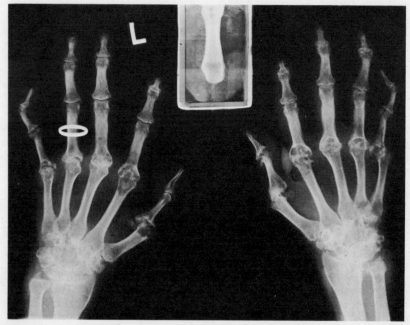

Fig. 30/1 Rheumatoid arthritis. X-ray of hands, showing destructive changes in meta-carpophalangeal joints and wrists.

Apart from the joints, there is usually a systemic upset, with malaise, anaemia and loss of weight. Tendons and their sheaths may be involved in the inflammatory process, and in the more severe case rheumatoid nodules may be present over bony prominences. Rarely, the inflammatory process may involve the arteries, giving rise to a *polyarteritis*; in such cases any system in the body may be affected by loss of blood supply—e.g. the peripheral nerves, giving rise to a *peripheral neuropathy*—and a fatal outcome may result.

The disease usually runs a variable course, tending to have periods when it is active (exacerbations) and periods of quiescence (remissions). With each exacerbation there tends to be a little more destructive change within the affected joints, so that over the years the patient usually becomes progressively more disabled.

The aims of medical treatment are:

To relieve pain.
To induce the disease to enter a phase of remission.
The prevention of deformity.
The restoration of function.

Pain may be relieved by a variety of drugs, some of which also possess anti-inflammatory properties. The most useful in rheumatoid arthritis are aspirin in its various forms, phenylbutazone (Butazolidin) and indomethacin (Indocid). Drugs used to induce the disease to enter a phase of remission are injections of a gold compound (Myocrisin), or the chloroquine group of drugs (e.g. Plaquenil). The steroid group of drugs has a remarkable effect upon the symptoms of the disease, but unfortunately they need to be used over a prolonged period and thus the dangers of their known side-effects prohibit their use in all except the most severe cases. However, in suitable cases a steroid preparation may be injected directly into the joint cavity, thus avoiding the dangers of systemic effects. *Deformity may be prevented by adequate nursing care and splintage of the affected joints, while restoration of function is the task of the physiotherapist.*

OSTEOARTHRITIS (Osteoarthrosis)

Unlike rheumatoid arthritis, osteoarthritis is purely a degenerative condition of the joints, and for this reason it has been suggested that the term osteoarthrosis should be used. Degenerative changes in the joints of

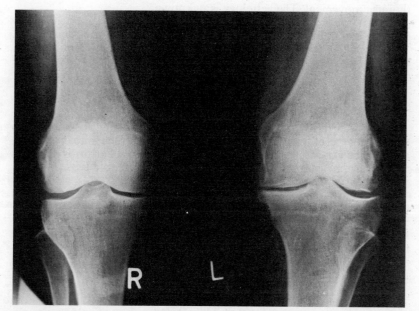

Fig. 30/2 Osteoarthritis. Right knee is normal, left knee shows thinning of cartilage and osteophytes at edge of joint.

greater or lesser degree are an inevitable result of the ageing process, though heredity, occupation, obesity or previous injury to joints may hasten the process of 'wear and tear'.

The articular cartilage capping the bone ends becomes fissured and thinned, so that the affected joint becomes somewhat stiff and may creak on movement. Except when it affects the hip joint, it is normally a benign condition, leading to little deformity or disability. The joints most commonly affected are the terminal joints of the fingers, giving rise to so-called Heberden's nodes on the joint margins, the knees (Fig. 30/2) and the hips, although any joint in the body may be affected. Similar changes in the cervical and lumbar spines affecting the intervertebral discs are usually referred to as 'spondylosis', since these are not true diarthrodial joints.

Reassurance of the patient, an adjustment of the way of life and simple analgesic drugs are usually all that is required in the treatment of osteoarthritis. The hip constitutes a special problem, since pain and stiffness may be severe when this joint is affected. Surgical treatment—e.g. replacement arthroplasty—may be called for (see p. 580).

ANKYLOSING SPONDYLITIS

This is a condition affecting young men much more commonly than women. An inflammatory arthritis starts in the sacro-iliac joints and tends gradually to spread up the spine, often giving rise to calcification or ossification of the spinal ligaments. Thus complete rigidity of part or whole of the spinal column may result. Occasionally the peripheral joints may be involved, particularly the shoulders and hips. The joints of the thoracic cage are also often affected, giving rise to much diminished thoracic movement. The aetiology is unknown.

Deep X-ray treatment to affected portions of the spine is often greatly helpful, but unfortunately carries a small risk of inducing leukaemia. *Anti-rheumatic drugs* such as phenylbutazone (Butazolidin) or indomethacin (Indocid) usually help to relieve the symptoms. *The patient should be taught to practise exercises to maintain good posture and spinal mobility.*

LESS COMMON FORMS OF ARTHRITIS

Psoriatic arthritis. A proportion of patients suffering from psoriasis develop a type of arthritis which closely resembles rheumatoid arthritis, and may be very destructive and disabling. This type of arthritis responds to the same measures in treatment as the true rheumatoid type.

Reiter's syndrome. This is sometimes considered to be a venereal disease, since it usually follows irregular sexual intercourse. Some cases, however, appear to follow bacillary dysentery. The classical triad of symptoms is a urethritis with a non-bacterial discharge, arthritis tending to affect predominantly the lower limbs, and, less often, conjunctivitis. A skin rash closely resembling psoriasis may also occur. The cause is unknown, though a viral infection has been suspected.

Still's disease. This is sometimes known as juvenile rheumatoid arthritis, since it is a disease of childhood with some resemblance to the adult form.

In the initial phase the swollen painful joints are usually accompanied by fever, leucocytosis, skin rashes and enlargement of the liver, spleen and lymph glands. The condition tends usually to be more benign than adult rheumatoid arthritis and the same measures may be used in treatment.

SOFT TISSUE RHEUMATISM

Non-specific inflammation of various soft tissues may give rise to pain and temporary disability. Muscles (myositis), fibrous tissue (fibrositis), tendons (tendinitis), and bursae (bursitis) are commonly affected. Psychological tension, injury or unaccustomed exercise, etc., may be the underlying causes of some of these. Rest of the affected part, the application of heat and simple analgesics will usually provide a cure.

GOUT

Gout is a metabolic disorder in which there is an excess of uric acid in the blood (hyperuricaemia), and in about 60 per cent of such cases the disorder is inherited. Hyperuricaemia may sometimes be secondary to other diseases—e.g. renal failure or leukaemia.

All members of a family with hyperuricaemia do not necessarily suffer attacks of gout, which are due to crystals of uric acid being deposited in joints. These crystals act as an acute irritant, and the clinical picture is of a sudden attack of severe pain in a joint (most often the great toe), which becomes swollen, red and exquisitely tender.

If untreated, the acute attack gradually subsides within 10 to 14 days, and the joint returns to normal. However, repeated attacks will gradually damage the joint, giving rise to permanent disability. In chronic cases uric acid may accumulate in and around joints and even in the cartilage of the ear, showing as chalky white deposits (tophi). Attacks of acute gout may occur at irregular intervals and affect any joint.

Hyperuricaemia may not only constitute a hazard to the patient from the attacks of joint pain, but may also be a danger, long term, to the life of the patient, for high levels of uric acid may not only give rise to renal damage, but are also known to be associated with arteriosclerosis. Fortunately, with modern treatment, not only can the acute attack be quickly relieved, but the hyperuricaemia can be controlled, thus preventing further attacks, and also protecting the patient from long-term dangers.

Treatment of acute gout. For many centuries, physicians have known that the drug colchicine, when given in adequate dosage, will quickly abort acute gout. Colchicine has the disadvantage of being a gastrointestinal irritant and has been largely replaced by either Butazolidin or indomethacin, both of which will promptly relieve the pain and swelling of acute gout.

Control of hyperuricaemia. There are several drugs (e.g. Benemid) which will cause the kidneys to excrete larger than usual quantities of uric acid, thus lowering the level to normal. More recently the drug allopurinol has been discovered, which suppresses the formation of uric acid, and this drug is of particular use where renal damage has already occurred. Whichever of these drugs is used, the level of uric acid will gradually be restored to normal, and attacks of gout will cease. Unfortunately, both drugs will usually need to be taken for the rest of the patient's life, but this is a small price to pay for the prevention of repeated crippling attacks of pain and the long-term dangers of renal damage or arteriosclerosis.

Chapter 31

Diseases and Disorders of the Skin

by G. M. LEVENE

*Introduction—terminology of lesions—itching—causes of skin disease
—nursing points—the eczemas—psoriasis—skin infections—parasitic
infestations—skin tumours—other common skin conditions, drug
eruptions, urticaria, acne vulgaris*

The skin is the largest organ of the body, making up about 15 per cent of
the total body weight. It comprises an outer cellular epidermis firmly
attached to a fibrous dermis containing blood vessels, lymphatics, nerves
and free cells (Fig. 31/1). It protects the body mechanically, keeps water
and bacteria out, prevents the undesirable loss of tissue fluid. It assists the
maintenance of a steady body temperature and is a most important sense
organ. Emotions are expressed via the skin, sometimes involuntarily, as in
the flushing of rage and shame, the pallor of anger and emotional sweating
in anxiety. The skin is liable to a large variety of disorders, most of which do
not harm the general health but cause distress because they are unsightly
or because they itch.

Several false notions regarding skin diseases are prevalent, particularly
that they are contagious, that they are caused by 'nerves' or by defective
diet and that very little can be done about them. In reality only a few skin
diseases are significantly contagious, the commoner ones being virus
warts, scabies, pediculosis, bacterial impetigo and syphilis. Genuine
examples of skin disorders caused directly by emotion or diet are uncommon and are usually fairly easily recognized. Many skin problems are
completely curable with treatment, some resolve spontaneously, and the
remainder can often be greatly alleviated by judicious therapy.

Terminology of skin lesions. Since skin diseases may have widely differing
appearances in different sites it is necessary to learn the definitions of the
various types of skin lesions.

> *Macule*, a flat spot of a different colour from the surrounding skin.
>   Freckles are macules.
> *Papule*, a small lump raised above the surface of the skin.
> *Nodule*, a more deeply situated lump.
> *Scale*, a flat mass of horny cells shed from the horny layer.
> *Crust*, a dried deposit on the skin. Usually refers to dried serum,
>   but occasionally the term is applied to thick keratin.

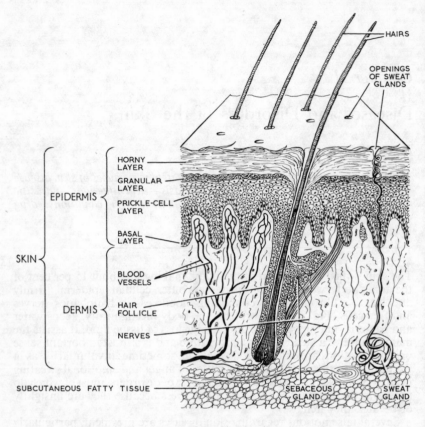

Fig. 31/1 The structure of the skin, showing salient points.

Blister, a skin bleb filled with clear fluid.

Vesicle, a small blister.

Pustule, a skin bleb filled with pus.

Excoriation, a scratch mark.

Plaque, a raised uniform thickening of a portion of the skin with a flat or rough surface and a well-defined edge.

Cyst, a deeply situated fluid-filled cavity.

Erythema, redness of the skin resulting from dilatation of dermal blood vessels.

Erosion, an area of superficial loss of skin.

Ulcer, an area of loss of the full thickness of the skin or mucous membrane.

The extent of lesions is indicated by terms such as sparse, scattered, extensive, profuse, and confluent. If the whole skin surface is inflamed the patient is said to have an *erythrodermia*. A skin disease is a *dermatosis* (plural, dermatoses).

ITCHING (Pruritus)

Itching is undoubtedly the most common symptom of skin disease. It can be a most intolerable and distressing sensation. General diseases such as obstructive jaundice and Hodgkin's disease may cause generalized itching, but most pruritus results from an inflammation arising in the skin. Skin diseases which usually itch severely are eczema (all types), scabies and pediculosis (see below).

CAUSES OF SKIN DISEASE

Skin disease may arise from agents which attack it from outside or from within. These agents may take the form of *damaging radiation* (e.g. severe sunburn), *irritants* (e.g. acids and alkalis), or *living organisms* (e.g. the virus of warts or the mite of scabies). Agents arising from outside the body may nevertheless be spread via the bloodstream, the usual effect being involvement of a wide area of skin in a symmetrical pattern; examples are the rashes of secondary syphilis, measles and those of many drug eruptions.

Genetic and *racial* factors are important since many skin disorders are inherited. *The climate*, especially the degree of sun exposure and the *humidity* may bring on skin lesions or modify existing ones. *Systemic disease* such as diabetes mellitus or malignant disease can make the skin more liable to infection by bacteria, yeasts and fungi. *Psychological upsets* undoubtedly influence skin disease but only rarely are they the primary cause.

GENERAL POINTS IN THE NURSING OF SKIN DISEASE

Patients with skin disease are often in considerable physical and mental discomfort, therefore the first task of the attendants, both nursing and medical, is to relieve discomfort and allay anxiety. The patient will be reassured by a calm confident approach and he should not be made to feel that his attendants are unwilling to come close.

The patient is usually most comfortable in a fairly cool environment. Rubber and plastic under-sheets are best removed. In the acute stages of skin disease *itching* may be a prominent feature and both daytime and night sedation with oral antihistamine or barbiturate drugs can be very helpful. Absolute bed rest is usually unnecessary and the patient can be allowed up for toilet purposes and for meals.

Baths. A morning bath daily or on alternate days often adds greatly to the patient's comfort *provided it is followed quickly by the appropriate topical therapy*. Bathing removes remnants of the previous topical applications together with any accumulated skin debris such as scales and dried serum. The water should be warm rather than hot and five minutes in the bath should be sufficient. After the bath the patient pats (not rubs) himself dry with a soft towel.

Bath additives are helpful in many skin diseases. *Emulsifying Ointment B.P.* 100 g in a bath of water helps to lubricate the skin and prevent dryness. Emulsifying ointment baths are used for patients with chronic dry eczematous dermatitis or any condition where dryness of the skin is troublesome. The emulsifying ointment is best dissolved in a small quantity (120 ml) of very hot water and added to the bath with stirring, otherwise it may remain as lumps floating on the surface. If the above material is found to be too greasy then a similar quantity of *Aqueous Cream B.N.F,* may be used.

Potassium permangate baths are used when bacterial infection is present. The correct concentration is achieved by adding 60 ml of potassium permanganate solution (1 in 8,000) to a bath of water. The not uncommon practice of adding potassium permanganate *crystals* to the bath is hazardous since small skin burns may be produced if some of the crystals which do not have time to dissolve settle on the skin.

Coal tar baths are used almost as a routine in the treatment of psoriasis. Sixty ml of strong solution of coal tar is added to a bath of water and the plaques of psoriasis are rubbed gently to remove loose scales.

Ointments and creams. *Topical corticosteroid preparations* have greatly improved the efficiency of treating many dermatoses, especially eczemas. The original preparation, hydrocortisone, although still useful in certain circumstances, has given way to more powerful steroids such as fluocinolone (Synalar) and betamethasone (Betnovate). Usually 1 in 4 dilutions give a satisfactory result. Often an antiseptic such as chinoform (Vioform) is added to treat or prevent infection. *Coal tar* ointments and *anti-fungal* ointments are also in common use.

Application. A thin layer is applied to the affected area of the skin and rubbed in gently but well with the fingers. Applying ointment with gauze swabs is inefficient since the essential 'rubbing in' phase is omitted. Although the ointment can be applied with bare fingers it is now common practice for a pair of disposable polythene gloves to be worn. *About 10 g of ointment is sufficient to cover the entire skin surface.*

If the appearance of the skin has changed for the worse since the treatment was prescribed, especially if pustules have appeared, then the doctor should be informed. *If in doubt it is safer to omit a treatment rather than persevere with unsuitable therapy.*

Dressings. The ideal covering for the skin after treatment is a single layer of stockinette gauze, since it is quickly applied, comfortable for the patient, and allows air to circulate freely. Corticosteroid ointments are sometimes used with *polythene occlusion;* an airtight layer of polythene over the treated skin is used to keep in moisture and aid penetration of the active constituents of the ointment to the deeper layers of the skin. For hands and feet polythene gloves and bags are employed; limbs and trunk may be wrapped in polythene sheeting. Unless otherwise ordered occlusion overnight only is employed.

Impregnated bandages are useful for wrapping affected limbs. The medicament contained in the bandage can be coal tar, ichthyol or a corticosteroid. An ichthyol paste bandage is especially useful for ulcerated legs. A common fault is to wrap the bandage too tightly, causing the patient much discomfort. If the bandage is cut across completely every 12 inches or so this problem will not arise. When the bandage has been thus applied in short strips it is held in place by a layer of stockinette gauze and a crêpe bandage. If an ambulant patient with leg ulcers or gravitational eczema is being treated in this way a firmer outside support is required and a stout elastic bandage is more effective than crêpe for this purpose.

Any *supportive* bandage should extend from the toes to the knee or higher, because if the foot is not included any tendency to oedema is aggravated.

THE ECZEMAS

Eczema is the term given to skin disease where there is a characteristic inflammation of the epidermis and dermis. In the *acute* phase the skin is itchy, red and weeping, but if the condition becomes *chronic* it appears mauvish-red, scaly and thickened like morocco leather (lichenification). *Dermatitis* is the same as eczema and the two terms are best regarded as interchangeable. Some common types are described below.

Eczemas of known cause. *Primary irritant contact eczema.* Repeated contact of the skin with irritating substances produces damage which may proceed to eczema. The situation arises commonly in industry when workers handle acids, alkalis, cooling oils and chemicals without protective clothing. Progress to eczema may then be further hastened by scrubbing the skin with harsh soaps and detergents in an effort to clean it. If contact with irritants continues, a disabling weeping eczema ensues which may take many weeks to heal.

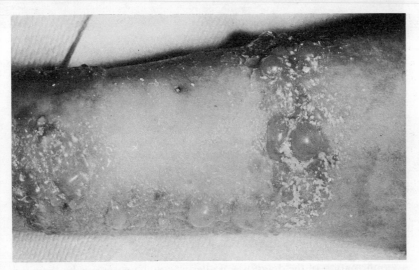

Fig. 31/2 Bullous allergic contact eczema of the forearm due to sticking plaster.

Allergic contact eczema (see Fig. 31/2). This important type of eczema differs from the foregoing in that the individual develops a specific allergy to a concentration of chemical substance which is normally quite harmless to the skin. A typical example of this phenomenon is allergic sensitivity to nickel. Any site where nickel-containing metal objects are in contact with the skin will develop an eczematous reaction in the sensitized person.

The sites involved are the suspender areas from contact with metal suspender clips, under bra rings and clasps, and sometimes on the wrists under metal watches and bracelets. Another cause of suspender dermatitis is allergy to a constituent of the rubber in the suspender (Fig. 31/3). Rubber sensitivity is a cause of hand eczema when rubber gloves are worn and also of a chronic foot eczema, since most shoes contain rubber. It must be noted that ointments used in treatment of skin conditions may also act as sensitizers so that inappropriate treatment may make the condition worse instead of better. Lanolin, contained in innumerable ointment bases, can act in this way as can some antibiotics when applied topically. Even plants may cause this problem, the common primula being a prime example.

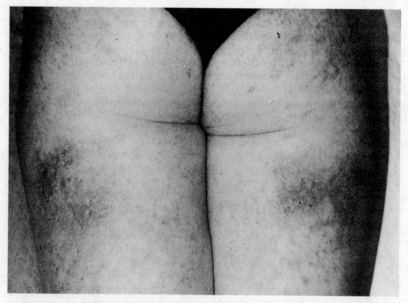

Fig. 31/3 Allergic contact eczema due to suspenders.

Allergic contact sensitization will affect only a small minority of people exposed to the sensitizer and it is a curious feature that an individual may be exposed to a chemical repeatedly for many years before sensitization occurs.

Confirmation of the diagnosis of allergic contact eczema is by the *patch test*. A suitable non-irritant concentration of the suspected chemical is made up in solution or in a bland ointment base and a small amount is placed on the back under an occlusive dressing. Forty-eight hours later the patch is removed and the site inspected. In normal individuals no change will be seen, but if the person is sensitive to the chemical a patch of inflammation will have developed at the site of application. *It is most important that any contact sensitizer be found, for avoidance of it will result in cure of the eczema.*

Gravitational eczema. The skin of the lower shins and around the ankles is liable to develop eczema, especially in people with varicose veins. An initial sign of gravitational change is brownish pigmentation where superficial capillaries have ruptured, and the skin may be indurated or oedematous (see Fig. 31/4). Even minor trauma can then result in a gravitational ulcer, and exudate from the ulcer and infection will further irritate the surrounding skin.

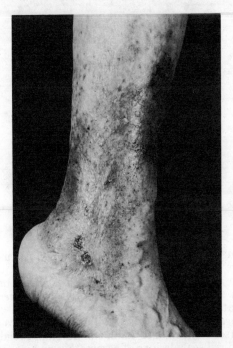

Fig. 31/4 Gravitational eczema.

Eczema associated with infection. Although infections of the skin due to fungi, bacteria and parasites may have a distinctive appearance in their early stages, the irritation of the skin and the scratching they provoke often leads to a picture which is indistinguishable from eczema.

Eczemas of unknown cause. *Atopic eczema.* There is an eczema-asthma-hay fever symptom complex which tends to run in families. The genetic make-up of the family renders each individual member liable to suffer from one or more of this trio of diseases and it is not uncommon for a parent with asthma to have a child with eczema. Atopic eczema is the commonest type of *infantile eczema*. Characteristically it starts as a generalized red itchy rash when the infant is a few months old. The eczema remains widespread until about the age of two years when it localizes preferentially to the distal flexures of the body (see Fig. 31/5) (i.e. the elbow, wrist, knee and ankle flexures), and to the face and neck. The severity of the eczema is variable during childhood, often becoming worse at times of psychological

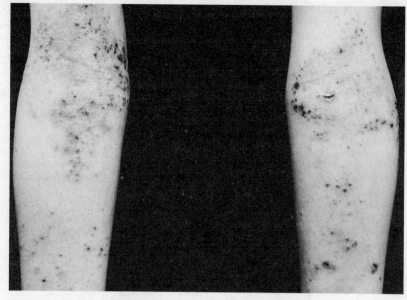

Fig. 31/5 Atopic eczema of elbow flexures, showing excoriations and lichenfication.

stress, but it usually responds well to treatment. Most cases clear by the time adolescence is reached.

Children with atopic eczema *should not be vaccinated* because vaccination 'takes' can spread all over the skin producing *eczema vaccinatum*, which may be fatal.

Seborrhoeic eczema. Individuals who have scaly scalps (dandruff) and a greasy skin (seborrhoea) are liable to develop eyelid inflammation (blepharitis) and red scaly lesions of eczematous appearance on the scalp, face, neck and trunk. A common infantile form is associated with thick adherent scales in the scalp (cradle-cap) or with a napkin eruption.

Palm and sole eczema. The palms and soles are liable to acute or chronic eczema which does not correspond to any of the eczema types described above. In the acute form crops of small tense vesicles appear on the palms, around the fingers and on the soles, pompholyx (see Fig. 31/6). The horny layer of the palms and soles is very thick; the blisters may attain a considerable size before they rupture. Pruritus is severe and infection is common, so prompt treatment is desirable. Effective emergency treatment consists of potassium permanganate soaks (1 in 8,000) several times daily. If this type of eczema becomes chronic the main features are hyperkeratosis with pruritus and painful fissuring.

Complications of eczema:
    (*a*) *Infection*: usually with staphylococci.
    (*b*) *Secondary spread* is a widespread symmetrical eczematous eruption which may develop suddenly in a patient with a

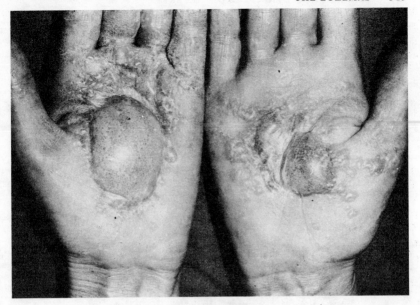

Fig. 31/6 Acute hand eczema (pompholyx).

localized area of active eczema. Gravitational eczema is especially liable to this complication.

(c) *Chronicity*. Acute eczemas become chronic if the cause is not removed or if treatment is delayed or inappropriate. If no cause is discovered it may be impossible to prevent.

Treatment. *Acute eczema* is intensely itchy and weeping and the patient is distressed. If the area involved is large, bed rest and sedation are essential. A potassium permanganate bath and normal saline or calamine lotion compresses will allay itching and help to remove accumulated crusts and serum. The oozing eczematous areas are encouraged to dry and heal by continued wet compresses or by application of a corticosteroid lotion or cream. Once weeping has ceased and the surface of the skin is dry, a process which takes 24 to 48 hours, the treatment becomes the same as that for chronic eczema.

Chronic eczema is also pruritic but the skin is dry and may be excoriated and lichenified. Emulsifying ointment baths are prescribed (see p. 313), daily in hospital, twice weekly outside. After bathing, a corticosteroid or other ointment is applied to all the affected areas. The corticosteroid reduces inflammation and the greasy base of the ointment prevents dehydration. Certain antihistamine drugs administered by mouth are sedative and are of value in relieving pruritus. Those most often used are promethazine hydrochloride (Phenergan), trimeprazine tartrate (Vallergan) and chlorpheniramine maleate (Piriton). Topical antihistamine preparations should not be used. Patches of eczema resistant to the above measures may yield to the same ointment under polythene occlusion, the application of coal-tar impregnated bandages, or irradiation with low-voltage X-rays.

PSORIASIS

Psoriasis affects between 1 and 2 per cent of the population of the United Kingdom and often runs in families. It is characterized by thick red scaly plaques on the elbows and knees (see Fig. 31/7). The plaques are clearly marginated from normal skin and are fairly symmetrically distributed. Scratching a plaque with a spatula demonstrates the typical silvery scales. The finger-nails are often pitted or deformed and a characteristic arthritis (psoriatic arthritis) may be associated with it. Psoriasis responds fairly well to topical therapy and itching is rarely severe, but recurrences are common and one cannot promise a complete cure.

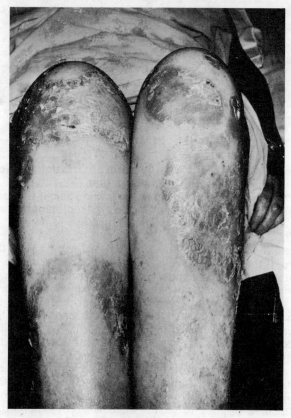

Fig. 31/7 Psoriasis of the legs.

Treatment. Ultraviolet light and coal tar baths are of value. Three topical preparations help: dithranol, coal tar and topical corticosteroids. Of these dithranol is the best treatment for large plaques. A low concentration (0·1 or 0·25 per cent) is used initially and a thin layer is applied strictly to the area of the plaque; it is renewed daily. Corticosteroid creams or ointments are the preferred treatment for flexural and facial lesions; they also work very quickly on large plaques, but unfortunately areas so treated often relapse in a short time after stopping treatment. Coal tar ointments work slowly but the beneficial effect lasts longer.

SKIN INFECTIONS (Bacterial, Yeast, Fungal and Viral)

Bacterial infections. *Staphylococcus aureus* and the beta-haemolytic streptococcus are the commonest pathogenic bacteria to cause skin disease. Low-grade infection of a large number of hair follicles is called *folliculitis*. A *septic spot* is an infection of a single hair follicle and if the inflammation is severe enough to cause a large pus-filled nodule it is called a *boil* (or furuncle). Boils are common in hairy areas such as the axilla and the back of the neck. Epidermal infection is called *impetigo contagiosa* (see Fig. 31/8); it appears, usually on the face in children, as inflamed weeping patches with accumulation of yellowish (honey-coloured) crusts. It lives up to its name, being readily transferred from child to child. A patch of eczema may become impetiginized as a result of bacterial infection.

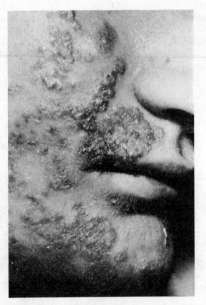

Fig. 31/8 Impetigo contagiosa of the face.

Treatment of small septic spots is by an anti-bacterial cream or paint. A crop of boils may require systemic treatment with penicillin or tetracycline. Impetigo can be cleared with a tetracycline ointment.

Yeast infections. *Candida albicans* (*Monilia*) is the common pathogenic yeast. It often affects the mouth in young babies ('thrush') as white patches, and the vulva in pregnant and diabetic women. It may cause intertriginous inflammation in the obese (i.e. in the groins and beneath pendulous breasts). Buccal and peri-anal monilial infection can occur following a course of a wide-spectrum antibiotic such as ampicillin. Treatment is with topical Vioform or Nystatin cream, or a paint such as gentian violet or magenta.

Fungal infections (ringworm). Pathogenic fungi feed and multiply in the horny layer of the skin and in the hair and nails. The diagnosis is made by taking scrapings of the skin, nails or hair, mounting them on a slide in caustic potash (potassium hydroxide) solution and examining them under the microscope. Fungal mycelia are observed to ramify amongst the horny scales as branching filaments and threads. The scrapings are then cultured on agar plates so that the exact fungal species can be identified.

Tinea capitis (fungus of scalp hair) is now rather uncommon; it causes rounded scaly balding patches in schoolchildren (see Fig. 31/9). *Tinea corporis* (fungal infection of body skin) may be contracted from animals and manifests itself as inflamed annular lesions (hence 'ringworm'). More chronic forms affect the groins, particularly in men (tinea cruris), the toe-webs (tinea pedis), and the nails.

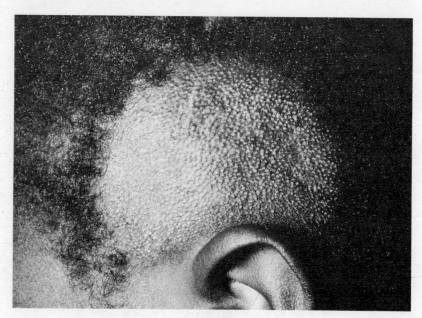

Fig. 31/9 Scalp ringworm in a child.

A simple and effective treatment for skin ringworm is compound benzoic acid (Whitfield's) ointment, but oral griseofulvin is necessary for scalp and nail ringworm. Griseofulvin is an antibiotic effective against most varieties of fungus.

Viral infections. The *common wart* (verruca) is caused by a virus. Warts are frequently found on the hands and the soles of the feet. They are contagious but prevention of spread is very difficult. They will eventually resolve spontaneously, but various destructive techniques are used to clear them with variable success.

Herpes simplex virus causes the 'cold sores' which erupt on the lips and occasionally at other sites as crops of small painful blisters during feverish episodes.

Herpes zoster ('shingles') is a virus infection which affects the skin in the area of distribution of one or more nerve roots. The infection is unilateral and the site affected depends on the nerve root involved. The usual appearance is a band of inflammation around one half of the trunk.

No reliable specific medication for viral infections is yet known but there is hope that one will soon be found.

PARASITIC INFESTATIONS

Scabies is caused by a mite, about half the size of a printed full stop, which burrows in the horny layer of the skin. It is contracted by close physical contact with a person suffering from the disease, and severe itching starts a few weeks later. Mite burrows are seen as raised lines and tiny individual vesicles especially on the hands. The mite can be seen on microscopic examination of scrapings from characteristic lesions. *Treatment* is by benzyl benzoate emulsion and it is important that all members of the household be treated, and that personal and bedclothing be washed and ironed when therapy is completed.

Lice may affect the scalp (pediculosis capitis), the body (pediculosis corporis) and the pubic hair (pediculosis pubis). With a magnifying glass scalp and pubic lice can be seen clinging to the hairs. Their eggs are visible as white specks ('nits') firmly attached to the lower hair shaft. Body lice characteristically inhabit the seams of clothing, which should be examined to make the diagnosis.

Flea-bites, appearing as itchy papules affecting the lower legs of children and adults are by no means uncommon. Pet cats and dogs carry the fleas and transmit them to humans.

Effective treatment for both lice and fleas is DDT powder or gamma-benzene hexachloride cream (Lorexane). Nits are removed with a fine tooth-comb. Other members of the household may have to be examined as possible sources of the trouble and appropriate disinfestation measures carried out.

SKIN TUMOURS

Of the very many tumours which affect the skin the **malignant melanoma** is the most dangerous. It begins as a spreading black spot and ulceration and bleeding may occur. Metastasis to lymph nodes is common and a fatal outcome is to be expected without prompt surgical treatment.

The basal-cell carcinoma is a slowly growing pearly tumour found on the light exposed areas of the face. Ulceration is common and at this stage it is often called a 'rodent ulcer' (see Fig. 31/10). When small it is easily removed surgically or by X-ray therapy and recurrence is very unusual.

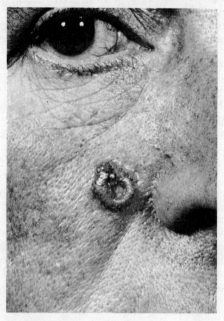

Fig. 31/10 Basal cell carcinoma of cheek ('rodent ulcer').

The **squamous-cell carcinoma** grows fast and is a dangerous tumour. The lower lip and the tip of the ear are common sites. Radiotherapy gives good results.

The above are malignant tumours. Benign tumours of various types occur more frequently and are harmless.

OTHER COMMON SKIN CONDITIONS
(Drug eruptions, Urticaria, Acne vulgaris)

Drug eruptions. Almost any drug can occasionally give rise to a skin rash which may be urticarial, erythematous, purpuric, eczematous or bullous. They are usually widespread and symmetrical but sometimes only a small skin area is affected. Pruritus is marked. Drugs which frequently cause skin eruptions are penicillin (see Fig. 31/11), especially ampicillin, and the sulphonamides.

Urticaria (nettle-rash) is diagnosed when itchy pale weals appear in crops all over the skin. *In the acute form*, which lasts a day or two, the attack may be the result of a food allergy (e.g. shellfish, strawberries, nuts) or a drug. *In chronic urticaria* attacks occur at frequent intervals over the course of months or years; in the majority of these patients no cause is ever found. Oral antihistamine drugs are the standard treatment.

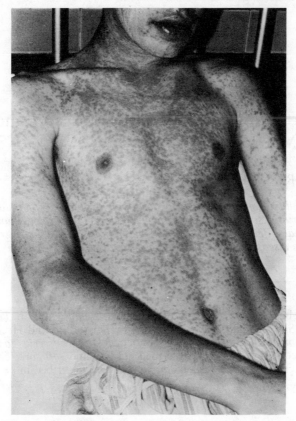

Fig. 31/11 Penicillin drug eruption.

Acne vulgaris is a disorder of sebaceous glands and hair follicles. The condition starts after puberty and affects young adults. The lesions are comedones (blackheads), red papules, pustules, nodules, cysts and scars, and the diagnosis is usually obvious by inspection. The tendency to acne subsides after a variable number of years, but since lesions often cause severe psychological stress and they leave scars, it is important that treatment is given.

Although conventional pathogenic bacteria are not found in acne lesions, antibacterial agents are of value in treatment. Excess greasiness in affected areas is washed away using an antiseptic soap (e.g. Cidal) or an antiseptic lotion (e.g. Phisohex). Topical agents which are antiseptic and which dry the skin and induce peeling are helpful: an example is Resorcinol and Sulphur Paste B.P.C. Ultraviolet light helps many cases. There is no evidence that diet influences acne for better or for worse. A medicated shampoo is used if there is associated dandruff.

For severe acne or that which responds poorly to topical therapy oral tetracycline is used in a dose of 250 mg taken once or twice daily.

Chapter 32

A Short Outline of Venereal Diseases and Their Management

by AMBROSE KING

> *Syphilis—gonorrhoea—gonococcal vulvo-vaginitis—ophthalmia neo-*
> *natorum—soft sore—lymphogranuloma venereum—non-specific*
> *genital infection—trichomonal vaginitis—other sexually communi-*
> *cable diseases—the spread of venereal disease—prevention*

The three best known venereal diseases are: *syphilis*, due to *Treponema pallidum* (*Spirochaeta pallida*) described by Schaudinn and Hoffmann in 1905; *gonorrhoea*, caused by the gonococcus or *Neisseria gonorrhoeae* (the diplococcus of Neisser), described in 1879; and *soft sore* (chancroid) due to Ducrey's bacillus (*Haemophilus ducreyi*), described in 1884.

SYPHILIS

Syphilis is a disease which runs a definite course, passing through several phases or stages. The *incubation period* is from 2 to 6 weeks with extreme limits of from 10 days to 3 months.

Infection is conveyed by sexual intercourse; in a few cases it may be conveyed by other close contact, such as kissing. In these instances the lips and mouth or any parts of the skin or mucous membrane are the sites of infection. It may also be contracted on rare occasions by doctors, dentists, nurses and midwives handling patients.

Syphilis may be *prenatal* (congenital) or *acquired. The first clinical sign of acquired syphilis* is usually the occurrence of a *syphilitic chancre* or sore at the site of inoculation—in men on the penis and in women on some part of the genital area. The lesion is described as *extragenital* when it appears elsewhere, as for example on lip or finger or in the ano-rectal region.

Treponema pallidum enters the body at the site of inoculation. It causes a local reaction which results in the appearance of the primary lesion (syphilitic chancre) and in most cases of some enlargement of the neighbouring lymphatic nodes. But the organism of syphilis not only invades the tissues, it also invades the bloodstream so that a general as well as a local infection is established from the outset.

Classification. For practical purposes syphilis can be divided into two stages—*early syphilis* which is infectious and transmissible, and constitutes a major public-health problem; and *late syphilis* which is not infectious but can be very destructive to tissue and may be dangerous to the patient's life and health.

Early syphilis may be found in primary or secondary stages or it may be hidden (early latent syphilis).

The *primary stage* is characterized by the initial reaction and appearance of the hard or syphilitic chancre usually 2 or 3 weeks after infection. Blood tests for syphilis become positive a week or 10 days after the appearance of the syphilitic chancre in most cases. In a few cases the tests take longer to become positive and in rare cases there is considerable delay.

The *secondary stage* commences 6 to 8 weeks after the appearance of the syphilitic chancre but it may be delayed. A rash may appear on the trunk and limbs, face, palms and soles and in the anal, perineal and genital regions. It may be pinkish or dull red and macular or papular—that is the spots may be within the skin or may project above it. The rash does not itch. When on the anal and genital regions it may take the appearance of large moist papules which slough on the surfaces and ooze serum—*condylomata lata. All nurses should be warned that erosions, sores, or wart-like growths over the genitalia or round the anus should not be touched; the matter should be reported to the head nurse or ward sister without mentioning the fact to the patient.* These lesions may be teeming with the organisms of syphilis and a source of infection by contact. The voice may be hoarse and there may be patchy loss of scalp hair.

The *constitutional symptoms* may be slight, mild or severe. In the majority they are mild and include headache, malaise, aching pains in the bones and muscles and a rise of temperature at night.

Mucous patches appear in the throat but give little or no pain. When some of these patches fuse and the surface slough separates, a serpentine erosion with shining floor is left; this is sometimes called 'a snail track ulcer'. Hoarseness of voice results from the presence of mucous patches in the larynx.

Late syphilis may be manifest or latent (hidden). The disease is said to be in the *tertiary stage*. The secondary stage merges into the tertiary, and lesions common to both may be seen occasionally at the end of the secondary and the beginning of the tertiary stage. More commonly, however, a variable period of latency, lasting months or years, intervenes between the secondary and tertiary stages. The division between *early latent* and *late latent syphilis* is usually fixed arbitrarily at the end of the second year after infection.

The manifestations of the tertiary stage are divided into:

(*a*) Those affecting the *covering and supporting structures of the body.* The characteristic lesion is called a 'gumma'. It may affect the skin, appearing as a nodule or group of nodules or as raised patches with scaling surface and rounded outline, usually confined to one part of the body. More commonly the gumma commences as a painless swelling in the *subcutaneous tissue* and breaks down to form a chronic ulcer or ulcers. This is most common on the lower legs and may be confused with varicose ulcers. Gummatous swellings also form in submucous tissue and ulcerate on *mucous membranes*. The ulcers may be very destructive and cause perforation of the palate or nasal septum and, on healing, much scarring and deformity. Destructive gummatous ulceration may involve the larynx. Diffuse gummatous inflammation of the tongue may cause *chronic glossitis* which is potentially a pre-cancerous condition.

Lesions of bone may be formative, or destructive with thickening and swelling of the long bones due to *periostitis*, and, in the flat bones such as those of the skull where destruction outpaces new bone formation, areas of erosion and perforation. In neglected cases involving the skull the condition has been called the '*worm-eaten skull*'. Inflammation of joints may cause gummatous arthritis but this is rare.

(*b*) Those involving the *viscera*. The commonest site is the first part of the thoracic aorta, giving the condition known as *syphilitic aortitis*. This is a very slow process proceeding over many years and the effects of it are seldom seen until 10 to 30 years after infection. Weakening of the wall of the aorta may cause insufficiency of the aortic valve, *aortic incompetence*, localized or generalized bulging of the aorta, *aortic aneurysm*, or narrowing of the openings of the coronary arteries, *coronary ostial stenosis*, with consequent damage to the heart which these arteries supply. Of the other viscera, the liver is the commonest organ to be involved with, sometimes, widespread gummatous destruction and much scarring on healing.

(*c*) Those involving *the nervous system*. (Neurosyphilis, see p. 266.) *Syphilitic meningitis* may occur. *Thrombosis* of cerebral or spinal arteries may follow syphilitic inflammation of the lining membranes (*endarteritis*). *Tabes dorsalis* (locomotor ataxia) may result from involvement of the spinal cord, and *general paralysis of the insane* (G.P.I.) from involvement of the brain, or a combination of these—*taboparesis*.

Congenital or pre-natal syphilis has decreased considerably in recent years owing to the early recognition and treatment of syphilis in adults and the practice of testing for syphilis the blood of all pregnant women, giving treatment if necessary.

When adequate treatment is given in the early months of pregnancy, infection of the fetus is almost certain to be prevented by penicillin given to the mother. When treatment is not given until later the infant may already be infected but may be cured through treatment of the mother.

In untreated cases the infant may be born with characteristic signs of syphilis or may develop them later. The signs are as follows:

Early signs include rashes, *snuffles* due to inflammation of the mucous lining of the nasal cavity, mucous patches in the mouth or on the genital organs, enlargement of the liver and spleen, inflammation of the long bones, particularly the growing ends (*osteochondritis*) and inflammation of the deep structures of the eyes (*choroido-retinitis*). These changes are likely to occur during the first two years of life.

Late signs, occurring from the beginning of the third year onwards, include *gummas* of the skin, mucous membranes and bones. Inflammation of the cornea of the eye, *interstitial keratitis*, is common and so is progressive deafness due to affection of the eighth or auditory nerves.

The stigmata. These are scars and disfigurements resulting from healed lesions, including corneal scars due to interstitial keratitis, depression or *'saddle shape'* of the bridge of the nose due to early inflammation of the bones of the nasal cavity, *Hutchinson's incisor teeth* which are peg-shaped and sometimes notched, prominence of the forehead, *frontal bossing*, characteristic scars at the mouth angles, so called *rhagades. Deafness* due to involvement of both auditory nerves may be absolute.

Latent syphilis. It is characteristic of syphilis in all its stages that the symptoms and signs of the disease may disappear with or without treatment and the condition can only be diagnosed by testing the patient's blood. Apart from the incubation period the disease may become latent during the early stages of infection but may continue to be infectious on sexual contact for one or even two years.

In the late stage it is the commonest form of the disease. Latency may at any time be followed by the development of late severe effects because the fact that the disease is hidden does not mean that it is inactive. On the other hand latency may continue for 30 or 40 years or even to the end of life.

Diagnostic tests for syphilis. Serum from the syphilitic chancre or from the open lesions of secondary syphilis usually contains the causative organism, *Treponema pallidum*, which may be seen as a delicate white spiral with characteristic movements, with high powers of the microscope using dark-ground illumination.

The original blood test for syphilis was the *Wassermann Reaction* (1906). An improved version of this is still used but many other blood tests are available. One of the most useful and most generally used is a precipitation test called the *V.D.R.L. (Venereal Disease Research Laboratory) test.* The ordinary blood tests for syphilis, including the Wassermann reaction and the V.D.R.L. test, are not specific for syphilis and may be positive due to other causes. In any case of doubt they must be confirmed by highly specific tests such as the *treponemal immobilization test,* the *fluorescent treponemal antibody test*, the *treponemal haemagglutination test* and the *Reiter protein complement fixation test.*

The treatment of syphilis

Treatment must be adequate and effective. The patient should be told the nature of the disease and the co-operation expected from him. The importance of regular attendance at a special clinic or surgery should be stressed. He should be informed that the history of his case and his record will be treated confidentially.

The *drugs* which have been employed in the past include preparations of arsenic, bismuth, mercury, and iodine.

Penicillin is the drug of choice and seems to have lost none of its effectiveness in the treatment of this disease. Low levels of the drug in the blood are fully effective but must be maintained continuously throughout the period of treatment which, for early syphilis, commonly lasts for about 10 days. Long-acting preparations are ideal for this purpose. 600,000 units of procaine penicillin in watery suspension injected intramuscularly gives adequate dosage for 24 hours and an effective method is to give one of these injections daily for 10 days. The same dose of procaine penicillin in oily suspension to which is added 2 per cent of aluminium monostearate (*PAM*) will prolong the effect for up to 72 hours and injections may then be given every 2 or 3 days. Even so, it is usual to give 10 injections.

In the cases of seamen and others unable to attend regularly, single large doses of benzathine penicillin, 2,400,000 units, may be given and will provide effective levels of the drug in the patient's blood for 2 weeks. Unfortunately, these injections are apt to cause pain.

Experience indicates that any of these methods of treatment will cure early syphilis in more than 95 per cent of cases. There are, however, occasional failures and it is essential that these patients should be under medical observation for 2 years after treatment. During this time patients are examined and their blood tested at intervals. The cerebrospinal fluid is also tested a year or more after treatment. Penicillin is also used for the late stages of syphilis, but usually for longer periods, the treatment being adapted to the individual case. With successful treatment of early syphilis the blood test becomes progressively less strongly positive and then negative. This is not necessarily so with late syphilis, and blood tests may remain positive for the rest of life in spite of successful treatment.

GONORRHOEA

Gonorrhoea is a highly communicable disease, due to the gonococcus which was discovered by Neisser in 1879. For this reason the disease is sometimes called 'Neisserian infection'. It is characterized by inflammation at the sites of infection, and frequently discharge of pus from the affected mucous surfaces. The incubation period is from 2 to 10 days.

Infection is nearly always transmitted in sexual intercourse. However, the conjunctivae are very susceptible to infection and the eyes of an infant may be infected when passing through the birth canal if the mother is infected at the time of delivery, *ophthalmia neonatorum*. Accidental infection of older children, particularly girls, also occurs occasionally.

Symptoms. In many early cases **in women** there are no symptoms or the symptoms are so slight that they are disregarded or attributed to some minor condition. In some cases there is copious vaginal discharge and inflammation of the vulva and thighs but this is nearly always due to an associated infection with the vaginal parasite, *Trichomonas vaginalis*. The sites of infection in uncomplicated cases are the urethra, the cervix uteri and sometimes the anal canal and rectum. Urethritis may give rise to some degree of discomfort or pain on passing urine. Possible *local complications* are inflammation of para-urethral ducts (*Skene's tubules*) or one or both *glands of Bartholin*, giving rise to a painful abscess at the vulval opening; but the main danger in undiagnosed and untreated cases is upward extension of infection giving rise to acute salpingitis, inflammation of the *Fallopian tubes*, with consequent acute illness due to pelvic peritonitis and the considerable possibility of subsequent sterility and perhaps recurring symptoms with chronic ill-health.

In men the disease presents with variable discomfort or pain on micturition and discharge from the urethra of yellow or greenish-yellow pus which is usually copious. *Local complications* may include infection of glands communicating with the urethra, such as the *prostate gland* and the *seminal vesicles* or extension by way of the *vas deferens* to the organ behind the testicle, the *epididymis*. Epididymitis on both sides may result in sterility. However, complications in men are now quite uncommon because the disease is usually evident at once and treatment is sought without delay owing to good propaganda.

General complications are now rare in both sexes because of the efficacy of modern treatment. They result from gonococcal septicaemia and include inflammation of joints (gonorrhoeal arthritis), pericarditis, myocarditis and endocarditis. There may be an associated purpuric rash of the skin.

Diagnosis. Diagnosis must be confirmed by identifying the gonococcus by microscopical examination of pus taken from sites of infection and by growing the organism in culture medium. Testing for specific antibodies in the blood by the gonococcal complement fixation test is of very little value in diagnosis.

Treatment. Penicillin remains the remedy of choice in cases of gonorrhoea but there is evidence that some strains of the organism have developed resistance to this drug so that larger doses are required to cure or the treatment may fail to cure. Common practice is giving long-acting penicillin, usually procaine penicillin in watery suspension, and a single dose given intramuscularly of 2 to 4 million units is still effective in most cases. Various preparations of penicillin given by mouth are also effective unless the organism is resistant. Other effective drugs are tetracycline and oxytetracycline by mouth and kanamycin and cephaloridine by injection. Good results have also been obtained with tablets by mouth containing a sulphonamide, sulphamethoxazole, and trimethoprim (Septrin: Bactrim). There is recent evidence that the tetracyclines may be less effective than formerly.

Tests for cure. Careful observation and tests after treatment are essential. Relief of symptoms does not necessarily mean cure, especially when the organisms are resistant. Patients may be examined and tested with microscopical and cultural tests, 2 or 3 days after treatment, then at weekly intervals for 1 month and then at monthly intervals for 2 months. With women a particularly good time for applying tests is shortly after the end of a menstrual period. The urethral and cervical secretions in women and the prostato-vesicular fluid in men should be examined.

Blood tests for syphilis should be done before treatment and at the end of the period of observation. The two diseases sometimes occur in the same patient and syphilis may be latent from the first.

Gonorrhoeal vulvo-vaginitis in children. Little girls may be directly infected by indecent assault, or indirectly by the use of contaminated towels or thermometers or by sharing a bed with an infected person.

Ophthalmia neonatorum. Inflammation of the eyes of the newly born is frequently though not always due to gonorrhoeal infection. It is treated by instilling penicillin solution, containing 10,000 units per ml, at very frequent intervals until cure is effected.

SOFT SORE OR CHANCROID

Soft sore is acquired by sexual contact. Ducrey's bacillus, *Haemophilus ducreyi*, is the causative organism. The incubation period is 3 to 5 days.

The disease presents as multiple, painful, localized ulcers on the genital organs, associated with tissue destruction and sloughing. The lymphatic nodes of the groin may become involved, resulting in the formation of abscesses which break down and ulcerate.

Treatment. Sulphonamides by mouth are effective; 2 to 4 g may be given at once and then 1 g every 4 hours until healing is well advanced or complete, which may take from 10 to 14 days. Streptomycin by injection and tetracycline and oxytetracycline by mouth are also effective.

LYMPHOGRANULOMA VENEREUM (L.G.V.)

Lymphogranuloma venereum, like chancroid, is uncommon in temperate climates but very common in tropical countries. It is due to an organism which is one of a group called *Chlamydia*, the members of which are intermediate in size and behaviour between viruses and bacteria. *The incubation period* is variable but usually less than a week. The disease presents as a small inconspicuous blister or ulcer in the genital organs and from there the infection may spread to lymphatic nodes in the groin and form abscesses which ulcerate. The patient may have a swinging temperature and be thoroughly ill for weeks and months if untreated. Late effects include stricture of the rectum, perianal and perirectal abscesses and lymphatic obstruction giving rise to gross swelling or 'elephantiasis' of genital organs or lower legs.

The *diagnosis* may be confirmed by finding the organism in pus from unruptured abscesses, by an intradermal test employing the killed organism, the so-called *Frei test*, and by a serological test, the *complement fixation test for L.G.V.*

Treatment. In early cases good results may follow the use of a sulphonamide, giving 5 g daily by mouth in divided doses, for 5 to 7 days. In later stages drugs of the tetracycline group may be more effective but treatment of all kinds is sometimes disappointing and the main effect of the antibiotics may be on secondary infection.

'NON-SPECIFIC' GENITAL INFECTION

This is a very common condition, perhaps as common as gonorrhoea and very like it in many respects. The cause of it is unknown, which accounts for the rather unsatisfactory name, but there is strong evidence that it is transmitted by sexual contact. The *incubation period* varies but is probably 10 to 14 days in most cases. *In men* it presents as urethritis with variable discomfort on micturition and urethral discharge which is usually a mixture of pus and mucus. No specific organisms can be found microscopically or on culture.

In women it causes cervicitis and urethritis and more often than not there are no symptoms in the early stages. Salpingitis is quite common and in both sexes there may be other severe complications such as *arthritis, conjunctivitis* and inflammation of the iris of the eye, *iritis*, a combination often called *Reiter's disease*.

Treatment. The disease responds only fairly well to broad-spectrum antibiotics such as tetracycline. Dosage may be from 250 to 500 mg by mouth every 6 hours for 1 to 3 weeks. Latent infection and relapse are common and many promiscuous people are harbouring this disease in infectious form.

TRICHOMONAL VAGINITIS

This is a common condition in women due to the vaginal parasite, *Trichomonas vaginalis.* Although not usually known as venereal disease it is certainly sexually communicable and often gives rise to no symptoms in men. In women it causes acute vaginitis with copious vaginal discharge of pus and often vulvitis and soreness of thighs. The organism is usually easy to find microscopically and also by culture.

Treatment. The condition responds quickly and well to tablets of metronidazole (Flagyl) by mouth, 200 mg three times daily for 7 days. As with the other sexually communicable diseases it is useless to treat one sexual partner and not the other.

OTHER SEXUALLY COMMUNICABLE DISEASES

These include *herpes genitalis*, an infection due to a virus closely allied to the cause of 'cold sores' which occur on the lips of many people. The genital form of this infection may be very painful and persistent and is subject to late relapse. Treatment is not very satisfactory.

Genital warts (Condylomata acuminata) are also caused by a virus and they tend to be recurrent. They are treated by applying strong chemical agents, such as solutions of podophyllin resin or trichloracetic acid. They tend to recur. If neglected they may form large 'cauliflower-like' masses and need to be removed with electro-cautery.

Molluscum contagiosum is a skin disease due to a virus which is mildly contagious and often affects the genitalia. It presents as a series of rounded small pinkish-grey swellings each with a depression or 'umbilicus' on the summit. Each lesion needs to be opened separately and the floor treated with strong antiseptic such as saturated solution of carbolic acid.

Candidiasis is a condition due to a fungus, *Candida albicans*, which causes vaginal thrush in women, resulting in vaginal discharge and vulval itching. It may cause balanitis and rarely urethritis in men. It is treated by the local application of an antifungal remedy, such as nystatin, but it is apt to recur.

THE SPREAD OF VENEREAL DISEASE

With the exception of 'non-specific' genital infection all the venereal diseases are due to known causes, and methods of treatment are effective. Nevertheless, there has been a world-wide increase in these diseases in recent years. The factor which is beyond medical control is, of course, human behaviour and various circumstances have determined a relaxation of standards of sexual behaviour for some years past. These include a decline in religious faith, and rejection of standards set by past generations. Other factors are increased movement of people by migration and for the purpose of holidays and business activities, easier divorce, modern methods of contraception which provide no barrier to infection and a general weakening of the strength and stability of family life. Greater independence of young people and, in particular, the removal of restrictions on girls and young women have also led to more sexual experiment and promiscuity.

THE PREVENTION OF VENEREAL DISEASE

From the individual point of view the obvious and only certain method of prevention is to avoid promiscuous intercourse. Those who are willing to have intercourse with a stranger or acquaintance on a casual meeting are likely to have had sexual experiences before and may be carrying disease. In the past reliance has often been placed upon the fact that men have worn rubber protectives or condoms, a method which has given some degree of protection. This method, of which the primary purpose was contraception, is now less used than formerly because so many women take the 'contraceptive pill' or are fitted with an intra-uterine contraceptive device. These give no protection against venereal disease.

From the public-health point of view the methods of prevention adopted in this country include the provision of special clinics throughout the country, staffed by experts who provide free diagnosis and treatment at convenient hours, the diligent tracing of 'contacts', that is those who have transmitted infection or to whom infection may have been transmitted, and education of the young in the dangers of promiscuity and the proper use of sexual function. It must be admitted that this last procedure is still in an early stage of development.

Chapter 33

Care of the Elderly

by JOHN MADDISON

Definitions—admission to hospital—observations—conditions met in the elderly—nutrition—hormone deficiency—incontinence—mental abnormalities—hypothermia—rehabilitation—prevention of accidents

---

Geriatrics is the medical care of the elderly.

Gerontology is the scientific study of ageing, including research into its causes.

Senility implies failure of body or mind in old age, and is a term best avoided.

Senescence is the natural process of growing old.

It is essential always to recognize that elderly people have dignity, self-respect and a spiritual value which must be respected. They are often far more sensitive to the atmosphere and attitudes of those around them than young people. In strange surroundings they may experience fear, anxiety and shyness. The feeling of dependence on others may render them inarticulate, afraid to express their wishes or feelings lest they be regarded as a nuisance. They respond more slowly and need to be given time to express themselves; memory for words is often impaired so they stumble in speech and repeat themselves. However, wisdom and judgement can more than offset the loss of memory and mental dexterity.

Elderly people should always be addressed properly with the correct prefix and the surname just as politeness requires everywhere; this regard for personal dignity is part of the treatment. Any discussion of serious aspects of the patient's illness should be avoided in front of him; words like cancer, growth, stroke, rheumatoid arthritis can have a sinister meaning.

ADMISSION TO HOSPITAL

There are dangers in admitting an elderly person to hospital: he may get a chest or bowel infection or be frequently disturbed by investigations and drugs. Moreover, the illness of an older person may quickly lead to rapid deterioration. It should not therefore be surprising when an elderly person is sometimes admitted who may be unkempt, neglected, confused and emaciated.

On admission *the history will be taken* as indicated in Chapter 2. In addition the physician will inquire about the patient's mode of life, habits, consumption of tobacco, alcohol and other factors which might lead to deterioration.

Maintenance of independence

The management of the health and sickness of older people should aim constantly at preserving the function of all faculties. *The preservation of the mental functions is of fundamental importance* for if these deteriorate the effect can be disastrous; therefore intellectual pursuits—work, study, reading, classes, conversation and hobbies—are essential. The constant attitude must be to encourage the patient to get back to full restitution of all his functions as quickly and as completely as possible in planned rehabilitation (see p. 343).

An elderly sick person is not necessarily best nursed in hospital; home often affords a better climate for recovery for him, where he can be more independent and more easily have certain minor defects corrected, especially of the feet, eyes, ears and teeth. Team work is essential and should aim at:

Preventing bedfastness.
Restoring mobility.
Preventing incontinence.
Developing a forward perspective towards full recovery.

Hospital nurses should work closely with doctors, social workers, physiotherapists, occupational therapists, chiropodists, health visitors, home nurses and the patient's own doctor. They should also co-operate with the voluntary helpers, the Red Cross and St John Ambulance Association, women's voluntary services and mobile library shop. The nurse should also aim at reducing the length of stay of patients in hospital and maintain links with the outside services—the staffs of the community physicians and welfare officers, the Department of Health and Social Security, Citizens' Advice Bureaux and the Old People's Welfare Association—in preparation for his discharge from hospital.

CLASSIFICATION OF CONDITIONS MET IN THE ELDERLY

A practical classification of the medical and nursing aims for older people can be summarized thus:

Healthy old people, especially husband and wife living together who support each other in all sorts of ways. Many seek no medical help at all; some need an occasional visit to a doctor, perhaps for a routine prescription. All of them should be seen for periodical screening examinations and they may need occasional attention in the home by a doctor or nurse for some temporary illness. Most people are fit and well to age 70 and beyond, but there are wide variations.

A proportion develop remediable states of ill-health such as malnutrition with anaemia and vitamin deficiency, hormone deficiency, obesity, arthritis and arterial disease and depression. They can be helped to lead independent lives by doctors and nurses, health visitors, home helps, a friendly visitor, laundry service, supervision, education, encouragement, a meal, clubs, classes, a day centre, occupational therapy, or remedial exercises.

Where a person is unable to climb stairs or needs fittings or adaptations to be able to live at home, the local authority can provide a ground-floor flat and make alterations and adaptations to suit particular needs. Ninety-five per cent of older people live at home.

When owing to frailty, *especially past age 80*, and where the person has become unable to look after himself properly at home, the local authority can provide a part III home (under part III of the National Assistance Act, 1946). These homes provide for the care by trained staff of frail elderly people who can dress themselves and be up and about and need very little personal attention. A special type of home is needed for frail people who are mentally confused; very few homes like this exist.

The tension created in a house by the presence of a partially demented old person, querulous, upsetting everyone, wandering around day and night and getting lost, can become intolerable and wreck the lives of relatives.

When frailty and disability are more severe, skilled attention and nursing care in a long-stay unit of a geriatric hospital or nursing home is needed. Devoted relatives will often undertake the nursing of a bedridden elderly relative at great self-sacrifice. They can be helped by short-term admissions to hospital alternating with periods at home, thus giving the relatives a temporary relief from strain.

Older people acutely ill or needing special investigation require admission either to the acute wards or the geriatric units of a general hospital.

Bedfastness is a grave danger in the elderly. A period in bed because of some acute illness may be essential, but prolonged bedfastness renders an elderly person very vulnerable as the bodily functions can rapidly deteriorate and some quite serious complications may arise.

Muscles lose strength, becoming weak and flabby.
Bones get thin and may break.
Joints stiffen and contractures occur.
Footdrop may result.
Control of bladder and bowel weakens and may fail.
Constipation with faecal impaction may result.
The desire to eat diminishes.
Pressure sores may occur.
Hypostatic pneumonia due to immobility may result.
Venous thrombosis and embolism, due to stagnation in the veins may occur.
The heart becomes weaker in the presence of heart disease.
A slipped intervertebral disc may occur.

Bodily functions lost during enforced bed rest are difficult to restore and patients must be safeguarded from deterioration due to inactivity (see note on rehabilitation, p. 343).

The care of paralysed or partially paralysed patients has been dealt with and also the care of the hemiplegic in Chapter 14, p. 135. It is sufficient to say here that a nurse when caring for any paralysed patient should move all the joints affected through their full range of movement at least twice a day.

Lessened vitality. Ageing people are less able to stand the stresses of life; minor upsets can produce serious consequences: a cold, indigestion or an emotional upset may produce a more serious illness and need longer time for recovery than in youth or middle life. Sudden changes of environment can produce confusion and incontinence. Variations in blood pressure can have serious effects from alterations in the blood supply to vital organs because of thickened and unhealthy arteries.

The diseases of old age are almost always multiple. In addition to the actual illness calling for urgent attention there is usually present also the *multiple deficiency syndrome*—malnutrition, anaemia, androgen or oestrogen deficiency, thyroid deficiency, arterial disease affecting heart, brain, kidneys, limbs, hypertension, defective teeth, vision, hearing, wax in ears, foot defects, arthritis and general weakness. There may be obesity, diabetes and infections of the urinary tract or lungs. The provision of correct glasses, a hearing aid, chiropody, can make all the difference between misery and happiness.

NUTRITION AND THE ELDERLY

For various reasons *the consumption of calories in food diminishes as age advances.* The body bulk becomes less—in both stature and cell mass—in muscle, bone, interstitial tissue, and internal organs. The basal metabolic rate also falls (possibly because of diminished activity of the endocrine organs). All these factors contribute to the reduced consumption of food.

Most men and women living alone seem to realize the importance of an adequate, well-balanced diet. The pages on understanding nutrition in Chapter 16 could now be read with advantage. Elderly people should have at least two protein-rich meals a day with about two ounces of meat, fish or cheese or an egg at each meal. The cheaper cuts of meat and offal, e.g. liver, are just as rich in protein as the expensive ones, but meat needs proper cooking and elderly people need well-fitting dentures if it is to be masticated properly. Cheap fish is just as nutritious as expensive cuts. Herrings, kippers and sardines are oily fish; they contain fat, vitamin D and plenty of protein and are very palatable.

Defects of nutrition can be responsible for many abnormalities such as the vitamin deficiency diseases: anaemia, diverticulitis of the colon, and, as we believe, artery disease. Vitamin C deficiency is common, leading specially to anaemia; the consumption of white bread leads to deficiency diseases due to lack of the wheat germ and bran removed in the milling. Constipation and diverticulitis of the colon and even depression can come from lack of the bulk-forming foods in the colon and deficiency of the B group of vitamins. There is much evidence to show that deficiency of unsaturated fatty acids such as corn oil or sunflower oil, and the heavy consumption of animal fats—butter, cream, beef fat, mutton fat and pork fat—all lead to artery disease. Overeating leads to obesity with serious consequences.

So the diet of everyone, and especially old people, should contain the prevention foods and we should abstain from eating dangerous foods. A preventive type of breakfast could be made up of some Weetabix, All-bran, Bemax, corn oil, dried separated milk, saccharin and hot water. This will make up a palatable porridge and would provide the roughage, unsaturated fat and vitamin B. A substitute for butter is Flora which contains a high proportion of unsaturated fat. Separated milk is better than full-cream cows' milk; a pint a day or the equivalent of dried milk provides essential calcium, especially if combined with cottage cheese which contains little animal fats. The lean cuts of meat are better than the fatty ones. An apple or an orange every day will provide vitamin C. A multi-vitamin tablet like Plurivite each day is a good safeguard against deficiency and a calcium and vitamin D tablet daily will help to protect against osteomalacia.

With improvements in pensions and supplementary allowances, provided people are aware of these benefits and see they get them, the malnutrition seen in former years has disappeared. There remains, however, certain groups who spend unwisely and those who turn to alcohol (which is expensive) for comfort. Others, due to apathy, frailty, confusion leading to forgetfulness and loneliness due to the loss of a marriage partner, eat less as their activity decreases and so their nutrition suffers.

Others again who have lived well-managed lives for years may meet with accident or illness which renders them vulnerable to deterioration. Nurses should be on the look-out for this type of cause and be ready to provide not only nursing but the ancillary aids available for shopping, cooking, cleaning, etc. For an elderly sick person the nurse must see that he gets the food and nutrients he needs in an attractive and appetizing form and that he eats it. She may have to help feed him but as soon as possible he should feed himself. Similarly old people with mental disability, confusion and depression often need help with their food.

Complete social breakdown may occur when the adverse factors are very severe. An elderly person may be found sitting in a chair semi-demented, very frail and undernourished, not having been to bed for days or weeks, without heating; the house may be filthy and he or she doubly incontinent. The outlook for such people is extremely grave.

DEFICIENCY OF OESTROGEN AND ANDROGEN

Consumption of good diets by older people is the rule, but good nutrition does not depend on food alone. Older men and women tend to have deficiency of androgens or oestrogens. The loss of these hormones leads to a deficiency in the absorption of protein into the tissues. The hormones have a trophic or protective effect; they help to maintain the healthiness of tissues and protect them from the degenerative changes of later life. They increase the muscle substance throughout the body and hence increase muscle strength. They have a protective effect on bones and prevent osteoporosis; this is a slow absorption of the calcium particles of bone into the bloodstream and their excretion in the urine; the protein matrix of the bone is also absorbed and metabolized as food. The bodies of the vertebrae become wedge-shaped, the spine becomes bent and the whole skeleton shrinks; thus we get the feeble little old man or woman. The process goes on for perhaps twenty or more years. The physician will be alert to these needs and will prescribe substituted hormones—androgens for men and oestrogens or anabolic steroids for women.

Obesity is due to a defect in the appetite-controlling centre in the midbrain. This subject has been dealt with in Chapter 16, Understanding Nutrition, and the dietetic treatment is outlined in Chapter 17.

As a rule elderly people should avoid increase in weight beyond what is average for their age and height. Reliable weight tables are available in many diaries and yearly calendars.

Deficiency of thyroid hormone. There is no place in the treatment of the elderly for the use of hormones as 'tonic' substances. The constant endeavour to relate the cause of ageing to hormone deficiency has failed. But where there is genuine hormone deficiency, clinically determined, then the correction of the deficiency can be very helpful.

Deficiency of thyroid hormone produced by the thyroid gland in the neck causes a slowing of all the body processes (see p. 292 for symptoms of myxoedema).

INCONTINENCE OF URINE
(see Chapter 25)

Loss of bladder control may occasionally happen to anyone after drinking a lot of fluid and where a toilet is not immediately available; this is specially so in later life. *Urgency and frequency* occur with infection or disability anywhere in the urinary tract. A mid-stream specimen (see p. 64) will be collected and examined for infection. Incontinence can occur from obstruction of the bladder causing retention of urine with overflow; in men usually from enlargement of the prostate, stone or stricture (see p. 242); in women from pelvic tumour or hypertrophy of the tissues round the neck of the bladder; in both elderly men and women from massive faecal impaction.

INCONTINENCE OF FAECES

Faecal incontinence in the elderly is often caused by defective diet leading to defective emptying and overflow from a solidly impacted overloaded bowel, assisted by diminished power of the abdominal muscles and lower bowel, by faulty habit, and the use of the bedpan. The bowel is never emptied properly; the contents harden into a solid mass which acts like a valve in the rectum, increasing in size all the time and allowing a small amount of faeces to get by at irregular and uncontrolled times. The patient gets bowel discomfort, feels the need to go to the lavatory and may get retention of urine. Digital examination of the rectum reveals the state of affairs. The bowel is emptied by inserting Fletcher's arachis oil retention enema in the evening, followed the next morning by either one of the phosphate enemas or Micralax enema. At the same time the patient should have by mouth 1–2 5 mg tablets of Dulcolax at night, or 2–4 tablets of Senokot, or 2 20 mg tablets thrice daily of Dioctyl-Medo or 2 teaspoonfuls once or twice daily of Normacol granules. The enema may have to be repeated frequently and the oral medicaments continued for anything up to three weeks before a severe case can be considered back to normal. The patient should be got out of bed onto a commode or be taken to the lavatory, if need be in a Sani-chair. He should take a book or newspaper and not be hurried. The nurse should remember that restlessness in a patient may indicate a desire to empty the bowel.

A group of patients with senile dementia may have a behaviour disorder with extensive loss of memory and sometimes aggressive outbursts. They pass the stools anywhere—in the clothing, in the ward or dayroom, or on the W.C. floor. They need to be dealt with in a psychiatric ward.

PRESSURE SORES

A bedsore or pressure sore is caused by unrelieved pressure on a part of the body for long periods of time (see Chapter 4 for prevention and treatment).

TUBERCULOSIS

A practical point for the nurse is to remember that pulmonary tuberculosis can be present, often with few symptoms. When handling an elderly 'bronchitic' the nurse should be careful to avoid getting herself infected.

MENTAL ABNORMALITIES IN OLDER PEOPLE

Most people have varying degrees of memory failure as they get older. Some find it difficult to remember names of people and places; some have difficulty in remembering recent events although the memory for events long past remains good. Older people also tend to get set in their ways and less inclined to adapt to changes; they feel out of place in new surroundings. The nurse will come across cases of more severe mental abnormality; for convenience they are classified under the following headings, but the types merge into each other and the symptoms often overlap.

Confusion varies from quiet disorientation to wild and noisy delirium. It usually starts acutely, fluctuates as the day goes on and is often worst at night. The patient is in a state of nervous agitation, is unable to talk rationally and may have incontinence. In between periods of confusion there are usually periods of complete lucidity. The causes are: any acute infection, drug accumulation or oversensitivity, malnutrition with vitamin deficiency or anaemia, heart failure, cerebral thrombosis, embolism or haemorrhage. The treatment is to get the patient back to normal health.

Senile dementia begins gradually, there is loss of memory, disorientation, lack of interest, relations are not recognized, the patient may wander about and get lost, especially at night. Lucidity does not return in spite of good bodily activity. As far as possible these patients should be kept busy by day and have a minimum of sedation. The condition is incurable.

Arteriopathic dementia usually comes on in the early sixties with erratic and noisy behaviour, uncontrolled emotions, delusions and aggressiveness. It is caused by repeated strokes from artery disease and high blood pressure leading to intolerable frustration and breakdown from aphasia and paralysis. The patient needs treatment in the psychiatric ward.

Reactive depression is seen in a patient with severe anxiety, sitting in a miserable attitude, unable to do things for himself, withdrawn and apathetic. He may have also insomnia, headache, anorexia, constipation and dreadful fears. The patient needs investigation in hospital to determine the presence of physical illnesses and to remove him from the environment with such painful memories. Treatment is needed for malnutrition, constipation and the concurrent illness. Electroconvulsive therapy is of value and antidepressant drugs are useful.

Psychotic depression is usually constitutional or inherited and is part of a manic-depressive psychosis. The patient has feelings of unworthiness, sinfulness and hopelessness, usually worse in the morning. There is a strong tendency to suicide. These cases are best dealt with in a psychiatric ward.

There are also patients with abnormal behaviour from mental defect, head injury, cerebral tumour, epilepsy or neurosis in early life. They may be aggressive, awkward, negative and suffer intolerable unhappiness. They are best dealt with in a hospital or a special home.

Restlessness in an elderly patient can be a serious problem for the nurse. The patient may go on all day and night with restlessness, noisiness or confusion. He may cry out or scream, tear the bedclothes, get out of bed and wander about upsetting everybody. He may even wander outside in his nightclothes. The acute phase may last only two or three days with intervals of lucidity; transfer to a mental hospital may be needed but not if recovery seems likely fairly quickly.

Before sedation is given the cause must be ascertained. Common causes are nervousness from fear; in hospital, change of bed or ward; from discomfort—too hot, too cold, thirsty, wanting to go to the lavatory; retention of urine, constipation from acute febrile illness, diabetes, malnutrition, heart failure or stroke; or from previous over-sedation causing drowsiness and inactivity during the day. Certain drugs can also cause confusion. Other measures needed may be examination of the rectum, catheterization or saline purge for dehydration. Simple measures of sedation are 2 aspirins and a hot drink of some kind. Bromides and barbiturates should not be used. Safe remedies are 2 tablets or 1 ounce of syrup of Welldorm; hypnotics include Indorm, Oblivon, or Mogadon. For great restlessness an intramuscular injection of 5 or 10 ml paraldehyde from a glass syringe is useful. For pain an injection of morphine sulphate, 10 or 20 mg in 1 ml of water may be needed. A valuable sedative for pain and sleeplessness is 5 or 10 ml of a mixture of Largactil 140 ml and linctus diamorphine 80 ml.

HYPOTHERMIA

The body temperature is controlled by a centre in the base of the brain. In later life this centre can get out of order, allowing the body temperature to fall. If an old person falls on the bedroom floor and is unable to get back into bed his temperature can drop to a dangerous level during the night. The nurse should equip herself with *a low-reading thermometer* (see p. 28) registering as low as 25 °C (77 °F), as the temperature in these cases can be well below 35 °C (95 °F). If the temperature falls below 32 °C (90 °F) the patient is in serious danger, for the mortality is high. Common causes are hypopituitarism, hypothyroidism, stroke, head injury, brain tumour, coma, paraplegia, arthritis, confusion, coronary thrombosis, severe infection, and drugs such as chlorpromazine and long-continued digoxin, which has a poisonous effect.

Try to ascertain the cause and treat it if possible. Get the patient into a warm room—22 °C (72 °F)—and slowly raise his body temperature, taking over 24 hours. Any attempt to raise it more rapidly may result in sweating which would further lower his temperature. Severe cases need oxygen and intravenous fluid like 5 per cent glucose. If the blood pressure falls very low noradrenaline may be required. Intravenous hydrocortisone and perhaps tetracycline may be needed every 6 hours.

REHABILITATION
(see Chapter 68)

Rehabilitation in the elderly means the complete restoration of the person's faculties after damage or illness, or making the most of any disability, such as defective sight or hearing, deformed feet, reduced activity due to stroke or arthritis or weakness after any illness. It aims to bring the patient back to independence, self-care and full or partial employment. The muscles, joints and other organs quickly lose their function if they are not kept active; and lying still in bed during the day-time is a most dangerous procedure in old age. In the hospital the nurse and doctor will often be assisted by a physiotherapist, but if one is not available, the nurse will have to supervise the rehabilitation herself.

In any illness it is important to get the patient up and about as much as possible from the very beginning. He should be encouraged by praise for every effort and improvement he makes.

The nurse should try to relieve his mind of worries about conditions at home and if need be call in a social worker. As far as possible the patient should do things for himself—get up and walk about, go to the lavatory, dress himself, put his shoes on, feed himself, take his own tray to the kitchen, join in ward activities and help with other patients. He can help to exercise his own fingers, hands, arms, legs and feet, and keep them moving. The atmosphere in the ward should be bright, cheerful and forward looking and without excessive discipline. The patient should not be put near those who are depressed, mentally disturbed or decrepit.

Good personal appearance is important so that both men and women should look clean and tidy when fully dressed; women should be given their cosmetics and have their hair seen to by a hairdresser. They should be advised to remove facial superfluous hair. All should be made to feel important. The relatives and visitors can be given instruction on how to maintain morale. In long-stay hospitals the patients should choose their own clothing. There are special adaptations of clothing to meet particular disabilities which are helpful.

PREVENTION OF ACCIDENTS

Accident proneness in later life is increased by the failing strength, general weakness, unsteadiness, diminished sensory perception and failing sight and hearing. The house should be made as comfortable as possible and kept warm by some means of good insulation. Bedroom windows should be closed at night in winter. The toilet should be near the bedroom and the way to it clear of clutter. A small bulb or a wax night-light can be left burning all night. The toilet can have hand-grips. Awkward steps, uneven floorboards, loose mats, worn linoleum, trailing flexes and polished floors should all be made safe. A non-slip rubber mat inside the bath prevents slipping. The feet should be washed daily, dried and the toe clefts powdered. Regular visits to the chiropodist are a safeguard. Socks, stockings and shoes should be well fitting. It is best to avoid hot-water bottles and use instead a correctly installed and adjusted electric overblanket.

Section 5

Communicable Diseases— Treatment and Nursing Care

Chapter 34

Introduction

by A. B. CHRISTIE

Bacteria—how germs cause disease—reactions of the body—diagnosing infections

Human beings and germs live very similar lives. They both depend for their existence on using the cells of other living things. Man eats the flesh of animals and the leaves and roots of plants. He breaks up their cells in his digestive tract and extracts substances from them to build new cells in his own body. Germs do exactly the same. Some of them live on plants, some on animals, some live on man. Many of the germs that live on man do him no harm. They are able to get the nourishment they need from substances on the surface of his body, on his skin, for example, or on his mucous membranes: some can live comfortably in his intestines, causing no trouble and even doing some useful work there. There are, unfortunately, other germs which, in their search for food, interfere with the life of the cells of the human body and so cause illness. The illness may consist of a local reaction to the presence of a germ, such as a septic finger or a sore throat, or the germ may get into the bloodstream and sweep through the body, causing septicaemia. Some germs can survive only if they get inside human cells, and, once inside, they upset the life of the cell and eventually kill it. The struggle between man and his germs is really a form of bacterial warfare.

Bacteria. This word comes from a Greek word meaning a staff or a rod and should refer only to rod-shaped germs. But it is nearly always used to mean any germs other than viruses.

Bacillus. This word, too, is often used to mean any germ, but it should be used only for rod-shaped germs, e.g. *Bacillus anthracis*, or the anthrax bacillus.

Coccus. This comes from a Greek word meaning a berry. Cocci are round germs like dots, e.g. streptococci, staphylococci, meningococci, gonococci. The word *strepto* means a chain, *staphylo* a bunch of grapes, while *meningo* means the brain covering, and *gono* refers to the genitals.

Virus. A virus is a very small germ; it cannot be seen under an ordinary microscope, whereas all the germs mentioned above can. The great difference between a virus and other germs is that a virus can multiply only *inside* a cell, whereas other germs can grow outside. In the laboratory, bacteria can be grown easily on various jellies which contain no living matter, but viruses can be grown only on living matter. Some are grown on developing hens' eggs, e.g. smallpox virus, others will grow only on animal or human cells kept alive in the laboratory: these collections of cells are called tissue cultures. They may be derived from the cells of rat kidney or human embryo lung and many other sources. Viruses can be made to grow in them and sometimes the viruses cause changes in the appearance of the cells, cytopathic or cell-damaging changes, which can be seen under a microscope. At other times their presence in the cells can be detected only by very sensitive tests.

Pathogenic. This word means 'causing disease', so a pathogenic germ is one which can cause disease in man. Many germs which live on man do not cause disease, many skin or bowel germs, for example: they are called non-pathogenic germs.

The mere presence of pathogenic germs on the body surface does not mean that disease will follow. Many people have streptococci, pneumococci or even meningococci on their throats without being ill at all. Such germs are called commensals: this words comes from *mensa*, a table, and commensals live together or share the same table. What makes commensals suddenly react with the body and cause disease is not exactly known: it may have something to do with changes in the virulence of the germ or in the resistance of the body.

How germs cause disease

Germs may react with the body in four main ways. They may cause local inflammation; they may spread over the lining cells of some body surface; they may produce a poison or toxin which enters the bloodstream; or they may themselves spread through the body.

Local inflammation. The germ irritates one part of the body and the body reacts locally. In a septic finger or boil there is a local tussle between the germ and the body's defences. White blood cells pour into the area to tackle the germs: the germs are destroyed and so are some of the white blood cells, and the resulting debris is called pus. Tonsillitis is a similar process; the attack takes place on the surface of the tonsils. There is often a general body reaction to these tussles, and the patient may feel ill, but the germs remain in the local area and do not get inside the body.

Surface cell inflammation. In this form of disease the germs get inside the cells of the surface linings of the body and spread from one cell to another, often destroying the cells as they spread. A typical example is the common cold in which viruses enter the cells of the nose and upper respiratory tract. Another is influenza where the influenza virus may spread through the lining cells of the greater part of the respiratory tract causing great distress.

Production of toxin. Some germs produce a poison or toxin which enters the bloodstream and causes damage to the internal organs. The germs of diphtheria, for example, do not themselves enter the bloodstream, but their toxin does and causes paralysis by poisoning the cells of the nervous system. The toxins of the germs of tetanus and botulism act in a similar manner. By contrast, the virus of poliomyelitis does not produce a toxin, but the virus itself gets into the bloodstream and enters the cells of the nervous system and destroys them.

Bloodstream invasion. The germ pierces the surface cells of the body and enters the bloodstream. It may multiply rapidly in the blood and be carried throughout the body. It may leak out of the bloodstream anywhere and cause disease in any organ, pneumonia or an abscess in the lung, for example, or meningitis, or an ulcer of the bowel as in typhoid fever. Viruses often spread in this way: the virus of rubella, for example, can spread through a pregnant woman's body, cross the placenta, enter the bloodstream of the fetus and cause serious damage to the developing organs of the infant.

None of these disease-forms is completely separate from the others. Germs may escape from a simple boil or tonsillitis and enter the bloodstream, and the virus of influenza, as well as causing a surface respiratory inflammation, usually enters the bloodstream, too, causing a viraemia.

How the body reacts

The body reacts to infection in three main ways: by a cellular response; a vascular response; and an antibody response.

Cellular response. The body pours out blood cells and fluids containing various substances to attack the germ. This is what happens in a boil or whitlow on the skin, but it also occurs inside the body in the form of abscesses of any organs—these are really internal boils. The same process may cause ulcers of the bowel as in typhoid fever and dysentery, or it may cause fluid and cells to accumulate in the air cells of the lungs as in pneumonia, or in the pleural spaces in pleurisy. Although these are defence mechanisms, they can seriously upset the body. The fluid in the air spaces in pneumonia prevents the passage of oxygen into the blood and so leads to cyanosis, and the ulcer in the intestinal wall may break down and cause severe haemorrhage or peritonitis; the fluid in pleurisy, though it is a reaction against a germ, can embarrass the patient by pressing on his lung and so interfering with respiration.

Vascular response. The blood vessels are often stimulated by germs or their toxins which cause them to swell or dilate. Such dilatation is the cause of the rashes seen in many infectious diseases. In some cases, the germ escapes from the blood into the rash, and causes destruction of the skin, as in smallpox and chickenpox. In others, the germ does not invade the skin but the toxin causes the rash, as in scarlet fever. A similar vascular response may occur inside the body: sometimes this is very severe as in meningococcal septicaemia where bleeding takes place in the adrenal glands and may cause the death of the patient.

Antibody response. Antibodies are substances formed in the body in response to a stimulus. The presence of a germ or its toxin acts as a stimulus and the body produces specific antibodies to the stimulus. By 'specific' is meant that the antibody reacts only with the stimulus that produced it: rubella antibody reacts only with rubella virus, streptococcal antitoxin only with the toxin of streptococci, typhoid antibody only with typhoid bacilli and so on. The body needs a little time to produce antibodies, so that the invading germ can multiply in the body for some time before it is attacked by antibodies. In rubella, for example, the virus multiplies in the body for over a week and then causes the rash to appear: but within a day or two of the rash, antibodies are poured into the bloodstream and the rash and symptoms of the disease then disappear. The outcome of a disease often depends on the struggle between the germs and the antibodies.

Diagnosing infections

A doctor diagnoses the presence of infection in two main ways: (1) by the symptoms in the patient, and (2) by tests to detect the germ. He learns to recognize certain features of the illness, studies the differences between the rashes of rubella and measles or between chickenpox and smallpox, for example, and can often be certain of the nature of the illness by clinical observation alone.

The Widal and other special tests. Special tests are of two kinds. The first is to find the germ itself: by taking swabs of the throat or the skin, samples of urine, sputum, faeces or blood and other fluids and trying to grow the germ in the laboratory. The second way is to examine the blood for antibodies. This is an indirect method but is sometimes the only one to use. Some viruses, for example, are difficult to grow, but if the bacteriologist can show that there has been a rise of antibodies against the virus in the patient's blood he can feel fairly sure that the virus has been the cause of the illness.

The laboratory tests for antibodies are of many different kinds. The easiest test to understand is the agglutination test in which serum from the patient's blood is mixed with fluid containing germs; if the serum contains antibodies to those germs, these cause the germs to clot or agglutinate and the clot can be seen quite easily. The Widal test is the best known agglutination test: it shows whether a patient's blood contains antibodies to typhoid and paratyphoid germs.

Complement-fixation tests are also done frequently: they are a little more complicated, but they test for the same thing—the presence or absence of antibody in the patient's blood. There is a complement-fixation test (C.F.T.), for example, for mumps, whooping cough and many other infections. Many similar tests are done, for example the haemagglutination-inhibition (H.A.I.) test for rubella; this is a rapid test for rubella antibody and, therefore, a most useful one to use in pregnant women who have been exposed to rubella. It is not necessary for nurses to know how the test is done: it is enough to know that it is a test for antibody in the patient's blood.

Summary

Germs are composed of one cell only, but they can cause much damage to the human body which is composed of many millions of cells. The reaction between the human body and the germs which attack it causes the symptoms and signs of infectious disease. Diagnostic tests try either to find the germ in the patient or to detect the antibody in his blood as evidence of that reaction.

Chapter 35

Epidemiology

by A. B. CHRISTIE

The cause of epidemics—how diseases spread—skin, respiratory and intestinal infections—fomites

---

The study of how disease spreads is called epidemiology. *Demos* is the Greek word for people, and an epidemic is something which descends on the people. 'Endemic' means *in* or *among* the people, and an endemic disease is one which is constantly present among a people. Smallpox, for example, is endemic in certain parts of India: there are always some cases. Every now and again the number of cases swells and India then has an epidemic of smallpox. In Britain, smallpox is not an endemic disease, for normally there are no cases: when the disease does reach Britain from abroad it is therefore always an epidemic, something that has fallen on the people, although the number of cases may be quite small.

'Sporadic' is another word applied to diseases. It comes from a Greek word meaning to sow or scatter: the Sporades are tiny Greek islands scattered in the Aegean Sea. A sporadic disease is one which is scattered in a population: cases keep occurring here and there throughout the country, but there is no concentration of cases in any one area. Meningococcal meningitis, for example, is a sporadic disease in Britain: there may be one or two cases in London, another one in Leeds, one in Bristol, two in Glasgow and so on, but no concentration of cases anywhere.

Measles, on the other hand, is an endemic disease in Britain: in any big city there are always cases, and every few years the numbers swell into an epidemic. Sporadic diseases, too, may increase unexpectedly but less commonly: the last epidemic of meningitis in Britain occurred 40 years ago.

One final word is pandemic: *pan* is the Greek word for all, and a pandemic is an epidemic that sweeps across the world, affecting *all* the peoples. The typical modern pandemic is influenza, which may start in China, spread across Asia and Europe to reach Britain and over the oceans to reach Australia and the Americas. In the Middle Ages plague, or the Black Death, was the great pandemic.

The cause of epidemics. There is much that is mysterious about epidemics. Why did the Black Death invade Europe in the middle of the fourteenth century, and why did Asian influenza sweep across the world in 1957? Two separate things are involved: one is the germ and the other is the human body. These are often referred to as the parasite and the host, and relation between the two is known as the host-parasite relationship. This host-parasite relationship keeps changing. Measles, for example, attacks mainly children. In a big epidemic of measles most of the young children catch the disease and, after their attack, become immune to the disease. The virus therefore finds itself with few children left to attack. It grumbles on for a year or two in the population, infecting a few of the children who escaped the epidemic. All this time many new babies are being born into the population. These babies have some antibodies in their blood which they get from their mothers and this protects them for about six months. After this time they lose their maternal antibodies and so have no protection against the disease. In this way a new young population of non-immune children builds up, the virus again finds it easy to spread among them, and another epidemic of measles breaks out. In this case, the changes have been in the hosts, the children, not in the virus or parasite. An obvious way of stopping this circle of events is to immunize children with measles vaccine as soon as they have lost their maternal antibodies. This makes them immune, and as the virus can multiply only in the non-immune body it must die out altogether in an immunized population, and there can be no more epidemics.

Sometimes the change is in the germ or parasite, and the nature of this we do not fully understand. The members of the influenza family of viruses, for example, are always circulating and they cause epidemics of influenza from time to time. People who suffer an attack from one of the viruses develop antibodies against the virus and are protected against it for varying periods of time: this tends to restrict the size and frequency of epidemics. Occasionally a completely new member of the family appears. This is what happened in China in 1957 when the new Asian influenza virus appeared, and again in 1968 when the Hong Kong virus appeared. No one had been infected with this virus before, so no one had any antibody against it. The result was that the virus found no opposition in the human hosts, and so spread rapidly across the world as a pandemic. What causes a new virus to appear, or whether it is really a new virus or an old one that has undergone some change, is just not known. The only way to stop a pandemic is for virologists to be constantly on the look-out for new strains of virus, and, as soon as one appears, to try to make a vaccine and immunize people with it before the virus can reach them. This is more difficult than it sounds, for germs spread quickly, but it takes time to make a vaccine and inject enough people with it.

How diseases spread. While there is some mystery about how epidemics come and go, there is none about how germs spread from one person to another. There are three main ways. The germs may be implanted on his skin; they may enter his body by the respiratory tract; or by the mouth and the digestive tract. Typical examples are impetigo or anthrax which infect the skin; influenza or the common cold viruses which are breathed in; and typhoid fever or food-poisoning, the germs of which are swallowed in food or drink.

Infection by the skin. A germ may pass from the skin of one person to the skin of another by direct contact. Children playing together in a sand-pit may spread germs on their hands to one another. Poliomyelitis and Sonne dysentery germs can be spread in this way, and so too may impetigo. Adult wrestlers have infected one another with the virus of herpes simplex in this direct method of contact, the somewhat fanciful name of *herpes gladiatorum* being given to this condition: herpes simplex is the virus which causes 'cold sores', and gladiators were unfortunate slaves who fought to the death with swords in Roman arenas.

Anthrax is a disease in which the germ is implanted on the skin, not from the skin of another person, but from animal hides, wool or hair while these are being handled in tanneries and wool-sorting factories (see p. 380). Syphilis is another disease which is spread by direct contact, usually on the genital mucous membranes but sometimes on the skin of the mouth or breast: the sores that then develop are known as extragenital chancres.

The method of skin spread that most concerns nurses is when germs are conveyed from the body of one patient in a ward to the skin of another patient. The germs may come from any part of the body of the first patient, from his nose and mouth, his skin, his eyes or his intestines. They contaminate his immediate surroundings, his pyjamas, his bedclothes, his crockery, his towels, the dust under his bed, everything around him. The germs can then be carried to the skin of another patient in one of two ways —across the ward in the air, especially after they have been stirred up in bedmaking or ward cleaning; or on the hands of a nurse who has been attending to the patient in any way. If the second patient has a recent operation wound or an ulcer or any break in the skin, the germs from the first patient can be implanted on, and cause secondary infection in, the skin of the second.

Infection by the respiratory tract. When a person breathes, warm moist air passes out of his nose and mouth into the air around him. This warm, moist air may carry germs from his respiratory tract contained in tiny moist droplets which float in the air for some time. When a person speaks, coughs or sneezes, far more of these droplets are discharged into the air. Some of the droplets fall quickly to the floor, but others remain floating for a long time. These floating droplets can be breathed in by another person and, if they contain pathogenic germs, the second person is infected with them and may become ill as a result. The commonest example of this form of infection is the common cold, but many far more serious diseases such as pneumonia and meningitis are also conveyed in this way. The droplets, as well as being breathed in, can settle on any surface. They may fall on the skin or the conjunctiva of a patient in a ward and cause inflammation and sepsis.

Dust is another source of infection by the respiratory route. The dust around a patient's bed is often heavily contaminated with his germs. Germs from urine, faeces, sputum, saliva and pus may all reach the dust around a bed, and as it is wafted on air currents across the ward, some of the dust may be breathed in by another patient. Most of the coarse particles of dust are caught by the cilia of the patient's nose and get no further, but very fine particles can escape the cilia and get far down into the respiratory tract, where they can then cause inflammation and disease.

Some dusts in industrial processes can also cause infection by the respiratory route. The dust in wool-sorting sheds is usually laden with anthrax germs and these are often breathed in by the workers. Fortunately man is very resistant to anthrax so that, in spite of the high exposure risk, respiratory anthrax, known as wool-sorter's disease, is a very rare disease. Dust from hay and grasses may also sometimes cause trouble: fungi and other germs are often present in such dust, and when they are breathed in they can cause serious disease in persons who are specially sensitive or allergic to them. One example is known as farmer's lung. But the kind of respiratory infection that a nurse must keep in mind is the silent spread of droplets through a ward, for this is constantly going on around her as she works.

Infection by the gastro-intestinal tract. Germs can enter by the mouth, be swallowed, pass through the stomach, into the intestines and out again in the faeces. This is always going on, and so long as no pathogenic or disease germs enter, there is no danger. But when pathogenic germs are swallowed, diseases such as gastro-enteritis, dysentery and typhoid fever may follow. It is important to know exactly how this happens.

First of all the germs must enter the mouth and be swallowed. Secondly, they can reach the mouth only from the rectum of some person or animal. This sounds crude, but gastro-intestinal infection *is* crude. When a nurse empties her bowels and uses toilet paper, intestinal germs can easily pass through the paper and contaminate her fingers. If she washes her hands at once, these germs are easily removed. If she does not, she can carry the germs directly to the mouth of a patient, or, more likely, she handles food, say bread and butter, and passes the germ onto the food, which the patient then eats. She can, of course, contaminate her hands just as easily when attending to the toilet of a patient, or indeed attending to the patient in any way, for intestinal germs spread over the perineum, thighs and abdomen of a patient and contaminate his pyjamas and bedclothes, especially if he has diarrhoea, so that a bed bath can be a very dangerous process for the nurse—a fact she may be inclined to forget. All nurses are very careful when handling bedpans, but bedclothes are just as dangerous in certain cases.

The nurse and the piece of bread and butter is an example of a simple direct little piece of epidemiology. In the processing, manipulation and distribution of food in the modern world of commerce the story can become very complex. There are vast food factories, vast bakeries, huge hotel and institutional kitchens, fleets of food vans, chains of great shops and multiple stores, and anywhere there may be a food-handler with dangerous germs on his hands, and these germs can get into the food. If the food is one on which the germs can grow quickly, as on cooked meats or cream cakes, the few germs on the food-handler's fingers can multiply into millions in the food, and a big outbreak of food poisoning, salmonella enteritis or typhoid fever results. Germs may in a similar manner get into milk or water supplies, and then a milk- or water-borne epidemic follows.

Animals often harbour intestinal germs, especially salmonellae. These germs can contaminate the meat in abattoirs, or the carcases in poultry plants. They are usually killed in cooking, but sometimes they survive, if the germs are deep inside the meat or a pie and the heat of cooking does not penetrate enough. Another danger is that cooked meat may be contaminated by germs from raw meat. Many outbreaks of salmonella enteritis have been caused in this way.

The epidemiological background of a food-borne outbreak may be very complicated, but the essential element is the spread of a germ from faeces to the mouth. A nurse is not concerned with the complex, commercial problems of food-borne disease. She does handle patients and she does handle food. She must be very careful.

Fomites is the name given to any articles around a patient that may be contaminated with his germs and then carried from his bedside to some other place. A towel, a cup, a powder tin, a piece of soap—all these can act as fomites, and if they are taken to the bedside of another patient, the germs are taken there also. Patients should, of course, always have their own toilet and other personal articles, so that fomites should never be carried from one bed to another.

Chapter 36

Food-borne Infections

by A. B. CHRISTIE

Food poisoning—bacillary dysentery—infantile gastro-enteritis—typhoid fever—botulism—brucellosis

FOOD POISONING

Food poisoning is not a very good name for two reasons: (1) most intestinal infections are caused by swallowing infected food or drink, e.g. typhoid fever, yet only a few are labelled food poisoning; and (2) the name is apt to cause undue alarm when the illness is mild. 'Enteritis', for example, does not worry the patient or his family, or excite the Press, but food poisoning gets the headlines: yet they are the same thing. The one merit of the name is that it draws attention to the fact that infection can be conveyed by food through carelessness somewhere.

Causes

Food poisoning can be caused by any poison that gets into the food. Zinc, lead and other metals may contaminate food or drink stored in unsuitable containers, and outbreaks of food poisoning have been caused in this way. But such outbreaks are now uncommon, because caterers know of these dangers, and in practice food poisoning usually means bacterial food poisoning. Bacterial food poisoning is usually caused by one of three groups of germs: salmonellae, staphylococci or *Clostridium welchii*. Two other germs, *Bacillus cereus* and *Vibrio parahaemolyticus*, are sometimes the cause: with changing food habits they may become commoner.

Salmonellae. There are over 1,000 members of the salmonella family. They inhabit the intestine of many animals, including man. Man and animals may become symptomless carriers of salmonellae after an attack of diarrhoea. No one who has had such an attack should be allowed to handle food until he or she has had faecal bacteriological tests. Salmonellae may get on food in the abattoir, food factory, shop or kitchen. They multiply rapidly on most foods at room temperature. They are usually killed by thorough cooking, but salmonellae in the centre of a sausage can survive light frying. Raw meat and cooked meat or other food should never be stored together, for salmonellae can be carried on knives and hands from the raw to the cooked food on which they will multiply rapidly.

Staphylococci. These are often present on the skin and in the noses of normal people. They are very common in sores and septic spots. No one with such sores should be allowed to handle food. There is a large number of different staphylococci, and not all are dangerous. It is necessary to type staphylococci in the laboratory when investigating an outbreak to prove that a staphylococcus grown from a food-handler is the same as one grown from food that has caused the illness. Some staphylococci produce a toxin, known as an enterotoxin, and it is this enterotoxin that causes food poisoning, not the staphylococci themselves. This toxin is not destroyed by heat, so that, if food is contaminated by toxin-producing staphylococci and then thoroughly cooked, the staphylococci will all be killed but the toxin will still cause food poisoning. This explains why in some outbreaks all specimens are reported negative for germs: dead germs cannot grow in the laboratory.

Clostridium welchii. This germ is a normal inhabitant of animal and human faeces and is often present in kitchen dust. Like staphylococci, it produces a heat-resistant toxin. It likes to grow and produce toxin in moist warm conditions where there is a little oxygen. It therefore flourishes in warm stews or meat covered with gravy and kept for a few hours before serving. Left-overs, too, suit it very well: it can multiply in the food as it cools, is not upset by a night in a refrigerator, and next day begins to grow again and produce more toxin when it is re-heated before being served. Food should never be kept warm for hours before being served. If it is to be kept till next day, it should be cooled rapidly and put in a refrigerator. But ideally food should be eaten as soon as possible after cooking. This is especially important in hospitals and institutions.

Food which is handled a lot before being served is most likely to carry the germs of food poisoning. Cold meats and cold chicken are likely sources, because the germs can be placed on them by food-handlers and they then multiply on the food if it is badly stored. Pies may be contaminated in preparation, and the heat of cooking may not penetrate the centre. Patties and rissoles are handled a lot, and often not thoroughly cooked. Trifles and creams and cream fillings are all favourite haunts of food-poisoning germs: they grow quickly on them if left in a warm room or on a warm food trolley. Canned food is very safe food because it is sterilized in the can: germs may get in through a defective can, but this is a very rare occurrence. Many people tend to regard canned food as dangerous, but this is quite wrong. After the can is opened, the food may be contaminated by a food-handler or by kitchen dust or dirt just like any other food. Freshly opened canned food can be eaten with complete safety.

Symptoms

The incubation period of staphylococcal food poisoning is short, from half an hour to six hours, of *Clostridium welchii* it is from 12 to 24 hours, and of salmonella infections from 12 to 48 hours. But the incubation period varies with the dosage of germs or toxins.

The three symptoms are diarrhoea, vomiting and abdominal pain. In salmonella cases the main symptom is usually diarrhoea, and the patients may have a little abdominal pain: vomiting is less common. In staphylococcal cases vomiting is the commonest symptom, for the enterotoxin irritates the stomach; diarrhoea is often slight or absent. In *Clostridium welchii* food poisoning, nagging abdominal pain is a typical feature, with diarrhoea, but rarely vomiting. All three symptoms vary in severity according to how badly the food is contaminated. The illness may be so mild as to pass unnoticed or it may be so severe, with vomiting, pain and diarrhoea, that the patient soon becomes prostrated.

Usually the germs stay in the intestines and cause symptoms there. Sometimes, especially in salmonella food poisoning, the germs enter the bloodstream and cause septicaemia. The patient may then have a long, hectic, febrile illness with such complications as bone abscess or cholecystitis. Some salmonellae seem more liable to invade the bloodstream than others, e.g. *Salmonella cholerae-suis* and *Salm. virchow*.

Salmonella typhimurium is one of the commonest food-poisoning germs: usually it stays in the intestines; occasionally it causes a bloodstream infection. It may depend on dosage.

Course of the disease

In most cases the illness is acute and short. In staphylococcal illnesses the patients may vomit repeatedly for a few hours and then the illness subsides, leaving the patient weak for a day or two. In salmonella cases, diarrhoea may be severe for a few hours, the patient going to stool every few minutes: it then eases off and the patient has a motion every 2 or 3 hours for 24 to 48 hours, and thereafter only two or three times a day for a few more days. In *Clostridium welchii* food poisoning abdominal pain may persist for several days: diarrhoea may be severe for the first hour or so, but usually it is less severe than in salmonella cases.

Most patients with food poisoning are back to normal within two or three days, but elderly, debilitated patients or young infants may be severely upset and ill for at least a week. Very occasionally in such patients the illness is fatal.

Diagnosis

The germ must be sought in the food, the vomit and the faeces, and specimens of all three must be sent to the laboratory. The bacteriologist and the Medical Officer of Health will try to trace the outbreak back to its origin.

Treatment

The main treatment is rest, nursing and fluids by mouth when the vomiting stops. Sometimes the patient becomes dehydrated and requires intravenous fluids. It is customary to give antidiarrhoeal medicines such as kaolin mixtures, but it is doubtful if they do any good. Sulphonamides and antibiotics are useless: they do not stop the diarrhoea, and they do not kill the germ, once it is inside the body. This is an important point, for the laboratory usually reports that the germ is sensitive to certain antibiotics *in vitro*: this means 'in glass', i.e. in jelly or broth in laboratory glassware. Unfortunately it is not true *in vivo*, i.e. in the living person. Nurses and doctors often feel that the patient must be *on* some drug treatment. But it is wrong to give drugs which have no effect *in vivo*.

Prevention

The prevention of food poisoning is simple in theory but complex in practice. Germs must not be allowed to get on food. This involves the personal hygiene of every food-handler from the slaughterer in the abattoir to the cook in the kitchen and the nurse on the ward. Food must be handled in such a way that germs are not given the chance to multiply in it. Meat should be eaten immediately after cooking, or if it must be kept, it should be quickly cooled and stored in a refrigerator. Raw and cooked food should not be handled together. Trifles, creams and all foods not requiring cooking should be stored at once in a refrigerator and kept there till served. Germs are not killed in a refrigerator, but they cannot multiply in the cold. All the principles of food hygiene are involved in the prevention of food poisoning.

BACILLARY DYSENTERY

Cause. Bacillary dysentery is caused by one of three germs, all members of the shigella family: *Shigella sonnei, Sh. flexneri* and *Sh. shigae.* (Sonne, Flexner and Shiga were the names of three doctors concerned with the discovery of these germs.) *Sh. sonnei* is the commonest cause of bacillary dysentery in Britain, but in tropical countries *Sh. flexneri* and *Sh. shigae* are commoner, and these two usually cause much more severe illnesses than *Sh. sonnei.*

Sonne dysentery is usually spread by direct contact. A child soils its hands at toilet and then touches another child's hand: the second child lifts its hand to its mouth and the dysentery germs enter. A very small dose of *Shigellae sonnei* is enough to cause infection. *Sh. flexneri* and *Sh. shigae* are usually spread by food or water. But, in all three types, infection means that the germ has been conveyed from the faeces of one person to the mouth of another.

Symptoms. The incubation period is from one or two days to a week. The main symptom is diarrhoea. This may be mild or very severe. Especially in Sonne dysentery, the patient may have only one or two loose motions. Nurses must be very careful about such incidents: they can so easily be infected, become carriers and not realize it. At the other extreme, especially with infections due to *Shigella flexneri* or *Sh. shigae,* the diarrhoea may be overwhelmingly severe, with much blood passed per rectum, so that the patient rapidly becomes prostrated and collapsed. Such patients have much abdominal pain and vomiting and become rapidly dehydrated.

Course. In Britain and most temperate countries, bacillary dysentery is a mild, often trivial illness over in a day or two. Only in young babies or in frail old patients is it a dangerous condition. In the tropics it is a severe, debilitating illness lasting for one or two weeks and sometimes fatal.

Diagnosis. Specimens of faeces or rectal swabs should be sent to the laboratory. If the disease seems to be food-borne, samples of the suspected food should also be sent.

Treatment. Mild cases require no special treatment and this refers to most cases of Sonne dysentery. Nurses must be very careful when disposing of faeces or soiled nappies, or even when changing bedclothes or washing the patient (see Chapter 35). For severe cases, especially in the tropics, treatment is by replacement of fluid, usually by intravenous infusions. Blood transfusions may be required for the worst cases.

If the patient can take liquid by mouth, he should be given drinks of glucose-saline flavoured with lemon or other fruit juices. Babies should be given plain 1/5 normal glucose-saline, but no milk till the diarrhoea has stopped. Diet must be built up gradually as the patient recovers.

Although sulphonamides and antibiotics do help to clear the bowel of dysentery germs, the germs can quickly become resistant to the drugs which are then useless. Moreover these resistant germs can transfer their resistance to other bowel germs. This transferable drug resistance is one of the great hazards of antibiotic therapy. It is better not to use antibiotics for dysentery except in very severe cases.

Prevention of bacillary dysentery depends on strict personal hygiene, aseptic nursing, good sanitation and careful food-handling. This can be difficult even in fully developed countries: in undeveloped tropical countries it is a major public-health problem.

INFANTILE GASTRO-ENTERITIS

This disease may be *caused by many different germs.* The commonest are the coliform germs, usually called *Escherichia coli* (Escherich was the name of a bacteriologist who described these germs). There are many different strains of *E. coli,* usually referred to by number, e.g. *E. coli 0111* or *E. coli 0126.* Viruses, too, may cause gastro-enteritis, especially the enteroviruses such as echoviruses and Coxsackie viruses. In many cases, no germ at all is found.

The disease is very infectious and can spread quickly round an infants' ward or nursery. The germ can be conveyed on hands and fomites (see p. 353).

The two main symptoms of infantile gastro-enteritis are diarrhoea and vomiting. In most infants, the disease is mild, but in others it can be severe or fatal. The third symptom, and the dangerous one, is dehydration. The signs of dehydration are sunken eyes and fontanelle, dry mouth and tongue, a pinched look of the face, and loss of elasticity of the skin. This last is best seen on the abdominal wall where, if the skin is pinched into a fold, the fold does not spring back, but only slowly subsides.

In most babies the symptoms disappear quickly with treatment. In some there is rapid deterioration with severe dehydration: unless this is corrected quickly, the baby may die. In a few cases, the disease runs a more chronic course with frequent relapses of the vomiting and diarrhoea: rarely, such babies die after weeks of illness.

Diagnosis is made clinically. Rectal swabs are sent to the laboratory but one cannot wait for the results before commencing treatment. Quite often bacteriological reports are negative, even in ill babies.

Treatment. All food is stopped. The baby is given 1/5 normal glucose-saline by mouth in small amounts frequently. On this treatment, vomiting and diarrhoea usually stop within the first day or two, and milk may be gradually added to the fluid till the baby is back to its normal feed.

Where there is any sign of dehydration, fluid must be given to the baby by intravenous drip. This is not often required for more than 24 hours, after which feeding by mouth can be restarted.

Antibiotics are of no value in the treatment of the disease. They may be of use in getting rid of the germ after the infant has recovered. The essential treatment is good nursing and fluid replacement, by mouth or intravenously.

Prevention. Infection spreads quickly among babies and strict isolation technique is essential. Feeds must be prepared with aseptic precautions and be sterilized. Nurses must scrub their hands carefully after handling an infant and before touching a feeding bottle. They must realize that everything in the ward may be contaminated with the germ—bedclothes, nappies, powder tins, wash bowls, beds, taps, floors. The germs can get there only from the intestine of an infected baby, but they can be conveyed on a careless nurse's hands.

Sometimes, in spite of all precautions, the disease continues to spread. It may then be necessary to close the ward and not re-open it till it has been disinfected and no new cases have occurred.

TYPHOID AND PARATYPHOID FEVERS

Typhoid and paratyphoid fevers are caused by *Salmonella typhi* and *Salm. paratyphi A, B,* or *C.* Only *Salm. paratyphi B* causes paratyphoid fever in Britain, but the other two paratyphoid germs are common in tropical countries. Typhoid or paratyphoid fever is always caused by infected food, milk or water. The source is always some human being, for typhoid and paratyphoid germs do not infect animals. Human beings may become symptomless carriers of the germ, and if such a carrier handles food or milk or is employed in water-works he may easily spread the infection to others. The germs leave the human body in the faeces in sewage: such infected sewage may contaminate water supplies, if there is any defect in sanitation.

Symptoms. *The incubation period* is 10 to 14 days. The onset is slow, with fatigue, headache and aching in the muscles. The temperature rises slowly in the first few days to reach 38·9 °C to 39·4 °C (102 °F to 103 °F). The patient becomes more and more ill and finally has to take to bed. If untreated, he may lapse into a state of semi-coma, the *typhoid state*. With early diagnosis and modern treatment, the patient should not reach this state. Typhoid fever is not typically a diarrhoeal disease: much more often the patient is constipated. The so-called pea-soup diarrhoea was probably often caused by a diet consisting exclusively of milk.

At the end of the first week, the abdomen may appear very slightly swollen. At this time the rose spots of typhoid fever are seen on the lower chest and upper abdomen. They are about 1 mm in diameter, pink, and flat, and they disappear when the skin is stretched. There are often not more than five or six such spots, so they are easily missed.

Course. On modern treatment, the disease is controlled within a week. Untreated, the patient may remain in the typhoid state for two or three weeks before gradually returning to normal. Sometimes, after the patient appears to be convalescent, typhoid germs re-invade the bloodstream, and all the symptoms, including rose spots, reappear. This is known as a relapse.

The commonest complications are haemorrhage from the bowel, or perforation of the bowel leading to peritonitis. Either of these may be fatal. Femoral thrombosis is also common, and less common complications include cholecystitis, pneumonia, nephritis, meningitis and bone abscess. None of these complications is common with modern treatment.

Paratyphoid fever resembles typhoid fever but is usually less severe. Sometimes it causes gastro-enteritis, rather than a febrile disease.

Diagnosis. Samples of blood, faeces and urine must be sent to the laboratory. *Salmonella typhi* or *Salm. paratyphi* may be grown from all three. Antibodies may also be found in the blood by performing the Widal test on the serum (see p. 347).

Treatment. A patient with typhoid fever requires devoted nursing. His mouth is often dry and crusted and needs careful toilet. His skin may be hot and clammy, and blanket baths give him great comfort. He has little appetite in the first few days and must be coaxed to take drinks: simple glucose drinks are best. Milk should be avoided: it is not easily digested by the febrile patient. As soon as the patient begins to recover, his diet should be increased and there is no reason why a patient with typhoid fever should not take a good mixed diet. The idea that meat and other foods cause haemorrhage and perforation by irritating the bowel wall is nonsense. These complications are caused by the inflammation in the bowel wall caused by the presence there of *Salmonella typhi*. Starvation may, in fact, encourage perforation and haemorrhage by reducing the resistance of the tissues to the germ.

Chloramphenicol is a very effective drug in the acute stage of typhoid and paratyphoid fevers. The dose for an adult is 2 g a day given for 7 to 10 days. Fever falls after 2 to 3 days usually, and the patient is comfortable and convalescent after a week. Sometimes corticosteroids are given as well as chloramphenicol. Relapses are treated in the same way as the acute attack. Co-trimoxazole (Septrin or Bactrim) is the only drug which can be compared with chloramphenicol in the treatment of typhoid fever.

Intestinal haemorrhage, if severe, must be treated by blood transfusion. Intestinal perforation usually requires a surgical operation, but sometimes the peritonitis can be treated with chloramphenicol by mouth, and the perforation is sealed off by natural tissue repair.

Typhoid carriers are treated with ampicillin by mouth: a course of treatment of at least one month is required. If this is not successful, cholecystectomy may be necessary. Renal carriers may require an operation on the kidney or renal tract.

Prevention. Immunization with TAB vaccine gives some, but not complete protection against typhoid and paratyphoid fevers. Effective prevention consists of rigorous public-health measures, aimed at preventing the contamination of food or drink by *Salmonella typhi* or *Salm. paratyphi*. This involves the installation of a water-carriage sewage system, the purification of water supplies, pasteurization of milk and the supervision of all forms of food production and distribution. Known carriers must be excluded from the handling of food and drink, and, when an outbreak occurs, every effort must be made to trace it to the source; this is always a human being excreting the germ from his body.

BOTULISM

Botulism comes from the Latin word *botulus*, a sausage; one of the first reported outbreaks of the disease occurred when 13 people shared one large sausage. The disease is caused by a germ, *Clostridium botulinum*, which is commonly present in earth and soil as a spore. If the spore gets into food it may under certain circumstances germinate and begin to multiply, and when it does so, it produces a very deadly poison or toxin in the food, a mere taste of which can be fatal. It does not grow in fresh food, but only in cooked, stored food in which there is very little oxygen. Most cases in man have followed the eating of cured sausages and hams, home-canned foods, or strange fermented fish and vegetable dishes. Commercially canned food is autoclaved at very high temperatures to make sure that any spores of *Cl. botulinum* are killed.

Symptoms. The toxin is rapidly absorbed from the stomach and reaches the central nervous system where it causes paralysis of the cranial nerves and of the nerves that control the respiratory muscles. The patient's vision becomes blurred, he finds it difficult to speak, he is unable to swallow and finally unable to breathe. He remains fully conscious and acutely aware of his danger. Death usually occurs within a day: some patients linger on for most of a week. Some patients do survive, probably because they have swallowed very little of the toxin.

Diagnosis. Specimens of the food, faeces, vomit and blood of the patient are sent to the laboratory for tests for toxin, but there is no time to await results. The diagnosis must be made clinically. If several patients are affected, the diagnosis is easy, for there is no other disease that causes such symptoms in several people at the same time. If only one patient is affected the doctor may think of poliomyelitis or encephalitis rather than botulism, for botulism is a very rare disease.

Treatment. Botulinum antitoxin should be given intravenously, though its effect is doubtful once the toxin has reached the cells of the central nervous system. Patients unable to swallow should be tube-fed and, if there is respiratory paralysis, they should be treated in an iron lung or by positive-pressure ventilation after tracheostomy. The difficulty is that the disease progresses so rapidly that it may not be possible to get the patient in time to a hospital where those facilities are available.

Prevention. Commercial canning can be relied on to kill *Clostridium botulinum*. Home canning of meat and vegetables should be done only if a pressure cooker is used: boiling the can is not sufficient. The germ does not grow in acid conditions, so that canning or bottling of fruit and jam is safe. Commercial production of smoked sausages, hams and other foods must be carefully controlled. The disease is rare, but carelessness could let the germ break through.

BRUCELLOSIS

Brucellae are germs called after Dr Bruce who first isolated them from the spleen of four patients who died of Malta fever in 1889. There are three types, *Brucella abortus*, *Br. melitensis* and *Br. suis*. They can all cause the disease brucellosis, other names for which are Malta fever, Mediterranean fever, abortus fever and undulant fever. The germ is very common in goats and sheep in Mediterranean countries and in cattle in Europe. Man is infected by drinking milk which may be teeming with brucellae, or by contact with infected animals, especially during lambing, kidding and calving.

Symptoms. Acute brucellosis is a febrile illness, with headache, joint and muscle pains and much sweating. This lasts for most of a fortnight and may then subside completely. Sometimes it passes into a subacute stage with recurring bouts of fever and pain. This is sometimes called undulant fever: undulant comes from the Latin word for waves, and the disease is characterized by 'waves' of fever. A few cases pass into the chronic stage, when the patient may have prolonged pains in the back and along the sciatic nerve and may suffer from depression and neurasthenia.

Diagnosis. Brucellae are present in the patient's blood or urine in the acute stage but they do not grow readily in the laboratory and reports are often negative. Agglutination and complement-fixation tests are done on the patient's serum, and they may lead to the diagnosis though the results are often difficult to interpret.

Prevention. Pasteurization kills brucellae, and only pasteurized milk is safe to drink. People who object to pasteurization do not know the dangers of brucellosis. Malta fever used to be a scourge in Malta: since pasteurization of goat and cow's milk was introduced in the island, the disease has become rare. The other method of prevention is to try to raise brucellosis-free herds of animals. This is done by carrying out tests on all animals, and removing and slaughtering those that are infected. In this way, brucellosis has been abolished in some countries, especially Scandinavia. It can be done elsewhere, but it takes time, perseverance and money.

Chapter 37

Some Acute Infections

by A. B. CHRISTIE

*Measles—rubella—mumps—whooping cough—scarlet fever—ery-
sipelas—acute rheumatism—diphtheria—glandular fever*

MEASLES

Measles virus does not survive long outside the human body: it depends for its survival on rapid spread from person to person in droplets.

Symptoms. The incubation period is 12 to 14 days. There is a prodromal period lasting 1 to 4 days in which the symptoms are catarrh, cough, croup and coryza: at this stage tiny white spots known as Koplik spots can be seen inside the mouth near the molar teeth. The temperature is between 37·2 °C and 38·9 °C (99 °F and 102 °F). At the end of the prodromal period the temperature rises, sometimes to 40 °C to 40·5 °C (104 °F to 105 °F), and the rash appears. The patient now has a persistent, harsh cough, and his respirations are increased. He looks and feels acutely ill. The rash consists of reddish-brown spots, mostly from a quarter to a half inch (6 to 12 mm) across, though some of them run together to form large blotches. The spots are slightly raised above the surface of the skin. They first appear along the forehead and behind the ears and quickly cover the face and the entire body. After two or three days the rash begins to fade, the temperature falls, the cough disappears, and by the end of a week the patient feels well again.

Complications. The two most important complications are pneumonia and encephalitis. Pneumonia is common, especially in some tropical countries, and may prove fatal in undernourished children. In most of Europe, pneumonia is much less common and responds rapidly to treatment with antibiotics. Encephalitis occurs in about 1 in every 1,000 cases. It occurs just as the rash is fading. The patient may pass rapidly into coma and remain in coma for weeks or months. When the patient comes out of coma he may be left with severe neurological defects or be mentally defective: but some patients return to normal health. Other complications are otitis media, enteritis and conjunctivitis.

Treatment. Most patients with measles recover without specific treatment; they require careful nursing and rest in bed during the acute stage, but most patients should be out of bed by the end of the week.

Drugs are not required in measles unless there are complications. Antibiotics do not prevent the onset of complications. When pneumonia sets in, penicillin is the best drug to use: the patient may also require oxygen. He needs very devoted nursing. There is no specific treatment for encephalitis. Corticosteroids are sometimes given, but their effect is very doubtful. The patient may be in coma for weeks. During this time he is fed through an intra-gastric tube: his skin must be carefully cared for and attention given to bowel and bladder. One should never give up hope with such a patient, even after long coma. Otitis media is treated with sulphonamides or penicillin.

Prevention. There are two ways of preventing measles. If a child is exposed to measles, he can be given an injection of gamma globulin which contains measles antibody. This may protect him completely for the time being, or he may develop modified measles. Modified measles is simply mild ordinary measles, and it leaves the child immune to measles for life.

The second method of prevention is to inoculate the child with measles vaccine. The vaccine is made from measles virus which has been weakened by being grown under special conditions in the laboratory; it is still live, but causes only slight symptoms in the vaccinated child, yet renders him immune, probably for life (see Chapter 42).

RUBELLA: GERMAN MEASLES

The disease is caused by the rubella virus which is spread by droplet. Patients are infectious for a few days before and a few days after the rash.

Symptoms. Rubella is a mild disease. The main symptoms are the rash, enlargement of the lymph glands in the neck, mild fever and slight malaise. Adult women sometimes have sore throat and arthritis, mainly of the small joints of the fingers. The rash is a fine, pink, flat macular rash: the spots are much smaller than in measles and do not run together to form blotches. The spots are sometimes so small that the rash looks like scarlet fever. The temperature is usually not higher than 37·2 °C to 37·8 °C (99 °F to 100 °F). The lymph glands are small and shotty. The rash fades quickly and the patient feels well within a few days.

Complications. Arthritis has already been mentioned. Encephalitis is a very rare complication and few doctors ever see such a case. The important complication is infection of the unborn baby, congenital rubella.

Congenital rubella. In the acute stage of rubella, the virus is present in the bloodstream, and if the patient is pregnant the virus can pass across the placenta and enter the bloodstream of the fetus. In the first three months of pregnancy vital organs are being formed in the fetus, and the entry of rubella virus into these organs can severely upset the formative process. The main organs concerned are the eye, heart and ear. Damage to these at this stage can result in cataract of the eye, with blindness, malformation of the heart, and deafness in the newborn child. There may also be damage to the liver causing jaundice, damage to the blood vessels causing purpura, and bone damage.

Diagnosis. It is not always easy to diagnose rubella clinically, for the rash may be slight and transient, and many other illnesses can produce similar rashes. Sometimes rubella occurs without any rash, and then it is impossible to make a diagnosis without help from the laboratory. The virus can be grown from a throat swab which must be taken to the laboratory in a small bottle of fluid (transport medium). The virus can be grown from the eye, the throat, urine and cerebrospinal fluid of a baby with congenital rubella. It is most important to make certain of the diagnosis in pregnancy, especially if there is any chance that the woman may be suffering from rubella without a rash. Blood tests for antibody may prove helpful.

Treatment. There is no specific treatment for rubella and most patients require none. Rest in bed for a day or two is all that is necessary. Babies with congenital rubella must be under the care of specialists from birth, for a good deal can be done in the treatment of cataract, heart malformation and deafness. Even if nothing curative can be done, the infants require specialized care to help them cope with their disabilities.

Prevention. When a pregnant woman in the first three months of pregnancy is exposed to infection with rubella it is vitally important to try to protect the fetus. A rapid blood test will show whether the mother is susceptible to rubella; if she is not, there is nothing to worry about—she cannot catch rubella and so cannot infect the fetus in her womb. If she is susceptible, she should be given an injection of gamma globulin: this contains antibody against rubella and *may* prevent the mother from getting the disease. It is not a certain preventative, and it may even lead to a false sense of security if the mother as a result gets rubella without a rash, for she may think she has escaped infection when, in fact, she has not, and may still give birth to a diseased baby. Blood tests can be taken to show whether or not she has escaped, but the results must be interpreted by an expert. If the mother in the first three months of pregnancy has been infected with rubella, the question of therapeutic abortion may have to be considered: after the fourth month there is no danger to the fetus.

The real solution to the rubella problem is a vaccine with which girls and young women can be made immune to the disease for life. Such a vaccine, made from rubella virus, is now available.

MUMPS

The disease is caused by mumps virus which is present in the saliva and in the throat for a few days before to a few days after the appearance of the swelling of the face.

Symptoms. *The incubation period* is usually between 14 and 18 days. The commonest symptom is swelling of one or, more commonly, both parotid glands. The swelling stretches from the front of the ear down over the lower jaw and into the neck. It is difficult to feel the lower jaw through the swelling: this is an important point, for swellings of the cervical glands are *below* the jaw, which can be easily felt by the examiner's fingers. The parotid swelling of mumps is painful and causes the patient great distress. The mouth is dry and the patient finds it difficult to open his mouth or swallow. His temperature is raised to between 37·2 °C and 39·4 °C (99 °F and 103 °F), and he feels very ill sometimes for several days till the swelling begins to go down. By the end of a week he is usually back to normal.

Complications. The commonest complication is orchitis, or epididymo-orchitis, an acute inflammation of the genital organs of the male. This occurs only after the onset of puberty—at least it is very rare in infants and young boys. The orchitis comes on three to five days after the onset of parotitis, just when the patient is beginning to feel the illness is over. It may occur without any preceding parotitis. The genital organs swell on one or both sides, and are very painful and tender. The patient's temperature soars to 40 °C to 40·5 °C (104 °F to 105 °F) and he appears toxic and feels very ill. The swelling and the illness last several days before they subside, and the patient is often exhausted with the pains and toxaemia. It used to be thought that sterility often followed mumps orchitis, but it is now known that this is an uncommon sequel, and patients can usually be reassured on this point.

The other common complication is *lymphocytic meningitis*. This comes on a few days after the parotitis but, like orchitis, may occur without parotitis. It is a mild form of meningitis and the patient usually recovers within a fortnight. Rare cases of meningo-encephalitis do occur, and this may leave the patient with severe neurological defects or even be fatal.

Oophoritis, or inflammation of the ovaries, and *mastitis* are both uncommon complications. *Pancreatitis* in a mild form is probably common, causing a little abdominal pain and vomiting. Severe pancreatitis with intense abdominal pain and much vomiting is rare; when it occurs, the doctor may have difficulty in distinguishing it from other forms of intra-abdominal inflammation.

Diagnosis. In patients with parotitis the diagnosis is easy. When complications occur without parotitis, only the history of contact with mumps may give the clue. Diagnosis can then be confirmed by blood tests for the presence of antibody.

Treatment. The patient with parotitis needs careful nursing for several days. Heat applied to the swelling sometimes gives relief, and the doctor may prescribe analgesics. When the swelling is intense, corticosteroids in high dosage for a day or two often give dramatic relief, but they are not required in most cases. The pain and swelling of orchitis are relieved by corticosteroids; 50 mg of prednisone, or similar preparation, daily for two or three days is required. The inflamed organs need to be supported on pads of cotton wool. There is no specific treatment for mumps meningitis; fortunately, in most patients, the condition resolves on its own. The patient needs all the nursing care given to other forms of meningitis.

Prevention. *Gamma globulin* is sometimes given in camps and institutions to try to stop the spread of mumps, but it is not a very successful form of prevention. *A mumps vaccine is available* but it is not yet known how useful this will be. Much depends on whether it will give protection for life. If it were only to postpone mumps from boyhood to adult life, it would be of no value at all, for complications are more common in the adult.

WHOOPING COUGH

The disease is caused by a germ called *Bordetella pertussis*, or simply the whooping cough bacillus. It is present in droplets in the expired air during the first two weeks of the illness but not often any later.

Symptoms. *The incubation period* is between two and four weeks. The illness begins like a common cold. This does not clear up and the cough becomes worse, till after a week or 10 days it becomes spasmodic. *The spasms consist of a succession of expiratory coughs without any indrawing of air between them*: there may be 20 or 30 coughs before the child is able to get a breath, and the air then has to force its way through the larynx which is still in spasm. This causes the crowing noise or whoop which gives the disease its name. The child becomes distressed during the spasm and often cyanosed, and after the whoop falls back exhausted.

The spasmodic stage usually lasts at least a fortnight, after which the symptoms gradually become less severe, but the child may continue to have a cough for many weeks. Many of the patients vomit after a spasm, and this and the exhausting effect of the spasms lead often to wasting and loss of weight.

Complications. The main complication is bronchopneumonia. When this sets in, the spasms often disappear but the child's temperature rises and he obviously becomes more ill. *Collapse of portions of the lungs* is also common, but rarely permanent. *Convulsions* and *coma* are very severe and sometimes fatal complications, but are rare. Minor complications due to increased pressure during spasms are haemorrhages under the conjunctiva, and umbilical or inguinal hernias.

Diagnosis. *The symptoms are usually themselves diagnostic.* The germ can be grown in the laboratory if pernasal swabs are taken carefully and sent quickly. A complement-fixation test can be done on the patient's blood, but this does not become positive until late in the disease.

Treatment. The essence of treatment is good nursing: the child needs reassurance more than medicine. In the very early stages, before the typical whoop has developed, antibiotics may be of some use, but later than this they are useless. Phenobarbitone or other sedatives may be prescribed, but they are of doubtful value. For bronchopneumonia antibiotics are of great value and it is their use in this complication which has led to the great drop in deaths from whooping cough. There is no specific treatment for the coma of whooping cough; devoted nursing is needed, often for weeks or months.

Prevention. The best hope of preventing whooping cough lies in the use of a vaccine. This is usually given along with vaccines against diphtheria, and tetanus in the so-called triple vaccine (see Chapter 42).

SCARLET FEVER

Scarlet fever is caused by haemolytic streptococci, a family of germs of which there are many strains. Some of them form an erythrogenic toxin which can cause the rash of scarlet fever. The germ is present in the nose and throat of carriers or patients.

Symptoms. *The incubation period* is from two to five days. The onset is abrupt with sore throat and vomiting: the temperature rises to 37·7 °C to 38·9 °C (100 °F to 102 °F) and the child feels ill and takes to bed. (In diphtheria the onset is slower and the child may mope about for several days before taking to bed, but is then much more ill.) The tongue is covered with a thick white fur through which the tiny red papillae project; soon the fur disappears leaving only the raw red surface stippled with the papillae. These two stages are known as the white and red strawberry tongues of scarlet fever.

On the second day the rash appears. There are two elements in it—a red flush or erythema and raised red specks or puncta on top of it, punctate erythema. It begins on the face but does not spread round the mouth: this circum-oral pallor is typical of scarlet fever, but it is also seen in measles and other diseases. The rash quickly spreads to the trunk and limbs. The fever usually falls after a day or two, the rash fades and by the end of a week the patient has recovered. This is the common course of the disease today, but in some countries it remains a severe disease with many complications and is sometimes fatal. At one time scarlet fever was one of the most serious epidemic diseases.

As the rash fades, the skin begins to peel, first around the clavicles, then in the groins and on the hands and feet. It is a fine pin-hole peeling or desquamation, but on the hands and feet the skin may separate in large flakes. Severe peeling is uncommon in the mild type of scarlet fever seen today.

Complications. There used to be many complications of scarlet fever, mostly of a septic nature due to the spread of streptococci from the throat to other parts of the body, e.g. otitis media, septic rhinitis, purulent cervical adenitis. Complications due to the toxin were acute nephritis and acute endocarditis. These are now rare, though they still occur in some epidemics. Acute rheumatic fever remains a danger, even in mild attacks, and this is why it is important to eliminate all the streptococci from the throat, for rheumatic fever is an allergic reaction to the presence of streptococci.

Diagnosis. The sore throat, the red stippled tongue and the rash are usually enough to make the diagnosis obvious. A throat swab may be sent to the laboratory to see if haemolytic streptococci are present. Skin tests are not used nowadays.

Treatment. The patient is kept in bed for the first few days and given plenty of fluids to drink. Gargles do nothing to soothe the sore throat: aspirin by mouth gives relief. Penicillin is the correct antibiotic; it can be given by mouth for a week, and then the patient can be given an injection of long-acting penicillin intramuscularly. This will make sure that all the streptococci are eliminated from the throat and helps to prevent the onset of acute rheumatism. Most patients can be up and about at the end of the first week; in the rare severe cases, the illness lasts several weeks and leaves the patient very weak for a long time.

Prevention. Active and passive immunization against scarlet fever are not now used, for they are unreliable and have unpleasant and sometimes dangerous side-effects. Oral penicillin may be given to contacts in institutions to try to prevent the disease spreading. Penicillin must be given daily for many years to children who develop rheumatic symptoms after scarlet fever in order to prevent recurrences.

ERYSIPELAS

This is another disease caused by haemolytic streptococci. It causes an erythematous or red rash, most often on the face but it may also appear on the legs. It is commonest in elderly people, but may appear on the legs in babies. The patient complains of tightness and discomfort in the face or leg, sometimes of severe pain. There may be some toxaemia with shivering and malaise. Usually the illness responds to treatment and one rarely sees severe cases nowadays, but sometimes a frail old patient is severely upset by an attack of erysipelas.

Treatment is by sulphonamides or penicillin. Local applications to the affected part may soothe the patient, but only simple ointments or lotions should be used. Penicillin cream should not be used, for patients may have acute local reactions to it.

ACUTE RHEUMATISM (Rheumatic fever)

Acute rheumatism and acute rheumatic fever mean the same—an acute disease which is an allergic reaction to a recent infection with streptococci. It may follow scarlet fever or acute streptococcal tonsillitis or even a streptococcal skin infection. It has nothing to do with painful muscle and joint conditions in adults, sometimes called 'rheumatism or rheumatics'. Nor has it anything in common with rheumatoid arthritis or osteoarthritis. It is an acute specific disease; fortunately it is becoming much rarer, but it used to be the commonest cause of serious heart disease in young people, especially of mitral stenosis.

Symptoms. The onset is acute, usually two to three weeks after an attack of tonsillitis or other streptococcal infection. The main symptoms are fever and joint pains. The joints are most often the larger joints such as the knees, ankles and elbows, but the small joints of the fingers and wrists may also be affected. The pain often shifts from one joint to another. The affected joints become very painful, and the overlying tissues become swollen and red. The child often sweats profusely.

The great danger of acute rheumatism is that the heart may be affected, usually the valves between the chambers of the heart. When this occurs, it may lead on to serious interference with the flow of the blood through the heart and eventually to heart failure.

The diagnosis is made on clinical grounds. A swab of the throat may grow streptococci and a serum test may show a rise of antistreptococcal (ASO) antibody.

Treatment. Salicylates are still the main drug treatment. They may be given as aspirin or as a salicylate mixture and they must be continued for a long time. Corticosteroids have been used but it is doubtful if they help much. *Good nursing is needed*; in the early stages the patient has a lot of pain and must be handled gently. The affected joints must be supported with pillows and the weight of the bedclothes must be lifted by cradles. The patient must be coaxed to take drinks during the acute stage, but when the pain is controlled he eats eagerly. The skin needs attention when there is much sweating; bed baths are required frequently, but it is doubtful if the old idea of nursing the patient between blankets is really of any value.

Prevention consists of preventing streptococcal infection. Streptococcal infections must be treated with penicillin in such a way that the drug is present in the patient's blood for at least 10 days. This can be done by giving him the drug by mouth for 10 days or by an injection of long-acting penicillin. A child who has had one attack of acute rheumatism must continue to take penicillin for the rest of childhood, for a second attack of streptococcal illness in a rheumatic child may have serious effect on the heart.

DIPHTHERIA

The disease is caused by Corynebacterium diphtheriae, commonly known as the diphtheria bacillus. It is present in the nose and throat of patients and carriers.

Symptoms. The incubation period is from two to six days. The onset is slow and insidious. Often the patient complains only of tiredness for the first day or two, and may have no sore throat. The tiredness becomes more marked and the patient begins to look toxic and ill. Examination of the throat at this stage reveals a membrane on the tonsils; this is at first white but rapidly changes to grey-green and finally to black. This differs from the membrane of glandular fever which remains white even after a week. The neck glands enlarge after a day or two and, in bad cases, the swelling may fill up all the space between the lower jaw and the clavicle—*the bull-neck of severe diphtheria.*

The severity of a case depends on the amount of membrane: if it is confined to the tonsils, the case is mild or only moderately severe and few such patients die. If it spreads on to the uvula, and beyond that on to the hard palate, the case is one of malignant or hypertoxic diphtheria and many such patients have extremely severe illnesses and death is a not uncommon end.

Complications. There are two sets of complications, *early cardiovascular* and *late paralytic complications.* Cardio-vascular collapse occurs in the first two weeks of the hypertoxic type of illness. The early symptoms are often abdominal pain and vomiting and the child turns pale and flops on the pillow, unable to hold his head up. The pulse is rapid, difficult to feel and irregular. There is a fluttering heart impulse visible on the chest, and when the doctor listens he finds the heart is in gallop rhythm.

The *first sign of paralysis occurs about the end of the third week of illness* and usually affects the power of the eye to accommodate, and the patient complains of blurred vision. The next paralysis is of the palate: the patient develops a nasal voice and cannot swallow without letting some fluid come back down the nose. Paralysis of the pharynx, larynx and the respiratory muscles occurs between the fifth and the seventh weeks, often when one is beginning to think that the worst is past. Paralysis of the limbs comes on even later.

These severe complications occur only in cases that are obviously severe at the outset. If membrane has not spread beyond the tonsils, the patient may suffer from paralysis of the eye and palate but will not get cardio-vascular complications or any of the more severe paralyses. All the paralyses of diphtheria are temporary and will disappear if the patient can be kept alive long enough.

Treatment. The main medical treatment is by the administration of antitoxin and penicillin. An average dose of antitoxin is 20,000 units intramuscularly; when more than this is required, some of it should be given intravenously.

For cardio-vascular collapse the main treatment is highly skilled nursing. The patient must be nursed flat with only one soft pillow, and the nurse must do everything for the patient. The doctor may decide to treat the patient in an oxygen tent and may prescribe intravenous glucose and also give corticosteroids, but there is no specific treatment. A great deal depends on the nursing.

Paralysis of the eye is usually fleeting and needs no treatment. When a child has paralysis of the palate he must be given fluids carefully but he can usually swallow solids without trouble. For paralysis of the pharynx and larynx tracheostomy may be required and the patient must be fed by intragastric tube. For respiratory paralysis artificial ventilation is essential. Paralysis of the limbs clears up with time.

Prevention. Diphtheria is a preventable disease. Diphtheria toxin is prepared in the laboratory from diphtheria bacilli; it is changed into toxoid by chemical treatment. This toxoid is not toxic to man, but still stimulates the production of antibodies when injected into his body. These antibodies confer active immunity on him.

This toxoid is given in various preparations; infants are given three injections of triple vaccine which contains diphtheria toxoid, whooping cough vaccine and tetanus toxoid, and protects the child against all three diseases, though booster doses are required later to maintain the immunity (see Chapter 42). *Older children and adults* are usually Schick tested first because many of them develop natural immunity; in a Schick test, a minute dose of diphtheria toxin is injected into the skin of the forearm; if the person requires to be immunized, a red patch develops at the injection site within two days, a positive reaction; if he is already immune, no patch appears, a negative reaction. False or pseudo-reactions occur in some people but the doctor can distinguish these from true reactions. A different preparation is used for immunizing older children and adults but the basis is still diphtheria toxoid.

GLANDULAR FEVER: INFECTIOUS MONONUCLEOSIS

The cause of glandular fever is probably the Epstein-Barr (EB) virus. Infection appears to follow close personal contact as in kissing.

Symptoms. *The incubation period* is probably about two to three weeks. The disease takes one of three forms—*anginose, febrile* or *glandular.* The anginose is much the commonest form. The patient has a sore throat and there is much membrane on the tonsils, often so much that the tonsils touch each other so that breathing and swallowing become difficult. The cervical glands swell and may stick out of the contour of the neck and can be seen like an egg under the skin. The glands in the axillae and the groins also enlarge but are never larger than small pebbles. The patient, most often a young adult, has a raised temperature of 37·2 °C to 37·8 °C (99 °F to 100 °F) and may be uncomfortable because of his sore throat and pharyngeal and nasal congestion, but he does not have the agonizing sore throat of streptococcal tonsillitis nor the severe toxaemia of diphtheria. The membrane in the throat remains white even after a week.

In the febrile type the patient has no definite symptom other than fever and malaise. His illness will be referred to by the doctor as P.U.O. until the diagnosis is settled. P.U.O. means pyrexia of uncertain origin. In the glandular type there is enlargement of the cervical, axillary and groin glands and mild fever: this type is commoner in young children. In all three types there may be enlargement of the spleen.

Complications. Glandular fever is not a serious disease and most patients recover within one or two weeks. Complications such as rupture of the spleen, meningitis and myocarditis have been recorded but they are all very rare and most doctors never see such a case during a lifetime of practice. Lay people seem to regard glandular fever with awe and as a severe debilitating disease, but there is no justification for this view at all. Nurses should be ready to reassure patients on this point.

The clinical diagnosis can be confirmed by examination of the blood. Abnormal monocytes, glandular fever cells, are seen in a blood film and the Paul-Bunnell test on the patient's serum is positive. This is a special antibody test.

There is no specific treatment for glandular fever. Antibiotics are useless. They are often prescribed because the throat looks as if streptococci must be responsible for the inflammation, but this is not the case. Ampicillin given to patients with glandular fever often produces an alarming and uncomfortable rash which leads to the patient's being sent into hospital.

When the swelling of the throat is severe and interfering with breathing, corticosteroids may produce a dramatic effect by reducing the inflammation, but they are required in only a few cases.

There is no way known of preventing glandular fever.

Chapter 38

Acute Infections (continued)

by A. B. CHRISTIE

Chickenpox—smallpox—herpes zoster—herpes simplex—poliomye-litis—encephalitis—influenza—rabies—anthrax—tetanus

---

CHICKENPOX (Varicella)

The disease is caused by the varicella-zoster virus. This virus can cause chickenpox in one patient but herpes zoster in another. The two diseases must be considered as different forms of the same infection.

Symptoms. In most cases the only evidence of the disease is the rash. This consists of crops of spots or macules which very quickly change into vesicles or blisters. The rash is heaviest on the trunk, less heavy on the limbs. On the limbs it is heavier above the elbows and knees than below. It is a rash therefore which 'seeks' the centre of the body. The rash of smallpox tends to fly away from the centre of the body. The rash of chickenpox is called centripetal or 'centre-seeking', that of smallpox is centrifugal or 'centre-fleeing'.

The rash of chickenpox dries up within two days, though it may be a week or more before the scabs begin to separate. The rash of smallpox takes at least a week to reach the scab stage. The two great differences between the diseases lie therefore in the distribution of the rashes on the body and the speed at which they develop.

Children are usually not ill with chickenpox but adults often have a fever and considerable malaise. A rare complication is pneumonia due to the virus. This is seen mainly in adults and can be very serious or fatal. Encephalitis is another very rare complication. Sepsis of some of the larger chickenpox spots is fairly common.

Diagnosis. This can usually be made clinically by examining the rash. In doubtful cases scrapings from the spots may be sent to the laboratory where the virus can be grown on tissue culture or seen under the electron microscope in a special virus laboratory.

Treatment. Most patients require no treatment. When itching is severe soothing lotions or powder may be applied. For virus pneumonia oxygen is needed and corticosteroids may be ordered. There is no treatment for encephalitis other than devoted nursing.

Prevention. There is no way of preventing the spread of infection other than by isolating the patient. Hyperimmune gamma globulin (see p. 399) may be given to neonates, for chickenpox can be very severe in newborn babies. This gamma globulin is derived from the blood of patients convalescent from chickenpox.

SMALLPOX (Variola)

The disease is caused by the smallpox virus of which there are two strains—variola major and variola minor viruses.

Symptoms. The incubation period is 10 to 14 days. There is a well-marked prodromal period before the rash comes out. This lasts two or three days and the patient is febrile, has a severe headache and severe backache; this prodromal illness resembles an acute attack of influenza. At the end of three days the temperature falls and the rash comes out, first on the face, then on the upper chest, the rest of the trunk, then on the arms and lastly on the legs. The rash consists at first of macules or flat spots, and these change slowly into vesicles, then into pustules and finally into scabs, the whole process taking at least a week. The rash is heavier on the limbs than on the trunk, and on the limbs it is heavier below the elbows and the knees than above. Both in distribution and development the rash is quite different from chickenpox. Atypical cases of both diseases occur and then the diagnosis can be made only by doctors with special experience of the disease.

The disease varies greatly in severity. A vaccinated person may have only a few spots and be scarcely ill at all. At the other extreme the patient's body may be covered from head to foot with a rash in which the spots have run together in one extensive eruption—confluent smallpox. Sometimes the early prodromal symptoms are so severe that the patient dies before the true rash comes. These patients have a purpuric or haemorrhagic rash and they often bleed from the body orifices. This is haemorrhagic or hypertoxic smallpox and all such patients die. The diagnosis can be very difficult, for the appearance of such patients is quite different from smallpox with the true rash.

Diagnosis. The diagnosis is made by a careful examination of the rash. It is nearly always confirmed by laboratory tests, as it is vitally important to be sure of the diagnosis, for in an outbreak of smallpox some patients always die. This is not true of variola minor in which the disease is always mild.

The virus can be grown inside fertile hens' eggs, or it may be seen under the electron microscope.

Treatment. There is no specific treatment for smallpox. The pustules look as if they must be full of staphylococci and other pus-forming germs which respond to antibiotics, but they are not. They contain only virus and dead cells. The patient needs careful nursing, with special attention to the eyes, the mouth and the skin. One must do everything possible to prevent the skin from breaking down, for secondary germs may then invade the broken pustules and cause sepsis. The illness may be long, and the patient must be coaxed to eat a nourishing diet.

Prevention. Vaccination prevents smallpox. Nurses and doctors should be revaccinated at regular intervals for they are liable to be exposed to unrecognized mild cases in their work. Contacts of cases must be vaccinated as quickly as possible; the theory that vaccination any time within four days of contact is safe is not 100 per cent reliable, and patients have caught smallpox even when vaccinated on the day of contact. An antiviral drug, Marboran, is of great value in dealing with close contacts; even when given five or six days after contact it may still prevent the onset of smallpox. Hyperimmune vaccinial gamma globulin is also useful. It is derived from the blood of recently vaccinated persons. Dangerous contacts of smallpox are always kept under surveillance by a doctor with special knowledge of the control of the disease. Marboran and gamma globulin are useless in the *treatment* of the disease. Their place is in prevention.

Vaccination itself can cause unpleasant and sometimes dangerous complications, such as *vaccinia gangrenosa* and *encephalitis*. *Routine* vaccination of infants is not now recommended in countries like Britain where smallpox has become a rare disease. But vaccination is still essential for contacts of smallpox patients, or for travellers going to countries where the disease is still common.

HERPES ZOSTER (Shingles)

This disease is caused by the varicella-zoster virus which is also the cause of chickenpox. Herpes zoster tends to occur in older people who have had chickenpox in childhood, and it seems that the virus settles down somewhere in their bodies and emerges years later in response to a stimulus. What that stimulus is, no one knows. Herpes zoster does sometimes occur in young children.

Symptoms. There are two symptoms—a rash and pain. The rash consists of a red base with fine vesicles or blisters on top of it. The rash creeps round the body—*herpes* means creeping, and *zoster* means the girdle. Often the rash creeps round a narrow band of the chest wall. Another common site is the forehead where the rash comes round the temple and on to the centre of the brow and the nose, but not across the centre line. This is because the virus follows the course of one nerve from its exit from the skull or spinal column to its end in the skin.

The pain of herpes zoster is sometimes severe and persistent. The only serious complication that is at all common is ulceration of the cornea of the eye, and patients whose eyes are affected should be under the care of an ophthalmologist. Quite often a patient with herpes zoster also develops a chickenpox rash elsewhere on the body. Paralysis of muscles supplied by affected nerves is a rare complication.

Treatment. Analgesics may be prescribed for the pain; in severe cases the doctor will try one after another. A solution of idoxuridine (IDU) applied locally on lint sometimes does good. The nurse's main task is to try to maintain the patient's morale by kindness and understanding, for the pain often lasts a long time especially in frail elderly people.

Prevention. There is no known way of preventing herpes zoster.

HERPES SIMPLEX (Cold sore)

The cause is the herpes simplex virus. It is quite distinct from the varicella-zoster virus.

Symptoms. The commonest symptom is the cold sore on the lips which so many adults suffer from. The virus is present in the cells of their body and comes to the surface every now and again. Sometimes a minor stimulus such as sunburn brings it out, sometimes a common cold, but some diseases, especially pneumonia and meningitis, also cause herpes to appear on the lips and mouth. These are all examples of recurring herpes, the virus having got into the body many years earlier. Primary infections can be much more serious. Young children get severe gingivo-stomatitis with primary herpes, and adults may get conjunctivitis or ulceration of the cornea. A very rare form of herpes simplex is encephalitis. Nurses sometimes get herpetic whitlows on the fingers from contact with herpetic patients.

Treatment. Most patients need no treatment. Corticosteroids are helpful in gingivo-stomatitis for they reduce the inflammation which causes so much of the child's discomfort. They must never be used in affections of the eye; patients with herpes of the eye must be under the care of an ophthalmologist. An anti-viral drug called IDU may be prescribed both for eye cases and for the rare cases of encephalitis. For the latter, the services of a neurosurgeon are required; he may decide to open the skull for decompression.

Prevention. There is no known way of preventing herpes simplex. Babies with eczema must be protected from exposure to adults with cold sores, for if the virus gets on eczematous skin it spreads rapidly as *eczema herpeticum*, and this is a serious and sometimes fatal condition.

POLIOMYELITIS

There are three strains of poliomyelitis virus called poliovirus 1, 2 and 3. The virus is excreted in the throat secretions of the patient for about a fortnight and in his faeces for up to three months.

Symptoms. The incubation is about a fortnight. The illness begins with a mild febrile episode when the patient has malaise, headache and perhaps a sore throat: this is called the minor illness and with most people the illness stops at this stage. In only a few the second stage sets in after three or four days. The second stage is the major illness and it is caused by the presence of the virus in the central nervous system: in the minor illness the virus is present in the bloodstream but does not penetrate the nervous system. The symptoms of the major illness are those of meningitis—stiff neck, headache and vomiting. Many of these patients recover after a week or 10 days with no further symptoms: their illness is called non-paralytic poliomyelitis. Only a very few develop paralysis. It is important to realize that paralysis is really an uncommon feature of the disease; out of 100 people infected, perhaps only one gets paralysis.

Paralysis may affect any muscle of the body. Those most often affected are the muscles in the front of the lower leg, the quadriceps in the thigh and the deltoid in the upper arm. In severe cases almost all the muscles in the body may be paralysed, including the muscles of swallowing and of respiration. The paralysis is of the floppy or flaccid type.

Course. Muscles which are only slightly paralysed tend to recover quickly, often within a month. Where paralysis is severe, recovery is usually only partial and the patient is left with some permanent paralysis. The doctor can usually give a fairly accurate forecast at the end of the first month of illness.

Diagnosis. There is usually no difficulty about the diagnosis except in very mild or non-paralytic cases. Then it may be necessary to attempt to grow the virus from the faeces or the throat secretions. Examination of the cerebrospinal fluid does not help a great deal, and most doctors do not like doing a lumbar puncture in a patient who may be suffering from poliomyelitis because of the danger of making the patient worse.

Treatment. Treatment requires the co-operation of physician, nurse, physiotherapist and orthopaedic surgeon from the start of the illness. Paralysed limbs must be rested and supported by light removable splints, and passive movements of the affected muscles are carefully carried out: the aim is to prevent deformity from the overaction of non-paralysed muscles. After the first three weeks patients are treated in the pool; the limbs are made to feel lighter in the water and the patient can move them more freely. If the paralysis does not disappear after a few weeks, the surgeon will probably arrange for calipers or other form of support and the patient is encouraged to make use of the supported limb. The last stage of treatment is rehabilitation, when the patient is taught to make the best use of his weakened muscles and to return to as normal a life as possible.

Where the muscles of swallowing or of respiration are paralysed, the patient must be treated by a team of people highly skilled in their management. Paralysis of swallowing is treated by postural drainage to allow saliva to drain out of the mouth, and the patient is fed by intragastric tube or by intravenous infusion. A nurse must be constantly at the bedside ready to deal with any difficulty. If the patient can be kept alive for a week or 10 days, the paralysis will probably disappear and recovery be complete. With respiratory paralysis the outlook is not so good, for the muscles of respiration do not recover well. Artificial ventilation is needed, and this is carried out in an iron lung or by some method of positive pressure ventilation after a tracheostomy has been done. The treatment may go on for months or even years. It is usually possible to get even the worst patients off their machines for at least part of the day, but this requires great skill and judgement on the part of the doctor, and sympathy and understanding from all the team.

Prevention. Poliomyelitis can be prevented. Polio vaccine does protect and if it can be given to enough people, especially children, the disease dies out in that population. This has happened already in America and Europe, but in less developed countries it is not so easy to get all the people vaccinated. Poliomyelitis is still therefore an important epidemic disease in these countries, and it can still break out in developed countries if there is any falling off in vaccination.

Live vaccine is better than killed virus vaccine. It is given by mouth, on sugar lumps, instead of by injection, and it gives better protection. All infants should be given three doses at monthly intervals, and it is probably wise to give a further dose at school entry. All nurses should of course be protected against poliomyelitis (see Chapter 42).

ENCEPHALITIS

Encephalitis is not one but several different diseases. The symptoms are similar in all, but the cause is different. Some forms are caused by viruses carried by mites, ticks and other biting insects: examples are Japanese B encephalitis, St Louis and Russian spring-summer encephalitis. Some forms follow common infectious diseases such as measles, chickenpox or smallpox. The virus of herpes simplex causes one rare form, but in many forms the cause is simply not known.

Symptoms. The commonest symptom is coma: it may be deep and prolonged or light and fleeting. There are usually some neurological abnormalities such as paralysis, and often there are personality changes or behaviour disorders. No two cases are exactly the same but all have similarities. The outlook is unpredictable. Some patients lie in coma for months yet make a complete recovery; others may recover consciousness but are mentally severely damaged or left with paralysis. Many die, yet in some the illness is so mild that the diagnosis can easily be overlooked.

Treatment. There is no specific treatment, except in herpes encephalitis (p. 376). The patient must be nursed through long periods of unconsciousness when attention must be paid to his nutrition, the care of his skin and the drainage of his bladder and emptying of his bowels. It is a long but often a rewarding task.

Prevention. The prevention of insect-borne forms depends on public-health measures based on the epidemiology of the disease in different parts of the world. If one can prevent measles and other diseases by immunization one would also prevent the encephalitis that sometimes follows them, though one must be sure that the vaccines themselves are safe. For many forms of encephalitis there is no known method of prevention.

INFLUENZA

Influenza is caused by one of the influenza viruses. There are three groups of these viruses, called A, B and C, and in each group there are several strains or types. Sometimes new types appear, such as the Asian type in 1957 and the Hong Kong type in 1968 (see also p. 350). Many illnesses are called influenza or 'flu, but only those caused by influenza virus are true influenza. It is, of course, not possible to do virus studies on every suspected case and it is only in epidemics that a clinical diagnosis can be made with confidence. There is probably no such thing as gastric 'flu, though this is a commonly used term: influenza viruses do not cause gastro-enteritis.

Symptoms. The onset is sudden. The patient is seized with feelings of weakness, headache, backache and general muscular pains. He often has a sore throat and pain in the eyes. His temperature rises to between 38·3 °C and 40·5 °C (101 °F and 105 °F) and he is often shivery or may have rigors. He is often prostrated by his illness but the symptoms begin to abate after a week and thereafter he rapidly regains a feeling of well-being, though it may be a week or two before he is back to normal after a severe attack. The disease can be quite mild, depending partly on the patient's resistance but also on the type of virus causing the illness.

Complications. The commonest and most dangerous complication is pneumonia. This may be caused by the virus itself and is a very severe and sometimes fatal form; or it may be caused by staphylococci, pneumococci or other germs. The staphylococcal form is very dangerous.

Encephalitis is a very rare complication—most doctors never see such a case. A good deal is heard of post-influenzal depression, but depression is no commoner after influenza than after many other illnesses: it depends more on the psychological make-up of the patient than on any effect of the influenza viruses. It is a term that should be dropped altogether.

Diagnosis. The diagnosis has usually to be made clinically. Throat secretions can be sent to the laboratory for virus culture, but in an epidemic no laboratory could cope with all the work. It is enough to do cultures on a sample of the early cases to find out which virus is concerned. The serum of patients can also be examined to see if there has been a rise of antibody to the virus.

Treatment. Patients with influenza must be kept in bed till their fever has settled. They require copious hot drinks during the fever and often need analgesics for their pains. Insomnia is troublesome and the doctor will order hypnotics as required. Antibiotics have no effect on the illness and should not be given simply because the patient has a raised temperature. Antibiotics act on germs, not on temperature charts; they have no effect on viruses or on fevers caused by viruses. Unfortunately, they are often prescribed without good reason.

Patients with influenzal pneumonia need expert treatment. If the pneumonia is due to bacteria (see above), antibiotics are certainly needed and the choice of antibiotic depends on which bacterium is the cause of the pneumonia. Oxygen will be ordered, and corticosteroids, noradrenaline or other drugs will be needed if the patient is shocked.

Prevention. Influenza vaccines give protection for only a few months at a time. They may be given in the autumn or winter when outbreaks are expected. They do not give complete protection but are worth giving to elderly persons or to those with heart or chest diseases, for in them influenza may be very dangerous. The difficulty with vaccines is that one does not know which strain of virus will cause the next outbreak. If it proves to be a new strain, a vaccine made from old strains will not protect. Special laboratories throughout the world try to track all new viruses and to prepare vaccines in advance of epidemics, but viruses travel quickly and vaccine preparation takes time.

RABIES

The cause of the disease is the rabies virus. This virus is a common cause of infection in small animals such as mongooses, minks, weasels and martens and even bats in many parts of the world. It does not cause severe illness in these animals but they can pass the infection to larger animals such as wolves, foxes and jackals, and these suffer severely and become rabid and then bite other animals, including dogs. The dogs in turn become rabid and bite man, giving him rabies.

Symptoms. The incubation period is between one and three months. This long period gives some chance of preventing the disease if measures are taken immediately after the bite (see below).

The symptoms are a mixture of nervous excitement and paralysis. Difficulty in swallowing is one of the commonest symptoms and this becomes so pronounced that the mere idea of swallowing terrifies the patient, especially of swallowing water: this fear of swallowing water is called hydrophobia, and the disease itself is often called hydrophobia. The progress of the disease is relentlessly downhill and the patient dies after a most distressing and terrifying illness.

Diagnosis. The saliva, urine, cerebrospinal fluid and faeces of the patient can be sent to the laboratory for virus culture, but the patient is likely to be dead before the results are known. After death the brain is examined for the presence of virus particles known as Negri bodies. In most cases the diagnosis of rabies is only too obvious during life.

Treatment. There is no specific treatment after the first symptoms have appeared. Sedation is the main source of relief from the worst aspects of the disease. Perhaps treatment with curare and artificial ventilation might keep the patient alive till the disease burned itself out; one successful case has been reported in America.

Prevention. A vaccine and a serum are both available. They must be given to the patient as soon after the bite as possible, and the course of treatment lasts at least a fortnight and is often successful. It is arduous for the patient and is not without risk, especially of vaccine encephalitis. People who are exposed to the risk of bites, for example those in charge of dog quarantine stations, can be actively immunized with vaccine. In island countries like Britain strict control of the entry of dogs from abroad prevents the importation of rabies, but in countries with common borders animals such as foxes can cross the frontier and the control of the disease is much more difficult.

ANTHRAX

The disease is caused by *Bacillus anthracis*. This is a germ which causes serious disease in animals, especially cattle, sheep and goats. The animals die and the germ escapes from their bodies and may contaminate any part of the carcase, wool, hides or bones. These may then be imported into countries thousands of miles away, and as the germ can survive months or years in the sporing stage, the disease can be carried to man in a distant country. Workers in the docks who handle the hides or in tanneries where the hides are cured may be infected; men who work in glue factories where bones are melted down are also at risk, as are people who handle bone fertilizers or the sacks containing them; and people who handle wool and hair in upholstery or carpet factories may breathe in some anthrax germs and so get the disease. Fortunately man is highly resistant to anthrax, so that though the risk of infection is very high, the number of workers who get anthrax is very small indeed.

Symptoms. The commonest form of the disease is the cutaneous form, often called malignant pustule: this is a bad name, for the sore is not malignant nor is it a pustule. The sore has a black centre (*anthrax* is the Greek word for coal) and a ring of purplish blisters around it. There is no pus in anthrax sore: this helps to distinguish it from boils and other septic sores. Lymphangitis often spreads from the sore to the nearest lymph glands. The commonest sites are the forearm and the head and neck. There is always a great deal of swelling of the tissues, often spreading far beyond the sore. The patient feels ill and has a fever and sometimes rigors, but cutaneous anthrax with modern treatment is rarely a fatal disease: the patient usually responds to treatment in a few days.

The pulmonary form of the disease, called often woolsorters' disease, is a highly fatal form of bronchitis with pulmonary oedema. It is fortunately much rarer. An intestinal form is rarer still.

Diagnosis. A swab from the sore can be stained and examined at once; the anthrax germ can be seen under the microscope. The swab is also rubbed on culture medium and the result of culture is known within 24 hours. Other laboratory tests include the inoculation of guinea-pigs, but the diagnosis of anthrax is usually easy clinically provided one thinks of the possibility of anthrax.

Treatment. The cutaneous form responds rapidly to penicillin, which must be given in high dosage. Local treatment of the sore is useless; the sore forms a scab which may take a few weeks to separate, but it is not infectious after the first day or two of treatment. For the pulmonary and intestinal forms penicillin is again the main treatment, along with all the emergency treatment needed to combat shock.

Prevention. The main line in prevention is to try to disinfect contaminated materials; this is easy with wool and hair but not so easy with hides. Control of exports in countries where the disease is common in animals is of great importance. A vaccine is available and should be given to all whose work involves the handling of contaminated materials.

TETANUS

The cause of tetanus is a germ called *Clostridium tetani* or the tetanus bacillus. It is very commonly present in soil and may easily get into wounds. It forms a very dangerous and powerful toxin which attacks nerve cells and causes spasms or convulsions of the related muscles.

Symptoms. The typical symptom of tetanus is spasm. This usually first attacks the muscles around the mouth and causes the twisting and grimacing of the mouth called trismus. Soon spasm appears in other muscles, especially those of the abdomen and the back, so that the patient's abdomen becomes board-like in hardness, and the back is arched. In the extreme form the whole of the back is lifted off the bed and only the shoulders and buttocks touch it—the condition is known as opisthotonos. In bad cases the patient may have violent spasms of the muscles of the limbs every few minutes, and this soon exhausts the patient. Spasm of the larynx or of the respiratory muscles can lead to sudden death unless immediately relieved. The disease lasts about three weeks, after which the spasms lessen and the patient returns to normal health. His care during these three weeks requires the highest nursing and medical skill.

Diagnosis. The diagnosis is usually painfully obvious at the bedside. Swabs may be taken of the wound and cultured for tetanus bacilli, but often tetanus follows trivial wounds and there is nothing to take a swab from.

Treatment. The essence of treatment is to abolish spasms by cutting out all stimulation of the patient. This involves absolute quiet in the sick room, and the minimum of interference with the patient as he lies in bed. It also involves the use of sedatives in doses which are very near the toxic limit. Many different drugs are used, the commonest being phenobarbitone and chlorpromazine; the dosage must be controlled by a doctor who is expert in their use. In very severe cases sedatives fail to control the spasms, and then the patient must be treated with curare, a drug which paralyses all the muscles in the body, including the muscles of breathing. This means that the patient must have a tracheostomy and be ventilated by a breathing machine. This treatment goes on for two or three weeks, and during that time a nurse must be constantly at the bedside and a doctor readily on call. If the patient can be kept alive for this time, recovery is eventually complete, but there are many hazards during the treatment with which only a well-trained team of doctors and nurses can deal.

Prevention. Tetanus is a preventable disease. Active immunization gives complete protection. Three doses of tetanus toxoid are needed, the first two at an interval of one month, the third after six months. This protects for many years; a booster dose should be given after 10 years. Infants are given this treatment when they receive triple vaccine, for this contains vaccine against diphtheria, whooping cough and tetanus (see Chapter 42).

ATS is anti-tetanic serum. It is important to understand the difference between this and tetanus toxoid. Tetanus toxoid is tetanus toxin changed slightly in the laboratory so that it is no longer poisonous but still stimulates the production of antibody against tetanus in the body of the person injected. This is his own antibody and therefore remains in his body and protects him for many years or even for life. ATS is serum derived from another animal that has been immunized with tetanus toxoid: it too contains antibody against tetanus, but it is animal, not human antibody, and the human body gets rid of it quickly, so that the protection it gives is only temporary, not more than a few weeks. Being a foreign substance, it can cause serious reactions in man, and its protective effect is uncertain, so that it is not used now so much as formerly. Serum can, of course, be obtained from another human being who has been immunized and this is free from the danger of side-effects, but it is in very short supply. ATS is still used in serious and dirty wounds but the real prevention of tetanus lies in active immunization with toxoid (see Chapter 42).

Chapter 39

Acute Infections (continued)

by A. B. CHRISTIE

Infectious hepatitis—enterovirus infections—meningitis—leptospiral infections—miscellaneous infections

---

INFECTIOUS HEPATITIS (Infectious jaundice)

There are two types of infectious jaundice—infectious hepatitis and serum hepatitis. Both are caused by a virus, but only the virus of serum hepatitis has been isolated. Infectious hepatitis is conveyed in the faeces of patients and carriers: it may spread by direct contact when hygene is poor, or it may be water- or food-borne. Serum hepatitis is conveyed mainly in blood: the virus gets into the human body in blood transfusions or in any injection where there is a danger that even the minutest trace of blood from some previous injection remains in the syringe. Heroin addicts are very liable to get this form of jaundice from sharing syringes. In medical and nursing practice disposable syringes should always be used for injections or for taking samples of blood.

Symptoms. The incubation period of infectious hepatitis is about one month; of serum hepatitis it is about three months. The onset is gradual with vague abdominal complaints. After about a week the patient's urine becomes dark with bile and soon the conjunctivae appear yellow; within a few days the yellowness spreads all over the body. The patient is febrile and feels very miserable, but the symptoms begin to clear up by the end of a week, though the jaundice persists often for several weeks. Patients with serum hepatitis are usually more ill than those with infectious hepatitis.

In some patients the disease is much more severe. The jaundice deepens and the patient's condition deteriorates. This is most liable to occur in women of child-bearing age. In some of these patients the jaundice begins to clear after many weeks, but in others the patient falls into coma and dies. In some the disease is overwhelming from the start with rapid ∂nset of hepatic coma. Once coma sets in, few patients survive.

Hepatitis may occur without jaundice—anicteric hepatitis (*icterus* is a Greek word meaning yellowness). But hepatitis must never be regarded as a trivial disease: it is one of the most severe infections, causing much debility and not a few deaths.

Diagnosis. The diagnosis is obvious from the jaundice. Various tests, including liver function tests, are carried out to help the doctor to distinguish the disease from other forms of jaundice, especially obstructive jaundice. Australia or SH antigen is found in the blood in serum hepatitis but not in infectious hepatitis.

Treatment. In the mild and moderate cases the essence of treatment is rest. This does not mean that the patient is confined to bed till every trace of jaundice has disappeared, but he should take things easily and have a long convalescence, not returning to work till he is thoroughly fit. The liver has enormous powers of recovery but it takes time to get back to normal.

The type of diet does not matter a great deal. High carbohydrate and high protein diet have both been used: the important thing is to maintain the patient's nutrition. In the early stages, the patient's appetite is poor and he usually dislikes fatty food, but after the first week he is hungry and there is no need to restrict any article of food. Care must be taken over drugs, for many are toxic to the liver, e.g. chlorpromazine and some hypnotics.

In very severe cases more strenuous methods must be tried. Corticosteroids sometimes help to reduce jaundice in subacute cases, but they are not life-saving in fulminating cases. When coma sets in, exchange transfusions may be tried and even perfusion through an artificial kidney machine or through animal liver; but these methods are rarely successful.

Prevention. When the virus of hepatitis is found it may be possible to have a vaccine against the disease. Until then prevention depends on personal hygiene, and on pure water and food supplies. Serum hepatitis can be reduced by cutting the number of transfusions: if the patient is given only one pint of blood, the question arises whether he really requires a blood transfusion at all. In other words, the risk of hepatitis should always be balanced against the need for blood. All injections should be given with disposable syringes. There is no way of preventing hepatitis in drug addicts, other than trying to cure their addiction.

ENTEROVIRUS INFECTIONS

The three groups of viruses called enteroviruses are the polioviruses, echoviruses and Coxsackie viruses. They are excreted in the faeces, hence the name enterovirus (*entero* is the Greek word for intestine). Polioviruses cause only poliomyelitis, but the other two groups cause a variety of diseases.

Both echo and Coxsackie viruses can cause *lymphocytic meningitis*. This is a form of meningitis in which the cerebrospinal fluid is usually clear and contains lymphocytes, whereas in meningococcal meningitis the fluid is turbid and contains polymorphonuclear or pus cells. One form of echo meningitis may be accompanied by a macular rash. Lymphocytic meningitis usually clears up without specific treatment.

Coxsackie viruses are the cause of *Bornholm disease*. (Bornholm is a Danish island, not a man's name: one of the early descriptions of the disease was of an outbreak on the island.) The illness consists of spasms of violent pain, usually round the lower chest or upper abdomen. It causes the patient to stop in his steps, sometimes he throws himself on the floor and gasps with the pain. The name 'devil's grip' has been given to it and emphasizes the agonizing character of the pain. In between spasms the patient is comfortable, though dreading the next bout of pain. The illness lasts only a few days and recovery is complete. It tends to occur in localized epidemics.

Another disease caused by Coxsackie viruses is *herpangina*. This is a condition in which there is inflammation of the throat, and tiny blisters or nodules can be seen on the tonsils and pharynx. The child is feverish and miserable but the condition settles in a few days. *Hand, foot and mouth disease* is also caused by Coxsackie viruses. Blisters occur on the mouth, hands and feet and the patient is feverish for a day or two. (The disease has nothing in common with foot and mouth disease of cattle.) Many vague febrile illnesses are caused by echo and Coxsackie viruses. The symptoms are those of an upper respiratory tract infection and the illness is often called simply *acute febrile catarrh*.

In young babies echo or Coxsackie viruses can cause severe generalized infections with destructive effects in many organs of the body. Myocarditis or pancarditis may occur in these babies and may cause death in neonates. Pericarditis is a rare form of enterovirus infection in adults.

LEPTOSPIRAL INFECTIONS

The two common leptospiral infections are Weil's disease and canicola fever. These diseases are caused by *Leptospira icterohaemorrhagiae* and *L. canicola*. There are many other leptospirae which cause different diseases in many parts of the world.

Symptoms. In Weil's disease the illness begins with a rise in temperature and malaise. After a few days in severe cases the patients become jaundiced, and a day or two later the kidneys begin to fail; the patient passes very little urine (oliguria), and soon no urine at all (anuria). At this stage haemorrhages appear in the skin and in the conjunctivae. The outlook for such patients is grave, but in most cases the illness is much milder and neither jaundice nor oliguria occur: such patients do well.

Canicola fever is a milder disease. The illness begins as a vague fever with headache and malaise, and sometimes the disease does not progress beyond this stage. In many patients signs of meningitis occur, and if a lumbar puncture is done the cerebrospinal fluid is found to contain lymphocytes; the illness is then a form of lymphocytic meningitis. This clears up after a week or 10 days and the patient recovers quickly. Jaundice and urinary failure are rare in canicola fever.

Treatment. Penicillin is effective against both the leptospirae and may be given for treatment of the disease. It is effective in canicola fever and in the early stages or milder cases of Weil's disease. When jaundice and renal failure are present, penicillin is no longer effective: the renal failure is caused by blockage of the renal tubules with dead kidney cells and other debris caused by an inflammatory reaction to the leptospirae, and penicillin cannot clear this away. The most hopeful treatment is by dialysis, a means whereby the function of the kidneys is carried out by the dialysing machine or artificial kidney in the hope that the patient's own kidneys will recover by the natural process of repair. The outlook is grave but not hopeless.

Prevention. Leptospirae are conveyed to man usually by some other animal. *Leptospira icterohaemorrhagiae* infects rats and is passed in their urine into water. Man is infected by exposure at work to infected water: sewer workers, miners and fish curers are liable to be attacked. Infection can also occur by bathing in contaminated water. *L. canicola* infects dogs (canicola means dog-borne). The dog is often not ill but becomes a carrier and passes the germ in its urine. It is easy to see how infection can then pass to man. Prevention consists in preventing the access of rats to working premises. Dogs can be immunized against canicola infection. An infected dog can be treated by penicillin but sometimes it is safer to have it destroyed.

MISCELLANEOUS INFECTIONS

Q Fever

This is a disease caused by a germ called *Coxiella burneti*. (Both Cox and Burnet were scientists connected with its discovery.) It is a disease mainly of sheep, goats and cattle, but the germ can spread to man. It can be spread in milk or by direct contact with the animals. Q means query: when the disease was first described in 1937, the cause was unknown and therefore queried. This happened in Queensland, but the Q means query, not Queensland.

The symptoms are those of an acute febrile disease with respiratory symptoms. X-rays often show extensive pneumonic consolidation of the lungs. The patient may have a high temperature for a week or 10 days but eventually the symptoms disappear and the patient recovers his previous health.

Treatment. The patient needs all the nursing given to patients with pneumonia. Tetracycline is the best antibiotic to use.

Prevention. The infection causes very little disease in the infected animals, and it does not affect their economic value. It is therefore difficult to introduce measures for its control in animals. Pasteurization of milk must be carried out thoroughly to destroy *Coxiella burneti* for it can survive at a temperature only a degree or two below pasteurization temperature. Vaccines for protecting workers with animals are under trial.

Psittacosis

Psittacosis is an infection of birds, mainly of the parrot family. (*Psittacos* is the Greek word for parrot.) The disease is caused by germs called Bedsoniae after the bacteriologist Bedson who first described them. Many birds other than parrots can be infected, including sparrows and pigeons. Most infections in man occur among those who handle parrots, budgerigars and pigeons. The Bedsoniae are excreted in the birds' faeces and so contaminate the cages and straw. When the cages are cleaned out, the dust is full of the germs and can be breathed in by the attendant.

Symptoms. The symptoms are mainly respiratory in nature. The patient has a cough and increased respiration, but often changes seen on X-ray are more extensive than the patient's symptoms suggest. There is considerable malaise and the temperature ranges between 37·7 °C and 38·8 °C (100 °F and 102 °F). The illness usually abates after a week or 10 days, but in severe cases it drags on much longer. Death is a rare occurrence in psittacosis; when it occurs it is due to respiratory failure.

Diagnosis. Blood, throat washings and sputum can all be cultured for the presence of the germ, and the serum can be tested for antibody. Post-mortem examination of birds can also help in the diagnosis.

Treatment. The patients need all the nursing treatment given to patients with pneumonia. Tetracycline is the best antibiotic.

Prevention. People who keep pigeons and birds of the parrot family should be made aware of the risks: wet methods in cleaning cages are safer than dry, for they keep down dust. Budgerigars are usually bred in large commercial plants, and they can be treated prophylactically with tetracycline. Such birds are safe to buy: birds from doubtful sources may be dangerous. Wild pigeons abound in cities but they have not been known to spread psittacosis to man.

Erythema multiforme: Stevens-Johnson syndrome

This disease is commonly seen in infectious diseases hospitals, but it is not certain that it is an infectious disease. Sometimes the patient has an attack of tonsillitis before the onset of this disease, but not always. Sometimes the patient has been treated with sulphonamides or other drugs and many doctors think the condition is an allergic response to the treatment. The cause is uncertain.

The patient reaches a fever hospital because he develops a rash which *looks* infectious. It is present all over the body, but is often much more marked on the limbs than on the trunk and can look very like smallpox. The spots vary in size and character—this is why it is called multiform: some are pustules, some are flat macules, some form big blisters or blebs, but the most characteristic appearance is the target spot, a large round blotch with rings of varying colour in it. The patient nearly always has a very sore mouth, often has conjunctivitis, and sometimes has vaginitis, urethritis or, in males, sores on the penis. The outlook is good, though some patients may be very toxic and have scarcely an inch of skin not covered with the rash. The disease is very rarely fatal.

The patient needs careful nursing, especially when the stomatitis is severe. In severe cases the skin must be treated very gently for it tends to break down easily. Corticosteroids are sometimes prescribed but their effect is doubtful. As we do not know the cause for certain, there is no known way of preventing this disease, but more care in prescribing drugs might cut down the incidence slightly.

Chapter 40

Some Tropical Infections

by A. B. CHRISTIE

Cholera—malaria—plague—typhus—leprosy—miscellaneous

CHOLERA

Cholera is caused by a germ called *Vibrio cholerae*; there are several different strains or types of vibrio, one of the most prevalent of recent years being the El Tor vibrio. The disease is spread by contaminated water or food, and carriers are important sources of infection.

Symptoms. The main early symptoms are diarrhoea and vomiting. The typical stool contains flakes of mucus in a watery fluid, the rice-water stool of cholera. The diarrhoea is often extremely severe and a patient can lose several litres of fluid from his body very rapidly in this way. Dehydration can occur quickly in a patient with severe diarrhoea and vomiting, and this leads to collapse and shock.

Mild and even asymptomatic cases occur, and some of these may become unrecognized chronic carriers.

Diagnosis. *Vibrio cholerae* can be seen under a dark-ground microscope in a fresh specimen of stool; this is best obtained on a rectal swab which is immediately broken off into a small bottle of special transport broth. The vibrio can also be grown on solid medium in the laboratory. The important diagnosis is the clinical one, for there is no time to wait for a bacteriological report when a patient is ill with cholera.

Treatment. The essence of treatment is rehydration. Fluid must be given intravenously in bad cases, and the first litre or two must be run in quickly. The lost salt and water must be replaced, and bicarbonate may also be needed to counteract the acidosis which is often present. As soon as the patient responds to this treatment and his pulse becomes stronger, rehydration can usually be continued by mouth. Children need special care, for it is more difficult to correct acidosis in them.

Tetracyclines and chloramphenicol are both effective in ridding the bowel of vibrios. Tetracyclines are much less toxic than chloramphenicol. A three-day course of tetracycline is enough in most cases.

Prevention. The most important part of prevention is good hygiene, especially in relation to food and water supply. Health education and sanitation are vital to any scheme of prevention. Vaccines are available against the disease and cut down the frequency of attacks, but the protection does not last long (see p. 403).

MALARIA

The disease is caused by the malaria parasite of which there are several varieties, each of which causes different clinical types of malaria. The parasites are carried by the anopheles group of mosquitoes which bite man to suck his blood and at the same time inject malaria parasites into the victim.

Symptoms. The symptoms are very variable, but in most attacks fever and rigors occur. The frequency of the rigors depends on the type of parasite in the patient's blood. But not all cases run true to type, and malaria can mimic almost any disease. Any febrile illness in a patient who has been in an area where malaria occurs should be regarded as possibly due to malaria and blood films should be examined for the parasites.

Diagnosis. This is made by the examination of stained films of the patient's blood. The examination takes only a few minutes. It should never be omitted in a febrile patient in or from a malarious country.

Types of malaria. *Benign tertian malaria* is characterized by rigors on alternate days. In spite of its name it is not always a mild disease (see chart, Chapter 3, p. 31). *Quartan malaria* causes rigors every third day. *Malignant tertian malaria* can cause a wide variety of symptoms. There may be high continued fever with little or no daily variation, or the patient may be cold and clammy and collapsed. Cerebral malaria soon leads to coma and death if not treated very quickly. Malaria is always a curable disease if it is diagnosed early enough; but after a certain stage is passed in the worst cases, death is inevitable.

Treatment. Anti-malarial drugs destroy or suppress the parasite in the patient's body. The correct drug must be selected according to the type of parasite in the patient's body. Some of the drugs are:

Proguanil monohydrochloride.
Pyrimethamine.
Chloroquine phosphate or sulphate.
Pamaquin.
Mepacrine.
Quinine.

Most of them cause some toxicity, and drug resistance tends to develop in the malaria parasite so that research is constantly going on to discover new drugs, and so keep ahead of the parasite's resistance.

The drugs are used both for prophylaxis and treatment. In prophylaxis the drug prevents the parasite multiplying in the patient's body and so prevents symptoms. The drug must be taken regularly all the time the person is in a malarious area and for some time after. Even if a person is in such an area for an hour or two, e.g. in port or airport, he should have suppressive treatment. Treatment of an attack requires bigger doses; the drug chosen depends on the type of parasite. In severe cases the drug must be given intravenously, and emergency measures include intravenous infusions and the use of various anti-shock drugs.

Prevention. Prevention can be considered under three heads—preventing the breeding of mosquitoes, preventing mosquitoes from biting man, and the use of suppressive drugs. The prevention of breeding depends on abolishing swamps and pools of stagnant water in which the larvae (young forms) of the parasite grow. The larvae can also be attacked by various sprays applied to collections of water, sometimes from aeroplanes. Prevention of bites means the wearing of special clothing and footwear when mosquitoes are about, and the use of nets over doors and windows and round beds. The use of suppressive drugs has already been discussed.

PLAGUE

Plague is a disease caused by a germ called *Pasteurella pestis*. This germ infects rats; sometimes it causes many deaths of rats, but often plague-infected rats remain well. Fleas feed on the rats' blood and if a flea then bites man, the germ is transferred to the victim and plague develops after two to six days.

Symptoms and treatment. There are three clinical types of plague. In *bubonic plague* there is a swelling or bubo in the patient's groin or axilla; this often breaks down, but the danger to the patient is from invasion of his bloodstream by the plague germ. *Pneumonic* and *septicaemic* plague are the other two forms. In the past all three forms were highly fatal diseases. The Black Death of the Middle Ages was almost certainly plague and it swept across continents, killing millions of people in its path. Today it is much rarer, though epidemics can still occur in conditions of poor hygiene; it has been common, for example, in Vietnam. Fortunately, today the disease can be successfully treated by sulphonamides and antibiotics.

Prevention. The prevention of plague depends on preventing rats and their fleas getting in contact with man. This is difficult in primitive conditions or during field warfare. In better conditions, rat-proofing of buildings and good hygiene in living quarters can be achieved. Ships must be de-ratted at regular intervals to prevent the importation of infected rats into ports, and Port Health Authorities carry out regular trapping and examination of dead rats to make sure none are carrying plague. Plague vaccine gives some protection (see p. 404). Insecticides are useful for killing fleas in dangerous areas.

TYPHUS

Typhus fever is caused by one of the *Rickettsia* germs: *R. prowazeki* is the commonest. The germ is spread by the body louse which passes it in its faeces. The patient scratches because of irritation caused by the presence of the lice and the rickettsia gets into the body through the scratched skin.

Symptoms. Typhus fever is a serious disease, and in the past caused many deaths wherever living conditions were bad and lice therefore common.

Such conditions used to be the rule in gaols, and typhus was often called gaol fever. The disease begins suddenly with fever and headache; soon the patient is racked with generalized pains, and often he is delirious at this stage. Finally he sinks into a mental torpor and dies in great misery. A red papular rash often appears on the chest and abdomen. The temperature is high throughout the illness, except towards the end when it may fall below normal.

Treatment. Chloramphenicol is a very effective drug; if given early enough, it saves the lives of most patients. The patient needs very careful nursing and all attendants must take precautions against lice passing from the patient. The patient on arrival must be covered with a sheet, and an attendant wearing protective clothing shaves the patient's body of all hair and an insecticide is used to kill lice. If there are no lice, there can be no typhus.

Prevention. The main part of prevention is to ensure good living conditions and cleanliness so that lice cannot infest man. This is easy in civilized areas, but not so easy under primitive conditions. Typhus vaccine gives some protection (see p. 403).

LEPROSY

Leprosy is caused by a germ *Bacillus leprae*, but close and prolonged contact seems necessary before a leper infects another person. Usually it is not possible to trace the path of infection, for years may pass before the the first sign of the disease appears.

Symptoms. The first sign in one form of the disease is a red or coppery patch on the skin of the hands or feet or on the face. This gradually thickens and forms a nodule in the skin. On the face almost the whole skin may be thickened, completely altering the features of the patient. Finally the nodules break down, forming large ulcers, often destroying the tissues of the nose or of the fingers and toes.

In the other form of the disease the nerves of the limbs are attacked. The first signs are pale patches on the skin in which there is no feeling. Gradually the nerves become thickened and large areas of the skin become anaesthetic or lack feeling, and sores form through injuries which cause no pain. Paralysis of limbs is common and adds greatly to the distress of the patient. In some patients both the nodular and the anaesthetic form of the disease are present. A patient in the late stages of the disease is a pathetic sight, with sores, paralysis and rotting stumps of fingers and toes. The patient with severe leprosy dies in the end from exhaustion, or from some added disease which he cannot resist in his grossly weakened state.

Leprosy has always been a dreaded disease, and the leper is conscious of this. He suffers from a *visible* disease and he knows the loathing it causes in those who see it. He is one of the untouchables of the ages. He needs understanding and sympathy.

Treatment. Sulphones and newer drugs have changed the outlook for leprosy, though there is still no speedy cure. The disease can, however, be arrested. Plastic and orthopaedic surgery can do a great deal to prevent or correct deformity.

MISCELLANEOUS INFECTIONS

Brief notes on some of the diseases prevalent in the tropics

Name	Causative organism	Mode of spread	Principal symptoms	Treatment
African Trypanosomiasis (sleeping sickness)	A trypanosome	Tsetse fly	Fever, erythema, oedema, drowsiness, finally coma	Chemotherapy to destroy trypanosomes in the blood. Measures to eradicate tsetse fly
Amoebiasis	Entamoeba histolytica	By food, water and carriers	Diarrhoea, later vague illness, fever	Chemotherapy, hygiene and sanitation
Ankylostomiasis (hookworm disease)	Ankylostoma, a genus of nematode round worms	Widespread in tropical and subtropical countries	Itching, anaemia, and epigastric discomfort	Chemotherapy, iron and good diet
Bilharziasis (schistosomiasis, or snail fever)	A parasite that lives part of its cycle in certain freshwater snails	Wading in, bathing in or drinking infected water	Light to severe, even fatal disease, with rashes and painful haematuria	Preventive by destroying snails with molluscacides—drugs entering the field aimed at killing the parasite in human blood are undergoing trial
Cholera	(See p. 388)			
Dengue (dandy, and also as breakbone fever)	Virus	Aedes mosquito	Mild to acute—headache, recurrent fever, rashes, malaise, intense joint and muscle pains	Analgesics for pain. Good nursing, rest and encouragement to raise morale

Disease	Cause	Carrier / Transmission	Symptoms	Treatment / Control
Dracontiasis (guinea worm disease)	Nematode (round worm)	Infected water. Embryos enter *water fleas* (Cyclops) and reach host in drinking water	Urticaria, blister through which worm extrudes	Remove worm by dragging it out where it extrudes. Avoid infection of worm track
Dysentery	(See p. 357)			
Elephantiasis Filariasis	Microfilaria, the developing worm, which is microscopic	Mosquitoes, often by *Culex fatigans*	Blockage of lymphatics in the tissues, with enlargement (elephantiasis) of the legs and external genitals with thickened scaly skin	Preventive; apart from controlling the breeding of mosquitoes, there is no known effective treatment
Leishmaniasis (kala-azar)	*Leishmania donovani*	Sandfly *Phlebotomus*	Spleen enlarged, anaemia, wasting leading to prostration. Dry rough skin, pigmentation	Intravenous injection of antimony, given early. Penicillin for secondary infections. Repellents, destruction of sandflies
Leprosy	(See p. 391)			
Malaria	(See p. 389)			
Onchocerciasis (river blindness)	Minute worm	By small black flies or gnats	Lumpy nodules appear in subcutaneous tissues over bony areas. In some cases the eyes are infected and destructive changes lead to blindness, partial or complete	Control measures to reduce number of flies. No known effective treatment. It is estimated that over 200 millions are affected by total blindness or economic blindness

Name	Causative organism	Mode of spread	Principal symptoms	Treatment
Paratyphoid fever	(See Typhoid, p. 359)			
Plague	(See p. 390)			
Sandfly fever	Virus	Sandflies	Similar to dengue (see p. 392) without a rash	Rest and analgesics
Smallpox	(See p. 374)			
Trachoma (granular conjunctivitis)	Virus-like body of the lymphogranuloma psittacosis group.	By tears, freely between children and families. Widespread infection in the Middle East, spread by flies	(see p. 646)	Local and systemic chemotherapy
Typhoid fever	(See p. 359)			
Typhus	(See p. 390)			
Undulant fever (brucellosis)	(See p. 361)			
Yaws	Treponema pertenue, a fine spirochaete	Organism present in skin sores rapidly spread by contact, as in families	Anaemia, infectious sores. Lesions occur in limbs, similar to gummata in syphilis, but yaws is a non-venereal infection	A single injection of long-acting penicillin can effect a cure
Yellow fever	Virus	Aedes mosquito	May be mild or severe, with headache and pains in the limbs, jaundice, nausea, vomiting, rigors and high fever, albuminuria	Good nursing, liberal fluids and alkalies. Protection by a special vaccine is available

Chapter 41

Tuberculosis

by A. B. CHRISTIE

*Introduction—the disease process—systems affected by tuberculosis—
symptoms—treatment—prevention*

Tuberculosis differs from most of the other infections described in this
book, except leprosy, in that it is a chronic, not an acute illness in most
cases. Although chronic, it is relentless, and has been one of the great
killing diseases both in developed and undeveloped countries. Life in
developed, industrialized countries has in fact provided the conditions in
which the disease flourishes, and tuberculosis has often been carried into
undeveloped countries by settlers from developed countries with dire
results for the native population. The disease is still one of the great
scourges of mankind, but modern treatment and prevention are leading to
its control. One day it may be conquered, but there are still vast problems
to be solved before that happens. Today man has the answer to many
diseases: the difficulty is how to apply the knowledge over vast tracts of
country and masses of scattered peoples.

The cause of tuberculosis is the tubercle bacillus, *Mycobacterium
tuberculosis*. It may enter the body by two main routes—the respiratory or
the gastro-intestinal: in other words, the bacillus can be breathed in or
swallowed. There are two main types of tubercle bacilli, the human type
and the bovine. Most infections with the human type enter by the respiratory tract; bovine bacilli are present in milk and are therefore swallowed.
Respiratory infections lead to disease in the lungs, while gastro-intestinal
infections cause disease in the tonsils and cervical glands and in the linings
of the intestinal tract and the mesenteric glands. Once into the body,
tubercle bacilli can spread to any part: human bacilli may spread to the
meninges, causing tuberculous meningitis, while bovine bacilli often cause
tuberculosis of the bones and joints.

The disease process. When the tubercle bacillus reaches any part of the
body, it sets up a slow form of inflammation. Lymphocytes and other cells
surround the germ and form a tiny nodule which encloses the bacillus,
though a few usually escape and reach the nearest lymph glands where they
are caught in another nodule. There may be a tiny nodule in the tonsil with
slight swelling of a cervical gland, a nodule in the lung and a swollen
mediastinal gland, or a nodule in the intestinal wall and an enlarged

mesenteric gland. The nodule and the gland form the *primary complex* of tuberculosis. In most infections the disease stops at this stage. The body defences clamp down on the invaders and seal off the complex by depositing calcium salts in it, which harden with time and imprison the bacilli. X-ray pictures of the lung or other organ show these complexes as dense small shadows. A nurse should not worry if she is told she has such a shadow in her X-ray: it means she has at some time been infected, but that the infection has been overcome and, as a result, she has become immune to the disease.

Occasionally the body's defences are not so successful. The nodule, or tubercle, as it is often called, instead of hardening, becomes soft and cheesy. This is known as caseous (i.e. cheesy) degeneration. Germs can escape from such tubercles in large numbers and spread to any part of the body. They may spread in the lung, causing *tuberculous bronchopneumonia*, or out into the bloodstream, causing small tubercles in almost every organ of the body, *miliary tuberculosis*. Sometimes they settle in one organ only, often the kidney where they cause *renal tuberculosis*; or they can reach the meninges and cause *tuberculous meningitis*.

All the above applies to infection of the body for the first time, or to primary tuberculosis; in the vast majority of cases, little damage is done. This is true of most infections with tubercle bacilli in childhood and in adults infected for the first time; such patients are tuberculin-negative before infection but tuberculin-positive after infection (see p. 403). They have become immune. Sometimes, however, this immunity breaks down, possibly because of bad working or housing conditions or malnutrition, and a tuberculin-positive person develops tuberculosis. The reasons for this are not understood, but the disease in such people takes a different course from primary tuberculosis. Instead of being locked up in hard tubercles, the bacilli spread widely in the lung causing caseous degeneration and great destruction of lung tissue. Cavities form in these areas of destruction and bronchi may be eroded by the advancing disease process. Patients may then expel tubercle bacilli into the air when they cough and this makes them dangerously infectious to other people. (Patients with primary tuberculosis by contrast are not usually infectious.) A blood vessel can be eaten into by the eroding process and then the patient coughs up blood, often in alarming amounts known as *haemoptysis*. This adult form of the disease is what is meant by the old term *consumption*, rarely heard today.

Sometimes the disease in the tuberculin-positive adult is not so severe as described above, probably depending on the patient's resistance, though no one is quite sure what that term really means. A patient may develop a pleural effusion with very little obvious disease in the lung itself. Sometimes there is disease in the lung but it is limited to a small area only. Sometimes there is no sign in the lung but the disease shows itself in the renal and genital tracts as *genito-urinary tuberculosis*.

All degrees of severity are met with, and even before the days of anti-biotics and chemotherapy many patients responded to treatment in sanatoria. The symptoms and treatment are also contained in various chapters according to the system affected, e.g. pulmonary tuberculosis in Chapter 21, p. 203, genito-urinary tuberculosis, Chapter 54, p. 530.

Symptoms. It is more important to understand the disease process as described above than to try to learn all about the symptoms of tuberculosis. There are two types of symptoms—those due to toxaemia and those due to local destructive disease. *Toxaemia* causes fever, tiredness, wasting, weakness, headaches, sweating and loss of energy. These symptoms may go on for months before local symptoms appear. The commonest local symptom is cough, slight at first and often attributed to 'a cold I can't shake off', but later becoming so severe and racking that the patient feels there must be something more serious the matter with him. Sometimes the appearance of blood in his sputum is the first sign that alarms him and takes him to his doctor. Pleurisy declares its presence by pain in the side, though often a pleural effusion develops painlessly. In *genito-urinary disease*, the earliest symptom may be no more than *polyuria*, but *dysuria* and *haematuria* are also common and more alarming. Often there are no suspicious symptoms at all, and the presence of tuberculosis of the lungs may be detected in a routine X-ray examination.

Diagnosis. The diagnosis depends on a complete examination of the patient. This includes X-ray of the lungs, bacteriological examination of the sputum and the urine, skin tests (see p. 204) and various blood tests which help to assess the activity of any disease present. If bone or joint disease is suspected, X-ray of the part affected is carried out.

Treatment. Three factors are concerned: adequate rest, adequate nutrition and drug therapy. Rest is necessary for the whole patient, but also special rest for the affected part. Rest of the lung can be secured by making part of it immobile; this is done by various surgical operations, but these are rarely carried out nowadays when drug therapy has so changed the outlook for patients. The patient himself should rest in bed till he is afebrile and has no other symptom of toxaemia. With drug treatment the period may be only a week or two, not months or years as in the past; many patients can have all their treatment at home, or can be sent home to complete their treatment after only a short time in hospital. With bone or joint disease, the affected part must still be rested for long periods, and splints or spinal frames are still required. But where milk is pasteurized this form of tuberculosis is almost unknown today, an immense change from 20 or 30 years ago when special hospitals were always full of children suffering from bone or joint tuberculosis. Many of these patients had to stay in hospital for years, often lying on a spinal frame all the time, and often after all the treatment they were still left with serious deformity of the limbs or spine.

Patients with tuberculosis need good food and good living conditions: a lot still depends on building up their strength and resistance. They require good nursing and, above all, understanding. Nearly every patient can be told he will make a fairly speedy recovery. Only those who live in poor underdeveloped countries now reach the late-stage disease before they get medical attention; *in such countries, tuberculosis is still an immense social and medical problem*.

The three main drugs are streptomycin, PAS (para-amino-salicylic acid) and INAH (isonicotinic acid hydrazide). These three drugs are usually given together; if the drugs are given singly, the tubercle bacilli may rapidly become resistant to them and this creates a serious problem both for the patient and for any person who may be infected by him with a resistant bacillus. When resistance to the three main drugs does occur, there are fortunately other drugs which can be used, such as ethionamide, pyrazinamide and thiacetazone. These are newer, but not better drugs than streptomycin, PAS and INAH. More drugs will probably be discovered, but the struggle between man and the tubercle bacillus will still go on.

Prevention. Prevention depends on three things: the early treatment of infectious patients to make them non-infectious as quickly as possible, and their isolation from other people, especially children, during the infectious period; the improvement of conditions of life for all people, including readily available medical services and a safe supply of milk; and immunization of all tuberculin-negative persons with B.C.G. (see p. 403). It is easy to write these recommendations: it is not so easy to carry them out, for they require immense organization, immense energy and vision, and a great deal of money. The last is the easiest, for it is a material consideration; the others depend on man himself.

Chapter 42

Prevention and Treatment of Acute Infections

by A. B. CHRISTIE

Antisera—vaccines—antibiotics—chemotherapy—immunization

ANTISERA

Serum is the clear liquid that separates out on the top of blood that has clotted. It contains the substances called globulins which carry the antibodies that have formed in the body in response to some stimulus. The commonest stimulus is a disease germ. When an animal or a man is injected with a fluid containing dead germs or some product of the germ such as toxin, antibodies form in his body against that germ or toxin, and this antibody will be present in the serum that separates from his blood. Such a serum is called antiserum because it contains these antibodies: if it contains antibodies to toxin, it is called an antitoxic serum or simply antitoxin. The name of the germ is also added, so that we get diphtheria antitoxin, tetanus antitoxin and so on.

Antisera and antitoxins are used less now than formerly. This is partly because some diseases, such as diphtheria, for which antitoxin is the correct treatment, have become less common, and partly because antibiotics have proved more effective in the treatment of some diseases, for example scarlet fever. Another reason is that antisera, if prepared from the blood of animals, often produce serum reactions when injected into man: for this reason tetanus antitoxin is now used much less than formerly (see p. 382). When the serum is derived from another human being, there is no danger of these reactions. Human tetanus antitoxin and human measles serum are both used in prevention, but, being produced from human blood, they are, of course, in short supply. Gamma globulin antibodies are carried in the globulin of serum, and gamma globulin is the antibody-containing part of the globulin extracted from the serum. It, too, comes from human blood and is in short supply. If the person has been recently immunized against a disease, for example smallpox, his blood will contain a lot of antibody against smallpox, and the extract may be called hyperimmune anti-vaccinial gamma globulin; this is used in protecting close contacts of smallpox (see p. 374).

VACCINES

Antisera, antitoxins and gamma globulin are all injected into the body to give it a ready-made supply of antibodies. These have not been manufactured *in* the body, and are, after a week or two, destroyed or eliminated by the body. They can therefore give the person only temporary protection, although this protection is immediate. A *vaccine*, on the other hand, does not contain antibody. It is composed of a lot of germs, live or dead, or of some product of germs such as toxin. When injected, these germs or toxin stimulate the body to produce antibodies against them. This process takes time, so the protection is not immediate; *but the antibodies, when they do appear, have been manufactured in the body* and therefore stay in the body for a long time, probably for life. One injection of vaccine just stimulates the antibody-producing mechanism and rarely results in enough antibody to give protection, but a second injection given a month later stirs the mechanism into active production of antibody, and a third leads to a great outpouring of antibody. This antibody may fall to a low level after the passage of time, but the mechanism remains sensitive and will respond to a similar stimulus even after many years. The stimulus may be another dose of vaccine, or it may be natural infection with the germ concerned. Thus if a person has had three injections of tetanus vaccine, *not* tetanus antitoxin, his body will react at once to the introduction of *Clostridium tetani* in a wound, or to the injection of more tetanus vaccine. In other words he has been actively immunized against tetanus and this gives him protection against the disease for many years, probably for life.

Some vaccines consist of live germs which have been grown in the laboratory in such a way that they no longer cause active disease but still stimulate the production of antibody. Examples are smallpox vaccine and live polio vaccine. Some contain dead germs, for example typhoid vaccine (TAB). Some contain no germs but only their toxins, and these toxins have been altered in the laboratory so that they are no longer toxic, but still provoke antitoxin; these altered toxins are called *toxoids*. Examples are tetanus toxoid and diphtheria toxoid (APT or alum-precipitated toxoid). In general, toxoids and live vaccines are better immunizing substances than dead vaccines.

ANTIBIOTICS AND CHEMOTHERAPY

Antibiotic is composed of two Greek words, *anti* and *bios*. *Bios* means life, and *anti* means against: an antibiotic is a substance derived from a living thing, usually a mould, and it acts against other living things, usually germs. But they are really just chemicals like many other medicines and are now often produced in chemical laboratories without the use of moulds at all. Chemotherapy means treatment with chemicals, for example sulphonamides, or quinine, and one tends to think that treatment with antibiotics is something quite different. In both instances we give the patient chemical substances in the hope that they will kill the germs that are causing his illness, or at least stop them multiplying: there is no essential difference.

The most important thing in treatment is to use the correct chemical, whether it is an antibiotic or not. This may sound obvious, but often a drug is prescribed before it is known which germ is causing the illness. Sometimes this cannot be avoided, as when the patient is seriously ill, and the doctor must make a clinical guess about the bacteriological cause; an experienced doctor usually guesses correctly, but he may have to change the treatment when the report comes from the laboratory. When a patient is not seriously ill, one can usually wait for the report before starting treatment with an antibiotic or other drug. This is much wiser than to put a patient on some powerful drug in the hope that it will do some good. The trouble is that drugs have toxic effects, and it is wrong to put patients on a toxic drug without good clinical reason. Another fault is to think that a new drug must be better than an old one, and patients are sometimes treated with a new drug when an older one would do him far more good. Penicillin was one of the first antibiotics to be discovered; it is still in many cases the best. This is true even of penicillin G, the one we can call 'ordinary' penicillin. Some of the newer penicillins, such as methicillin or cloxacillin, are essential in certain circumstances; but if the germ is sensitive to ordinary penicillin, this is a much more potent or powerful drug than the newer ones. One should always know exactly why one antibiotic or other drug is used in preference to another. Tetracyclines can attack some germs that resist penicillin; this is a correct reason for using tetracycline. Chloramphenicol, on the other hand, is the best drug by far in the treatment of typhoid fever and must be used in that disease: but it has no advantage over other antibiotics in the treatment of most other diseases. Moreover, it is a very toxic drug and it is therefore wrong to use it except in typhoid fever and a few other uncommon diseases.

It is much better for a nurse to understand the general rules for the use of drugs in infections, rather than to try to learn the specific drugs and doses for each disease. That is the doctor's job. Sometimes a patient is better without any drug at all. Nurses sometimes try to persuade the doctor to put the patient on some drug: they like to feel their patient is *on* something. They should remember that nature itself can often deal better with an infection than any drug.

IMMUNIZATION

Immunization is a process of imitating nature. Instead of undergoing natural infection, the patient has injected into him either a vaccine to stimulate the production of antibody, or ready-made antibody as described on p. 399. The first form is called active immunization, because the body has to actively produce antibody; the second form is called passive immunization, because the body passively receives antibody manufactured in some other body. We must now consider the forms of immunization available for various diseases.

Diphtheria, whooping cough and tetanus

These three diseases are taken together because the vaccines against them are usually mixed together and given as one injection, usually called *triple vaccine*. This contains diphtheria toxoid, tetanus toxoid and dead whooping cough bacilli. The first dose is given to infants at 6 months old, the second 4 to 6 weeks later and the third after 6 months. A booster dose of diphtheria and tetanus toxoids should be given when the child goes to school, but whooping cough vaccine is not given because by then the most dangerous age for that disease has passed. Another dose of tetanus toxoid should be given when the pupil leaves school at 15 years old or later.

These are the recommendations the Department of Health and Social Security (old Ministry of Health) made in 1972. They can be altered to suit conditions in other countries, and immunization can, of course, be carried out against any of the three diseases separately.

Poliomyelitis

Two vaccines are available, killed or live: the killed is often called Salk, and the live Sabin, after the doctors who did the early work on the vaccines. The killed must be given by three injections at one-month intervals; the live is taken by mouth on sugar in three doses once a month. The live vaccine gives slightly better protection and is much easier to give, especially in mass immunization campaigns. The only advantage of the killed vaccine is that it can be mixed with other vaccines, e.g. triple vaccine, and immunization against four diseases given in one injection.

Live polio vaccine can be given at the same time as triple vaccine, and again at school entry and leaving. Poliomyelitis has been almost banished from many countries by the use of vaccine, and it is most important that anyone leaving such a country for one where polio virus is still common should be well immunized against the disease.

Measles

Live measles vaccine is given by one injection; it should be given some time in the first two years of life. Babies under 6 months old may have antibody derived from their mothers' blood in the womb, and measles is rare under 6 months of age. In countries where measles is still a deadly disease, vaccine should be given in the first few months of life, but in other countries it may be given in the second year.

Gamma globulin is often given to prevent measles in children exposed to the disease who have not had measles vaccine. This is done most in hospitals and residential institutions. The gamma globulin protects the child only for a week or two; it is passive, not active immunization. Sometimes after gamma globulin the child gets an attack of very mild measles, called modified measles. This, like an attack of ordinary measles, leaves the child immune for life, but it is difficult to judge the timing and the dose of gamma globulin to produce this result. One snag is that modified measles is still infectious for other children in the institution.

Rubella

A live vaccine against rubella is now available. Vaccination against rubella is now being offered to all girls between 11 and 14 years old, and it will soon be possible to immunize all females against rubella before they reach child-bearing age, and so the problem of congenital rubella will be solved.

Smallpox

Smallpox vaccine is a live vaccine. It is given into the skin of the arm and produces there a sore which is really like a highly modified form of smallpox called vaccinia. This is an infectious disease and can be spread from one person to another by contact, accidental vaccinia; it stimulates the production of antibodies against vaccinia and smallpox. The vaccine is usually given to children in the first two years of life: in countries where the disease is common it should be given in the earliest months. Smallpox vaccination protects for a long time, sometimes even for life, but people vary in their response to it, and it is safer to re-vaccinate people who are at special risk, either because of their work, e.g. doctors and nurses, or because they live in a country where smallpox is common. Doctors and nurses in fever hospitals should be vaccinated every two years, people in smallpox countries at least every 10 years. In a country like Britain where smallpox is uncommon, routine vaccination is not required; when the disease does occur, the Medical Officer of Health takes charge of the vaccination situation and he confines his attention mainly to close contacts of the disease. It is rarely necessary to call for mass vaccination though the uninformed Press and Radio often do so.

For close contacts hyperimmune gamma globulin is also available (see p. 375). This can be given the day after vaccination, and an anti-viral drug (Marboran) may be given as well.

Tuberculosis

If a person is immune to tuberculosis, his skin reacts to the injection of tuberculin into it; this is shown by an area of redness. There are several different ways of doing the skin test (Mantoux test, Heaf test) but they measure the same thing. If a person is negative to the test he should be immunized against the disease. Newborn babies can be assumed to be negative. The vaccine consists of a live but weakened strain of tubercle bacillus, and is injected into the skin. This makes a tuberculin-negative person tuberculin-positive, a process known as tuberculin conversion. The Department of Health and Social Security in 1972 recommended immunization of all children between 10 and 13 years old if still tuberculin-negative, but some doctors prefer to immunize as a routine in early infancy. The practice varies according to the incidence of tuberculosis in any area. The vaccine is usually referred to as BCG, after the doctors Calmette and Guerin who first produced it. (See also tuberculin tests, pp. 204–5.)

Typhoid fever

The vaccine used to protect against typhoid and paratyphoid fevers is composed of dead typhoid and paratyphoid A and B germs: it is usually called TAB. Two doses are given subcutaneously at an interval of 4 or 6 weeks. This gives some, but not complete protection. A careless nurse can easily infect herself with typhoid fever when nursing a typhoid patient, even though recently vaccinated with TAB. The vaccine is certainly worth giving to anyone going to a country where typhoid is common. It gives some protection, but if a vaccinated person does get typhoid fever, the TAB does not guarantee that the attack will be milder.

Cholera

Cholera vaccine consists of several strains of dead *Vibrio cholerae*, the germs of cholera. Two doses are given by injection at an interval of 4 to 6 weeks. Protection lasts for only 6 months, so that anyone going to an area where the disease is common requires a booster dose every 6 months. The vaccine can be mixed with TAB vaccine, as indeed can tetanus toxoid.

Yellow fever

This is a live virus vaccine. Only one injection is required, and the protection lasts for 10 years.

Typhus

Typhus vaccine consists of dead rickettsiae, the germs which cause the various types of typhus. Three injections are given at intervals of 10 days, and a booster dose should be given every year in typhus areas. The vaccine may not protect against catching the disease, but it does lessen the severity of the attack and lowers the mortality from the disease.

Plague

This vaccine consists of dead *Pasteurella pestis*, the germ which causes plague. Two injections are given at an interval of 4 weeks, and a booster dose is given each year to persons living in an area where plague is common.

There is, of course, no limit to the number of vaccines which can be made, provided the germ or virus of a disease can be grown in the laboratory. A mumps vaccine is already available but it is not yet clear whether it is wise to use it (see p. 366). A common cold vaccine could be made, but there are about 100 different common cold viruses, all of which would have to go into a vaccine. This would mean an enormous injection or a very large number of smaller ones, a vast amount of laboratory work, and yet the protection might be poor and of short duration. Another difficulty is that the strains of viruses tend to change from time to time; this is especially true of influenza virus (see p. 379). In spite of many difficulties, both theoretical and practical, the development of vaccines against so many diseases has been one of the triumphs of twentieth-century preventive medicine.

Section 6

Surgical Conditions, Their Treatment and Nursing Care

Introduction to Surgical Nursing

by MICHAEL HOBSLEY

No exact definition of surgery is possible. On the whole, the hall-mark of surgery as distinct from medicine is that the techniques of treatment involve the doctor's manual dexterity, i.e. a surgical operation. In times past, the distinctions between surgery and medicine were clear-cut: today, they are becoming much more blurred. Diagnosis, the preparation for a surgical operation, the management of the postoperative period and its many possible complications, are all features that loom large in the sum of surgical activity: the operation itself is just an incident in the total treatment. At the same time, physicians are becoming increasingly adept at various skills requiring extreme manual dexterity: gastroscopy (the inspection of the interior of the stomach through a telescope passed via the mouth and gullet) and needle-biopsy of the liver (needling the liver from the exterior to obtain samples of tissue for microscopical examination) are two examples.

The best working definition is probably that surgery is what surgeons do. Convention and tradition play an important part in defining the field of surgery. Acute symptoms due to stones in the urinary tract and stones in the gall bladder are not usually treated by a surgical operation in the first instance, but patients with these conditions are nonetheless admitted in most hospitals to surgical wards. By contrast, acute bleeding from the stomach often requires a surgical operation, but patients with this problem are usually admitted to medical wards.

The new patients whom a nurse meets on their admission to a surgical ward fall into two distinct categories: the emergency admission and the elective or routine admission. The patient admitted as an emergency is nearly always apprehensive, usually in pain or afflicted with other distressing symptoms, and often bewildered. The nurse will find it particularly distressing at first that her seniors and the medical staff seem to be unaccountably reluctant to treat the patient's symptoms. Even severe pain demanding treatment by morphine may appear to be allowed to continue unheeded. This is not due to carelessness or any worse cause: opiates may mask important signs of disease and should not be given, for example, to a patient with an acute abdominal emergency until he has been examined by the surgeon whose immediate responsibility it is to decide whether to operate at once. *The patient in pain cannot usually understand such a consideration and the nurse's responsibility to the comfort of her patient is accordingly heavy* (see also, p. 126).

Patients admitted from the routine waiting-list are quite different: usually they appear fit and healthy, and they may joke about their impending experience. Nonetheless, most are apprehensive and need reassurance; and even if they do not, they will want to know the answer to a multitude of questions, such as how strict is sister about visiting hours, what time does the newspaper trolley come round, what are the arrangements for posting letters? *The nurse will find these questions trivial, and sometimes irritating, but she must not reveal these feelings to her patient to whom the answers are important.*

Complete nursing care thus involves considerations like the above as well as the technical aspects. A nurse cannot be taught how to support the patient, though she can profit from example. The *technical aspects* can be taught: they are the methods whereby she aids the surgeon to achieve his objectives. These aims are threefold: *to preserve life*; *to repair damage*; and *to relieve symptoms.* The order in which these aims have been stated is significant; there is no point in relieving symptoms if the measures taken to relieve the symptoms jeopardize the patient's life.

Symptomatic treatment will be mentioned where indicated throughout the chapters on surgical conditions. The preservation of life and the repair of damage are so important as general principles that the next two chapters are devoted to the conditions that threaten life and damage the tissues.

Chapter 43

Life-threatening Conditions

by MICHAEL HOBSLEY

> *The respiratory cycle—disturbances of pulmonary gas exchange—*
> *disturbances of oxygen transport—disturbances of tissue respiration—*
> *management of life-threatening conditions—cyanosis—shock*

THE RESPIRATORY CYCLE

Life depends upon a series of complex chemical reactions, *metabolism*, occurring in the cells of living matter. The energy needed to drive all these reactions is ultimately derived from a particular reaction called *tissue* or *cellular respiration*. The combustion of the carbon in compounds such as glucose, with the gas oxygen, produces the gas carbon dioxide with the evolution of heat and *chemical energy*. The vitality of the organism therefore depends upon a supply of oxygen and glucose and upon the removal of carbon dioxide.

Oxygen is present in the atmosphere in the proportion of one part in five, the remaining four parts being the inert gas, nitrogen. The rhythmic movements of the chest wall and the diaphragm, that we call breathing, produce a mass movement of air between the atmosphere and the lungs—*ventilation*. Oxygen in the inspired air passes through the walls of the microscopic air sacs, *alveoli*, in the lungs, and through the walls of the blood vessels, *pulmonary alveolar capillaries*, that lie in close proximity and thus into the blood. The process of permeation of gas is called *diffusion*. The process whereby a balance is maintained in all parts of the lungs between the volume of air ventilating the local alveoli and the volume of blood perfusing the local alveolar capillaries is called *distribution*.

Oxygen transport to the tissues is a function of the *blood circulation*. The oxygen gas is carried in the blood to a small extent dissolved in the plasma, but mostly in the red cells in chemical combination with the protein, *haemoglobin*. The oxygenated compound with haemoglobin, *oxyhaemoglobin*, is bright red and gives its characteristic colour to arterial blood which is saturated with oxygen since it has passed through the pulmonary alveolar capillaries.

The arterial blood is pumped by the heart to the tissues, and its excess oxygen content diffuses into the tissue cells together with glucose that is ultimately derived from food. Excess carbon dioxide that has accumulated in the cells moves in the opposite direction, into the blood, and continues by way of the veins to the heart and then on in the pulmonary circulation to the pulmonary capillaries.

The venous blood is tinged with a dark blue colour, which is the colour of haemoglobin as distinct from bright red oxyhaemoglobin. The pulmonary capillary blood gives up its excess carbon dioxide to the air in the alveoli, and this air is then expired. The whole process of ventilation, gaseous exchange in the lungs by diffusion and distribution, and transport of gases to and from the tissue cells by the circulation and cellular respiration is called, simply, respiration.

The acute life-threatening conditions all interfere with cellular respiration. Either there is not enough oxygen in the blood reaching the tissues, or there is too much carbon dioxide; or the circulation itself is inadequate; or there is not enough fuel (glucose) reaching the cells.

Human cells are not all equally sensitive to the effects of inadequate respiration. The cells in muscle, for example, can manage with an in-adequate supply of oxygen for long periods because they have an alternative chemical source of energy to respiration. During violent exercise much more energy is needed than can be provided by the circulation in the form of oxygen. The alternative source results in the production of lactic acid, and the accumulation of this material ultimately poisons the cell. The exercise cannot be continued indefinitely, because the destruction of the excess lactic acid itself demands oxygen. The muscle is said to have accumulated an *oxygen debt* during the exercise, and must rest and repay this debt to rid itself of the lactic acid.

Many tissues have no alternative to respiration, but their metabolic activities (and hence their demands for oxygen) are small. Such tissues, like skin, tendon, and bone, can endure a disturbance of tissue respiration for long periods. Other tissues or organs, however, are very sensitive to such disturbances because their metabolic activities are very great and the importance of their efficient functioning to the whole organism is critical. The three most important organs in this context are the *brain*, the *heart* and the *kidneys*.

The brain is the most sensitive to the effects of anoxia (absence of oxygen): its delicate mechanisms, the seat of consciousness and intellect, emotion and volition, everything that distinguishes man from the lesser orders of life, crumble irreversibly if they are deprived of oxygen for as little as four minutes. This is the length of time available to the bystander if the acute emergency of cerebral anoxia develops. Long before four minutes the consciousness is impaired. The patient's vision goes dark, he feels sick and becomes dizzy as his mechanisms of balance falter, and then he loses con-sciousness and falls to the ground. Recovery is nonetheless usually com-plete if an oxygen supply is restored to the brain before four minutes have passed.

The heart is a little less delicate: its anoxia-time is *of the order of eight minutes.* After this period the electrical activity in the cardiac muscle fibres that is intimately associated with their ability to contract becomes dis-orderly and the circulation ceases, so that circulatory arrest is added as another cause to whatever caused the primary anoxia.

The kidney is less clear-cut in its sensitivity, but it is usually said to be able to recover from acute anoxia which does not last longer than about

30 minutes. The flow of urine may cease (i.e. *anuria* may occur) before this time, but provided tissue oxygenation is restored before 30 minutes, eventual recovery can be expected.

One problem peculiar to the kidney is that even if the damage is still reversible it may be so severe that the kidney cannot start functioning adequately for several days after the anoxic incident. During this period the kidney can secrete only a very dilute urine, so that waste products like urea which are normally excreted by the kidney accumulate in the body and poison the patient. To tide the patient over this period of renal in-efficiency and to keep him alive until his own kidneys start working properly again, various techniques have been devised to remove the poisons from the patient, e.g. the artificial kidney, Chapter 25, p. 246.

The various acute conditions threatening life, and simple measures used in their treatment are discussed in more detail below.

DISTURBANCES OF PULMONARY GAS EXCHANGE

The following factors may interfere with this process.

(1) **Oxygen deficiency in the atmosphere.** This situation usually arises in mines or caves or in the smoke and fumes of a fire. Always try to get the patient into fresh air as soon as possible.

(2) **Inadequate ventilation.** The patient cannot breathe effectively, either because there is an *obstruction* in his *upper respiratory passages* (mouth, nose, pharynx, trachea), e.g. inhaled vomit, or because there is some interference with the *movements* of his chest wall and diaphragm or with the *nerves* supplying the muscles of the respiratory system. Inadequate ventilation results not only in anoxia but also in the accumulation of carbon dioxide in the blood; but the reduction in oxygen (*hypoxia*) is more important in the acute situation.

(3) **Impaired diffusion.** A reduction in the rate at which oxygen diffuses from the pulmonary alveoli into the blood occurs in certain chronic diseases of the lungs or as a result of exposure to some inhalant poisons like mustard-gas.

(4) **Impaired distribution.** In surgical wards the most important example of an interference with this process is the condition of segmental collapse of parts of the lungs which may occur as a complication after surgical operations (Chapter 49, p. 462). In those parts of the lung which are collapsed, no air is entering the alveoli. In consequence, the blood in the pulmonary capillaries of these areas fails to be oxygenated and contributes a quota of reduced haemoglobin to the peripheral arterial blood so that less oxygen is available for the tissues.

DISTURBANCES OF OXYGEN TRANSPORT

(1) **Haemoglobin.** Since most of the oxygen in the blood is carried in chemical combination with haemoglobin, a diminished concentration of haemoglobin in the blood, *anaemia*, reduces the availability of oxygen to the tissues. The normal blood haemoglobin concentration is 14 to 15 g

per 100 ml, but in severe chronic anaemia the figure may fall to less than 5 g per 100 ml. All the tissues and organs of the body are chronically starved of oxygen and they are therefore peculiarly sensitive to any sudden insult: in these circumstances a blood transfusion meant to correct the anaemia may overload the damaged heart and provoke cardiac failure and death.

The haemoglobin may also be present in normal concentration, but not available for carrying oxygen because it has combined with *carbon monoxide* gas. Carbon monoxide has an even greater chemical affinity for haemoglobin than has oxygen. This property accounts for the dangers of poor ventilation in buildings such as garages where an accumulation of carbon monoxide (from the exhaust gases of a car's engine) may be expected.

(2) **Circulation.** Interference with the circulation may be *complete*, when it is due to the heart stopping, *cardiac arrest*. It is important to remember that only a few seconds after the heart stops, the part of the brain that controls the respiratory system, *the respiratory centre*, is damaged and ventilation ceases. Complete stoppage of the circulation is better called *cardio-respiratory arrest* to emphasize this point. *Incomplete* interference with the circulation, usually called *circulatory failure*, results from a variety of causes.

(i) *Failure of the pump.* This may be called *central circulatory failure*. When the heart is damaged by disease or by poison so that it cannot cope with pumping onwards the whole of the blood being brought back from the tissues by the veins, the *venous return*, the chambers of the heart and the great veins which are responsible for the venous return dilate. The pressure rises in the great veins, the *superior* and *inferior venae cavae*, which enter the right side of the heart within the thoracic cavity: this raised *central venous pressure* is diagnostic of a failing heart.

(ii) *Failure of the venous return.* The heart, no matter how strong, cannot pump out to the tissues any more blood than it receives. An inadequate cardiac output may therefore be due to an inadequate venous return. Since the cells receive an inadequate supply of blood despite the efforts of a normal heart, this situation is sometimes called *peripheral* (as distinct from central) circulatory failure. It is important to realize, however, that central circulatory failure reduces the cardiac output and hence the arterial supply to the periphery and to this extent the two terms are confusing.

Failure of the venous return has two possible causes: a reduction in the volume of the circulating blood, *hypovolaemia*, and a dilatation of the small vessels, *arterioles, capillaries*, which bring the blood closest to the tissue cells. Of these two types, hypovolaemia is the more important in surgery because it is frequently due to a loss of blood, *haemorrhage* (see p. 420). It is obvious that haemorrhage results in a reduction in the venous return, and hence in a reduction in the cardiac output. But a dilatation of the arteriolar-capillary bed means that at any given moment there is more blood in these small vessels than usual, so that if the cardiac output into the arteries is normal in volume there *must* be less blood in the veins.

The classical example of a diminished cardiac output due to vasodilatation is the simple fainting attack, in which the small blood vessels of the muscles dilate—usually as a result of an emotional disturbance; another important example is the vasodilatation produced by toxic substances derived from bacteria growing in the bloodstream, a condition known as *septicaemia*.

The important distinction between failure of the venous return and failure of the pump is that in the former the central venous pressure is low instead of high.

DISTURBANCES OF TISSUE RESPIRATION

At cellular level, the oxygen brought by the blood may still be ineffective in supporting respiration because the chemical processes involved have been poisoned (cyanide produces its fatal results in this way), or because there is not enough food in the cell to react with the oxygen. Glucose, as already stated, is the primary fuel, but metabolism in many types of cells can make do with other chemicals as food for the reaction of respiration. The brain, however, is completely dependent upon glucose molecules, and if the level of glucose in the blood is greatly reduced (for example, by an overdose of insulin) unconsciousness and even death are produced just as by cutting off the blood supply to the brain.

MANAGEMENT OF LIFE-THREATENING CONDITIONS

From the foregoing remarks, it is clear that the aim of treatment must be to maintain a good supply of well-oxygenated blood to the tissues. To remember that tissue oxygenation depends on gas-exchange in the lungs, on transport to the cells, and on efficient chemistry within the cells makes it easy to adopt a logical approach to these problems.

Is the airway clear? This point is particularly relevant to the unconscious patient. The most common cause of airway obstruction is the patient's own tongue, which may flop backwards when the unconscious patient is lying on his back and obstruct the entrance to the larynx. Other common obstructing agents are inhaled false teeth and vomitus. Treatment is to inspect the mouth and pharynx, remove any foreign body or hook forward the tongue with a finger, and then if possible turn the patient into the semi-prone position so that the jaw and tongue fall forwards rather than backwards. If the patient must for other reasons be nursed on his back, then the lower jaw (to which the tongue is attached) must be held well forwards by finger-tips behind the angles of the jaws.

Is the patient breathing? If there are no definite spontaneous movements of respiration visible, artificial respiration must be undertaken (see below and p. 447). If there is an embarrassment to respiratory movements, every effort must be made to put it right. Possible embarrassments are open pneumothorax, tension pneumothorax, and flail chest (p. 591). The management of disorders of diffusion and distribution are beyond the province of the nurse.

Is the patient's heart beating? This question must be settled *rapidly* by reference to the pulse at the wrist or in the neck, or by listening for heart beats through the anterior chest wall with a stethoscope. Remember that:

1. When the heart stops, only four minutes are available for resuscitation before the brain suffers irreversible damage
2. Respiratory movements also stop.

Therefore, management includes the rapid institution of both artificial respiration and *external cardiac massage* (p. 448) so that some reasonably well oxygenated air inflates the pulmonary alveoli and some circulation of blood is maintained. *Since these measures and further treatment aimed at re-starting the heart are too complicated to be undertaken single-handed, the nurse must call for help as soon as possible.*

Is the patient bleeding externally? Of the many causes of a diminution in the cardiac output mentioned previously, the only one which the nurse can tackle directly is obvious blood loss, *external haemorrhage*, from an accessible site on the surface of the patient. The bleeding must be stopped so that the cardiac output is not further reduced. The most effective method in nearly every case is direct pressure on the bleeding point with the cleanest agent available in the emergency—preferably, a sterile dressing. Haemorrhage is further considered on p. 420.

Are the kidneys functioning? After a period of circulatory arrest, the doctor usually requires a urethral catheter to be inserted in order to obtain early warning of renal failure: cessation of urine flow, *anuria*, or a reduction of flow rate to less than 350 ml in 24 hours in an adult, *oliguria*.

CYANOSIS

Cyanosis means a blue colour of the skin and mucous membranes (i.e. the linings of body cavities such as the mouth) due to an increase in the concentration of reduced haemoglobin in the capillaries above the level of 5 g per 100 ml. This increase may be due to some defect of oxygenation in the lungs, or to the removal of more oxygen than normal as the blood passes through the tissues. If the primary defect is one of oxygenation, the blue colour is independent of any effect produced during circulation through the tissues: the cyanosis is therefore present in the mouth, which retains a good blood supply despite a diminished cardiac output. Such cyanosis is called *central*.

An excessive removal of oxygen by the tissues is basically due to an inadequate blood supply to the tissues (low cardiac output), and the resultant cyanosis is therefore seen best where the circulation is poorest, namely in the hands and feet, and is often called *peripheral cyanosis*. Cyanosis is thus a useful sign that something is wrong with pulmonary gas exchange, or else with the circulation. However, it is unwise to rely on this sign because it may be absent despite severe cardiopulmonary disturbances.

SHOCK

This word in its medical sense is difficult to define; it should probably never be used without a modifying adjective such as *haemorrhagic, hypovolaemic* (low circulatory volume), *septicaemic, cardiogenic*, and so on.

The concept of shock arose from the observation of wounded men and animals. Even though the nature of the wound might vary widely from one individual to another, a clinical picture developed which in many respects was similar in all.

Nowadays, we understand this common reaction with increasing clarity. *The concept of shock is becoming identified with the effects of a diminished circulation to the tissues*: these effects are partly the impairment of functions of sensitive organs, and partly reactionary responses of the subject which are aimed at minimizing the consequences of the injury. In particular it must be emphasized that shock in a medical context has no relation to the emotional disturbance referred to as shock in everyday speech.

The earliest features of shock are due to the sensitivity of the brain to a reduction in blood supply: agitation, inability to concentrate, nausea, giddiness, dimness of vision, prostration, unconsciousness. As the cardiac output diminishes, the arterial blood pressure falls; as the renal blood flow drops, the urine output ceases.

The compensatory measures are that the *heart-rate increases* and the *blood vessels* in areas that are insensitive to the blood-lack, particularly the skin, *constrict*. The narrowing of the skin blood vessels produces the pallor and coldness typical of inadequate cardiac output. These effects are partly produced by an increased liberation of the hormone *adrenaline* from the adrenal gland, and because this agent also has an effect upon sweat glands the subject breaks out into a (cold) sweat. The compensatory changes of vasoconstriction and an increase in the heart-rate bolster up the arterial blood pressure for a time. Ultimately, this phase of compensation can no longer be maintained and there is a precipitate fall in blood pressure and a marked deterioration in the patient's condition.

The key to management is the state of the veins. If the *central venous pressure* is high the heart is failing and drugs to increase the efficiency of the heart are indicated. If the central venous pressure is low (in which case peripheral veins such as those in the back of the hand look collapsed) then the circulatory failure is due to a diminished blood volume or to a dilatation of the capillary circulation.

The surgeon may place a fine catheter via the veins of the neck or the arm into the large veins entering the heart within the thorax, and order a slow infusion of normal saline solution to be maintained to keep the catheter patent. From time to time this infusion can be stopped and the central venous pressure measured by noting the height above the sternum to which the column of saline in the tubing falls. In cases of reduction in the venous return, the surgeon will set up a second intravenous infusion through which the circulation can be restored with blood or other fluids.

Chapter 44

Damage to Tissues

by MICHAEL HOBSLEY

> *Damage to living tissues—classification of damage to tissues—external physicochemical factors—external biological factors: infection—intrinsic factors—defences against damage: inflammation, immunity—consequences of external physical trauma—management of wounds of soft tissues*

DAMAGE TO LIVING TISSUES

The aim of every doctor is to understand the nature and causes of damage to living tissues so that he can try to repair the damage. *The nurse, as the doctor's most important assistant, must have a clear conception of the various ways in which living matter may be damaged and the natural mechanisms of repair and defence.* The present chapter concentrates on items of particular interest to surgeons, but the opportunity is taken to present a classification of all types of damage to the organism. The role of surgery is best appreciated by viewing it in relation to the wider field of the rest of medicine.

Damage to a living organism may be *somatic* (affecting the physical structure and functioning of the body) or *psychic*. Many types of physical damage have mental effects, and it is sometimes more important to deal with the psychic rather than with the somatic effect of the problem. Psychological factors will not, however, be considered further here.

Trauma and *injury* are synonymous with *damage*, and in the following sections no special significance is to be attached to the use of one of these words rather than the others. *Trauma* in particular is often given a more restricted meaning, such as damage by external mechanical factors, but this practice can be confusing.

CLASSIFICATION OF DAMAGE

External physicochemical factors:

> Mechanical.
> Thermal.
> Chemical.
> Electrical.
> Radiant.

External biological factors:

Infection.
Foreign protein.

Intrinsic factors:

Degeneration.
Metabolism.
Nutrition.
Neoplasia.
Auto-immunity.

EXTERNAL PHYSICOCHEMICAL FACTORS

Agents

Mechanical trauma may be produced by the *pressure* of blunt objects, by *cutting* done by sharp objects, by *friction* (which produces results very similar to burns), and by *perforation* due to pointed objects. *High-velocity missiles*, e.g. bullets, are a special case of perforation: they set up shock waves in the tissues which are disrupted and destroyed over a large region around the missile-track.

Thermal trauma can be produced by the application of heat (a *burn*), but also by the application of *cold*. The heat may be generated by *flame*, a *high environmental temperature*, or the application of *hot liquids or vapours* (a *scald*). These injuries and their management are described in Chapter 67.

Chemical damage can occur in two ways. Tissues lining the external or internal surfaces of the body, i.e. skin or alimentary tract, may be harmed by contact with substances that react chemically with living tissues; such surface damage is similar to burning. Alternatively, the chemical agent may damage the organism only after being absorbed—*poisoning*. Poisons and their treatment are discussed in Chapter 28.

Electrical damage consists of burning of the area which comes into contact with the source of electricity, and electric 'shock'. The latter describes the disturbance in the functioning of nerves and muscles which may be expressed as a jerking movement of the local muscles, or in severe cases by cessation of the heart beat and death.

Radiant damage depends not only on the dose but also on the wavelength of the rays. Visible light produces thermal effects (sunburn). X-rays also have some thermal effect, but in addition produce long-term changes in blood vessels that reduce their calibre, and subtle alterations in the cell nucleus that result in disorders of cell-replication or even malignant transformation (see Chapter 64).

Another way of classifying trauma by external physicochemical factors is according to the nature of the injury.

Types of injury produced

Injuries produced by mechanical forces may be *open* (*compound*) or *closed* (*simple*). The distinction is that in an open injury there is a break in the continuity of the protective surface of the organism, either skin or mucous membrane (a *wound*), while in a closed injury there is no such break. The major importance of this classification is, of course, that the open wound may become infected.

Types of wound.

(1) An *incision* is a clean-cut wound, made with a sharp instrument such as a surgical scalpel.

(2) A *contused* wound is bruised: the force of a blunt object has broken the skin over the resistance of the underlying bone, but in the neighbouring areas the force, while insufficient to break the skin, has damaged blood vessels which have bled into the tissues.

(3) In a *laceration* the edges of the wound are jagged because the structures have been torn rather than incised neatly.

(4) A *punctured* wound is one which is much deeper than its area at the surface. It has been made by a sharp narrow object.

(5) A *burn* is produced by dry heat, a *scald* by wet heat. Friction produces a lesion very similar to a burn. Burns and their treatment are described in Chapter 67.

Types of closed injury.

(1) A *contusion* or *bruise* has already been described as part of the lesion known as a contused wound.

(2) *Disruption* of an organ far from the surface can be produced by external pressure.

(3) Bones may break (*fractures*) and joints and ligaments may suffer, respectively, *dislocation* and *spraining*. These injuries are described in Chapter 56.

EXTERNAL BIOLOGICAL FACTORS

Infection. The invasion of an organism by other living organisms which are nearly always so small as to be visible only under the microscope, and the subsequent growth of the micro-organisms within the tissues of the host with consequent damage to the host is called *infection*. The problem of infection dominates the practice of surgery, because most *pathogenic* (*disease-producing*) micro-organisms only constitute a problem when they gain access to the tissues through a break in the continuity of the skin such as the surgeon must make to perform an internal operation.

The classification of infective unicellular micro-organisms is a complex matter. Basically they are subdivided by size as *filterable* (i.e., so small that they can pass through filters of the smallest pore-size that we can construct)—this group includes the *viruses*; and those which are *non-filterable*. Among the latter are *bacteria*, which are further subdivided into the round forms (*cocci*) and the rod-shaped forms (*bacilli*). Larger than the bacteria are *yeasts* and *fungi*, which are for example responsible for many cases of vaginal discharge, and larger again are the multicellular organisms (some of which are visible to the naked eye) known as *metazoa*, e.g. worms that *infest* the intestinal tract.

Foreign protein. Harm may also result from the introduction into the body of foreign (usually protein) material which is not necessarily alive.

This usually occurs only in such artificial situations as tissue- and organ-transplanting, but the damage produced can be widespread. This aspect of the subject will be considered later in the section on immunity (p. 418).

INTRINSIC FACTORS

Degeneration. This word designates the ageing process. Familiar as we are with the general appearance of the changes produced by ageing, we as yet know practically nothing about the reasons for the inevitability of ageing, why it should happen at different rates in different individuals, or—most important—why it should occur prematurely in some.

Metabolism. Sometimes the chemical processes occurring in some or all cells take a wrong pathway and result in the formation of a new substance —or more usually in the accumulation of one present normally in very small concentration—which has a toxic effect on the cells. The accumulation of lactic acid in exercising muscle is an example that can be readily cured by resting the muscle; however, in gout the accumulation of *uric acid* in soft tissues around joints is not so easily corrected.

Nutrition. In order to survive, cells must receive the raw materials for their metabolism, and their waste-products must be removed. Disturbances affecting blood supply or respiratory gas exchange in general are important and may threaten life (Chapter 43). Localized disturbances may also occur, due to obstruction of the local blood vessels supplying or draining the area.

Neoplasia. This word literally means new growth. It is synonymous with the layman's term 'cancer'. The essential characteristic of neoplasia is that certain cells grow in an inappropriate and disorderly fashion. It is important to recognize that even in a fully grown adult almost every cell in the body is growing by dividing into two new cells (the exceptions are the cells of the central nervous system). This process is essential because cells are also dying. In health there must be mechanisms (although we know practically nothing about them) that balance the rate of growth against the rate of destruction. In neoplasia, certain cells escape from the restriction of these mechanisms and grow unchecked. The extent of this escape can vary within very wide limits. Often the new growth (tumour) increases in size only for a limited period and then remains static. Such tumours are called *benign*, because they hardly disturb the rest of the body.

At the other extreme are fast-growing tumours which spread inexorably either by *local continuity* or by discontinuous spread to a distance (*metastasis*) in the bloodstream, the lymphatics, or across body cavities like the peritoneum, and finally kill the patient by the interference that the widespread deposits of tumour (*metastases*) exert on the vital functions of such organs as liver, lungs or brain.

Malignant tumours are subdivided into: (*a*) *carcinomas* derived from the skin lining the external surface of the body or the mucous membranes lining the digestive, respiratory and urogenital tracts and their related glands; and (*b*) *sarcomas*, derived from the connective tissues such as bone, muscle, cartilage, fascia, etc.

Auto-immunity. This phenomenon is described with immunity (p. 419).

Advances in the last 100 years have gone far towards solving the problems posed by external physical and biological agents that cause injury. The problems of degeneration and neoplasia, and to a less extent the errors of metabolism, now dominate the thoughts and efforts of medical scientists.

DEFENCES AGAINST DAMAGE

Inflammation

The local response of the tissues to damage, no matter how the damage is caused, is called *inflammation*. The features of inflammation are *redness*, *warmth*, *swelling* and *pain*, and because of these an *impairment of function* of the wounded area. When living tissues are damaged, chemical substances are liberated in the area and produce a dilatation of the local small vessels, arterioles, capillaries and venules, and a corresponding increase in the local blood supply (redness and warmth). The distended venules also become more permeable so that plasma leaks through their walls and floods the wound (swelling or *oedema*). Certain white blood cells (*polymorphonuclear leucocytes*) in the plasma act as scavengers, destroying any foreign material in the wound and any tissues damaged beyond repair, while other cells with the help of the plasma proteins construct new tissues to repair the defect. Pain is produced by the action of the chemical substance on the nerves, as well as by the original trauma. *Acute inflammation* may have several outcomes:

1. *Resolution*—when complete return to normality occurs occasionally, as in lobar pneumonia
2. *Healing* by fibrous (scar) tissue, as in wounds
3. *Chronic inflammation* when the changes take a long time to settle down
4. *Death of tissue* (*necrosis*)—a word which applies to the death of relatively small numbers of cells—or *gangrene*, which applies to the death of a large area such as a digit or even a limb

Immunity

Immunology may be defined as the study of the ability of the tissues of an individual (*host*) to recognize and subsequently react to foreign substances (*antigens*).

The *immune response* comprises:

1. Recognition that the material is foreign (an antigen)
2. Primary reaction against the antigen
3. Stored memory in the tissues of contact with the antigen
4. Specific and altered (usually enhanced) reaction to the antigen upon subsequent exposure

The whole response is a function of the host *lymphoid tissue*, by which is meant the tissues in which white blood cells other than the polymorphonuclear leucocytes are formed. Lymphoid tissue occurs in lymph nodes, spleen, thymus, tonsil and intestine.

Recognition. During fetal life, the individual is thought to learn not to react against its own tissues. This phenomenon is called *tolerance*. Under certain circumstances individuals can be made tolerant of foreign antigen. One way of inducing tolerance is by giving repeated injections of very small amounts of antigen: an example is the process of *desensitization* by a course of injections of the offending pollen for sufferers from hay-fever.

The primary reaction may be mediated by serum *antibodies* or by *cells*.

Some antigens stimulate the *plasma cells* in the lymphoid tissue to secrete antibodies, which are special proteins (*immunoglobulins*) which circulate in the plasma. Antibody reacts with specific antigen, in such a way that the antigen is more easily eliminated from the body by polymorphonuclear leucocytes.

Examples of antibody-mediated immunity are the protection of normal people against tetanus or typhoid by the injection of weakened forms of the organisms that produce these diseases, leading to the development of circulating antibodies. The immune response takes several days to develop, and is called *active immunity*.

Another way in which antibody-type immunity can be used is to protect the individual by injection of antibody (e.g. plasma, or a concentrate of the appropriate fraction of the plasma protein) from another immunized individual—*passive immunity*. This technique is used to treat diphtheria and tetanus.

Cell-mediated immunity is a form of immune response in which no circulating antibodies can be detected; it is probably a function of the small lymphocytes. Classical examples are the response of the body to tuberculosis, e.g. the Mantoux test, p. 204, and the rejection of grafts from foreign donors. In a period of about a week after grafting, the neighbouring lymph nodes swell and show a rapid increase in their content of small lymphocytes; then similar white cells invade the graft and it is destroyed by an inflammatory reaction. A subsequent graft from the same foreign donor is rejected much more rapidly because the host is now sensitized (immune).

Auto-immunity. Failure of *tolerance* results in an individual attacking his own tissues by making antibodies to them. This phenomenon of auto-immunity is known to be implicated in a variety of diseases including Hashimoto's thyroiditis, rheumatoid arthritis, myasthenia gravis, and probably many others.

Surgical applications

(1) *Immunization*. The production of active or passive immunity against various infective organisms has been discussed above (see also p. 401).

(2) *Blood transfusion*. The importance of the antigens which define human blood-groups, and the cross-matching techniques that are used to determine whether a particular donor's blood is suitable for transfusion into a particular recipient are discussed in Chapter 48.

(3) *Tissue- and organ-grafting*. Recent advances in this field have been spectacular. The transplantation of a kidney is now quite a common procedure; several liver transplantations have been performed, as well as the more controversial cardiac transplants. New hope has been given to sufferers from chronic diseases of essential organs.

The technical problems of the surgical operations required have been largely solved. There remain the inter-related problems of providing suitable donor-organs and avoiding rejection of the graft by the host.

There are no problems of immune responses between *identical twins*, but grafts excite such a response with increasing strength as one proceeds from closely related donors (brothers, sisters) through unrelated human donors to donors of different species. The immune response can be diminished by three measures: (i) certain chemicals such as azathioprine (Imuran); (ii) corticosteroids such as cortisone or prednisone; and (iii) X-rays. One or more of these measures must be applied vigorously in the first few weeks after the grafting has been done, and because *all* immune responses are depressed including the defence against infection, special precautions must be taken against sepsis in the operating theatre and the recovery ward.

If the donor is a near-relative, the usual situation is that he is a volunteer and the operations for removing the donor-organ and transplanting it into the host can be done synchronously. In these circumstances the problem of *preserving* the donor-organ is relatively minor, because there is no delay. If the donor is not related, the necessity of removing the donor-organ very soon after the death of the donor to minimize ischaemic damage to the organ usually results in some delay before the host can be brought to operation, and methods of *organ-preservation* are being explored. If successful methods are found, it will become possible to organize organ-banks in the same way that we now have blood-banks, and the fact that a suitable organ has just become available due to the death of the donor will no longer make it necessary for the surgeon to operate in a hurry on the host.

CONSEQUENCES OF MECHANICAL TRAUMA

Local consequences

Bleeding (*haemorrhage*) occurring as a direct and immediate consequence of trauma is called *primary haemorrhage*. It is rapid and pulsatile if large arteries are cut, a less rapid ooze at a low pressure if the capillaries are involved, and non-pulsatile and bluish in colour if the larger veins are breached. Bleeding must be stopped as soon as possible. The blood pressure in the veins is so low that venous bleeding can be stopped simply by raising the affected part above the level of the heart: firm local pressure is necessary for arterial and capillary bleeding, and if these measures do not suffice the surgeon occludes the open vessels with stitches (sutures) or by tying ligatures round them.

There is a danger of bleeding recurring in the wound during the first 24 hours, *reactionary haemorrhage*. During the operation to stop the bleeding the patient's blood pressure may have been low (due to haemorrhagic shock, or perhaps to the anaesthetic administered); on his return to the ward the blood pressure recovers and small holes in the vessels which were temporarily sealed with blood-clot start leaking again. Another danger period occurs 7 to 14 days after the infliction of the wound: this *secondary haemorrhage* is caused by infection which softens the clots that repaired the holes in the vessels.

Infection. If bacteria in sufficient numbers or of sufficient virulence enter the wound, they multiply. In three or four days it becomes clear that the signs of inflammation produced by the injury are increasing rather than subsiding. The debris of the battle between the invaders and the defenders—dead germs and dead leucocytes—are liquefied by enzymes manufactured by both sides, and the resultant yellow liquid is called *pus*. A wound cannot heal if it contains pus, because new tissue cannot grow into the dead, oxygen-lacking material. Moreover, the pressure exerted by the pus embarrasses the local circulation and hinders the arrival of fresh leucocytes. For these reasons, the oldest surgical dictum, 'where there's pus, let it out', applies just as strongly today in the antibiotic era as it ever did.

Systemic consequences

Traumatic shock is one of the varieties of *hypovolaemic shock* (Chapter 43, p. 412). The reduction in circulating-blood volume is due partly to loss of blood and partly to the exudation of plasma from the dilated damaged small vessels. Injuries provoking a particularly large loss of plasma (such as burns) result in an increased ratio of red cells to plasma in the blood (*haemoconcentration*). Normally the red cells occupy about 45 per cent (*haematocrit* or *packed cell volume*) of the total blood volume, but this figure may exceed 50 per cent in haemoconcentration.

The metabolic response to trauma. With all but trivial injuries, there is a profound alteration in the chemical processes (metabolism) of the injured patient. For 24 to 48 hours after the injury (or surgical operation) the kidneys have difficulty in excreting *water* and *sodium ions*. The water effect is stronger than the sodium effect so that the small volumes of urine passed tend to have a higher concentration of sodium ions and a higher specific gravity (they weigh more per unit volume because of the higher concentration of dissolved solids) than normal. On the other hand, for three to four days there is an increased elimination of *potassium ions* in the urine. The normal breakdown of old cells that occurs all the time is accelerated for a very variable time (at least four days), and the amount of nitrogenous products derived from protein that is discharged in the urine is greater than the intake of protein (negative nitrogen balance). The changes in water and electrolyte (sodium and potassium) excretion are important because they affect the management of intravenous fluid therapy after major operations. The negative nitrogen balance affects the availability of protein for the re-building of the damaged tissues. To minimize this factor, it is essential that a full diet with a liberal allowance of protein is taken as soon as possible after operation.

The systemic response to infection. If the local defences are overwhelmed, spread of the infection may occur via the lymphatic channels (lymphangitis), recognized by red streaks running under the skin towards the heart, or into the bloodstream (*septicaemia*), whereupon the patient becomes much more ill with a high fever, rigors, flushed skin, sweating, headache and prostration.

Infections, in common with other external (or even internal) agents may provoke the *immune response*. This is considered separately (p. 418).

MANAGEMENT OF WOUNDS OF SOFT TISSUES

Reduce the risk of infection. All foreign material is removed from the wound—clothing, grit, etc.—because it is potentially contaminated with bacteria and because all such material increases the work demanded of the scavenging leucocytes. Dead or dying tissue ranks as foreign material. In certain instances, antibiotics such as penicillin will be prescribed.

Facilitate the reaction of inflammation. Nothing must be allowed to interfere with a good blood supply to the wound. *Bandages* must not be too tight. *Haematomas* (collections of shed blood) must not be allowed to form since they separate the healing edges of the wound as well as increasing the local pressure in the tissues, hence interfering with the inflow of blood. Another useful measure to prevent a build-up of tissue pressure is *elevation* of the part so that gravity may assist in the drainage away of venous blood and tissue fluid.

Prevent subsequent infection and limit plasma loss. The surgeon tries to achieve skin cover for the wound as soon as possible. Where the area of loss of skin is extensive, this is the province of the plastic surgeon (see Chapter 67). With lesser degrees of loss it is usually possible to *approximate the skin edges* so as to facilitate healing.

Repair damaged structures, and restore function. Function is more important than the precise anatomy, although cosmetic considerations are naturally important. Some structures and organs are not vital, e.g. the spleen, the gall bladder, and when these are severely damaged they may be removed. Minor damage of an important structure can usually be repaired by direct suturing. When there is loss of a large part of a structure or organ with important functions, the alternatives are to make good the deficiency with the patient's own tissues from elsewhere (some form of *autograft*, e.g. nerve or skin graft), or to use a transplant from another individual of the same species (*allograft*) or another species (*xenograft*); or else to use an artificial replacement (*prosthesis*) such as an artificial limb.

For Healing of Wounds see Chapter 49, pp. 465–7.

Special injuries of soft tissues

Internal haemorrhage. Bleeding through an external wound is a menace, but at least it is obvious. Bleeding into one of the great cavities of the body —*cranium, thorax* and *abdomen*—is not obvious. Intracranial bleeding produces characteristic effects through disturbance of the brain long before the amount of blood lost assumes serious proportions as a cause of peripheral circulatory failure. Intrathoracic bleeding may be diagnosed with the help of X-rays. The great problem in diagnosis for the general surgeon is intra-abdominal haemorrhage such as may occur with a *ruptured spleen.* The surgeon follows the safe rule that if there is evidence of blood loss in a patient who has had an accident and there appears to be no blood loss anywhere else, then the bleeding is intra-peritoneal and requires an operation to look inside the abdomen (*exploratory laparotomy*). *The main evidence of such hidden losses is likely to be the rising pulse rate and the falling blood pressure which the nurse measures and records.*

Peritonitis. Both closed and open injuries may tear a hole in one of the hollow viscera of the abdomen, especially the gastro-intestinal tract or the bladder. The contents of these viscera are acidic or alkaline and hence irritant to the peritoneal cavity: in the case of the gut, the contents habitually contain pathogenic micro-organisms. *A severe inflammation of the peritoneum ensues, abdominal pain is intense and widespread, and the muscles of the abdominal wall are rigid. Treatment must include a laparotomy and suture of the perforation.*

Bites and Stings

Animal bites are treated like any other wound. Anti-tetanus precautions are usually advisable (p. 382), and the wound is cleaned of foreign material and dead tissue. The question of *rabies* is considered on p. 380.

Snake bite. In Britain the only venomous snake is the adder. The colour varies between black and reddish brown, there are zigzag dark markings along the back, and it is rarely longer than 20 inches. Management of an adder-bite should be rest, reassurance and the relief of pain and anxiety. The injection of antisera, and local measures such as incising and sucking the wound, probably do more harm than good.

Wasp and bee stings. The bee sting should be removed from the wound by wiping it out with a handkerchief. Wasps do not leave their sting behind. The best local application for both types of sting is an antihistamine cream, but alkalies (sodium bicarbonate, soap) for bee stings or weak acids (vinegar) for wasp stings are satisfactory.

Chapter 45

Surgical Techniques

by MARJORIE MATTHIAS

Introduction—preparation of a patient for operation—prevention of infection—steam sterilization of equipment—tests for efficiency of steam sterilization—dry heat sterilization—disinfection and disinfectants—swabs and sponges—sutures and ligatures—surgical needles—set of instruments for laparotomy

Operating theatre experience is not considered essential today as part of the student nurse's educational programme, and its place is often taken by a short period of observation in the theatre. This is regrettable as the experience does demonstrate some aspects of nursing to a degree not approached elsewhere.

The operating team consists of surgeon, anaesthetist, nurses and other auxiliary workers—male and female. The person in charge of a suite of theatres should be a nurse. Her responsibility is to co-ordinate the duties of all members of her staff and to link up their functions with the rest of the hospital and to achieve a safe environment for the patient's surgery.

Each nurse should become familiar with the layout of an operating theatre or theatre suite in her training school. Every nurse who prepares and accompanies a patient to the theatre for operation should be conversant with the method of preparing him for surgery.

THE WARD PREPARATION OF A PATIENT FOR A GENERAL ANAESTHETIC

In some hospitals the patient to have a general anaesthetic for an elective operation will already have had a preliminary examination by an anaesthetist (see p. 445). This routine examination may also reveal dental caries, which should be dealt with before the patient's surgery to remove a possible septic focus. The patient will be advised to restrict smoking and alcohol, if necessary. Certain exercises to improve lung function may be ordered.

On admission to the ward the patient is asked to sign a form giving *consent for anaesthetic and operation*. This is usually done by the house surgeon who also signs the form indicating that he has given the patient an explanation of what his operation will entail, and who will do it. This helps to allay the patient's natural anxiety about the ordeal ahead of him. It is usual to fit an identity bracelet to the patient's wrist at this stage.

Routine procedures should be explained to the patient by the nurse, who is able to reassure him that he will be given an injection (having made sure that this is so) and that he will be drowsy or asleep before he is taken to the theatre. Should the patient be having an operation under a local anaesthetic this procedure must be explained to him.

The nurse should also see that the patient's relatives are aware of what is going to happen, and she should advise them to telephone before visiting for the first time.

Routine preparation for *bowel surgery* usually includes an enema or colonic wash-out.

The patient should be assured of a good night's sleep before the day of the operation. A sedative is usually ordered. All preliminary X-rays, blood examinations and routine urinary examinations, and other investigations necessary will have been carried out.

The morning of the operation the patient should, if possible, have a shower. If the operation is to be on the head, trunk or lower limbs, shaving of the operative site is necessary. Whether this is done by nurse, medical student or barber, the nurse is responsible for seeing that it is correctly done. This should preferably be done immediately before the operation. The earlier it is done, the greater the danger of the small abrasions becoming septic foci. If a bath is impossible, the operative site must be thoroughly cleansed and shaved while the patient has a bed bath. Usually this is all the skin preparation the patient is given in the ward. Some orthopaedic units still require limbs to be cleansed with antiseptic soap and lotion on two occasions in the ward pre-operatively after which the area is covered with a sterile towel or sterile stockinette which is only removed before the final preparation in the theatre.

Probably the most important single point in the preparation of the patient for general anaesthetic is to ensure that the stomach is empty for at least four hours before the anaesthetic. Some anaesthetists insist on six hours starving. This is to avoid the danger of the patient vomiting or regurgitating the stomach contents during anaesthesia, when the fluid could quite easily be aspirated into the lungs. *For emergency surgery* it is usual to pass a stomach tube in order to aspirate the gastric contents.

The bladder and bowel should be emptied. Before gynaecological, or genito-urinary surgery the patient is catheterized in the theatre. The urine is measured and tested for sugar, albumin, ketones and the time of catheterization is noted. This is important in cases of bladder-outlet obstructions when the surgeon will wish to know the amount of residual urine.

It is usual for the patient to wear an easily removed gown. Sometimes hospital policy dictates a cap and stockings, but these are not necessary. Jewellery should be removed for safe-keeping and also because a large ring or bracelet could cause bruising if there is slight pressure on the arm. A wedding ring should be covered with a small piece of strapping.

Make-up should be removed as lipstick can mask signs of cyanosis, and also it is unpleasant for the anaesthetist when manipulating tubes and masks. *Hair slides and pins* should be removed as they could injure the head, particularly the ears. Long hair in both sexes should be confined by adequate covering. *Dentures* should be removed and placed in the patient's locker in a clearly marked container. Any large dental crowns, inlays or loose teeth should be noted and reported to the anaesthetist.

The final step in the pre-operative preparation is the pre-medication. This is ordered by the anaesthetist when he examines the patient after admission to the ward. It is usually given intramuscularly and the time of administration should be recorded by the nurse after she has given it.

The pre-medication has three chief functions: to relieve pain, to allay anxiety, to abolish parasympathetic effects such as increased bronchial secretions, salivation and cardiac irregularities.

The nurse should explain to the patient that the pre-medication is not the anaesthetic, that he will feel drowsy but will not be asleep, and that his mouth may feel uncomfortably dry. After the pre-medication has been given the patient should be left quietly to rest.

Meanwhile the nurse should be assembling the articles which should accompany the patient to the theatre. These are:

All the relevant notes and charts.

X-ray films and reports. Care should be taken that these include the most recent ones which may not have been returned to the ward from the radiodiagnostic department.

The consent form.

The drug chart upon which the pre-medication should be recorded.

The patient should be lightly and warmly covered for transit to the theatre. The pillow should have a protective covering on it. Whatever policy the hospital has for checking the identity of the patient should be meticulously observed before the patient leaves the ward.

Who accompanies the patient to the theatre, and whether he goes to the theatre on a trolley or in his own bed depends on the individual hospital. The nurse responsible should supervise these procedures carefully. Theatre porters, although they are instructed in the lifting and management of sick patients, cannot know about each patient's individual problems and hazards. It is the nurse's responsibility to protect the patient from injury.

On arriving in the theatre the patient is welcomed by a member of the theatre staff who checks his identity and ascertains that all the preliminary preparations have been completed by the ward staff. The patient is then wheeled into the anaesthetic room.

The anaesthetic room should be quiet, with the minimum number of people about. There should be no glaring overhead lighting beamed directly into the patient's eyes. Care should be taken by doctors, nurses and their assistants not to talk unnecessarily, and to have no conversation that does not include the patient. It should be remembered that the pre-medication often alarmingly distorts what he hears.

The patient is anaesthetized on a trolley or operating-table, and wheeled into the theatre where he is put into the appropriate position for his operation.

The patient is only moved under the anaesthetist's supervision, and it is important for the theatre staff to treat the unconscious patient with the same respect, and even more care, than they would if he were awake.

For easy lifting the patient should lie on a stretcher cover into which lifting poles can be threaded. This avoids danger to the patient, and back strain for the attendants doing the lifting.

To give the surgeon adequate access, various positions are used; in all of them there are inherent dangers for the patient:

> *Temporary or permanent paralysis* caused by undue pressure on or sudden stretching of nerves. This can be avoided by gentle movement, adequate support of limbs and suitable padding of bony prominences.
>
> *Venous thrombosis* caused by pressure. This is particularly liable to occur in the vessels of the calf. Pressure can be removed from this region by a foam cushion placed under the patient's heels.
>
> *Postoperative back pain* caused by lack of support and careless movement of the legs.
>
> *Dislocation of a joint or even fracture* if the arm is allowed to slip between trolley and table when lifting.

The patient is placed in the correct position on the table and the operating lights accurately focused on the operative site.

PREVENTION OF INFECTION

Wound infection is caused by *bacteria*, single-celled organisms of microscopic size. These organisms may be derived from the *patient* himself, or from his *surroundings* including the *operating theatre staff*.

Bacteria are normally found growing on the surface of the skin, and in body cavities close to the skin such as the mouth, nose, vagina and anal canal. There is also a normal population of bacteria in the alimentary canal, particularly the large bowel. In their normal habitat, these organisms cause no harm to the individual. However, should they gain access to the tissues via an external wound in numbers sufficient to overcome the natural defences of the body, some of these bacteria can *cause disease* (they are then said to be *pathogenic*). *The pre-operative skin-toilet and shaving, and the final skin-preparation in theatre* (see p. 428) *are designed to reduce the danger to the patient from himself.*

The *surroundings* include the air, the surfaces, and the equipment of the operating theatre, as well as the staff. Air-conditioning systems are used in many modern theatres to reduce, by processes such as filtration, the contamination of the air. Surfaces are designed to be easily and efficiently cleaned. Any member of the staff with a septic condition such as a sore throat or a skin infection must report sick and keep away from the operating theatre. The wearing of masks reduces contamination of the atmosphere by infected droplets of moisture from the nose and mouth, while all external clothing is replaced before entry to the operating room by freshly laundered garments designed to reduce dispersion of organisms from the body surfaces. The operator and assistants thoroughly cleanse hands and forearms, and wear sterile gowns and gloves. The theatre equipment used during an operation falls into two groups. First, there are instruments, linen and other supplies that come into direct contact with the open wound and must be sterile. The second group consists of the larger equipment in the theatre, such as table, lamp, diathermy, suction consoles and trolleys, which are not sterile, but which should be thoroughly cleaned.

The following definitions are important:

Spores, a dormant, highly resistant form into which some organisms can change when environmental factors (heat, cold, chemicals) threaten their life.

Asepsis, freedom from infection, or the absence of organisms. Aseptic techniques cover a wide variety of practices which, if carried out correctly, reduce the incidence of infection.

Sterilization, a physical or chemical process which destroys all bacteria and their spores. It is the basis of all aseptic techniques (see below).

Disinfection, the physical or chemical process by which most organisms are destroyed, but not the more resistant spores and viruses.

Antisepsis, the process by which most bacteria are destroyed or their growth prevented. Antiseptics are usually preparations designed for application to living tissue.

Sanitization, a good cleaning process or boiling which is used to destroy bacteria. It is ineffective against spores.

Sterile, completely free from bacteria and their spores. It is an absolute term; either an article is sterile or it is not. It is never 'almost sterile' or 'partly sterile'.

Skin preparation in theatre

This is the final preparation of the operative site. A wide area is cleansed with the antiseptic of the surgeon's choice following the method adopted by the hospital. All *antiseptics used for skin-cleansing should be coloured, so that the area that has been cleansed can be clearly defined*, and so that they cannot be mistaken for any solutions used internally.

All sponges used for skin-cleansing should be different from those used during the operation, so that they can be discarded immediately after use and not included in the count. Cubes of plastic foam are more effective and more economical than gauze swabs for this purpose.

This cleansing of the patient's skin may be done either by the 'scrubbed team', who must avoid contaminating themselves, or by a non-scrubbed member of the team who wears sterile gloves. In either case, sterilized sponges and forceps are used.

METHODS OF STERILIZATION OF EQUIPMENT

Physical means:

(i) Heat (*a*) moist, (*b*) dry.
(ii) Irradiation.

Chemical disinfection and sterilization:

(i) Liquid.
(ii) Gaseous.

When a population of bacteria is exposed to any sterilizing influence, the death of the cells does not occur instantaneously. In order to achieve sterility it is necessary to calculate the exposure period necessary to destroy the whole bacterial population.

Moist heat destroys bacteria at a relatively low temperature by coagulating the protein in their cells. When moisture is absent higher temperatures and longer exposures are required, because destruction of the bacteria cells by dry heat is primarily by a slower process of oxidation.

Moist heat in the form of boiling water will destroy only vegetative bacteria and not spores. *It is not an adequate method for sterilizing surgical instruments*, and should be used only if no other method is available.

Steam sterilization

Steam sterilization or the exposure of articles to saturated steam under pressure is the most dependable method. The temperature of atmospheric steam is that of boiling water, 100 °C (212 °F). Like boiling water it will destroy vegetative organisms but not spores, and like boiling water it has no value for the sterilization of surgical instruments. To raise the saturated steam to the required temperature the steam pressure has to be increased. It is important to remember that pressure itself has no part in the destruction of microbial life—it is merely a method of raising the temperature of the steam. *Saturated steam is that which has in it the maximum content of water vapour.* This increases the moisture and improves its penetration.

Steam sterilization is achieved by the use of an autoclave. This is an instrument usually consisting of two concentric shells, the outer one known as the jacket. Steam under pressure is first admitted to the jacket. This heats the walls of the inner chamber so that no condensation forms on these walls. Articles to be sterilized are placed in the inner chamber, from which the air has to be evacuated before steam can fill it. This evacuation may be by a vacuum pump, or the air may be expelled by the pressure of the entering steam. There are thus two types of autoclaves:

> The high vacuum autoclave.
> The gravity displacement autoclave.

The high vacuum autoclave is considered to be the more satisfactory instrument, and is in general use in this country.

Steam under pressure has the property of heating materials and permeating porous substances by a process of condensation. Steam gives up its heat in sterilizing by condensing back into the water from which it came. This means that every fibre of a porous article undergoing sterilization will absorb a quantity of moisture from the steam. This moisture is necessary (see p. 428), for the destruction of microbial life. When the entire mass of fabric in the sterilizer has been heated, the temperature of the fabric will remain constant at the temperature of the surrounding steam. At the end of the prescribed time the steam is evacuated and the load is subjected to a vacuum in order to dry it, followed by an intake of air through a bacteriological filter.

Time-temperature ratios for steam sterilization

°C	°F	Time Minutes
132	270	2
125	257	8
121	250	12
118	245	18
116	240	30

These are figures for *direct exposure to saturated steam* and do not provide for the additional time factor required for steam penetration through porous coverings.

It is possible to prescribe a shorter period of sterilization for unwrapped instruments than for fabrics which require time for penetration. *Knowledge of this principle is of importance to the nurse, as articles for sterilization in an autoclave, if wrapped at all, must be enclosed in a covering or wrapping through which steam can easily penetrate.*

Tests for the efficiency of steam sterilization

Charts. Recording thermometers should be standard equipment on all autoclaves. They should register the temperature at the discharge (the coolest point in the chamber) and the length of each exposure.

Bacteriologically. Resistant spores (*Bacillus stearothermophilus*) are placed at the centre of the autoclave load. They should produce a negative culture if the requisite temperature has been reached.

Chemically. Browne's tubes (Black spot) are also placed to the centre of the load. These contain a red fluid that turns green on exposure to heat. If the fluid turns an intermediate colour of orange or amber it denotes that the necessary temperature has not been reached.

Engineering efficiency. The Bowie test. A sheet of heat-sensitive paper is placed at the centre of a large pack of linen. The markings should be uniformly dark. A pale pattern in the centre denotes an inadequate penetration of steam, due to the presence of air in the chamber, which prevents the temperature reaching the necessary level.

Applying indicating tape to the outside of a pack does not guarantee the sterility of its contents—it merely indicates that the *outside* of the pack has been subjected to steam at the stated temperature. This method should only be used in conjunction with the other tests.

Klintex. Coloured papers will turn white when exposed to steam at 129 °C (265 °F). They too should be in the centre of a pack.

Preparing articles for steam sterilization. *Packs* have now taken the place of drums, and many types of wrapping can safely be used in a high vacuum sterilizer. There should *always be at least two wrappings or covers for a sterile article. Each pack should be loosely, but securely, wrapped. It should be folded with protective cuffs so that it can be unwrapped by ungloved hands without contaminating its contents.* When opened the wrap should be large enough to serve as a sterile working surface. The following articles may be employed.

Cotton fabric. It must be strong and of a fine weave, is still the easiest to handle, but the sorting and checking is time consuming and any worn area or hole is a hazard.

Paper. There are now many types of paper on the market for wrapping. A heavier paper is generally used as an outerwrap for greater protection, while a lighter one is used as the innerwrap. Paper has the greater advantage of being disposable, but though improvements are continual, it still lacks the good draping qualities of cloth.

Paper bags are suitable for small items, but they should be folded in such a way that the contents can be extruded past the edge without being contaminated. Cutting or tearing a bag open is not acceptable practice.

Nylon and polypropylene film. These have the advantage of being strong and waterproof, though permeable to steam under pressure. Packs wrapped in film need a fully effective vacuum autoclave as it is more difficult for air to be extracted from a pack wrapped in nylon than from one wrapped in paper or cloth. There is an additional hazard from increased static electricity if nylon film is used which has not been specially treated.

Dry heat sterilization. *Dry heat sterilization* is used when direct contact of the material to be sterilized with saturated steam is impossible. It is well suited for keen cutting instruments, and glassware. The action of dry heat on objects is that of conduction, the heat being absorbed by the exterior surface of an article and transmitted to the interior.

The dry sterilizing unit is similar to an ordinary oven, but it should have a fan to circulate the air to provide an even temperature in all parts of the chamber. *The time-temperature ratio* is higher than that for steam sterilization. As there is no moisture a higher temperature is also needed. A temperature of 160 °C (320 °F) for one hour will guarantee microbial destruction.

Tests for the efficiency of dry heat sterilization.
Charts. Recording thermometers should be standard equipment on all hot air sterilizers.

Bacteriological tests. Resistant spores should be placed at the centre of each load.

Chemically. Browne's tubes (Yellow spot) specially designed for dry sterilizers; their red fluid turns to green when subjected to a temperature of 160 °C (320 °F). *As with the steam sterilizer checking tubes,* p. 430, *intermediate colours denote inadequate sterilization.*

Preparing articles for dry heat sterilization. Linen and paper are unsuitable as they will burn at 160 °C (320 °F). Nylon will melt at that temperature. The most suitable containers are metal or glass as heat can readily be conducted through to their contents. These can be completely sealed before being put into the sterilizer.

Irradiation

This can only be carried out commercially. It is the most satisfactory method of all as it guarantees the total destruction of microbial life on materials in almost any kind of container or wrapping. It is particularly suitable for articles which will not withstand heat such as some forms of plastic, or delicate instruments. It is not suitable for some plastic materials, glassware or lensed instruments as it causes a brown discoloration of the glass.

The recommended dose of radiation for the sterilization of surgical equipment is 2·5 megarads. This amount is achieved by exposing articles to be sterilized to a radioactive cobalt 60 source by means of a conveyor system. No residual radiation remains in the article at the completion of this process.

Chemical disinfection

Before any chemical disinfection or sterilization is attempted the instrument should be physically clean. Organic soiling will absorb the germicidal molecules and inactivate them, and also make penetration by the chemical agent more difficult.

Whereas steam under pressure and gamma radiation can sterilize rapidly, only a few sporicidal chemicals can be relied on for sterilization, and these require a long exposure at high concentration. This is the case with 8 per cent formaldehyde, 2 per cent glutaraldehyde and 11 per cent ethylene oxide which when adequate exposure times are used are sporicidal. Only under these conditions is sterility achieved, the micro-organism being destroyed in much the same way as it is by moist heat. In other conditions chemical disinfection does not achieve this.

Liquid disinfectants

Quaternary ammonium compounds. These have the advantage of being bland in use, and can therefore be used as skin antiseptics.

Iodines. Iodine is a good germicide but has the disadvantage of staining. The staining can be reduced by combining the iodine with a detergent; this combination is known as an iodophor.

The alcohols. Ethyl and isopropyl alcohol (70 per cent) are much more useful as antiseptics than as disinfectants. Disinfectants can act only as long as they are in solution and this means that alcohols become ineffectual as soon as they evaporate.

Formaldehyde. This chemical in aqueous solution is known as formalin and is usually used in a 20 per cent solution. This is a powerful germicide and its activity is further increased by adding alcohol.

Gaseous disinfectants

Formaldehyde vapour. Sterilization by formaldehyde vapour is only possible in a moist atmosphere within a heated cabinet. If there is adequate moisture for the sterilization process, it tends to cause corrosion of metal. This limits the usefulness of the process. It is difficult to measure the concentration of the vapour, and as its penetration is doubtful because it is not under pressure, it is impossible to calculate its sterilization time. Formaldehyde has great toxicity so it is necessary that articles be thoroughly rinsed before use. *Attention should be paid particularly to any lensed instruments with eye pieces which, if not properly rinsed, can seriously affect the operator's eyes.*

Ethylene oxide. This gas is toxic, and in high concentrations it is flammable. It can penetrate through a mass of dry material with ease and can be used to sterilize articles which will not withstand heat, but there is a danger of some residual gas being left in the load at the completion of the sterilization process. Authorities vary in the lengths of time they suggest for the clearance of this. It may be from two or three hours for a small article to several days for a large one. For this reason, ethylene oxide sterilization is not popular in this country unless it is done commercially on a large scale with equipment fully tested to deliver the gas at the correct concentration, in the most effective humidity, and for the right length of exposure. Absence of residual gas must also be guaranteed.

Articles to be sterilized by gas should be wrapped in paper or cloth which is permeable to the vapour. Some plastic films also are suitable.

SWABS AND SPONGES

At present most swabs and packs used in surgery are made of cotton fibre. Various synthetic materials are also available which are equally absorbent and less expensive to use. *All swabs used should be disposable. They should be absorbent, and non-traumatic to the tissues, soft but not friable in use and have no loose fibre.* Most swabs can be bought ready made, many of them conveniently tied into bundles ready for use. The time-consuming and expensive way of hand-making swabs from rolls of gauze is now almost abandoned.

All swabs used for operation in the theatre should contain a radio-opaque thread. Swabs used by the anaesthetist or for minor procedures, such as catheterization, in the theatre should be of a different colour, to distinguish them from those used by the surgeon.

It is recommended in the Joint Memorandum published by the Medical Defence Union and the Royal College of Nursing that swabs be counted for 'every operation, however trivial', and a procedure is laid down for the swab count. All the points in this procedure should be carried out, and the theatre superintendent should prepare an even more detailed procedure to be carried out in her particular department. Nowadays, with staff constantly changing, it is imperative that all members of the theatre team be fully instructed in and scrupulously observe a printed procedure.

Although in many cases swabs are supplied already tied in bundles of five, *it is necessary for these to be checked by at least two people* at the following stages of the operation:

> Before the incision is made.
> Before the closure of any hollow viscus within the abdomen, chest or pelvic cavities, e.g. hysterectomy, cystotomy.
> Before the pelvic peritoneum is closed, e.g. sigmoid colectomy, hysterectomy, etc.
> Before the posterior parietal peritoneum is closed, e.g. aortic procedures, anterior spinal operations.
> In orthopaedic cases before any fixation device is inserted, e.g. plate, graft.
> In cases when a prosthesis is used, e.g. valve, vascular or joint.
> Before the first layer of the main wound is closed, e.g. peritoneum, joint capsule, pleura.
> After the final muscle closure and before the skin is sutured.

The surgeon should ascertain by direct inquiry, before the completion of the operation, whether all swabs have been accounted for. The 'scrubbed nurse' and her assistant should sign the record at the end of the operation that the count is correct.

There should also be a written procedure with the rules to be followed, should there be any discrepancy in the count. The radio-opaque thread in each swab is an additional safeguard as the patient can be X-rayed if there is any doubt.

All tapes and other materials used for retracting vessels etc. should also be included in the count. These, too, should be radio-opaque, but at present they are not available in this form.

Various types of score boards for swab counts are available; *metal boards* are the most satisfactory. Clear printed numbers can be mounted on an adhesive rubber magnetic backing. Cancellation signals, for used swabs, are convenient and accurate.

SUTURES AND LIGATURES

A *suture* is a stitch, a length of material threaded on a needle for sewing two surfaces together.

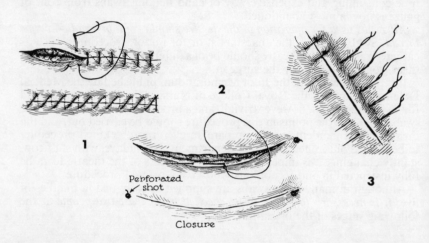

Fig. 45/1 Common types of skin suture. 1. Two types of continuous suture: their particular merit is speed. 2. The subcuticular suture, invisible after insertion apart from where it is anchored at its two ends. There are no stitch marks and the resultant scar may be cosmetically perfect. 3. Simple interrupted sutures have the advantage that individual sutures can be easily removed at different times, for example, to drain pus from an infected area.

There are many types of suturing used in surgery, each of them designed for a particular purpose. All types fall into two classes.

> *Interrupted.* A suture line consisting of separate sutures, each of them tied and cut individually. This type of suture line is usually considered to be the strongest. It is used for tissues where the blood supply is not plentiful, e.g. for large bowel anastomosis, etc., and for fascia which needs maximum support during healing.
>
> *Continuous.* The suture line consists of one running stitch tied at each end. It is haemostatic and non-leak, and is used for closing the peritoneum, and for the anastomosis of bowel and blood vessels.

Ligatures. One of the most common ways of establishing haemostasis during surgery is by ligature. By definition a ligature is a length of material tied round a blood vessel, or a leash of blood vessels, to prevent bleeding.

There are two main classifications of ligature and suture materials:

1. Absorbable
2. Non-absorbable

Absorbable materials become part of the host's body by being 'digested' by the tissues into which they are implanted. They are usually of animal origin. A synthetic absorbable suture material is now available.

Catgut.
Ribbon gut.
Fascia.
Kangaroo tendon.
Polyglycolic acid filament.

Non-absorbable. These materials may be of vegetable or mineral origin, or may be synthetically produced. All can be left buried in the body as well as on the surface. If left buried they will disintegrate in time.

Silk.
Nylon and other synthetics, Dacron, Mersilene, Orlon, Terylene.
Linen thread.
Wire—silver, stainless steel, tantalum, vitallium.
Cotton.
Silver clips.
Adhesive strips and Michel clips for skin closure.

Non-absorbable sutures

Silk. This is the most commonly used of all suture materials. It is usually supplied braided, but can be obtained twisted, or in a floss. It can be coated with wax or other substances to ease its passage through tissues. Silk is used extensively for buried sutures and ligatures, and for skin sutures. It has good tensile strength and handles well.

Nylon, Mersilene, Terylene, Orlon and Dacron. These are all synthetically produced forms of a polyester fibre. The various names are trade names of different firms. All these fibres can be coloured for easy identification. They are practically inert to the body and have great tensile strength, but do not handle quite as easily as does silk.

Other sutures include *wire, silver and tantalum clips and Michel clips*. These are used to close the skin of clean wounds in the lower abdomen, breast and neck. They have the advantage of leaving little scar and, unlike the suture, no part of the clip has to pass through the subcutaneous tissues.

Transverse adhesive strips are placed across the line of incision to approximate the skin edges. They are often used instead of skin sutures, particularly for children.

Most suture materials are supplied sterile and are governed by stringent Board of Trade controls. They should be in a double-peel-pack and be conveniently labelled and colour coded. The size range is constant throughout all types of materials and has to conform to standards of the British Pharmacopoeia. This size range has been adjusted to the metric scale.

SURGICAL NEEDLES

Surgeons' needles are many and varied. They are nearly all made of finely tempered steel, most are stainless and others are plated. They can be classified in various ways.

(i) By the type of point.
(ii) By the type of eye.
(iii) By shape.

Generally speaking:

> For (i) the surgeon's choice depends on *what* he is suturing.
> For (ii) the surgeon's choice depends on *how* he is suturing.
> For (iii) the surgeon's choice depends on *where* he is suturing.

The amount of trauma which a needle causes in the tissues is determined by its thickness and not its length. The part of the needle causing most trauma is the eye, where there are two thicknesses of suture material. To avoid this, *atraumatic or eyeless needles* have been devised.

The shape. Needles may be:

1. Straight
2. Half-curved
3. Half circle
4. $\frac{3}{8}$ circle or curved
5. $\frac{5}{8}$ circle

There is a vast range in all of the types and shapes of needles. A needle is measured by the length of its shaft. This can vary from about 3 mm to over 100 mm. All needles used should be counted and checked at appropriate stages of the operation.

INSTRUMENTS

The nurse should be familiar with the basic instruments needed for surgery. It is important that she should learn the instruments and their function at the same time.

Most surgical instruments are made of stainless steel. They are precision tools and should be used only for the purpose for which they were designed. They are expensive, as many are hand made. A basic set for an abdominal case will cost well over £200, while the instruments for a cardiac operation will cost in the region of £2,000.

Ideally, instruments after use should be cleaned by a mechanical washer, followed by immersion in an ultra-sonic cleaner. If they are cleaned by hand they should be scrubbed under cold, running water with a stiff nylon brush.

Instruments should never be oiled, but should be lubricated regularly, preferably after each washing, with a special non-organic lubricant.

Most instruments are best sterilized in an autoclave. The instruments for an operation are assembled together on a tray for sterilizing. The instrument tray may be combined with the rest of the sterile materials needed for the operation and sterilized as one unit (the pre-set tray system). The instruments may be sterilized in the theatre preparation room and added to the case pack in the theatre 'lay-up' room. The method used is governed by the space available, the number of cases and the types of surgery catered for. Special instruments with delicate points or finely tempered edges remain in a more satisfactory condition if they are sterilized in a hot-air oven.

Laparotomy, or alternatively abdominal section, is making a surgical incision into the abdomen. It may be for exploratory (or elective) purposes. The instruments required for a laparotomy are shown in Fig. 45/2.

The procedure of a laparotomy and the instruments needed for each stage.

What the surgeon does	*The instruments he needs*
1. Cleans the skin.	Sponge holding forceps (1), mounted with foam sponge.
2. Places the sterile towels in position and keeps them in place.	Towel clips (2).
3. Makes the incision.	Scalpel—consisting of handle with detachable, disposable blade (3).
4. Controls haemorrhage.	Artery forceps, straight (4) or, curved (5), used with diathermy electrodes and lead (6); or insulated diathermy dissecting or artery forceps (7) and lead.
5. Dissects and further incises tissue.	Dissecting forceps, toothed or plain (8); and dissecting scissors, straight (9) or curved (10) *(see also p. 438)*

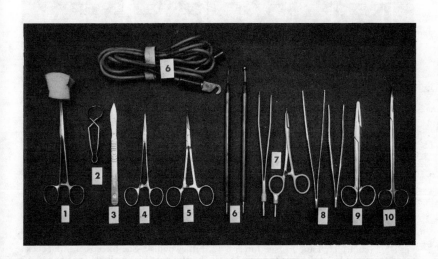

Fig. 45/2 Instruments for a laparotomy. 1. Sponge-holding forceps, mounted with foam sponge. 2. Towel clips. 3. Scalpel handle with detachable, disposable blade. 4 and 5. Straight and curved artery forceps. 6. Diathermy electrodes and lead. 7. Insulated diathermy dissecting forceps and artery forceps. 8. Dissecting forceps, toothed and plain. 9 and 10. Straight and curved dissecting scissors *(see also p. 438)*

6. Exposes operation site.

Tissue forceps—Lane's (11); Littlewood's (12); Babcock's (13); Allis' (14). Or retractors—hooked (15); blade (16, 18); bar (17).

7. Isolates and ligates blood vessels and pedicles.

Grooved dissector (19), or curved dissector. Aneurysm needle (20).

8. Removes any blood or peritoneal fluid.

Suction nozzles and tubing (21).

9. Repairs tissue layers.

With needles on holders— long and short (22).

10. Final closure of wound.

Michel clips (23). Introducing forceps (24).

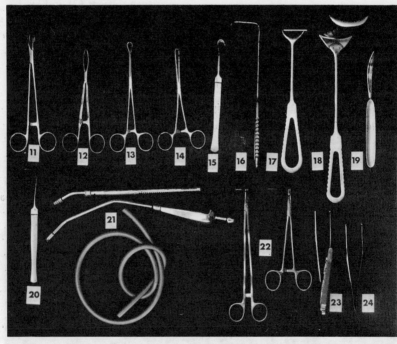

Fig. 45/2 (cont.) 11. Lane's tissue forceps. 12. Littlewood's tissue forceps. 13. Babcock's tissue forceps. 14. Allis' tissue forceps. 15. Hook retractor. 16. Small blade retractor. 17. Bar retractor. 18. Large blade retractor. 19. Grooved dissector. 20. Aneurysm needle. 21. Suction nozzles and tubing. 22. Long and short needle-holders with needles. 23. Michel clip-carrier forceps. 24. Michel clip-introducing forceps.

Chapter 46

Anaesthesia
Basic principles and the duties of the nurse

by W. K. SLACK

Introduction—general anaesthesia—muscle relaxants—local anal-
gesia—pre-medication—immediate pre- and postoperative nursing
care—cardiac arrest and its treatment

Anaesthesia is artificially produced loss of feeling or insensibility to pain.
Before the discovery of anaesthetics surgical operations were very limited
in scope; intra-abdominal and intra-thoracic operations were impossible,
and amputations of limbs were performed expeditiously by the surgeon but
with great suffering to the patient. Patients were often given sufficient
alcohol to produce virtual unconsciousness before operation. The earliest
recorded anaesthetics were in America and were the administration of
ether in 1842 and nitrous oxide in 1844, in both instances for extraction of a
tooth. Ether was first used in England at University College Hospital on
21 December 1846. The father of modern anaesthesia and the first full-
time anaesthetist in England was John Snow (1813–58). In 1853 he
anaesthetized Queen Victoria for the birth of her eighth child, Prince
Leopold.
   The science of modern anaesthesia has advanced since those early days,
and description of physiological effects and technical intricacies are
beyond the scope of this chapter. *The nurse should understand the principles*
of anaesthesia and the ways in which she can help both patient and anaesthetist.
Anaesthesia divides into:

> *General anaesthesia*, which implies production of total incapacity
> for feeling pain coincident with induction of unconsciousness.
> *Local analgesia*, which is production of incapacity for feeling pain
> in part of the body but without induction of unconsciousness.

GENERAL ANAESTHESIA

This is produced by intravenous or inhalational agents. All general
anaesthetic agents, whether administered intravenously or by inhalation,
reach the brain via the circulating blood and are absorbed into the brain
cells where they interfere with the metabolism of these cells, to produce
sleep and inability to feel pain. Speed of onset and recovery from anaes-

thesia varies from the quick-induction, quick-recovery intravenous agents to the slow-induction, slow-recovery volatile inhalation anaesthetic, ether. Although recovery of consciousness is rapid from the short-acting intravenous barbiturate anaesthetics, elimination of the agent from the body is much slower as these agents are rapidly redistributed in the fat stores of the body, thus reducing their concentration in the brain cells, and then broken down by liver enzymes.

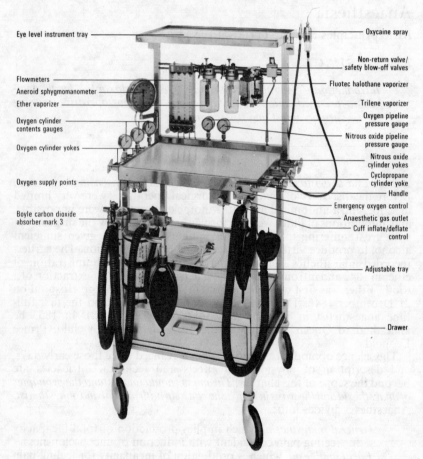

Eye level instrument tray

Flowmeters
Aneroid sphygmomanometer
Ether vaporizer
Oxygen cylinder contents gauges
Oxygen cylinder yokes
Oxygen supply points
Boyle carbon dioxide absorber mark 3

Oxycaine spray
Non-return valve/ safety blow-off valves
Fluotec halothane vaporizer
Trilene vaporizer
Oxygen pipeline pressure gauge
Nitrous oxide pipeline pressure gauge
Nitrous oxide cylinder yokes
Cyclopropane cylinder yoke
Handle
Emergency oxygen control
Anaesthetic gas outlet
Cuff inflate/deflate control
Adjustable tray
Drawer

Fig. 46/1 Boyle's machine.

For short operations, the barbiturates thiopentone and methohexitone, or the non-barbiturate Propanidid, administered intravenously are sometimes used alone. *For longer operations*, anaesthesia is usually induced by intravenous administration of one of the short-acting drugs mentioned above and maintained by inhalational agents, either nitrous oxide and oxygen gas mixtures alone, or more often supplemented by passage of these gas mixtures over a volatile liquid anaesthetic agent, such as halo-

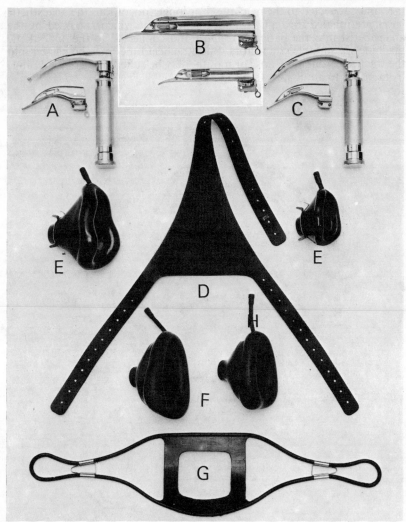

Fig. 46/2 Laryngoscopes. (*a*) Macintosh laryngoscope with Macintosh blades. (*b*) Magill blades. (*c*) Hook-on laryngoscope with Macintosh blades. (*d*) Clausen harness. (*e*) Anaesthetic face masks (anatomically shaped pad). (*f*) Anaesthetic face masks (flat pad). (*g*) Cornell harness.

thane, trichlorethylene or ether. Chloroform, once used frequently, is used little today because of its rare but serious hepatotoxic effects. Cyclopropane, a purely gaseous agent, is used occasionally in combination with oxygen for induction and maintenance of anaesthesia. The inhalational anaesthetics are usually administered from anaesthetic machines; the most popular is the Boyle's machine (see Fig. 46/1).

For simple short operations inhalational anaesthetics are administered via a face mask (see Fig. 46/2), which is held or strapped on the patient's face and connected to the machine. For longer operations the anaesthetic gases are inhaled through an endotracheal tube which is passed by the anaesthetist into the patient's trachea and connected to the anaesthetic machine via suitable connectors. Endotracheal tubes may be passed into the trachea through the nose or mouth, may be cuffed or plain, and range from infant to adult sizes (see Fig. 46/3).

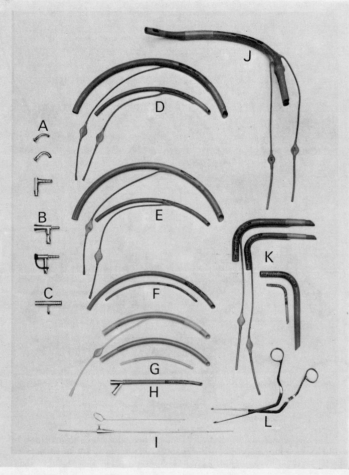

Fig. 46/3 Endotracheal tubes, cuffed or plain, infant to adult sizes. (a) Magill (oral and nasal) and Rowbotham connections. (b) Magill and Cobb suction unions. (c) Ayre T-piece. (d) Magill cuffed endotracheal tubes. (e) Magill 'streamline' cuffed endotracheal tubes. (f) Magill endotracheal tubes (plain). (g) Nylon reinforced latex endotracheal tubes. (h) Magill flexometallic tube. (i) Stilette and malleable introducer. (j) Robertshaw endobronchial tube. (k) Oxford non-kinking tubes cuffed and plain. (l) Magill forceps.

The cuff on the endotracheal tube is inflated following passage of the tube into the trachea and seals the external wall of the tube to the internal wall of the trachea, ensuring that the patient breathes only gases from the anaesthetic machine. The cuff is also effective in preventing regurgitated material from the stomach passing down the trachea into the lungs where it could cause dangerous complications, such as aspiration pneumonia. For some intrathoracic operations it is necessary to collapse one lung, the patient breathing exclusively with the remaining lung. To achieve this the anaesthetist uses endobronchial tubes or 'bronchial blockers'. Sometimes double lumen tubes are used which allow one or both lungs to be inflated at will. A selection of these tubes is shown in Fig. 46/3.

MUSCLE RELAXANTS

For intra-abdominal operations, relaxation of the abdominal muscles is necessary. Before the introduction of muscle relaxants the only way of achieving this with a general anaesthetic was to deepen anaesthesia with ether or other inhalational agent. Unfortunately, this often caused prolonged postoperative nausea and vomiting. *The introduction of muscle-relaxant drugs revolutionized anaesthesia, permitting attainment of adequate muscular relaxation by drug-induced paralysis of the skeletal muscles, in association with only light general anaesthesia.* Muscle relaxants also made possible major intra-thoracic operations as, when the chest is opened, controlled artificial ventilation of the lungs is necessary and this can be achieved satisfactorily only in a completely relaxed patient.

The first muscle-relaxant drug, introduced in the early 1940s, was tubocurarine chloride or curare, which is a purified form of the South American arrow poison derived from the plant *Chondodendron tomentosum*. This drug acts by blocking the transfer of nerve impulses from the nerve to the muscle at the motor endplate where the nerve joins the muscle. Other drugs acting in a similar manner are gallamine triethiodide (Flaxedil) and pancuronium bromide (Pavulon). The drugs of this group have a duration of action from 20 minutes for gallamine, to 45 minutes for curare. Where only brief muscular relaxation is required (as for introduction of an endotracheal tube, manipulations under general anaesthesia or for endoscopies) a short-acting muscle relaxant is used, most frequently suxamethonium chloride (Scoline) which acts for only 3 to 6 minutes and produces muscular relaxation in a different way pharmacologically than the 'curare-type' drugs. Curare and similarly acting drugs produce muscular relaxation by competing with—or blocking—the action of acetylcholine at the motor endplate (neuromuscular junction) thus preventing the muscle contracting in response to impulses passing down its motor nerve. Acetylcholine is the chemical substance which is released at the motor endplate and causes the muscle to contract following electrical depolarization of the motor nerve when an impulse passes down it to tell the muscle to contract.

The paralysis produced by drugs of the curare family is reversed at the end of an operation by the intravenous injection of a suitable dose of neostigmine (Prostigmin) which is an anticholinesterase and blocks the action of cholinesterase, which has the normal function of destroying unwanted acetylcholine. Thus, acetylcholine builds up again at the motor endplate and overcomes the action of the curare. Atropine 1·2 mg is always given intravenously shortly before, or with, the normal 2·5 mg dose of neostigmine, to prevent the undesirable actions of neostigmine which are cardiac slowing and production of profuse salivary and bronchial secretions.

The short-acting muscle relaxant suxamethonium chloride (Scoline) acts by causing prolonged depolarization of the motor nerve and excessive release of acetylcholine at the motor endplate. This causes an initial twitching—or fasciculation—of the muscle (this generalized twitching following the initial intravenous injection of Scoline must have been observed by most nurses assisting anaesthetists), followed by a flaccid paralysis for 3 to 6 minutes until the enzyme plasma pseudocholinesterase has destroyed the excess acetylcholine, allowing 'tone' to return to the muscle.

Pseudocholinesterase, the antagonist to suxamethonium, is produced in the liver and there is no commercially available similar substance, so in patients with liver disease in whom there may be a deficiency of pseudocholinesterase, the anaesthetist will usually avoid the use of suxamethonium because of the danger of producing prolonged apnoea from paralysis of the respiratory muscles (Scoline apnoea). Rarely, patients are encountered who, although otherwise healthy, have an inherited pseudocholinesterase deficiency and, if given suxamethonium, suffer prolonged paralysis, sometimes necessitating artificial positive pressure ventilation for several hours before they regain normal muscle tone and can resume spontaneous breathing. Once detected, it is normal to warn these patients that they are 'sensitive to Scoline and subject to Scoline apnoea', and it is usually prudent to test their near relatives for similar pseudocholinesterase deficiency.

LOCAL ANALGESIA

Abolition of pain is produced by the injection of solutions of local anaesthetic agents, which block impulses in motor and sensory nerves. Local analgesia is divided into:

> *Local infiltration*, used for such procedures as the excision of a small wart on the skin.
>
> *Regional analgesia.* An example is brachial plexus block, where the tissues round the main nerves to the upper limb are infiltrated with local analgesic solution either in the supraclavicular region or in the axilla. Operations can be performed on the upper limb without the patient feeling pain.
>
> *Spinal analgesia*, which renders the patient insensitive to pain below the level of the block and provides muscular relaxation for major operations on the lower limbs or abdomen. When spinal analgesia is given, the local anaesthetic solution is introduced into the cerebrospinal fluid in the subarachnoid space and blocks both sensory and motor nerves at their roots in the spinal cord.
>
> *Extradural analgesia*, which also is used for operations on the lower limbs and abdomen, and again the local analgesic solution is introduced near to the source of the motor and sensory nerves but, in this instance, not into the cerebrospinal fluid but into the extradural (epidural) space, which is the space between the outer surface of the dura mater (the outer layer of the spinal meninges) and the inner surface of the ligaments joining the laminae of the

vertebrae. This space extends from the foramen magnum to the sacrum.

The drugs mainly used for the production of local analgesia are lignocaine hydrochloride, which is used for local infiltration, regional nerve blocks and extradural blocks, and heavy cinchocaine (that is, cinchocaine 1/200 in 6 per cent glucose solution), for spinal analgesia. Both lignocaine and cinchocaine solutions can be used plain or with the addition of adrenaline to delay their absorption following injection. *An important duty of a nurse assisting an anaesthetist is to cross-check with him or her the strength of adrenaline added to the solutions as, if too much adrenaline is added, it can cause cardio-vascular disturbance and even death.*

PRE-MEDICATION

The nurse's duties relating to patients about to have an anaesthetic and operation start long before the patient goes to the operating theatre.

Preparation for anaesthesia and operation usually starts the previous day when a visit is made by the anaesthetist to assess the patient's general condition. He, or she, will need the patient's notes and relevant X-rays and will examine the patient with particular reference to heart and lungs and note any deformities of nose or mouth which could interfere with the fit of face masks or with the introduction of endotracheal tubes. If spinal or extradural analgesia is contemplated, it will be necessary to examine the patient's back for deformities which could interfere with the introduction of spinal or epidural needles. Stethoscope, sphygmomanometer, torch and spatula will be needed for the examination.

Pre-medicant drugs prescribed by the anaesthetist are given before operation for sedation and to depress reflex activity, which may be excessive in a nervous patient. The common sedative drugs used for pre-medication are Omnopon, morphine and pethidine. Scopolamine is often combined with Omnopon, as the former has a central sedative action as well as its depressant action on vagal reflex activity which helps to dry up salivary and bronchial secretion. Atropine, which also dries up salivary and bronchial secretions and protects the heart against vagal reflex activity, is often used in combination with pethidine or morphine. *In children* the common pre-medicants are Nepenthe and atropine, Vallergan and atropine, or graded doses of Omnopon and Scopolamine. *Anti-emetic drugs* are often given in combination with the pre-medication to prevent postoperative nausea and vomiting. Such drugs are Haloperidol (which is also a tranquillizer) and the antihistamine Promethazine. The pre-medication is given by the nurse by subcutaneous or intramuscular injection half to one hour before operation except in the case of Vallergan which is given to children according to body weight as a small volume oral dose of a syrup about 2 hours before operation. The sites for injection are the deltoid muscle in the arm or the upper and outer quadrant of the buttock (see Fig. 9/1, p. 85). After pre-medication the patient should be made comfortable and encouraged to sleep.

PRE-OPERATIVE NURSING CARE

Other important nursing duties in pre-operative care include withdrawal of food and drink from the patient for at least four hours before general anaesthesia. If the stomach is full, regurgitation of its contents can occur on induction of anaesthesia. Anaesthesia abolishes the normal protective laryngeal reflexes which prevent inhalation of stomach contents if vomiting occurs. *Inhaled vomit can cause aspiration pneumonia*, the development later of lung abscess or, in gross inhalation, even drowning and death. *It is doubly important that a careful watch is kept following pre-medication as the patient may be disorientated and forget earlier instructions not to eat or drink*. Dentures or other artificial aids must be removed before the patient goes to the operating theatre.

All patients are afraid of anaesthesia and operations, however much they may attempt to hide it, and *a compassionate pre-operative nursing duty is to allay fear and promote tranquillity*. The ward nurse should accompany the patient to the operating theatre, ensuring minimum mental or physical disturbance, and should remain in the anaesthetic room until the patient is anaesthetized.

In the operating theatre. The nurse's duties as assistant to the anaesthetist vary in different hospitals. In some, the anaesthetist is assisted by operating theatre technicians. In others, a sister or staff-nurse helps; in small hospitals particularly, the ward nurse who brings the patient to the operating theatre is the person to assist the anaesthetist during the induction of anaesthesia.

When assisting the anaesthetist in the theatre, the nurse should ensure that the necessary drugs, syringes and intravenous drip sets are available and prepared. Syringes and needles are usually disposable or supplied sterilized from a central sterile supply department. Syringes should not be boiled to sterilize them as boiling does not eradicate sporing bacteria or the virus of serum hepatitis; 20 ml or 10 ml syringes are usually used for the injection of thiopentone, and 2 ml or 5 ml ones for the injection of muscle relaxants and other drugs.

The induction of anaesthesia. The intravenous injection to induce anaesthesia is usually given into a vein on the back of the hand or in the ante-cubital fossa. The former site is preferred as accidental intra-arterial injection is possible in the ante-cubital fossa because of the occasional presence of aberrant branches of the brachial artery. If thiopentone is injected intra-arterially, it causes intense arterial spasm and subsequent ischaemic contractures in the arm. Aberrant arteries are rare on the dorsum of the hand and thus it is the safest site for the injection.

To give an intravenous injection it is necessary to distend the selected vein. *The wrist or arm is encircled by the nurse with both hands and gripped with a pressure sufficient to occlude the venous return from below the site at which the arm is held but insufficient to occlude the arterial supply.* It is important to encircle the arm completely as otherwise collateral veins will allow emptying of the vein which it is wished to distend.

After intravenous induction of anaesthesia and injection of the appropriate muscle relaxant, the anaesthetist will inflate the patient's lungs with oxygen from the anaesthetic machine and, using a laryngoscope to visualize the larynx, will insert an endotracheal tube. The laryngoscope used will probably be a Macintosh or Magill, or a variation of these types (see Fig. 46/2) and these instruments should be ready. Other instruments sometimes required to facilitate intubation are Magill's endotracheal intubation forceps, and malleable directors which, when inserted down the endotracheal tube, vary its curvature (see Fig. 46/3, p. 442).

For oral or nasal operations, it is necessary to pack the throat to prevent blood or operative debris passing into the trachea or oesophagus, and a pack should be available. The throat can be packed round the endotracheal tube with sterile two-inch ribbon gauze soaked in sterile normal saline solution and then wrung out, or soaked in sterile liquid paraffin and very thoroughly wrung out. *It is important that the paraffin-soaked throat pack should be wrung dry as liquid paraffin, if aspirated into the lung, can cause severe pneumonia.* Some anaesthetists prefer to pack the throat with intravaginal tampons placed in the pharynx each side of the endotracheal tube.

Duties of a nurse during anaesthesia. He or she may assist with setting up intravenous drips and should ensure that the supply of syringes and drugs is adequate. It may be necessary to use suction to clear the mouth, throat and trachea of accumulated secretions while the operation is in progress, and appropriate sterile suction catheters will be required. At the end of the operation a clean laryngoscope, sucker and swabs will be needed by the anaesthetist to ensure the patient's airway is clear, and a clean oral airway must be available to place in the patient's mouth.

POSTOPERATIVE NURSING CARE

Under ideal conditions the patient will then be moved from the operating theatre to a recovery room within the theatre suite, to await return of consciousness before transfer to the ward. A nurse will normally be left to watch the patient during this period when consciousness has not fully returned. The most critical moments in anaesthesia are during induction and recovery.

During the recovery phase particular care is necessary to ensure that the airway remains clear, that respiration is adequate and that pulse and blood pressure are steady. Any changes should be notified immediately to the anaesthetist. The patient's colour should be observed and any cyanosis reported immediately. It is particularly important that patients who are carriers of the 'sickle cell trait' (see Chapter 23, page 219) should not be allowed to suffer even the most minor degree of hypoxia in the recovery period from anaesthesia, as such hypoxia can precipitate a fatal sickle cell crisis. Usually, patients who are sickle cell positive are given 100 per cent oxygen or oxygen-enriched air by inhalation during the postoperative period until they are fully awake. These patients should not be allowed to become hypotensive, chilled or to suffer any local circulatory impairment (e.g. obstruction of the circulation caused by pressure on a limb because of bad positioning), as hypotension, chilling or circulatory obstruction cause circulatory stasis, metabolic acidosis and tissue anoxia, which factors may precipitate a sickle cell crisis. It is also important to prevent dehydration as this also can cause a sickle cell crisis, so intravenous infusions must be watched carefully and if they stop, this must be reported immediately.

Finally, patients must not be allowed to harm themselves by unconsciously assuming abnormal positions during recovery from anaesthesia.

Cardiac arrest may occur during induction of, and recovery from, anaesthesia and when this happens it is almost always due to hypoxia and again illustrates the paramount importance of keeping the airway clear. If the patient suddenly becomes cyanosed or grey in colour, with dilated pupils and absence of peripheral pulses, *cardiac arrest should be suspected and immediate remedial action taken. The time of the cardiac arrest should be noted.* The lungs should be inflated with oxygen using the anaesthetic face mask and rebreathing bags connected to the oxygen supply (which should be available in all recovery rooms), and immediate *external cardiac massage* commenced at a rate of 60 per minute, after first ensuring that the airway is clear. Time must not be wasted. Irreversible brain damage occurs in three to four minutes if an adequate circulation of oxygenated blood is not restored to the brain. Each second that is wasted before the institution of effective external cardiac massage and artificial ventilation adds to the possibility of subsequent brain damage even if the patient recovers. Medical assistance must be summoned immediately. Rhythmical sternal compression should be commenced at once and after every 10 pressures on the lower end of the sternum with the flat of the hands, the patient's lungs should be re-inflated. If no oxygen equipment is available, then mouth-to-mouth breathing must be performed.

It is important that the technique of external cardiac massage and artificial ventilation with mouth-to-mouth breathing for the treatment of cardiac arrest, should be taught to nurses by practical demonstration as soon as possible after starting their training.

During normal recovery from anaesthesia the patient rapidly regains consciousness and can then be returned to the ward. Even then the nurse's duties relating to the care of the anaesthetized patient have not ended. The patient may still have a labile blood pressure from disturbance of the autonomic nervous system during anaesthesia or because of postoperative pain. *Pulse, blood pressure and respiration must be watched carefully. A rising pulse rate may indicate postoperative bleeding or may, of course, just be a response to pain. Concurrent rise in pulse rate and fall in blood pressure are more likely to be due to bleeding.*

The patient must be encouraged to breathe adequately and to cough, to help to clear accumulated bronchial secretions and thus diminish the risk of postoperative pulmonary atelectasis or pneumonia. Pain after abdominal operation often prevents adequate deep breathing or coughing, and effective analgesics are necessary. *Movement of the limbs,* especially the legs, should be encouraged, whenever possible, to prevent postoperative venous thrombosis which predisposes to pulmonary embolism. *Any significant or unexpected change in the patient's condition should be reported immediately.*

After operation on the mouth, nose or throat, when particular care is necessary to ensure maintenance of a clear airway and that no blood is inhaled, the patient is placed on his or her side in the postoperative 'tonsil' position (see Fig. 8/3, p. 80) until full reflex activity has returned.

Postoperative intravenous infusions should not be allowed to run too quickly, which may overload the patient's circulation, or too slowly, which may result in an inadequate fluid intake (see also Blood Transfusions, p. 455. If subcutaneous swelling occurs at the site of an intravenous drip, it should be stopped and the doctor informed, as such swelling indicates that the drip is running outside the vein.

Chapter 47

Oxygen and Hyperbaric Oxygen Therapy
Indications and hazards in relation to nursing care

by W. K. SLACK

> *Uses of oxygen therapy—methods of administering oxygen—hyperbaric oxygen therapy—the hazards of oxygen therapy and of hyperbaric oxygen therapy.*

Oxygen, a gas forming 20 per cent of air, is necessary for virtually all mammalian metabolism and without it human life cannot continue. When air is breathed, haemoglobin is only 97 per cent saturated with oxygen, but if 100 per cent oxygen is breathed instead, haemoglobin becomes fully saturated and nitrogen, which forms 80 per cent of air, is washed out of the lungs and replaced by oxygen. Excess oxygen is dissolved in the plasma and thus reaches the tissues in greater than normal amounts and gradually eliminates all nitrogen.

Oxygen deprivation is most disastrous initially to highly developed tissues and organs. Thus, the brain, the most specialized organ, dies if deprived of oxygen for more than four to five minutes, and brief cerebral hypoxia, as occurs in common syncope or fainting, causes temporary unconsciousness. Conversely, the less highly developed tissues of the limbs can stand more prolonged oxygen deprivation, which is demonstrated by their resistance to hypoxia following application of tourniquets to cut off blood supply during orthopaedic operations.

Oxygen administration helps in conditions featuring hypoxia, occurring:

(1) *When breathing is impaired.*
   (*a*) In partial obstruction of the airways, as may occur in tumours or inflammation of the larynx or trachea.
   (*b*) In respiratory inadequacy from muscular weakness, which occurs in some diseases of the nervous system.
(2) *In disease of the lungs* which diminishes diffusion of oxygen to the blood. Examples are severe bronchitis, chronic bronchitis with emphysema, acute pneumonia, or heart failure with consequent pulmonary oedema. In the treatment of these conditions it is important that the inspired air should not be enriched with more than 30 per cent oxygen without specific medical instructions, as inhalation of higher concentrations of oxygen can cause respiratory arrest because of abolition of the anoxic drive from the chemoreceptors in the patient's carotid sinuses.

(3) *In impairment of oxygen transport by the blood* to the tissues.
   (*a*) In severe anaemia, where there is deficiency of haemoglobin.
   (*b*) In severe haemorrhage where, again, there is deficiency of haemoglobin plus loss of circulating blood volume.
   (*c*) In carbon monoxide poisoning, where haemoglobin combines preferentially with carbon monoxide rather than with oxygen.
   (*d*) In congestive heart failure, where slowing of the circulation occurs in addition to the diffusion defect in the lungs mentioned earlier.
(4) Finally, when oxygen may fail to reach the tissues because of degenerative disease of the blood vessels.

METHODS OF ADMINISTRATION OF OXYGEN

One hundred per cent oxygen can be administered alone or the inspired air can be enriched with varying amounts of oxygen. In the ward, oxygen is supplied from cylinders or pipe-line and after passage through pressure-reducing valves and flow-meters, is usually breathed by the patient via a

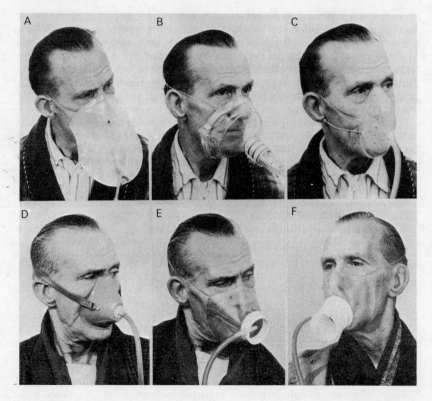

Fig. 47/1 Face masks. (*a*) Polymask. (*b*) Vickers Ventimask. (*c*) Harris mask. (*d*) BOC mask. (*e*) Edinburgh mask. (*f*) Edinburgh mask with extension.

face mask (see Fig. 47/1). Most face masks are relatively inefficient because of poor fit and consequent leakage, and the patient usually does not receive more than 60 per cent oxygen.

Another now rather out-dated method of oxygen administration is by means of special spectacles, worn by the patient, and carrying fine tubes, the ends of which pass into the patient's nostrils and through which a stream of oxygen is delivered to enrich the inspired air.

The patient can be placed in a plastic tent which is supplied with 100 per cent oxygen, but is unlikely to receive more than 40 per cent oxygen because of leakage of air into the tent and oxygen out of it.

Humidification. During long-term administration of oxygen it is necessary to humidify the gas to prevent irritation of the respiratory mucosae by the dry oxygen supplied from cylinders or pipe-line. The basic principle of humidification is to pass the dry gas through a waterbath before it reaches the patient so that it will pick up water vapour. Various commercially produced humidifiers are available.

HYPERBARIC OXYGENATION

Hyperbaric oxygenation can be defined as the inhalation of oxygen when the surrounding air, oxygen or other gases are at a pressure greater than atmospheric (atmospheric pressure = 760 mm mercury or 14·7 lb per sq. in. at sea level). In clinical practice this means that the patient breathes 100 per cent oxygen while within an air or oxygen environment at greater than atmospheric pressure. When breathing 100 per cent oxygen under hyperbaric conditions, more oxygen is dissolved in the blood plasma than when

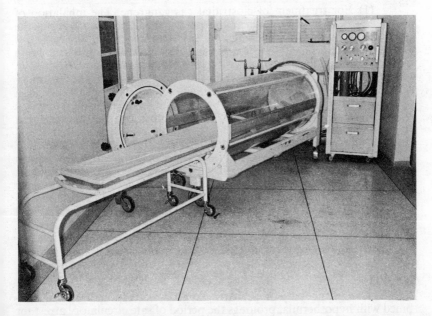

Fig. 47/2 Vicker's hyperbaric oxygen single-patient clinical chamber in hyperbaric oxygen unit at Whipps Cross Hospital.

breathing air or oxygen at normal pressure, so extra oxygen is available to the tissues.

There are two methods of giving hyperbaric oxygen therapy. In the first the patient is enclosed in a single-person hyperbaric oxygen chamber (see Fig. 47/2), which is filled and ventilated with 100 per cent oxygen at a pressure greater than atmospheric, usually two or three atmospheres absolute (atmospheric pressure equals one atmosphere absolute). Thus the patient breathes oxygen at this increased pressure. In the second method, the patient and medical and nursing staff are enclosed within a large chamber which is filled and ventilated with air compressed to similar pressure. The patient, however, breathes 100 per cent oxygen from a mask or via an endotracheal tube (depending on whether conscious or anaesthetized), while the medical staff breathe compressed air. In these conditions the oxygen breathed by the patient is at the same pressure as that to which the air in the chamber is compressed.

INDICATIONS FOR HYPERBARIC OXYGEN

Hyperbaric oxygen therapy is indicated for treatment of conditions featuring deficient tissue oxygenation or certain infections in which oxygen at high pressure inhibits growth of the causative organisms. Hyperbaric oxygen therapy also is used concurrently with radiotherapy for the treatment of some malignant tumours where there is evidence that results are better when the two regimes are used simultaneously.

Although still relatively experimental, hyperbaric oxygen therapy is used clinically:

(1) For treatment of clostridial gas gangrene. The inhalation of 100 per cent oxygen at increased ambient pressure prevents the growth of *Clostridium welchii* (a true anaerobe), the causative organism of the disease, and also prevents clostridial toxin production.

(2) For treatment of carbon monoxide poisoning. Carbon monoxide combines with haemoglobin much more readily than oxygen. Oxygen, when breathed at high pressure, competes with carbon monoxide for attachment to the haemoglobin molecule and 'drives off' the carbon monoxide.

(3) In conjunction with radiotherapy, as mentioned above.

(4) For treatment of surface infections caused by aerobic organisms which are sensitive to oxygen at increased pressure. Patients with infected varicose ulcers, pressure sores and burns may benefit. Hyperbaric oxygen therapy also seems to reduce infection and increase the rate of healing in split skin grafts and ischaemic pedicle skin grafts.

(5) In haemorrhagic shock.

(6) In the treatment of coronary thrombosis.

Its use in the treatment of these last two conditions is still very experimental.

Again experimentally, hyperbaric oxygenation, especially when combined with hypothermia, prolongs the period of safe circulatory arrest for cardiac surgery, and clinical experience with this technique in the surgery of congenital heart disease in infants is encouraging.

THE HAZARDS OF OXYGEN THERAPY AND HYPERBARIC OXYGEN THERAPY

The greatest risk during oxygen and hyperbaric oxygen therapy is that of *fire*. Oxygen supports combustion much more readily than does air, because air consists of approximately 80 per cent nitrogen, an inert gas, which has a smothering effect on fire. Combustion occurs 1,000 times more readily in a 100 per cent oxygen atmosphere than in air, and after ignition the fire burns five times more rapidly in oxygen than in air. Furthermore, *fires in oxygen have special characteristics and will flash over the surface of the body and, indeed, actually set light to the skin or the nap of the body and cannot be smothered. They require a very dense water spray to extinguish them.*

It is essential that any possible fire risk is eliminated whenever a patient is receiving oxygen therapy. All sources of ignition, such as matches, cigarette lighters, electric bell pushes and frictional or sparking toys should be excluded from oxygen tents or hyperbaric chambers. No clothing made of nylon or man-made fibre should be worn by patients or nurses entering hyperbaric oxygen chambers, as these materials accumulate static electrical charges which cause sparking. No grease should be used on the valves of oxygen cylinders as this can cause fire when the valves are opened.

Special hazards of hyperbaric oxygen therapy. A limited number of nurses are expected to work in hyperbaric oxygen units and they should appreciate the special hazards involved. Some nurses are expected to enter the large compressed-air hyperbaric chambers in which patients have operations. Nurses entering these chambers run the risks common to all workers in a compressed-air environment. These are:

Otitic barotrauma. This is the damage which may occur to the eardrums if blockage of the Eustachian tube by catarrh prevents air from entering or leaving the middle ear when the environmental pressure is changed.

Decompression sickness. This occurs if decompression is carried out too rapidly following exposure to compressed air. Bubbles of nitrogen form in the body tissues. In *simple bends* (or Type I decompression sickness) the bubbles collect round the large joints and cause pain. In Type II decompression sickness the bubbles may collect in the pulmonary circulation causing 'the chokes', a feeling of intense shortness of breath; in the cardiac circulation causing symptoms similar to those of coronary thrombosis; or in the blood vessels supplying the brain and spinal cord, causing neurological disturbances often referred to as 'the staggers'. *The last is the most serious type of decompression sickness which, unless treated very rapidly by recompression, may cause permanent paralysis or death.*

Rupture of lung cysts and emphysematous bullae during decompression. Lung cysts or bullae may fill with compressed gas which expands during decompression of the chamber causing rupture of the cyst. Patients and staff should have routine X-ray examinations to exclude this possibility.

Nitrogen narcosis. Nitrogen, when breathed at high pressures (and remember, air contains 80 per cent nitrogen) becomes a mildly narcotic gas and can cause slight disturbances of intellect. This shows itself in an inability to perform complicated tasks satisfactorily unless they have been learned thoroughly beforehand. *This means that a doctor or a nurse in a compressed-air environment meeting a complicated emergency for the first time may not be able to think so clearly and thus may be unable to cope with the situation as satisfactorily as if the same emergency had occurred at normal atmospheric pressure.*

Avascular necrosis of bone. This is a sinister hazard, as it can have a latent period of development from three months to 10 years after exposure to compressed air. The aetiology is still not completely clear but is probably related to nitrogen bubbling in the blood vessels of the bone during decompression, the pressure of the bubbles cutting off the blood supply to areas of bone and causing avascular necrosis. If this occurs at the end of a bone beneath the articular cartilage at a joint, the joint surface collapses and this subsequently causes crippling arthritis.

In hospitals where there are single-person hyperbaric oxygen chambers, the nurses operating them will not be exposed to the hazards accepted by those who enter the larger chambers. It is important, however, that they also appreciate the *hazards to the patient* of hyperbaric oxygen therapy. These are:

(1) *Oxygen toxicity.* Pure oxygen, when breathed for prolonged periods and especially if breathed at high partial pressure, is toxic to all living cells. During hyperbaric oxygen therapy it is necessary to watch especially carefully for the neurological effects of oxygen toxicity. Initially these take the form of a feeling of unease, sweating and palpitations, and rapidly progress to twitching and a major convulsion. If this occurs the patient has to be decompressed rapidly and returned to breathing air, when no permanent sequelae are likely to occur.

(2) *Otitic barotrauma and aural atelectasis.* This occurs if there is blockage of the Eustachian tubes. Oxygen is absorbed from the middle ear much more rapidly than air, so aural atelectasis occurs more rapidly when breathing oxygen than air.

(3) *Pulmonary atelectasis.* This can occur if the patient has a chest infection and a main or subsidiary bronchus becomes blocked by a mucous plug. Oxygen is rapidly absorbed from the alveoli beyond the block, and collapse of the blocked segment of lung occurs.

It must be realized that oxygen is a useful therapeutic agent, but its use presents hazards to both patients and nurses.

Chapter 48

Blood Transfusion

by A. J. E. BRAFIELD

*Introduction—blood groups—preparation for transfusion—the trans-
fusion—the ill-effects of blood transfusion—the Rhesus factor—
exchange blood transfusion—blood donors—other infusion fluids*

The idea of transfusing blood is not a recent one. A German surgeon in the
seventeenth century proposed a reciprocal transfusion of blood to recon-
cile the parties of an unhappy marriage. Mollison quotes Dennis (1667)
who described a transfusion given to a man who had fallen into a 'Phrensy
... occasioned by a disgrace he received in some Amours.' It was hoped that
the calf's blood used for the transfusion, 'by its mildness and freshness,
might possibly delay the heat and ebullition of his blood.' Yet at the turn
of this century, the means of transfusing blood successfully was unknown.
In 1901 Landsteiner described the ABO blood groups, and the First World
War gave considerable impetus to the study of this problem.

For a successful blood transfusion, two things are essential—the blood
must be of the correct group, and it must be sterile.

The components of blood. Blood consists of plasma (water plus protein)
in which are suspended red cells, white cells (leucocytes) and platelets. The
function of the red cell is to carry oxygen; leucocytes form the first line of
defence against bacteria; platelets assist in the coagulation of blood;
plasma proteins provide us with antibodies against disease and with clotting factors, and also help to maintain the blood pressure. Knowing this
we can understand the reasons for giving a blood transfusion. These are:

> *To increase the oxygen-carrying capacity* when this is very low, as
> in anaemia.
> *To maintain the blood pressure and blood volume* when these have
> been reduced by haemorrhage.
> *To provide platelets and clotting factors* when necessary, as in
> haemophilia.

BLOOD GROUPS

The red cells contain substances (antigens) which have been designated
A, B and O. Upon the presence or absence of these depends a person's
blood group. In the plasma occur other substances (antibodies) which are

able to clump (agglutinate) red cells. Each antibody can react with only one group of red cells, and are therefore referred to as anti-A, anti-B, etc., antibodies. Red cells of group A, and plasma containing anti-A antibody are said to be 'incompatible'. It is obvious that an antigen and its corresponding antibody would never normally occur together in the same blood. The antigen/antibody composition of the different blood groups is shown in the Table below. It is not difficult to see why A blood, for instance, cannot be given to either group B or group O patients: the blood of both these groups contains anti-A antibodies.

Blood group	Red cell antigen	Plasma antibodies
A	A	anti B
B	B	anti A
AB	AB	nil
O	O	anti A and anti B

There are many other blood groups, e.g. M, N, S, P, etc., which are of minor importance in transfusion. The Rhesus system has some special features and is described on p. 459.

Maintenance of sterility. When the blood is withdrawn from a donor, full sterile precautions are observed. All equipment and bottles are pre-sterilized. Any bacteria which might gain entrance are discouraged from growing by keeping the blood in a refrigerator. Every hospital should possess a special blood bank refrigerator with a built-in alarm system to warn the staff if the temperature rises above 6 °C (42·8 °F) or falls below 2 °C (35·6 °F). All forms of domestic refrigerator used in the wards are unsuitable for this purpose.

PREPARATION FOR TRANSFUSION

To ensure that the patient is safely transfused meticulous attention to detail is necessary from the moment the transfusion is ordered. The *request form* must be filled in (by the doctor) carefully and clearly. The *specimen of the patient's blood which accompanies the form to the laboratory must be clearly labelled.* Ample time should be allowed to the laboratory to find blood of the correct group and to carry out a cross match. When ready the blood will be retained in the laboratory until required for use. When the blood is collected check all details carefully. Compare the information given on the label tied to the bottle (i.e., the bottle number and group, the patient's full name and hospital number, and the ward) with that shown in the blood register, and also in the patient's case notes. On return to the ward re-check all details with a second person—nurse or doctor—before the transfusion is set up. Sometimes special measures are adopted to identify the patient when unconscious, as during an operation, by writing his name or hospital number on the skin, or attaching a label to wrist or ankle. Whatever the local requirements the nurse should know them, and carry them out carefully. Note that the colours of the bottle labels are different for each group:

Group A is yellow.   Group B is pink.
Group O is blue.   Group AB is white.

Rhesus negative blood is distinguished by having the writing on the labels in red.

Do not warm the blood before use unless specifically instructed to do so by the doctor. Raising the temperature will encourage the growth of bacteria. If you are instructed to warm the blood, stand the bottle in water at blood heat, no more.

Finally set out the appropriate instruments, sterile towels, etc., needed for a minor operation, and include a straight splint and some bandages.

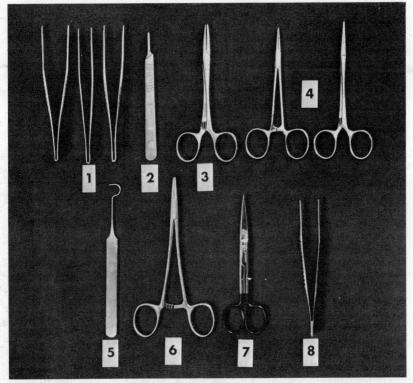

Fig. 48/1 Articles for intravenous 'cut down' blood transfusion. 1. Three five-inch plain dissecting forceps. 2. Bard Parker knife (handle only shown). 3. One five-inch Spencer Wells forceps. 4. Two Halstead Mosquito forceps. 5. One aneurysm needle. 6. One needle-holder. 7. One pair of stitch scissors. 8. One pair of toothed dissecting forceps. In addition a curved needle and suture of the doctor's choice, Kleenex folded towels, stitched swabs and gallipots with wool swabs should be supplied.

The transfusion is set up by the doctor himself. Using a sterile technique the special needle is introduced directly into a suitable vein. This is usually in the upper forearm, but may be in the leg or hand. In infants, scalp veins are occasionally used.

In difficult cases it may be necessary to 'cut down'; the instruments required are seen in Fig. 48/1. The skin is first cleansed, then incised; the vein is exposed and a cannula is introduced and tied into the vein. The skin is then sutured. Once the blood is running in freely the needle or cannula is secured in position with sticking plaster; the limb may be lightly bandaged to a splint—do not obstruct the blood flow—and secured to the side of the bed. *The patient is now kept under very close supervision for 15 to 20 minutes, and intermittently thereafter until the transfusion is complete.* The same pattern of supervision should be followed with each new bottle. The *speed of the transfusion* is usually about 20 to 40 drops per minute, but may be required to be much slower, as in cases of long-standing anaemia in which the heart muscle is weak, or very fast, as when there has been severe haemorrhage.

When the transfusion is completed the bottles should be sent back to the laboratory. *Do not wash the bottles, nor detach their labels.* Finally, a precise record of the transfusion is made in the patient's notes.

For care of the administration of an infusion postoperatively, see p. 461.

THE ILL-EFFECTS OF BLOOD TRANSFUSION

When a patient receives blood which is in any way unsuitable he may suffer a *reaction*. This usually occurs within 20 minutes of commencing the transfusion. *There may be backache, hot flushes, sweating, rigors, headache, or a rise in temperature. Urticarial weals may appear, and rarely, there is rapidly developing severe shock.* When a reaction is noted, stop the transfusion and inform the doctor immediately. He may require the blood to be returned to the laboratory for checking, together with a fresh specimen of the patient's blood and a sample of his urine. The ill-effects of transfusion may be the result of the following.

Incompatibility—i.e., blood of the wrong group. The red cells become agglutinated in the patient's circulation and are rapidly destroyed (haemolysed). Symptoms may appear early, or they may be delayed. Haemoglobin may appear in the urine, and later the patient becomes jaundiced. Rarely, the kidneys may fail and the flow of urine cease.

Allergy—the patient being sensitive to substances in the plasma. Symptoms are usually mild and skin manifestations common.

Bacterial contamination. If bacteria have been able to grow in the blood the reaction is likely to be very severe and even fatal, sometimes after only a few ml of blood have been given.

Transmission of disease. Virus hepatitis, syphilis, and (in the tropics) malaria are commonly transmitted if the donors are not carefully screened.

Circulatory overload, due to too rapid transfusion.

Air embolism. If pressure is being used to hasten the transfusion air may get into the vein with serious consequences. Never apply air pressure in an effort to relieve a blockage in the needle.

THE RHESUS FACTOR

In the red cells of some patients there occurs an antigen which has also been found in the blood of the rhesus monkey. These patients are said to be *rhesus positive*. Unlike the ABO system, rhesus antibodies are not normmally found in the plasma, not even in those who are rhesus negative.

When a rhesus negative person receives a rhesus positive transfusion for the first time, no reaction occurs, but the patient develops *anti-rhesus antibodies*. If a second transfusion of rhesus positive blood is now administered the result is precisely the same as with an ABO incompatible transfusion (see p. 456) though the symptoms are usually milder.

When a rhesus negative mother carries a rhesus positive fetus the effect is the same as if she had a rhesus positive transfusion, viz. no immediate effect, but antibodies will develop in her blood and these will react against any subsequent rhesus positive fetus or blood transfusion.

A fetus so affected suffers from anaemia which may be severe, and is due to the anti-rhesus antibodies from the mother entering the fetal circulation and destroying the red cells. *There may be deep jaundice and severe brain damage.*

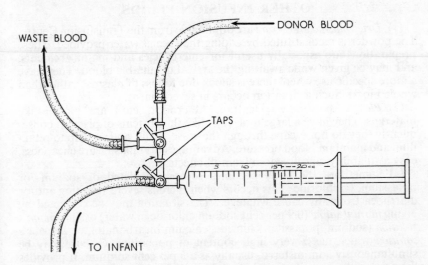

Fig. 48/2 Exchange transfusion equipment. The taps may be positioned to allow donor blood to be drawn into the syringe and then introduced into the infant. Mixed blood is then withdrawn from the infant and expelled through the waste tube.

Early exchange transfusion is the only recourse in such cases. Ideally this consists of administering a transfusion of rhesus negative blood into a vein, and simultaneously bleeding the infant from an artery. In practice the whole procedure is usually carried out through the umbilical vein. Into this a plastic catheter is inserted, and by attaching a three-way tap and a syringe (Fig. 48/2), rhesus negative blood is introduced, and an equal volume of blood is withdrawn and discarded. The discarded blood contains the infant's damaged red cells together with the offending antibody. In this way the content of new, undamaged rhesus negative red cells is gradually built up within the infant's circulation and the amount of antibody is reduced. *The most stringent sterile precautions are necessary throughout in order to prevent infection entering via the umbilical cord.*

The lesson of all that has been said is, that no rhesus negative female person, child or adult, under the age of 50, should ever be given a rhesus positive transfusion.

Blood donors. Normally all blood is obtained from the Regional Blood Transfusion Centre. Occasionally, in an emergency, volunteers may be asked to provide fresh blood. Having had the prospective donor checked for anaemia and general health, he is bled lying down in a comfortable position and employing full sterile precautions. Sterile 'taking sets' and bottles for this purpose are normally stocked by the laboratory. After the donation the donor is kept lying down for five minutes and thereafter permitted to rise, but must be observed for signs of fainting which may occur in the inexperienced. Ensure that the puncture wound is dry and dressed. The blood bottle is carefully labelled with the donor's full name, and placed in the blood refrigerator until required.

OTHER INFUSION FLUIDS

(1) *Dried plasma* and *serum* are obtainable from the Transfusion Centre. The powder is reconstituted by adding the special water provided. These preparations are especially useful for emergencies and major accidents, and may be given while awaiting the arrival of suitable blood. They have a more specific use where there is shock due to loss of plasma, rather than whole blood. Such a situation occurs in severe burns.

(2) *Plasma substitutes* (Dextran, Macrodex, etc.) are plasma-like materials. They have a large molecule, like the proteins of plasma; consequently they do not escape through the vessel walls, and so help to retain fluid and maintain blood pressure. Advantages over plasma are cheapness, easy availability, and freedom from ill-effects.

(3) Sometimes the body becomes severely depleted of sodium, or potassium, or chloride. This occurs when there is severe vomiting and/or diarrhoea from any cause whatever. The situation may be corrected by giving *normal saline* (0·9 per cent sodium chloride in water) or *Hartmann's solution* (sodium, potassium chloride, calcium bicarbonate), or *Darrow's solution* which has a very high content of potassium. *Glucose* may be simultaneously administered, usually as a 5 per cent solution. It provides the body with a source of easily metabolized food, and forms an essential part in the treatment of diabetic comas. Also in this condition the blood may become too acid, and solutions of sodium *lactate* or *bicarbonate* may be administered. Finally it may be desirable to produce vigorous diuresis in a patient, as in some cases of poisoning. Solutions of *urea* or *mannitol* may be given intravenously for this purpose.

(4) *Fresh frozen plasma* (FFP) is plasma which has been separated from the red cells, and immediately deep frozen. This preserves the clotting factors, some of which disappear rapidly at room temperature. FFP is usually infused when there is uncontrolled haemorrhage.

Chapter 49

Postoperative Care. Complications of Surgical Operations

by MICHAEL HOBSLEY

Care of the unconscious patient—the circulatory system—the chest—fluid and electrolyte balance—the wound—thromboembolism—urinary problems—review of postoperative pyrexia

---

CARE OF THE UNCONSCIOUS PATIENT
(see also Chapter 62, p. 665)

When the patient arrives back in the ward from the operating theatre he may still be unconscious; an anaesthetist's plastic airway will be present in the mouth, hooking the tongue forward, and he will probably be in the semiprone position. *The pulse rate is recorded every 15 minutes and the blood pressure every half-hour until his level of consciousness lightens so far that he no longer tolerates his airway.*

Pressure-points are particularly vulnerable in the unconscious patient. For details about this and other points in the nursing care, see Chapter 4.

Once normal consciousness is regained, the routine care involves the circulation, respiration, fluid balance, the wound, and thromboembolism.

THE CIRCULATORY SYSTEM

The specific responsibility of the nurse is to chart pulse rate and blood pressure at the intervals ordered. An average routine after major surgery is that pulse rate is noted hourly for 24 hours, and then every 6 hours till recovery is well advanced, while blood pressure is measured every 6 hours for 24 to 48 hours only.

The point of this charting in the first 24 to 48 hours is to assist the doctor in the early diagnosis of internal *reactionary haemorrhage* (p. 422). *The nurse should therefore be alert for signs and symptoms of a low cardiac output, giddiness, faintness, sweating, pallor, etc., and be prepared to report these.*

Care of blood transfusions. A blood transfusion is commonly given in the first 24 hours to complete the restoration of any operative blood loss. *Pyrexia is particularly common as a reaction to transfused blood, and many hospitals require the temperature to be taken at regular intervals, often hourly, during the transfusion.*

THE CHEST

A common complication of major surgery is *pulmonary segmental collapse*. In this condition the respiratory rate rises sharply, breathing becomes laboured (the nostrils twitch and the patient contracts his neck muscles to assist the effort of breathing in), and the temperature rises about 1 °C or 3 to 5 °F. These changes commonly occur during the first 24 to 48 hours. In severe cases the patient becomes cyanosed and the condition may even be fatal. The mortality was quite high until about 20 years ago when the cause was discovered.

The problem concerns the *removal of mucus* from the respiratory passages. Mucus is a sticky colourless liquid secreted by the *mucous glands* in the lining of the trachea and bronchi. Its function is lubrication of the airway, to make it easier for the *cilia*, microscopic hair-like structures arising from special cells in the lining, to waft particles of foreign material (soot, dust) out of the lungs and upwards to the pharynx. In health, only just sufficient mucus is secreted to perform this function, and the individual is not aware of having any sputum to expectorate.

After a surgical operation there may be an increased formation of mucus because of the irritation of inhaled anaesthetic gases and of the presence during many operations of a tube in the trachea (endotracheal tube).

Anaesthesia also depresses the activity of the cilia. The mucus is often stickier than normal because the patient may be short of water (the preoperative period of starvation for at least four hours to ensure an empty stomach is an important factor here) and because the injection of *atropine*, which is an important part of the anaesthetist's pre-medication, has this effect upon the nature of the mucus. For all these reasons, it becomes more difficult for ciliary activity to keep the airways clear.

The body's defence mechanism in such circumstances is cough, a very forceful expiration produced, after a deep inspiration, by the contraction in particular of the upper abdominal muscles. Stimulation of the nerves in the bronchial lining by the presence of an excess of mucus (or a foreign body) excites the cough reflex via pathways in the brain, and the forceful expiration ejects the offending material as *sputum*.

Coughing is *painful* after an operation on the chest or abdomen, particularly the upper abdomen. The patient becomes reluctant to cough heartily, and the sensitivity of the cough reflex may be impaired by drugs such as morphine given to relieve the pain of the wound.

The patient may fail to expectorate all his mucus, and sticky plugs of mucus may finally block completely some of the smaller bronchi or even occasionally a main bronchus. No air can then enter the alveoli in the segment of lung beyond the block, and the stagnant air trapped in these alveoli soon becomes absorbed into the blood so that the empty alveoli *collapse*.

This condition is known as *pulmonary segmental collapse*, or often in medical jargon simply as the *postoperative chest*. The blood in the pulmonary capillaries of the non-aerated parts of the lungs passes through into the systemic arteries with its reduced content of oxygen so that the patient is hypoxic and often cyanosed. Mechanical stimuli from the collapsed areas affect the respiratory centre of the brain and produce *laboured rapid respiration*. Infection in the stagnant area produces *pneumonia* and a *pyrexia* of rapid onset.

Patients at risk. The rate of production of mucus and its viscosity are increased by local irritation. Irritants include *acute infections* (influenza, acute bronchitis), *chronic infections* (especially the very important and common group of *chronic bronchitis*), *smoking*, and *inhaled foreign material*. Patients with *bronchial asthma* have a tendency towards spasmodic constriction of the bronchi when these are irritated, and this may make it difficult to dislodge mucus. *Inhaled foreign material* includes stomach contents: acid gastric juice produces a particularly virulent inflammatory response when inhaled, and the danger of this happening is the most important reason why the anaesthetist tries to ensure the patient's stomach is empty before he depresses the guarding cough reflex by inducing anaesthesia.

Management of pulmonary segmental collapse. Prophylaxis before operation is vital. The importance of coughing must be explained to the patient, and he must be instructed how to cough with his two hands supporting the wound to reduce pain. Since coughing depends for its effects upon first taking in a deep breath, and since surprisingly frequently the patient has little idea how to use his lungs to maximal effect, *deep breathing exercises are taught and the patient must be encouraged by the nurse to practise these.*

Patients producing sputum (i.e. those with chronic bronchitis) should have their operations deferred if possible to the healthier summer months. If operation is urgent, the physiotherapist uses *postural drainage* (the patient is placed in a succession of different postures to assist by gravity the drainage from all parts of the lungs) in combination with *percussion* of the chest wall to assist in dislodging sticky plugs of mucus. *The patient should be encouraged to give up, or reduce, smoking.* The value of *prophylactic antibiotics* is disputed, but if a pathogenic organism is isolated from the sputum before operation a suitable antibiotic is usually prescribed.

All these measures are continued after operation, and patients may need bullying as well as cajoling into coughing. *Signs and symptoms suggestive of a pulmonary segmental collapse must be reported immediately: remember that this complication can be lethal.* Early mobilization is an important weapon in the fight against this condition. If further vigorous physiotherapy and antibiotics are unavailing, the doctor may undertake some procedure to allow a direct bronchial toilet (aspiration of the mucus from the bronchial tubes): either by the once-only tiding-over procedure of *bronchoscopy* (p. 585) or by the construction of a *tracheostomy* (p. 628) which remains in place for a few days till the patient recovers the ability to cough.

FLUID AND ELECTROLYTE BALANCE

Postoperative interference with feeding. Many patients are unable to drink and eat normally for several days after a surgical operation. The reason may be simply that after a very major operation they feel too tired and ill. A specific reason, however, is any operation involving much *handling* of, or a *large incision* into, the *gastro-intestinal tract*. A large incision requires repair by suturing (e.g. after a *resection*—removal of a length of gut—and *anastomosis*—the joining together of the two free ends), and healing is aided by rest, so the surgeon limits the food intake to avoid the stimulus which food in the gut gives to *peristalsis*.

Even without an incision of the gut, food intake must be limited after major abdominal surgery because the handling of the bowel and other less well understood factors during the operation temporarily depress the activity of peristalsis, *paralytic ileus*. If food and drink are given in these circumstances, they collect in the stomach and upper small bowel, and the consequent *distension* of the gut has a further depressant effect upon peristalsis.

Even if nothing is given by mouth, the normal *secretions* of the upper alimentary canal, *saliva, gastric juice, bile, pancreatic juice*, and the *succus entericus* of the small intestine continue and *it must be appreciated that these amount to no less than 9 litres in 24 hours*. Normally these secretions are almost completely reabsorbed by the terminal part of the small bowel (the second half of the *ileum*) and by the large bowel, but in the absence of peristalsis they accumulate in the upper part of the gastro-intestinal tract and thereby perpetuate the *ileus*. The patient's *abdomen becomes distended*, he feels *nausea*, and ultimately the collected liquids distend the stomach so severely that copious *vomiting* occurs.

Management. The essentials of management are therefore *gastric aspiration* to keep the stomach empty, and feeding by some route other than the digestive tract, *parenteral*, usually *intravenous alimentation*.

Gastric aspiration. After an abdominal operation the surgeon may leave a tube in the stomach, bringing one end out to the surface through a hole in the stomach and a hole in the abdominal wall below the left ribs (a *gastrostomy*). More often, before operation the tube is passed through a nostril (occasionally the mouth), and then swallowed by the patient's own efforts until its tip lies in the stomach—a *nasogastric tube*.

Passing a nasogastric tube. Choose the wider nostril (test by asking the patient to sniff while one nostril is closed by external pressure). Moisten the tip of the tube in ice-water, hold it three inches from the tip, and pass it into the nostril straight backwards till the patient feels it in his throat. Encourage the patient to swallow vigorously and allow the tube to be taken in: do not push forcefully or the patient will retch. When the second mark on the tube nears the nostril, the tip should be in the stomach.

Aspirated liquid should turn litmus red. If no liquid is obtained, ask the patient to drink 20 ml of water and try to aspirate again. If there is still no aspirate, or only air, or if the aspirate turns litmus blue, it is possible that the patient has inhaled rather than swallowed the tube (coughing may be surprisingly minor): withdraw the tube till its tip is in the throat and start again.

Postoperative handling of gastric aspiration. Aspiration may be ordered by continuous pump or (more usually) intermittently. Intermittent suction by syringe should be performed at the intervals requested, usually hourly in the first instance. Since abdominal distension is controlled by this routine, water may be given by mouth, usually at first in a dose of 30 ml hourly, immediately after each aspiration.

Chart the oral intake and gastric aspirations very carefully: the surgeon relies on your figures for evidence that peristalsis is beginning; when the aspirate becomes less than the intake, positive oral balance, he will order an increased intake (60 ml hourly, 90 ml hourly) and a reduced aspiration-frequency (every 2 hours, every 3 hours) until it is clear that the tube can be dispensed with and oral feeding started.

Always chart the nature of the aspirate—whether it contains blood or bile or looks faecal. *Never be satisfied with a zero aspirate from an intact stomach: some liquid can always be obtained from an intact stomach, unless the tube is in the wrong place or blocked.*

Intravenous feeding is carried out by a drip-infusion. Provided that the disturbance of feeding only lasts the usual three or four days, and that the patient's nutritional state before operation was normal, it is only necessary to maintain water and salt (sodium) balance. A normal intake of water is 2 to 3 litres per 24 hours, according to the size of the adult. If half a litre is given as *normal (physiological) saline*, 0·85 g per 100 ml, this provides sufficient sodium for 24 hours; the rest may be given as 5 per cent dextrose.

Each 12 hours the surgeon prescribes the intravenous fluids for the subsequent 12 hours; his guidelines are to give the basal requirements calculated from the figures above, plus the previous 12 hours' abnormal losses from the gut—gastric aspirate, diarrhoea, fluid discharge from a *fistula*. The abnormal losses are replaced as normal saline, because they approximate to this fluid in constitution.

The nurse will appreciate that her accurate keeping of fluid intake—and output—charts is the basis of efficient management of fluid and electrolyte therapy after operation. Apart from the points already made, the best guide to the adequacy of replacement is a satisfactory volume of urine output with a low specific gravity (but see p. 245 for disturbances in urine output in the first 24 to 48 hours).

Care of an intravenous infusion. The nurse will ensure that the correct fluids are given, and at the rate specified. Signs of *inflammation at the drip site* or evidence that the *fluid is running into the tissues* (*swelling, failure to stop the drip by encircling pressure on the limb nearer the heart*) *must be reported promptly. Attention must be drawn swiftly to a tendency for the rate of flow to slow down or stop. Most important of all, a bottle of infusion-fluid must never be allowed to empty, as air might then be sucked into the veins and travel round the circulation as an air embolus. An air-lock may thus be produced that prevents blood reaching the brain or the heart muscle, and this condition can be rapidly fatal.*

THE WOUND

The uncomplicated clean incision

Most surgical incisions are made with clean sharp instruments through well-prepared skin and with extreme precautions against contamination with pathogenic organisms. Such wounds, in which the gap between the opposing edges is minimal, *heal by a process called 'first intention'*, with *a minimum of scarring*. Apposition of the edges is maintained by sutures or metal clips. These must remain in place until the strength of healing of the skin is sufficient by itself to prevent the wound opening.

The length of time necessarily varies, mainly according to the richness of the blood supply to the area. Sutures may be removed from wounds of the scalp, face and neck *in three or four days*, while it is advisable to leave *the stitches in a wound on the leg or foot for a minimum of 10 days*. If the edges appear to gape as the nurse removes the first few stitches, the nurse should report this and await further instructions.

Dressings of clean wounds are largely a matter of surgical idiosyncrasy. Within a few hours of sewing up the wound, the tissue exudate solidifies into a firm barrier which external agents cannot easily penetrate. Some surgeons therefore use no dressing except a light coating with a liquid that dries to form an artificial skin—e.g. Nobecutane. Others use an occlusive dressing of gauze, held in place by adhesive strapping.

Dressings should be changed as infrequently as possible; *indications for changing the dressing are that it has become soaked with blood (and therefore a source of nutrition to external bacteria), or that it has become necessary to inspect the wound because there is a suspicion of haemorrhage or infection.*

Wound drains, usually of corrugated rubber or in the form of a tube to which suction may be applied, are inserted for two different indications: to remove blood or exudate which is expected to form in the wound (usually only up to 72 hours); or to act as a route to the exterior for fluid leaking from some hollow organ as a result of the breaking down of a suture line in the organ. In the latter case, the drain is left in place for 7 to 10 days until the risk of leakage is past, or until the surgeon is confident that a track has formed round the drain which will itself act as a conduit to the exterior.

Complications of wounds

Reactionary and *secondary haemorrhage* have already been described (p. 420).

Infection of a clean wound usually becomes manifest about the fifth day. *A complaint by the patient that the wound is becoming more rather than less painful must always be taken seriously as it usually indicates infection. Pyrexia may have a similar significance.*

The wound must be inspected, and *tenderness* and *swelling* sought. Even if no other local signs are present, the surgeon may note that the tissues immediately deep to the incision feel soft rather than firm. He will then order some or all of the skin sutures to be removed and the wound opened gently with sinus forceps to allow the liquid out. The liquid may appear to be a collection of non-infected stale blood, *haematoma,* or it may be frank pus. In either event, a wound swab should be well soaked in the fluid and sent to the bacteriology laboratory for culture so that any organisms present can be identified and their sensitivities to antibiotics determined.

Care of open wounds. The surgeon must ensure *free dependent drainage* from the wound, or discharges will accumulate in pockets and initiate or perpetuate infection. Apart from opening the skin incision as much as necessary, some measure to *prevent premature healing of the skin* (leaving a slower-healing pocket of infection in the subcutaneous tissue) must be adopted. The *dressings* used must perform this function; they must also in their deeper layers *absorb* the discharges to prevent them contaminating the neighbouring skin of the patient, his bed, and the whole environment of the surgical ward; and in their more superficial layers they must be *occlusive* to prevent any new infection getting into the wound.

Finally, *anti-infection chemicals* (*antiseptics*) are usually used with the dressings: an example in common use is sodium hypochlorite solution (eusol). Some surgeons use antibiotics, local or systemic, while others reserve these drugs for patients with evidence of spread of the infection (lymphangitis, septicaemia).

Notes of warning. *Wounds should not be too tightly packed, in an effort to* *absorb discharges, as this would result in the edges being kept apart and delayed healing.* Too frequent changes of dressings can be as harmful as too infrequent; the dressing should be changed only as often as necessary to prevent saturation of the outer (occlusive) layers of the dressing with discharge. *Nurses dressing the wounds of several patients in a ward may become potent instruments of cross-infection: only the strictest precautions in non-touch techniques, disposal of infected materials, sterilization procedures and personal hygiene will prevent this occurring.*

Burst abdomen. This is a serious complication of abdominal surgery. It may occur at any time up to about 10 days after the operation. Warning of this catastrophe may be given by a *discharge of salmon-pink liquid from the wound,* and *the nurse should report such a discharge as a matter of great urgency.* She should reassure the patient, and prepare saline soaks and an abdominal binder for the surgeon's use (see below). In the fully developed case, the patient suddenly feels the wound give way and coils of intestine erupt from the wound to lie in the bed. The medical staff must be summoned urgently, and the intestines must be manipulated as far as possible back into the abdomen (the supine position helps) and kept in place with moist (saline-soaked) sterile dressings and an abdominal binder until the patient can be taken to the operating theatre for re-suture.

Healing by second intention. This is a much slower process than healing by first intention. The gap between the wound edges fills with exudate, and then blood vessels gradually grow into it from the wound margins. White blood cells and proteins exude into the tissue space and solidify (organize) into a bright red lumpy or granular material known as *granulation tissue.* When this has completely filled the gap up to the surface, the surface layer (skin or mucous membrane) can grow across the granulation tissue to complete healing.

Sometimes when a wound has become fairly clean (always in the case of a burst abdomen because of the necessity of containing the abdominal viscera) the surgeon sews it loosely together to minimize the granulating process, *secondary suture.*

THROMBOEMBOLISM

Thrombosis

Pathology. Thrombosis is the formation within the blood vascular system of a solid mass derived from the constituents of the circulating blood. The solid mass formed is called a *thrombus.*

Thrombosis may occur in arteries (see Chapter 52, p. 506) or in veins, *venous thrombosis* or *phlebothrombosis.* The earliest stages in the process are the deposition of the blood *platelets* (particles much smaller than the red cells or the white cells) and fibres of the protein *fibrin* (derived from the fibrinogen of the plasma) on the wall of the blood vessel. Similar changes occur to seal a hole in a blood vessel, or when blood clots, *coagulates,* after being shed from the body, but the deposition is inappropriate in thrombosis.

Venous thrombosis is a common phenomenon in the veins of the pelvis or the lower limb in patients who have been put to bed for any cause. It is probably at least as frequent in medical as in surgical wards. Recent estimates of its incidence in surgical patients suggests that it may occur in about one-quarter of all patients undergoing major surgery. Contraceptive pills of the type that contain much *oestrogen* predispose towards venous thrombosis, but pregnancy is a more potent cause.

Clinical features. The classical description is that about the seventh to tenth day after operation a rise in temperature to about 37·8 °C or 100 °F occurs, and the patient complains of pain and tenderness in the calf. Recent work, however, suggests that most cases are well established by the second day after operation, and that most are symptomless and demonstrated only by special investigations, e.g. *phlebography* (the outlining of the veins and their contained thrombi by radio-opaque material injected into the veins on the top of the foot).

Consequences of venous thrombosis. The thrombus may gradually be dissolved by agents, *fibrinolysins,* in the blood that dissolve fibrin. Recovery may be complete, but if the valves in the veins are destroyed *varicose veins* and *gravitational ulcers* may occur years later (Chapter 52, p. 518). Alternatively, the thrombus may break off the wall of the vein and is then known as an *embolus*—any mass lying free in the circulation. The current carries the embolus back to the right side of the heart, through the right atrium and right ventricle, and on through the pulmonary artery to the lungs. The embolus sticks here as the pulmonary artery and its branches divide successively into smaller vessels, giving rise to a *pulmonary embolism.*

Pulmonary embolism. Most cases are probably symptomless, just like venous thrombosis in the lower limb. *Clinical signs and symptoms* occur in about one per cent of surgical patients. In *severe* cases, the patient has a sudden call to stool, then becomes shocked as the obstruction to the outflow from the heart to the lungs reduces the venous return to the left side of the heart. Cyanosis is prominent, and the veins in the neck that drain into the obstructed right side of the heart are engorged. Death may follow immediately, or after some hours. *Less severe* cases are characterized by the patient complaining of pain in the affected area of the chest, worse on breathing, and the coughing up of bloodstained sputum.

Management of venous thromboembolism. *Predisposing factors. Stasis* or stagnation in the veins of the calf is produced by bed rest. *Damage to the walls of the calf veins* may occur by pressure on the calves during the unconsciousness of anaesthesia, and the traumatized area may initiate the thrombosis. *Changes in the coagulability of the blood* are also involved. The concentration of the platelets in the blood increases after splenectomy and this operation is followed by a very high incidence of thrombosis compared with most others. Patients with disorders of the blood and with neoplastic disease may owe to a hypercoagulable state their greater susceptibility to this complication.

Prophylaxis. Early ambulation should reduce stasis, and many surgeons use accessory measures such as raising the foot of the bed slightly to aid by gravity the venous return from the legs, or the wearing of elastic stockings to obliterate the superficial veins and hence force all the blood flow through the deep veins at a greater velocity. *Leg exercises are taught before operation and supervised afterwards by the physiotherapist.*

The *calves* are protected from pressure during the operation by suitable supports and cushioning, while a cradle under the bedclothes may be used to prevent their weight lying on the legs. *Anticoagulant* drugs like *heparin* and *Dindevan* have been used by some surgeons to reduce the coagulability of the blood, but their prophylactic use carries a danger of excessive haemorrhage during the operation. However, encouraging results have recently been obtained with very small doses of heparin that do not cause abnormal bleeding.

Treatment of venous thrombosis. Apart from redoubling the prophylactic exercises, etc., anticoagulants are usually prescribed. A large clot obstructing the main vein draining the limb in the region of the thigh is so likely to produce complications that some surgeons advise a direct operation to remove the clot, *phlebothrombectomy.* Operations are also available to *interrupt the inferior vena cava,* the main vein carrying blood from the lower half of the body back to the heart, to reduce the risk of pulmonary embolism.

Treatment of pulmonary embolism. Anticoagulants and drugs to support the embarrassed heart, together with oxygen, are the main lines. In very severe cases, when death does not immediately occur, the heroic operation of opening the chest and directly removing the clot from the pulmonary vessels (*Trendelenberg's* operation; not to be confused with Trendelenberg's operation for varicose veins—p. 518) has been performed with success. In most cases the functions of the lungs and heart are taken over by some artificial machine (an *extracorporeal circulation*) while the pulmonary artery is isolated and opened and the clot sucked out.

Urinary problems

Retention of urine, and infections of the urinary tract, especially cystitis, are quite common problems after a surgical operation. They are discussed in Chapter 54, p. 533.

REVIEW OF POSTOPERATIVE PYREXIA

The following comments may be useful. *During a blood transfusion,* pyrexia is probably due to the blood transfusion.

Otherwise, *during the first 48 hours* the likely cause is pulmonary segmental collapse; at the *fifth to tenth day* it is infection of the wound; at *any time,* pyrexia may signify *thromboembolism;* while if a catheter has been passed previously (and especially if the rise in pulse rate is small compared with the rise in temperature) *it may signify a urinary infection.*

Chapter 50

Surgery of the Alimentary Tract (Excluding Disorders of the Large Bowel)

by MICHAEL HOBSLEY

Mouth and salivary glands—the oesophagus—the stomach and duodenum—the liver, gall bladder and bile ducts—the small intestines —intestinal obstruction—the appendix—hernia

MOUTH AND SALIVARY GLANDS

The parotid salivary glands lie one in front of each ear. Characteristically they are enlarged in *mumps*.

Postoperative parotitis. Painful swelling of both parotid salivary glands, with local heat, pyrexia and malaise, may occur as a result of infection spreading from the mouth up the ducts that drain the glands. The weak patient whose general resistance is lowered, and whose attention to oral hygiene is distracted, is at risk both in surgical and in medical wards. This used to be a common condition but with the modern appreciation of the importance of oral hygiene it has largely disappeared. The occasional case nowadays must be considered a nursing failure.

Intermittent swelling of salivary glands. The parotid, and also the submandibular salivary glands which lie one on each side of the neck, immediately under the jaw, may swell from time to time for a few hours, usually starting while the patient is eating a meal. The common condition causing such swelling is an obstruction by a stone of the duct through which the secretions of the affected gland drain into the mouth. Usually the stone is accessible through the mouth. An incision is made through the mucosa immediately over the stone and the latter extracted. The wound in the mouth is usually left unsutured and the patient can leave hospital 24 to 48 hours later. It is surprising how little discomfort there is with eating after this time, but for the first one or two days a bland liquid diet is offered. If the stone is not accessible through the mouth because it is far back in or near the gland, there is no alternative to removing the gland itself—the operation of *submandibular sialadenectomy* or *parotidectomy* (see Fig. 50/2, p. 472).

Tumours of the parotid. A lump arising in the region of the parotid salivary gland is usually a neoplasm of the parotid. The exact nature of the lump cannot be determined by external examination, and the surgeon usually undertakes to remove the whole or most of the gland, with a wide margin of apparently healthy tissue all round the lump, in the hope of eradicating the tumour completely. A common form of tumour which responds well to this treatment is called the 'mixed parotid tumour'. It may appear at any age and grow very slowly for many years, but there is always a risk that eventually it will change into carcinoma of the parotid, which is much more malignant.

The operation of parotidectomy is often qualified by the adjectives *conservative* and *radical*. These adjectives apply to whether the surgeon conserves the *facial nerve*, which is at risk during the operation because it runs through the gland. If the nerve is sacrificed, the muscles of facial expression which it supplies become completely and irrevocably paralysed. The resultant deformity of the face is shown in Fig. 50/1. Such a deformity may also occur temporarily as a result of dissecting close to the nerve during a conservative operation, but if the nerve has not been cut recovery in a few days or weeks is certain.

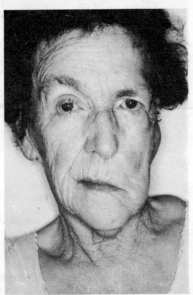

Fig. 50/1 Complete left facial nerve palsy. The main trunk of the facial nerve was involved in a carcinoma and had to be excised. The left eye, unprotected by blinking, is prone to conjunctivitis. The whole of the left side of the face has dropped compared with the right.

The nurse should be particularly on her guard if patients wish to discuss facial paralysis, the likelihood of its occurrence, and the chance of its recovery. All such queries should be referred to her superiors or to the medical staff.

Reactionary haemorrhage is a serious problem after operations on very vascular areas like the face and neck, and suction drainage is commonly used for 48 hours after the operation. Fig. 50/2 depicts one form of suction drainage using a Canny-Ryall bulb syringe.

Operations in the mouth

Operations such as removal of nodules and ulcers of the cheeks or tongue do not require special nursing care apart from their effects on feeding and oral hygiene. Stitches inserted in the mucous membrane lining the mouth are usually catgut (absorbable) and therefore do not need

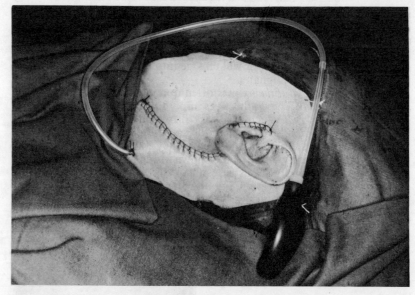

Fig. 50/2 Parotidectomy. The S-shaped incision is well posterior so that the main trunk of the facial nerve can be found as soon as it emerges from the skull, and followed through the gland. Note the method of suction drainage.

removal. If the lesion removed turns out to be neoplastic, subsequent treatment is usually by radiotherapy.

THE OESOPHAGUS

Most operations upon the oesophagus are performed by thoracic surgeons (see Chapter 58).

Achalasia of the cardia

In this condition the lowest few inches of the oesophagus fail to relax to allow the swallowed bolus of food to pass on into the stomach. In consequence the oesophagus above the affected area dilates and elongates giving the dramatic appearance shown in Fig. 50/3. The patient complains of *dysphagia* (difficulty in swallowing) and often *regurgitates* the stagnant food in his oesophagus.

Cause. There is an abnormality of the *plexus* (network) of nerves in the wall of the oesophagus that is supposed to co-ordinate the passage of the peristaltic wave that propels the bolus down the oesophagus.

Treatment. **Oesophageal dilation** at regular intervals with bougies may keep the patient comfortable, but many have to have **Heller's operation**. In this procedure, an incision is made longitudinally in the wall of the lower few inches of the oesophagus and the upper few inches of the stomach, and deepened down to, but not through, the mucous membrane lining the inside of these organs. The mucous membrane bulges out between the

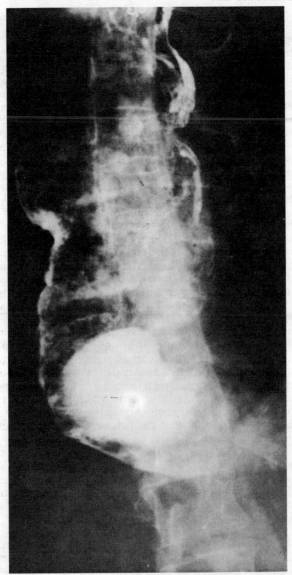

Fig. 50/3 X-ray (barium swallow) of achalasia of the oesophagus. There is a tremendous dilatation of the oesophagus
above a smooth tapering lower end.

edges of the incision in the muscle as these edges part, and the calibre of the
lower end of the oesophagus is greatly increased. The chief complication
is *peritonitis*, which may occur if the mucous membrane is punctured
without the surgeon realizing this.

THE STOMACH AND DUODENUM

Curative operations for peptic ulcer

Aim. These operations are designed to reduce the output of gastric juice. Gastric juice is important in the disease of *peptic ulceration* (see p. 226) because a peptic ulcer never occurs in those people who show an inability to secrete gastric hydrochloric acid (*achlorhydria*), because patients with *duodenal ulcer* (but not *gastric ulcer*) often secrete more gastric juice than normal subjects, and because experience has shown that any measure resulting in a reduced secretory power leads to healing of a peptic ulcer.

Types of operation. Gastric secretion of acid and pepsin takes place from the two-thirds of the stomach above the pyloric antrum. It is under the control of two mechanisms, *nervous* and *hormonal.* The *nervous mechanism* is mediated by the two *vagus nerves,* which originate in the brain, and pass down the neck and thorax into the abdomen in the region of the oesophagus. The left nerve lies in front of the lowest inch of the oesophagus, the right lies behind. They continue downwards to innervate not only the stomach and duodenum but also the liver, gall bladder, pancreas and intestines as far as the middle of the transverse colon.

The sight, smell and taste of food, and its presence in the stomach, all stimulate the vagus nerves. When the surgeon cuts the vagus nerves (*vagotomy*) in the region of the upper end of the stomach, acid production is reduced by about a half to two-thirds, but is not destroyed completely because the hormonal mechanism remains. The *hormonal mechanism* is activated by distension of the stomach or the presence of food within the stomach: these stimulate certain cells in the *pyloric antrum* to secrete a hormone, *gastrin.* This substance is carried right round the circulation till it returns to the stomach, where it excites the gastric glands of the part of the stomach above the antrum to secrete acid. The alternative operation to vagotomy is therefore *partial gastrectomy,* which is meant to reduce the acid-producing area of the stomach. About two-thirds of the stomach is removed, and it is important that the pyloric antral area is removed so that gastrin is not produced.

Operative details (see Fig. 50/4). Vagotomy may be performed through the abdomen, *abdominal vagotomy,* or through the chest, *trans-thoracic vagotomy.* The abdominal operation may be *total,* or *selective;* in the latter the surgeon tries to preserve the vagal nerves supplying the other abdominal organs.

The vagus nerve also carries motor impulses to the muscle of the stomach wall, and for a variable time after vagotomy there is a paralysis of the stomach and the organ empties only very slowly by gravity into the duodenum. For this reason the surgeon always combines vagotomy with a '*drainage procedure*'—some operation to increase the rate of stomach-emptying. The procedures usually employed are either a plastic operation to enlarge the pylorus (*pyloroplasty*) or a by-pass between the stomach and the small intestines (*gastro-jejunostomy*). After *partial gastrectomy* the continuity of the alimentary tract is restored by joining the stomach remnant either to the duodenum (*Billroth I type*) or to the jejunum (*Billroth II* or *Polya type*).

Nursing care. Accurate charting of fluid intake and output is vital after such operations. Suture lines in the stomach or intestines must be given a

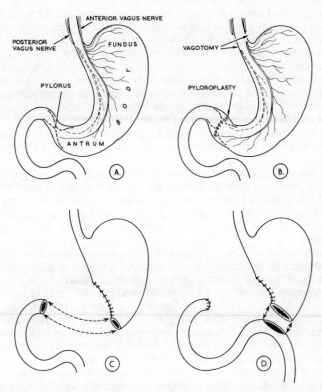

Fig. 50/4 Operations for peptic ulcer. (*a*) Normal anatomy and physiology. The fundus and body secrete acid and pepsin, the antrum secretes gastrin. The vagus nerves influence all the secretory activities of the stomach. (*b*) Vagotomy and pyloroplasty. Vagotomy slows stomach emptying; this effect is counteracted by enlarging the pyloric channel. (*c*) Billroth I partial gastrectomy: gastroduodenal anastomosis. (*d*) Polya partial gastrectomy: gastrojejunal anastomosis.

chance to heal and liquid must not be allowed to accumulate in the slowly emptying stomach or the gastric remnant, so intake will be restricted to small volumes of water at first, and gastric aspiration will be frequent (p. 464). The surgeon will anxiously await the news that *bile* has appeared in the gastric aspirate after a Polya gastrectomy: in this operation the duodenal loop may kink at its junction with the stomach remnant (see Fig. 50/4) and the build-up of bile and pancreatic juice in the duodenum may burst the sutures closing the cut end of the duodenum—the surgical catastrophe known as a '*burst duodenal stump*' which produces the severe pain and prostration of a rapidly spreading *peritonitis* due to the escape of the highly alkaline irritant secretions. When bile appears in the gastric aspirate it is clear that the kinking has not occurred and this catastrophe is unlikely.

To lessen the dangers of a burst duodenal stump, the surgeon may place a large drain down to that region. When the stump leaks, the fluid drains to the exterior instead of flooding the peritoneal cavity. The situation is still serious because this *fistula* (an abnormal communication between a hollow organ and another or between a hollow organ and the surface of the body) is a source of massive loss of water and electrolytes, and because the alkaline nature of the liquid and its high concentration of digestive enzymes encourage the digestion of the abdominal wall around the drain. Some arrangement of an adhesive bag, perhaps combined with suction drainage, must be devised to reduce the contact of the fistula-fluid with the patient's skin and to enable the volume of fluid to be measured so that water balance can be maintained. The skin must be coated liberally with a protective material like aluminium paint or a buffer jelly.

Gastric operations are carried out in the *upper* abdomen, and are therefore followed by a high incidence of pulmonary segmental collapse.

Later consequences of gastric surgery. Patients are encouraged to think of their digestive system as normal and to take a *normal diet*, with one proviso: they should avoid citrus fruits (oranges, lemons, etc.) because the pith of these is difficult to digest when gastric acid production is reduced, and a mass of pith may pass on into the intestines and produce an obstruction.

Iron-absorption is slightly impaired, and patients should be advised to eat plenty of iron-containing foods to avoid *anaemia* in later years. They may also need inorganic iron, such as ferrous sulphate.

The *capacity for food* may be limited, and patients may complain that taking a meal may produce *abdominal distension* and *rumbling noises* (borborygmi), *tiredness* and a *desire to lie down*, and *sweating*. These symptoms comprise the *dumping syndrome*, and are due to the too rapid emptying into the intestines from the stomach remnant, or from the whole stomach after the delaying effect of vagotomy has worn off. The same tendency *of the intestinal contents to hurry* may result in *diarrhoea*, especially after vagotomy. Later complications are *difficulty in absorbing calcium* from the diet, so that many years later *a bone disease, osteomalacia*, may develop; and occasionally malabsorption of vitamin B.

Emergency operations for peptic ulcer

Haemorrhage from a peptic ulcer produces the vomiting of blood, *haematemesis*, or the passing of tarry black liquid stools, *melaena*. It is treated by medical measures in the first instance, but if the bleeding persists, recurs or is very severe the surgeon operates. The operation performed is partial gastrectomy if the ulcer is in the stomach, and for a duodenal ulcer either a partial gastrectomy including the ulcer or a vagotomy and drainage procedure after stopping the bleeding vessel with sutures through the ulcer.

Perforation of the ulcer produces a widespread peritonitis, and an operation is performed to close the leak with sutures.

Malignant change ocasionally takes place in a peptic ulcer of the stomach, but never in duodenal ulcer.

Pyloric stenosis is a contraction at the outlet of the stomach due to the scarring and spasm of a nearby duodenal ulcer, or to a carcinoma of the stomach. The obstruction produces copious vomiting of stomach contents, a mixture of stagnant food and hydrochloric acid together with some sodium and potassium. *Preparation for surgery includes gastric aspiration with a nasogastric tube or a larger oesophageal tube if the stomach is full of solid or semi-solid material, and gastric lavage.* The fluid and electrolyte deficits are replaced over the course of a few days by intravenous infusion, and when the gastric distension and inflammation have worn off and the stomach is relatively clean an operation is performed, the nature of which depends upon the cause of the stenosis.

Operations for carcinoma of the stomach

By the time the patient comes to operation a curative procedure is seldom possible because obvious spread of the growth to distant sites has already occurred. Some form of *palliative partial gastrectomy* is usually performed, but occasionally *a total gastrectomy* is attempted in the hope of achieving a complete removal of the tumour. The spleen is usually removed as part of the latter operation, and the incidence of subsequent venous thrombosis is high (see p. 517).

THE LIVER, GALL BLADDER AND BILE DUCTS

Operations for liver diseases

Occasionally a portion of the liver is removed, *partial hepatectomy*, to excise a tumour or cyst. Cirrhosis of the liver is one cause of portal hypertension (see p. 520); the surgical management of this condition is described in Chapter 52.

Operations on the gall bladder

Cholecystectomy. The usual reason for removing the gall bladder is that it contains *gallstones*. Patients with gallstones frequently complain of *flatulent dyspepsia*, but even in the absence of such symptoms the surgeon usually advises cholecystectomy because of the high frequency of serious complications.

Cholecystectomy is performed through an oblique incision below the lower right ribs in the anterior abdominal wall, *Kocher's incision*, or through a vertical incision near the midline, *right paramedian incision*. The operation does not disturb the patient as much as a gastrectomy, and nasogastric aspiration and intravenous infusion are usually unnecessary. Liquids may be offered the next morning, and a rapid return to a normal diet can be anticipated. *Patients with gallstones have usually been advised to avoid fatty foods while awaiting surgery, and it is important that they be reassured that there is no need to maintain this restriction after cholecystectomy.* The wound is always drained for a few days because small bile ducts on the surface of the liver may have been opened during the removal of the gall bladder and the leaking bile must be guided to the exterior or it might irritate the peritoneum, producing *biliary peritonitis.*

Management of acute cholecystitis. Acute inflammation of the gall bladder is usually due to the obstruction of the exit from the gall bladder, the *cystic duct*, by the impaction of a gallstone. The severe pain and tenderness in the upper abdomen radiate through to the back between the shoulder blades, and there are nausea, vomiting, and usually pyrexia.

Some surgeons are inclined to perform immediate cholecystectomy, but most adopt a conservative routine of a fluid diet, bed rest, and often antibiotics, and the symptoms usually settle down so that elective cholecystectomy can be performed a few weeks later. Sometimes the condition does not respond, and there is evidence suggesting that septicaemia, or rupture of the gall bladder with a consequential very severe peritonitis, are impending. *The nurse's accurate charting of a rising pulse rate and a rising temperature, and early reporting of the patient's complaint of increasing pain and spreading abdominal tenderness, will be important in assisting the surgeon to forestall these complications by the operation of cholecystostomy*—the insertion of a tube-drain, often a Foley catheter into the gall bladder through a small abdominal incision. This procedure relieves the tension in the gall bladder and allows the inflammation to subside. Cholecystectomy is always undertaken a few weeks later.

Gallstones in the common bile duct. This complication may be suspected if a patient known to have gallstones has attacks of rigors (due to infection in the bile passages of the liver, *ascending cholangitis*), or *jaundice*. The ordinary X-ray of the gall bladder, the cholecystogram (p. 692), is efficient for demonstrating stones in the gall bladder, while the special investigation called an *intravenous cholangiogram* (p. 480) is good at demonstrating stones in the duct. *Jaundice* in these circumstances is due to impaction of a gallstone in the lower end of the common bile duct with obstruction to the outflow of bile, so that the greenish-yellow pigments of the bile cannot reach the intestines and therefore reflux through the liver cells back into the blood, thereby staining the tissues. This form of obstructive jaundice is therefore due to large duct obstruction.

Diagnosis of jaundice. *The nurse plays an important part through testing the urine.* In patients with *obstructive jaundice* the bile pigments accumulating in the blood have previously been excreted through the liver cells and only afterwards have come back into the blood: as a result of alterations effected in the liver cells, these pigments, *posthepatic bilirubin*, can be excreted in the urine. By contrast, pigments, *prehepatic bilirubin*, which have accumulated in the blood faster than the liver can excrete them because of excessive destruction of the red blood cells, *haemolytic jaundice*, do not appear in the urine—hence the term *acholuric jaundice*. Further, if obstructive jaundice is complete then no bilirubin gets into the intestines and therefore none is reabsorbed into the body and therefore none is excreted in the urine. *Absence of urobilinogen in the urine* is most valuable as an indication of complete obstruction. Finally, if in a succession of urine samples (instructions are usually given that every sample voided should be separately tested) urobilinogen is sometimes present and sometimes absent this suggests that the cause of the obstruction is slightly intermittent and likely to be a stone which can become disimpacted at times; whereas unremitting absence in all samples is likely to indicate a constant obstruction such as malignant disease at the lower end of the common bile duct which is most often carcinoma of the head of the pancreas.

Preparation of the jaundiced patient for surgery. The most important consideration is *haemostasis*. Bile in the intestine is essential for the absorption of fat. In obstructive jaundice fat is therefore poorly absorbed. *Vitamin K* is fat-soluble and therefore also poorly absorbed: in its absence the liver cannot synthesize *prothrombin*, which is an essential ingredient of the blood-clotting process. The bleeding tendency produced by obstructive jaundice would make surgery in such patients hazardous. Fortunately there are preparations of vitamin K that can be injected intra-

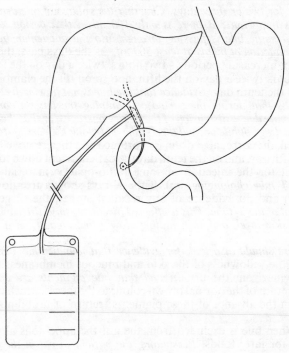

Fig. 50/5 T-tube drainage of the common bile duct after exploration of the duct. The T-tube acts as a safety valve to drain bile to the exterior if spasm at the lower end of the common bile duct prevents free flow into the duodenum.

muscularly (Synkavit) or intravenously (Konakion) to make good the deficiency, or a transfusion of *fresh* blood can be used since the prothrombin content of freshly shed blood is high.

Exploration of the common bile duct. The surgeon makes a small incision, *choledochotomy*, in the common bile duct as it runs between the liver and the duodenum, and he explores the duct with various instruments. Any stones found are removed, *choledocholithotomy*. Sometimes a plastic procedure to enlarge the sphincter at the lower end of the duct is thought advisable, *sphincterotomy* or *sphincteroplasty*. Afterwards the surgeon closes the opening in the duct around a special plastic tube-drain shaped like the letter T (Fig. 50/5). The T-tube is usually advisable because after exploration the sphincter at the lower end of the duct may be irritable and contract, causing an obstruction to the flow of bile into the duodenum; if this happens the raised pressure of bile in the duct may burst open the sutured wound in the duct and cause biliary peritonitis. The short segment of the T-tube allows bile to flow down into the duodenum if the lower end of the duct is patent, but the long stem, which is usually brought out through the same stab incision in the abdominal wall as the corrugated drain, acts as a safety-valve to the exterior if necessary.

Nursing care after operations on the bile duct. *The T-tube. The surgeon usually requests that the T-tube be allowed to drain freely into a sterile* *plastic bag for two or three days. Charting the volume of bile draining each 12 hours is important: if there is only 100 ml in that period it is almost certain that some bile is passing through into the duodenum because the 12-hour production of bile is at least 300 ml.* As the days pass, the T-tube is clamped for increasing periods—two hours, twice a day on the fourth day, for four hours twice a day on the fifth, and so on till the clamping is continuous by the tenth day. *Evidence that the bile is not flowing freely into the duodenum is that during the period of clamping the patient complains of abdominal pain due to distension of the biliary passages, or that there is a considerable leakage of bile around the T-tube and along the corrugated drain.* If all goes well, the corrugated drain is shortened and then removed about the fourth to fifth day, and on the tenth day the patient is sent down to the X-ray department for the injection of some radio-opaque material along the T-tube (a *T-tube cholangiogram*). If the X-rays show a free flow into the duodenum and no evidence of any residual stones, the surgeon orders the *removal of the T-tube. This is effected by cutting any stitch anchoring the T-tube at skin-level, and then pulling slowly and steadily in a downward direction.*

The nurse should also look for evidence that jaundice has been relieved (fading of the yellowness of the skin and mucous membranes; absence of bile pigments from the urine); *and that bile pigments are entering the intestine* (return of the normal brown colour to the faeces, which were putty-coloured in the absence of these pigments; return of urobilinogen to the urine).

Diet. When bile is excluded from the gut the appetite is always poor, especially for fatty foods. *Persuading the patient to eat in the early days after the operation is unrewarding: it is better to reassure him that his appetite will return as soon as the flow of bile is restored.* Meanwhile, fluid drinks with plenty of carbohydrate (dextrose) should be encouraged: a high carbohydrate intake protects the liver from some of the biochemical injury produced by obstructive jaundice.

THE SMALL INTESTINES

The only common operation is *resection* (excision) of a length of small bowel, followed by the *primary* (immediate) *anastomosis* (joining together) of the remaining cut ends. Primary anastomosis is possible, even in cases of intestinal obstruction, because the blood supply of the small bowel is excellent. This is quite the opposite of the situation in the less well perfused large bowel (see Chapter 51). Occasionally the reason for resection is some disease of the small bowel itself (e.g. Crohn's disease, p. 230, or rare tumours). More often, the reason is that the affected part has been involved in an obstruction of the small intestine.

INTESTINAL OBSTRUCTION

Types
The *paralytic* form, *paralytic ileus*, has already been described as a sequel to major abdominal operations (p. 464). As the bowel is not contracting, the abdomen is silent when a stethoscope is placed on the anterior abdominal wall. The condition itself is painless, although it may be produced by a painful condition such as generalized peritonitis.

In the *mechanical form,* the bowel above the obstruction reacts by contracting more vigorously but still in the normal pattern of peristalsis in waves with periods of relaxation between the waves. The intense contractions of peristalsis are associated with a typical pain, *colic,* which is diffuse, symmetrically placed or in the midline, makes the patient press his abdomen for relief, and above all is *intermittent.* The word *colic* is most confusing because it was originally used for any abdominal pain. In its modern specific usage, it means any pain due to excessive peristaltic activity in a hollow muscular tube, and identical symptoms arise from the genital tract (labour pains) and in the ureter (ureteric colic due to a stone in the ureter, see p. 530). The confusion is further exaggerated by the fact that certain pains are traditionally called colic that are not in fact colicky: the pain of a stone in the common bile duct is usually called biliary colic even though it is usually *constantly* present for hours or days. A safer term to use than colic is therefore *intermittent* abdominal pain. The increased peristalsis is associated on *auscultation* with an *increased frequency of bowel sounds* and a change in their character.

Both forms of obstruction produce *abdominal distension, nausea and vomiting,* as the intestinal secretions above the obstruction are dammed back, and after the contents of the colon beyond the obstruction have been evacuated, *constipation.* A good guide to the level of a mechanical obstruction is provided by the relative preponderance of these symptoms: in a case of *high* obstruction vomiting is early, whereas in *low* obstruction (e.g. large bowel obstruction) distension is prominent and vomiting a late feature.

Small bowel obstruction. Mechanical obstruction can be classified by its *cause.* In the small bowel, the obstructing agent is occasionally *in the lumen* (e.g. a bolus of orange-pith after a gastrectomy—p. 476), or *in the wall* (tumours, etc.); in the majority, however, the obstructing agent is *outside the wall.* Such external pressure is commonly due to *kinking by bands and adhesions* of fibrous tissue in the peritoneal cavity, a sequel to a previous abdominal operation, or by trapping a loop of bowel in the sac of a *hernia* (p. 485).

An interesting type of obstruction is the condition of *intussusception,* in which a length of bowel telescopes into the bowel beyond. Intussusception is common in infants about nine months old; its cause is unknown. Much less commonly, it occurs in adults and is then usually associated with a tumour projecting into the lumen of the bowel from its wall: the tumour becomes gripped by peristaltic waves and forms the apex of the intussusception.

External pressure on the entering and leaving limbs of a loop of bowel trapped in a hernia or between adhesions can produce the serious complication of *strangulation* (Fig. 50/6). The blood vessels supplying and draining the loop are vulnerable to the external pressure at the base of the loop. The veins, with their low internal pressure, collapse first while the arteries are still patent: in consequence the loop distends with trapped blood, and its capillaries dilate and leak protein-rich fluid into its wall, into the lumen, and into the peritoneal cavity. There is a contraction of the blood volume due to this loss of plasma, and an increase in the haematocrit, see p. 421, just as occurs with the loss of plasma in severe burns. Finally there is a damming back of the arterial inflow, and the congested sodden plum-coloured bowel becomes deprived of oxygen, turns black, and dies. Per-

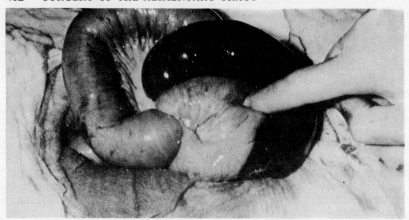

Fig. 50/6 Strangulation. The finger points to a peritoneal adhesion which has ensnared a loop of bowel. The strangulated bowel is dark and has lost its surface lustre; the changes are irreversible, and the loop must be excised.

foration and general peritonitis ensue. *Strangulation is a potentially lethal complication of intestinal obstruction and must be diagnosed promptly.* The important clinical features are that the intermittent abdominal pain becomes *continuous*, and that the patient becomes rapidly more ill (due to the onset of hypovolaemic shock).

Treatment of small intestinal obstruction. *Operation* to remove the obstructing cause, and if necessary to remove devitalized bowel and restore intestinal continuity, is mandatory if strangulation is present or suspected. Otherwise, the surgeon may operate or he may try *conservative management,* being prepared to resort to operation if there is no definite improvement in 24 hours.

Preparation for surgery. Decompression of the stomach and proximal small bowel is essential, in order to reduce the risks of (i) inhalation of stomach contents during the induction of anaesthesia and (ii) perforation of the distended bowel before the operation can be started. A state of depletion of water and electrolytes (and in the case of strangulation, plasma) exists, and will be corrected by *intravenous infusion.* The medical assessment of fluid balance is greatly assisted by information from the *urine. The first sample that the patient passes after admission is of crucial importance: its volume and specific gravity should be measured, and it should be kept in case further tests are required.*

The conservative management is exactly the same as preparation for surgery, except that some surgeons pass a special intestinal tube (e.g. Miller-Abbott tube) instead of an ordinary nasogastric tube. This two-lumen tube has a weighted tip which is guided through the pylorus under X-ray control. Then a balloon near the tip is inflated through one lumen, in the hope that peristaltic activity in the bowel will grip the balloon and carry it on to the point of obstruction while continuous aspiration is maintained through the second channel. The reason behind using such a tube is that deflation of the bowel just above a kink may itself encourage the kink to smooth itself out, thereby releasing the obstruction. *Once the tip of the tube is within the duodenum the nurse must fasten it to the nose or forehead with a free loop of about 12 inches (30 cm) always available to be taken up by the onward movement of the tube.*

Postoperative care is as for gastrectomy (p. 474).

Large bowel obstruction. The important differences from small bowel obstruction are that *constipation* and *distension* are more prominent than colicky abdominal pain and vomiting. Constipation can be a difficult complaint to interpret: the significant feature is a complaint that no flatus has been passed. A diagnosis of large bowel obstruction is confirmed by the appearance of X-radiographs of the abdomen: gas and fluid levels are seen in large bowel up to the point of obstruction, as well as in small bowel.

The common lesion producing large bowel obstruction is carcinoma of the left side of the colon, and the common sites are the upper rectum and the lower sigmoid colon so that the lesion is often revealed by digital examination of the rectum or sigmoidoscopy. Other causes are diverticular disease and volvulus of the sigmoid colon (see Chapter 51, p. 505).

Treatment of large bowel obstruction. The essential preliminary is that the patient should be given an *enema. The nurse in reporting the result of the enema must pay particular attention to whether the patient passed much flatus.* If the abdomen can be deflated to some extent, the obstruction may be temporarily relieved and the urgency is taken out of the situation; routine investigations can be performed to make an accurate diagnosis, and in the absence of obstruction the surgery to remove the lesion is relatively straightforward.

If the enema yields a poor result, *emergency surgery* is necessary. The urgency of the situation is that the high pressure building up in the colon may perforate the bowel (this often occurs at the caecum): large bowel has a poor blood supply and the risk is greater than in small bowel obstruction. The primary concern of the emergency operation is to diagnose the site and (if possible) the nature of the obstruction and to deflate the obstructed bowel. It may be possible to remove the lesion at this time, but anastomoses in *obstructed* large bowel are very prone to leak and so it is unlikely that the surgeon will be able to restore continuity at this emergency operation.

The patient therefore usually returns to the ward with a colostomy somewhere proximal to the obstruction, usually a left iliac or transverse colostomy, and the carcinoma of the recto-sigmoid is still *in situ.* Occasionally a carcinoma high in the sigmoid can be excised at the first operation, and the two cut ends of the bowel brought out in the left iliac fossa as a double-barrelled colostomy, *Paul-Mikulicz operation.* The rarer carcinoma of the right side of the colon may be treated by immediate right hemicolectomy with primary anastomosis of the terminal ileum to the transverse colon: this procedure is reasonably safe because one of the pieces of bowel being anastomosed is small intestine.

Details of the operations on large bowel and the care of a colostomy are given in Chapter 51.

THE APPENDIX

The only common condition is *acute appendicitis*: *subacute appendicitis* also occurs, but *chronic appendicitis* is a doubtful entity. Occasionally, when an acutely inflamed appendix is examined histologically it is found to contain a tumour called *carcinoid tumour*.

Acute appendicitis

Acute inflammation is usually consequent upon a blocking of the lumen of the appendix by means of a hard concretion in the faeces—a *faecolith*. The common initial symptoms are central colicky abdominal pain with nausea or vomiting (as in any intestinal obstruction), but later when the organ is grossly inflamed and swollen the inflammation may spread to the neighbouring parietal peritoneum and the pain shifts down to the right lower quadrant of the abdomen and becomes continuous.

The *treatment* of acute appendicitis is appendicectomy as soon as possible, to avoid the serious risk of perforation of the organ with an ensuing general peritonitis. The usual incision is called a 'grid-iron' incision because the various layers of skin and muscles are divided in different directions, and it lies in the right lower quadrant of the anterior abdominal wall.

Postoperative complications include *infection* in the subcutaneous layers of the wound; *pelvic abscess*, heralded by mucous diarrhoea and diagnosed by feeling a bulge into the rectum on rectal examination; *and subphrenic abscess*. All these complications are associated with a swinging temperature and a high leucocyte count in the blood. Pus under the diaphragm may be particularly difficult to diagnose: X-rays of the chest, and screening of the diaphragm to demonstrate that its movements are impaired, may be helpful. Abscesses must be *drained* by appropriate surgery: in the case of pelvic abscesses, it is fortunate that they usually drain themselves by spontaneously bursting into the rectum or vagina.

Subacute appendicitis

Sometimes an inflamed appendix becomes wrapped around with omentum and coils of small bowel so that the infection becomes sealed off from the general peritoneal cavity. This situation is recognized by the palpation of a mass in the right lower quadrant of the abdomen. An attempt at appendicectomy in these circumstances is unwise: it is better to let the inflammation subside, and then remove the appendix two or three months later (*interval appendicectomy*), rather than risk spreading pus around the peritoneal cavity by breaking down the adhesions surrounding the appendix.

The nurse plays the most important role in the management of a patient with appendicitis with a mass. The nursing observations decide whether an expectant policy can be continued or whether an operation to drain the mass is necessary. Complaints of increased pain or spreading of the pain will probably be made in the first instance to the nursing staff, and are important indications for immediate surgery. The other indications include enlargement of the mass, redness of the overlying skin, increases in the white count, rigors, and a swinging temperature. All these factors suggest that pus is forming under tension, with septic absorption (septicaemia) and a threat of rupture to produce general peritonitis.

Chronic appendicitis

Recurrent attacks in young adults of mild pain in the right lower quadrant of the abdomen, continuing for months and years, and often associated with nausea, are commonly ascribed to chronic inflammation of the appendix. Appendicectomy is often performed, but histologically such appendices are rarely abnormal and the clinical results are often disappointing. This is a matter of opinion, but the author doubts whether there is such a pathological state as chronic appendicitis.

HERNIA

A hernia is a protuberance of part of the contents of a body cavity beyond the usual boundaries of the cavity. The common hernias arising from the abdominal cavity are the inguinal and femoral hernias in the groin, umbilical and periumbilical hernias, incisional hernia, and gastro-oesophageal (hiatus) hernia.

Hernias in the groin

These present as a lump at the medial end of the groin. The two major varieties are the inguinal and the femoral. An *inguinal hernia* passes along the inguinal canal and emerges into the superficial tissues through the superficial inguinal ring, *medial to the pubic tubercle.* A *femoral hernia* passes along the femoral canal and emerges through the fossa ovalis, *lateral to the pubic tubercle.*

The inguinal hernia is usually at first reducible by manipulation, or may disappear spontaneously when the patient lies down. Anything that raises the intra-abdominal pressure increases the protrusion; for example, if the patient coughs a momentary bulging of the lump is seen—a *cough* impulse. Apart from the discomfort associated with the lump, hernias should preferably be repaired by surgery to avoid the complications of irreducibility, strangulation and intestinal obstruction. If the patient refuses surgery or there is some medical contra-indication, a truss may be prescribed. It must be emphasized, however, that a truss is designed to keep the hernia reduced, and therefore the hernia must be reducible and the patient must be taught how to reduce the bulge (usually lying down) before applying the truss. A truss that does not keep the hernia reduced is valueless at preventing the complications, and may damage by pressure the coverings of the hernia.

The *femoral hernia* for anatomical reasons does not usually have a cough impulse and is usually not reducible; for this reason it cannot be treated by a truss and surgery is indicated because of a high risk of strangulation.

Umbilical hernias

True umbilical hernias through the point of weakness produced by the umbilical cord are common in infants, especially of African race. They usually require no treatment: the risk of complications is small, and the hernias usually disappear spontaneously during the first three years of life.

Para-umbilical hernias arise at a point of weakness in the abdominal wall just at the margin of the umbilicus itself. They occur in obese elderly patients and are very prone to the complication of strangulation, so they should be repaired surgically.

Incisional hernias

A weakness and a bulge may occur in any abdominal incision, though vertical incisions are more at risk than transverse or oblique ones. Repair of these can be technically very difficult, and if the hernia is easily reducible the surgeon may advise an abdominal belt rather than operation.

Gastro-oesophageal (hiatus) hernias

A portion of the stomach moves upwards into the chest, through the hole in the diaphragm (the *oesophageal hiatus*) through which the oesophagus normally enters the abdomen.

This condition occurs particularly in middle-aged obese patients. The common symptoms are acid regurgitation into the mouth, and heartburn, a burning sensation experienced behind the lower end of the sternum. The symptoms are due to reflux of acid gastric juice into the lower end of the oesophagus, the mucosa of which was not designed to resist the acid-peptic digestive effect of the gastric juice. The reflux is due to the herniation upwards of the *cardia*, the junction between oesophagus and stomach, and may interfere with its valve-like action. Symptoms are exacerbated by anything that raises the intra-abdominal pressure: obesity, tight corsets, bending forwards. *Conservative management* is described in Chapter 24, p. 224, but should conservative measures fail and complications of the oesophagitis (stricture-formation, ulceration, bleeding) threaten, an *operation* may be advised to reduce the stomach into the abdomen and narrow the hiatal orifice. Such operations may be carried out through the abdomen or through a low left thoracotomy: the results are sometimes disappointing.

Chapter 51

Surgical Conditions of the Colon, Rectum and Anal Canal, and Their Nursing Care

by PETER F. JONES

Introduction—diagnosis—examination—sigmoidoscopy—procto-
scopy—haemorrhoids—anal fissure—ano-rectal abscess—injuries—
rectal prolapse—carcinoma of colon and rectum—abdomino-perineal
excision—colostomy—polyps of colon and rectum—ulcerative colitis
—colectomy—ileostomy—diverticular disease of colon

The surgical diseases of these regions are a fruitful and satisfying field of work for both nurses and surgeons. Patients often have acutely distressing symptoms and are embarrassed about their complaints. Gentleness and sureness of touch both in the general care and local treatment of these patients are very important, and nurses have a particularly good opportunity to show tact and understanding as well as technical skill. The major surgery of the rectum and colon can be as demanding as any, both in the operating theatre and in pre- and postoperative care. The distress patients feel before treatment seems to make them the more pleased and satisfied as they find their troubles being resolved.

Diagnosis. Most patients are first seen in the out-patient department. They are referred by their family doctors because their symptoms and signs suggest rectal disease. The presentation of colonic disease is often very similar to disease in the rectum and the surgery of the two regions cannot usefully be separated.

History. Most patients say they have 'piles', but the exact complaint must be clarified—whether it be bleeding, pain on defaecation, rectal discharge, diarrhoea or prolapse—to reach an accurate diagnosis.

EXAMINATION

General and abdominal examination. All surgeons must also be physicians taking a wide view of the general health of their patients. Anaemia is commonly present in rectal patients and needs recognition and treatment. Conditions such as heart and lung disease, incipient prostatic obstruction and latent diabetes must all be detected before undertaking a major operation. In a disease such as ulcerative colitis collaboration with an interested physician will be important so that the medical and surgical aspects of care may be co-ordinated.

Abdominal examination may reveal signs of intestinal obstruction in colonic carcinoma, or the presence of a palpable mass. Enlargement of the liver may suggest that a carcinoma has metastasized.

Digital rectal examination. The patient lies on his left side with hips and knees fully flexed, and the body sloped across the couch so that the buttocks hang over the edge. This position enables the surgeon to have a good view of the area and to manœuvre a sigmoidoscope.

Inspection is the first step. A good light is necessary. An anal fistula or fissure, or prolapse of haemorrhoids or a polyp, or peri-anal dermatitis may be seen.

Palpation. The right index finger protected by a finger cot or a disposable glove is introduced slowly through the anal canal into the rectum. Painful spasm of the sphincter suggests the presence of a fissure. Haemorrhoids are not usually palpable. The rectal mucosa is searched for the hard nodular feel of a carcinoma and note is taken of the size and consistency of the prostate or cervix. On withdrawing the finger the character of faeces adhering to the glove is noted, especially the presence of blood, and a sample is often smeared on filter paper and tested for occult blood.

Sigmoidoscopy. This is a most valuable out-patient examination. If the 1·3 cm diameter Lloyd-Davies sigmoidoscope is used a useful examination can nearly always be performed without previous preparation. If gently done, this examination need not upset the patient.

If the sigmoidoscope is passed to its full length of 25 cm the whole of the rectal and the lower sigmoid mucosa can be examined. Over 50 per cent of all large bowel carcinomata occur in this area so there is a good chance of a positive diagnosis being made and a biopsy obtained on the first visit to out-patients. If the signs of proctitis or colitis are seen, these will also be vital in making an accurate diagnosis. The materials needed for sigmoidoscopy are clearly shown in Fig. 51/1.

Proctoscopy is usually performed last because it is necessary to know that there is no major disease such as rectal carcinoma or proctitis before treating haemorrhoids, which are only visualized through a proctoscope.

The proctoscope generally used is 2 cm in diameter and 8 cm long. It is passed as far as possible with the obturator in place and this is then removed. The mucosa of the rectal ampulla is seen and the proctoscope slowly withdrawn. If haemorrhoids or polypi are present they will prolapse into the lumen and so can be seen. Internal haemorrhoids can, if suitable, be injected there and then. At the end of these four steps the surgeon will often have made his diagnosis; in the case of haemorrhoids he may well have completed treatment by injection. In some patients, however, there will have to be further investigation.

Further investigation usually means the performance of a barium enema commonly arranged to take place a few days later. The *aim of the barium enema* is to show up abnormalities which lie more proximal in the colon than the point in the sigmoid inspected by the sigmoidoscope. Neoplasms

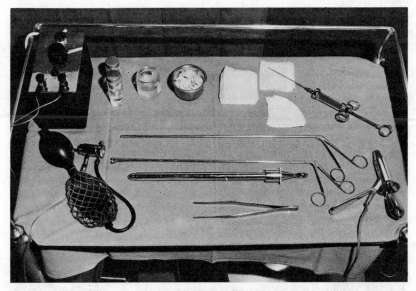

Fig. 51/1 Trolley set up for rectal clinic. The apparatus needed for digital examination, sigmoidoscopy, proctoscopy and injection of haemorrhoids is laid out. 1. Finger cots, gauze and lubricant for digital examination. Pieces of filter paper are ready for smearing with faeces and for testing for occult blood. 2. The small-bore (1·3 cm) Lloyd-Davies sigmoidoscope, together with the viewing lens, light and bellows are ready. Here the bulb is lit from an adjustable mains transformer. Immediately above the sigmoidoscope is the 40 cm biopsy forceps with which a small specimen of a tumour can be punched out. This is placed in one of the universal containers, which contains fixative. The other 40 cm forceps are used for holding small cotton-wool or gauze swabs for mopping away faeces. 3. On the right lies the Naunton Morgan proctoscope with its light. The long blunt dissecting forceps are used for mopping down the proctoscope. The Gabriel haemorrhoidal syringe and needle lies ready for injection of haemorrhoids. It is filled with 10 ml of 5 per cent phenol in almond oil (PAM solution). On the lower platform lies a long receiver for the dirty instruments. Nowadays, most hospitals would illuminate the sigmoidoscope and proctoscope by means of a flexible fibre-optic cable connecting the endoscope to a powerful light source.

of the colon, ulcerative colitis and diverticulitis, produce characteristic deformities during the filling of the colon with barium (Fig. 51/2).

The development of the flexible fibre-optic bundle has led to the production of the *colonoscope*, which can be guided up the curves of the colon, allowing the operator to view the whole of the colonic mucosa. This is a specialist procedure and requires screening control in an X-ray department.

HAEMORRHOIDS

Internal haemorrhoids are due to varicosity of the rectal veins. They lie in the lowermost part of the rectum and upper part of the anal canal and are covered by mucous membrane. They are the commonest rectal abnormality and are due to dilatation of the branches of one or more of the three superior rectal veins. These venous swellings become congested when the patient strains and are very liable to bleed during defaecation. Constipation is much the commonest cause of bleeding from haemorrhoids so treatment should always include advice on regulation of the bowel.

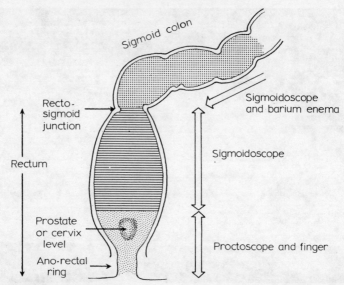

Fig. 51/2 This diagram shows the areas of lower bowel which can be examined by the four main methods. The anal canal and lower rectum are examined with the finger and the proctoscope; through the sigmoidoscope can be seen the whole of the rectum and a variable distance up the sigmoid colon. A barium enema does not give reliable information below the recto-sigmoid junction but above this point becomes the principal method of examining the colon.

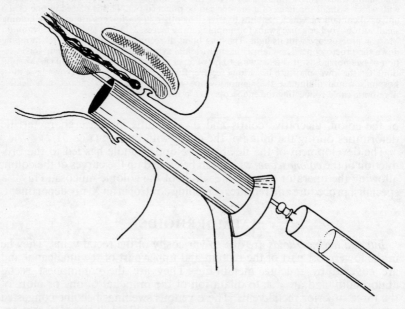

Fig. 51/3 Injection of internal haemorrhoids with PAM solution. The injection is placed just under the mucous membrane at the upper end of the haemorrhoid. The lower end of the haemorrhoid is kept compressed by the proctoscope.

When haemorrhoids are small, *of the first degree*, they bleed but do not prolapse and are well treated by injection with 5 per cent phenol in almond oil (PAM solution). If this solution is placed at the upper end of the pile it sets up an aseptic inflammatory reaction which causes the haemorrhoid to shrink by progressive fibrosis. This is a most effective treatment of small haemorrhoids (Fig. 51/3).

When haemorrhoids increase in size they elongate and prolapse outside the anus during defaecation, returning within the anal canal afterwards. These *second degree* haemorrhoids can often be successfully treated by injection.

When the haemorrhoids protrude through the anus all the time, causing discomfort and irritation (*third degree*), they can only be cured by operation.

'*Strangulated piles*' are internal haemorrhoids which have prolapsed suddenly and been caught by a strong anal sphincter. This obstructs the venous return from the haemorrhoids, they swell and become very congested and so look dark blue. This acute prolapse is very painful and the pain is relieved if the piles can be replaced within the anal canal by firm pressure. In these circumstances it is wise for the patient to stay in bed until oedema has subsided. It is most important to replace the piles if they prolapse again at defaecation.

If the attack is severe, with much oedema and sloughing, manual reduction is not possible. These patients usually need admission. They should lie flat with the foot of the bed raised. The perianal area should be shaved. Frequent lead lotion compresses are soothing. An olive oil enema may be needed if the bowel does not move.

Some surgeons have recently advocated emergency haemorrhoidectomy for this and it can be a valuable way of terminating an unpleasant condition.

Operative treatment of internal haemorrhoids. The patient is admitted on the day before operation and the bowel emptied with a Veripaque wash-out (see p. 93). A low-residue diet is given. Careful shaving of the operative area is carried out. Most surgeons prefer that no wash-out is done on the day of operation.

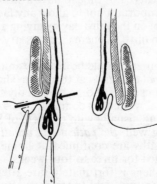

Fig. 51/4 Operative ligation of a third-degree haemorrhoid. The pile is drawn down with a forceps. The left-hand arrow shows the plane along which dissection passes, and which removes some peri-anal skin and the peri-anal plexus. The two arrows show the point at which the pile is ligated.

The *operation* consists of the dissection of the haemorrhoids so that a ligature can be placed around the base of the pile (Fig. 51/4). This ligature is tied very tight and so the haemorrhoidal tissue distal to it sloughs, the ligature usually coming away between seven and ten days after operation. This process of ligation to produce sloughing is liable to cause some post-operative pain and the area is necessarily septic, so frequent dressings are needed. A firm pad and T-bandage is applied at operation and the operative site must be carefully watched postoperatively; bleeding is not common but occasionally—perhaps once in 50 patients—there will be obvious soakage of blood into the dressings. This is hardly ever due to a ligature slipping but usually comes from the subcutaneus plexus where the skin has been incised. *It is important to report this to the house surgeon because this bleeding, though rarely rapid, can be very persistent and lead to considerable blood loss.* This type of reactionary haemorrhage usually has to be treated by returning the patient to theatre and tying off the bleeding point.

Many patients find it difficult to pass urine after haemorrhoidectomy. Men should be helped to stand up, when they will usually manage to micturate. Women should have their T-bandage loosened and be placed on the commode. If urine is not passed carbachol may be prescribed.

No dressing is needed on the day after operation and it is usual to leave the packs which were inserted at operation until the third morning. Some make a practice of removing these under a general anaesthetic but most surgeons give a laxative such as Senokot on the second evening and let the packs soften in a warm bath on the third morning, after which they come away when the bowel moves. An olive oil enema is given if the bowel fails to open. Some surgeons favour irrigation of anal wounds with eusol, others use twice-daily baths. The main point is that the area should be kept clean with plenty of water, and the wounds dressed with half-strength eusol.

Opening the bowel for the first time after haemorrhoidectomy is something of an ordeal. It is a mistake to allow the patient to get too worked-up, because the easiest way is to wait until there is a clear call to evacuate a stool. Straining just because it is time to have a stool is not helpful. On the other hand, it is most important not to allow any faecal impaction to build up. Try to secure a stool on the third day by giving a laxative on the second evening and by using an olive oil enema if necessary. A Beogex suppository can be very helpful.

On the fifth day the patient should be gently examined digitally and many surgeons commence *anal dilatation* at this time. The patient is shown how to pass the dilator and uses it at home twice daily for three to four weeks until healing of the anal wounds is complete.

If the bowel is moving, usually with the help of Senokot or Normacol, and dilatation is going well, *the patient can usually be discharged on the sixth day.* Frequent baths are continued at home. Review at the rectal clinic is usually arranged for three to four weeks after discharge.

Secondary haemorrhage is fortunately rare after haemorrhoidectomy, especially as it occurs around eight to ten days after operation when most patients have returned home. It is usually of a minor character. Very occasionally haemorrhage is more profuse and this is an important indication for immediate re-admission.

External haemorrhoids. This term is applied to two separate conditions which share the common features that they are covered by skin, and are therefore very sensitive.

External anal haematoma is a haemorrhage under the peri-anal skin. This is an acutely painful condition, usually due to rupture of a peri-anal vein during defaecation. It causes a characteristic tense, blue, acutely tender swelling to one side of the anus. Immediate relief is obtained if the haematoma is evacuated by incision; this can be done under local anaesthesia in the out-patient department.

Peri-anal skin tags are usually the remnants of previous peri-anal haematomata. They can cause considerable discomfort and may need operative removal. This is often done when the internal haemorrhoids which are often co-existent are ligated.

ANAL FISSURE

This is a common and distressing condition which is often endured for a surprisingly long time before the patient comes to hospital. It is also a common cause of rectal pain and bleeding in infancy. *A fissure is a persistent crack in the peri-anal skin*, usually in the midline posteriorly. This is very sensitive skin and every time the crack is disturbed by defaecation acute pain is caused, which can persist for some hours. Defaecation is made difficult not only by the pain caused but by the very marked internal sphincter spasm which is always present. A fissure can always be seen and usually it is also palpable. However, very great care is needed in doing this because this examination is acutely painful. Patience and gentleness are outstandingly important in examining patients with this condition. *A sigmoidoscopy must always be done at some stage*; a fissure can hide a more important lesion of the rectum such as a polyp or carcinoma.

The **treatment** of a very acute and painful fissure is to *dilate the anal sphincter under general anaesthesia*. This temporarily paralyses the sphincter and is followed by a remarkable relief of pain and quick healing of the fissure. When the fissure has been present for months it is usually necessary to add an excision of the fissure and division of the lower fibres of the internal sphincter—*internal sphincterotomy*—which is a most effective operation.

ANO-RECTAL ABSCESSES

Considering the rather septic nature of the area, it is perhaps surprising that abscesses are not more common in the ano-rectal area. These abscesses occur twice as frequently in men as in women. They are of two main types.

Peri-anal abscess. A subcutaneous abscess under the peri-anal skin. It is for that reason an acutely painful condition and is therefore usually incised fairly early and causes few complications.

Ischio-rectal abscess. This is a deeply sited abscess in the fat of the ischiorectal fossa. Its start is more silent and the external signs are few so that when it causes symptoms it is already well established. There is diffuse swelling out into the buttock and a much deeper and more careful incision and drainage procedure is needed if it is to heal without difficulty.

The main thought which dominates the treatment of these patients is to avoid the production of an anal fistula.

ANAL FISTULA

A fistula is an abnormal granulation-lined track connecting two epithelial surfaces. In this region a fistula runs between the rectum or anal canal and the skin of the peri-anal area and causes a constant discharge. It is the consequence of an ano-rectal abscess which has been inadequately treated.

If the fistula follows an ischio-rectal abscess, it is likely to run through the sphincters and its cure will mean division of some of the sphincter muscle. This is not serious provided some of the sphincteric ring is left intact. The aim of surgery is to leave a flat triangular wound which will heal by granulation tissue, meanwhile leaving part of the sphincter intact to preserve anal continence.

A high anal fistula will require a careful and lengthy operation of some difficulty for its cure, and recovery will considerably depend on the care with which this large operative wound is dressed postoperatively.

Crohn's disease of the colon (see p. 230) is especially likely to be associated with fistulae of the peri-anal area.

INJURIES

It is fairly unusual for the colon or rectum to be injured in civilian life. Very rarely the rectum is torn by a sigmoidoscope. The anus and rectum may suffer injury by impalement when a patient falls onto a sharp object. These are serious wounds because a perforation of the rectum may lead to pelvic cellulitis, and there is always a danger that the bladder or small bowel may be injured. Very careful operative exploration is needed and a temporary colostomy may have to be established while the rectum heals.

RECTAL PROLAPSE

This is a condition which is more or less confined to infants and to women beyond middle age. It is due to a disturbance of function in the sphincters of the anal canal. In infancy it tends to improve with age but the reverse is true in older patients, who suffer increasing distress and tend to become house-bound as their prolapse worsens. Complete rectal prolapse in older patients is a form of abdominal herniation, and in this state conservative measures can achieve very little—although there is now fresh interest in the possibility of long-term electrical stimulation of the sphincters to overcome this disability.

Most patients with severe rectal prolapse require operative treatment and the number of methods available makes it evident that none is wholly successful. There are two different approaches. In one the aim is to narrow the anal canal so that the prolapse cannot emerge—this is useful in old and unfit patients but the major problem here is that defaecation is also made difficult. The other method aims to fix the lower rectum in the pelvis so that it cannot prolapse: this is much the more promising method because it allows the cure of the abdominal hernia which is a major part of the problem. The hernial sac, which pushes between rectum and vagina, is completely removed. The rectum is then fixed in the pelvis and a repair performed to prevent recurrence of herniation.

CARCINOMA OF THE COLON AND RECTUM

Malignant disease of the colon and rectum is one of the major neoplasms. It is second in order of frequency of occurrence (carcinoma of the bronchus being the commonest neoplasm) and is much the most promising malignant neoplasm treated by surgery. In early cases cure is almost invariable following radical resection.

About half of the carcinomata of the colon and rectum occur in the rectum and the lowermost part of the sigmoid colon, the other half occurring fairly evenly over the remainder of the colon, with a small preponderance in the caecum. In the proximal colon carcinomata tend to be polypoid and to bleed readily but they obstruct the bowel late. As a consequence, patients become anaemic and do not usually have symptoms referable to the bowel.

Carcinomata in the distal colon are more likely to be annular and to cause some mechanical upset of the bowel, so the patient may complain of diarrhoea or of increasing constipation. In the sigmoid colon and rectum a carcinoma often bleeds and the patient notices fresh blood on the stool. It is characteristic that there is a frequent call to defaecate which produces blood and mucus but little or no faeces. The correct diagnosis is, therefore, likely to be made more quickly in the distal colon neoplasms. Abdominal palpation may reveal a lump in the line of the colon, digital examination of the rectum will allow a low rectal neoplasm to be felt, sigmoidoscopy allows visualization of tumours within 20–25 cm of the anal canal, while barium enema examination, if expertly performed, will reveal a carcinoma anywhere in the colon (though not in the rectum) by showing a constant filling defect in the barium shadow.

The surgery of carcinomata in the colon and rectum is based on the principle that a wide local excision of the primary should be combined with block excision of all the lymph nodes into which it may have metastasized. There is little that can be done about spread through the portal vein to the liver (although a few successful cases of partial hepatectomy for secondary carcinoma from the colon have been recorded).

Pre-operative preparation. The most important preliminary to large bowel surgery is mechanical cleansing to reduce the faecal content to the minimum. *For this reason patients are usually admitted three or four days before operation, given a nourishing diet without roughage, and daily colonic wash-outs are carried out, Veripaque, which has a direct stimulant effect on the colon, is much used for these wash-outs. Correction of anaemia before operation* is important. Most surgeons attempt to sterilize the bowel before operation by giving oral sulphonamides or antibiotics. These are probably of value in diminishing wound infections but have no other useful effect. If the operation proposed involves the likelihood of a colostomy, this must be discussed with the patient (see below).

Operation. *Carcinomata in the caecum and ascending colon* are removed by the operation of *right hemicolectomy*: this includes removal of terminal ileum, right colon, and the whole of the mesentery of the right colon, with all glands around the ileo-colic vessels.

Carcinomata in the transverse colon require removal of the transverse colon and the transverse mesocolon along with the whole of the middle colic vessels. The hepatic and splenic flexures are mobilized to allow anastomosis.

Carcinomata in the descending colon require removal of the affected bowel and as much as possible of the associated left colic vessels and lymph nodes.

Carcinomata in the sigmoid colon require removal of the sigmoid loop and some of the upper rectum, together with the sigmoid and the inferior mesenteric vessels and nodes. The descending colon is mobilized and joined to the upper rectum.

All these procedures are concluded by intraperitoneal end-to-end anastomosis of the two open ends of bowel.

It is a rule that all colonic anastomoses are drained so that, in the event of a leak, there is a line of drainage. If this happens, there is a strong tendency to healing after a few days.

Carcinoma of the rectum is treated by two different operations, depending on the level at which the neoplasm occurs in the rectum. If it lies low, within easy reach of the finger at rectal examination, then it will be impossible to remove the carcinoma radically without also taking out the anal canal. This is done by *abdomino-perineal excision* and necessarily this operation must leave the patient with a terminal colostomy.

If the carcinoma lies in the upper part of the rectum there is a reasonable

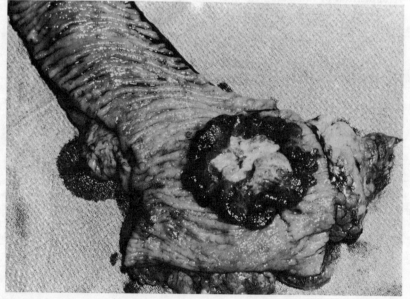

Fig. 51/5 A typical carcinoma of the rectum, showing the rolled raised edge of the ulcer and its sloughy centre. This opened specimen has been removed by anterior resection.

chance that the surgeon will be able to resect enough rectum below the neoplasm to achieve radical clearance and still to leave a part of the rectum to which mobilized sigmoid colon can be anastomosed. This procedure is usually called an *anterior resection* (see Fig. 51/5).

Abdomino-perineal excision. This operation is now universally performed in the lithotomy-Trendelenburg position devised by Lloyd-Davies in 1939. The essential point is the use of special stirrups which hold the legs apart to give access to the perineum but which hold the thighs only slightly flexed so that the abdominal operator has free access to the lower abdomen. Before the operation starts an indwelling catheter is inserted to keep the bladder empty during and after the operation and an intravenous infusion is set up in a wide vein in an arm so that blood can be transfused quickly when required during the excision. Lloyd-Davies devised his position so that a *synchronous combined operation* could be done by one surgeon working in the abdomen while another freed the anal canal and rectum through the perineum. This is still often practised but when a surgeon has to work single-handed the position is still very useful.

When rectum and anus have been removed the perineal skin is closed around a tube which drains the large raw area left in the pelvis. The abdominal wound is closed and the terminal colostomy formed through a cylindrical incision in the left iliac fossa. The colon edge is sutured to the skin edge: this rapidly heals and prevents subsequent colostomy stenosis. The colostomy is immediately covered with a disposable adhesive bag.

An **anterior resection** (see Fig. 51/6) proceeds in exactly the same way

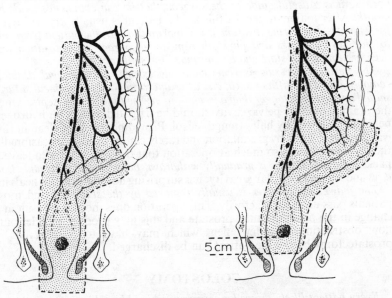

Fig. 51/6 The tissue removed in abdomino-perineal resection (*left*) and anterior resection of the rectum (*right*). The lymph nodes along the superior rectal artery—in which metastasis may occur—are equally radically removed in both operations. If the lower rectum is preserved by anterior resection it must be divided 5 cm below the lower edge of the neoplasm.

as the abdominal dissection in a combined excision but it stops when the rectum has been mobilized for about 10 cm below the carcinoma. After thorough irrigation with a cytotoxic agent such as perchloride of mercury, the rectum is divided at least 5 cm below the lower edge of the carcinoma and continuity restored by end-to-end anastomosis. This can be technically quite difficult but it is worth taking trouble to achieve a join because this will allow normal defaecation.

Postoperative care

Any operation for excision of the rectum involves working deep in the pelvis where it is difficult to see and tie off every major blood vessel before it is cut. Consequently blood loss at operation is variable but can be considerable—up to 1,500 ml—and this loss may continue postoperatively. Great care is taken to secure as dry a field as possible during operation but it is quite possible for *reactionary haemorrhage* to occur in the very large area of tissue exposed. *Close observation of the patient's condition, pulse rate and blood pressure and of drainage from the perineum is therefore particularly important so that extra blood can be infused if necessary.* In *colectomy* it is usually possible to tie off all major vessels before they are cut, but a watch on the drainage tube and on the circulation is still important because unexpected intra-peritoneal bleeding occasionally occurs.

No food or drink can be taken for two or three days and fluids will be given intravenously during that time. All patients have an indwelling catheter left in the bladder and this should be checked for satisfactory drainage.

The colostomy is likely to be inactive for several days, although flatus may be seen to collect in the bag after 48 hours. *It is important to report this because it is a useful guide to the surgeon that he can commence fluids by mouth.* After major surgery of this kind a patient is usually *kept lying flat for 24 hours, but during this time it is important to turn the patient from side to side several times and physiotherapy to encourage expectoration and deep breathing will start and be continued for some days.*

The perineal dressing is renewed as necessary. The perineal drain is removed about the fifth or sixth day after operation and the perineal sutures should not be left in longer than a week—otherwise they become septic. Once the drain is out, the pelvic cavity should be irrigated daily with hydrogen peroxide followed by half-strength eusol. Providing it is kept clean in this way it heals steadily by granulation and rarely causes trouble. Occasionally the perineum bleeds so much at operation that the surgeon has to leave a pack in position. *This is gradually withdrawn between the third and sixth days* and leaves a fairly large cavity; it is surprising how quickly this heals in.

The indwelling catheter is usually removed by the sixth day and most patients pass urine satisfactorily. This operation does, however, result in a change in the position of the prostate and this may produce bladder outflow obstruction in a few men, which may have to be relieved by prostatectomy before the patient can be discharged.

COLOSTOMY

Every patient likely to need a colostomy should be told of the possibility, and every patient given a colostomy must understand that the removal of their rectum was the only way to health. Some accept the idea of a colostomy more easily than others: it is often helpful to arrange a meeting with a patient who has managed a colostomy successfully for some time. It is important to remember the fear of 'a side passage' in the lay mind. Gossip among patients can distort and magnify the problems. The best antidote is the personal experience of a wise former patient.

Types of colostomy. Most colostomies are constructed at the end of an abdomino-perineal excision of rectum when the cut end of the sigmoid colon is brought out through a small incision in the left iliac fossa as a *terminal colostomy*. The other major type of colostomy is a *loop colostomy* and this is made in two circumstances:

1. *In an emergency operation for large bowel perforation or obstruction due to a carcinoma in'the distal colon or rectum*. The right side of the transverse colon is mobilized and two or three inches of bowel brought through a short incision in the right rectus muscle and retained in position by a short length of tubing passed under the colon, through the mesentery. The incision closes snugly round the bowel, an incision is then made into the wall of the colon and through this faeces will emerge onto the surface, so relieving the obstruction. In a loop colostomy there are therefore two openings—the *proximal opening* discharging faeces and flatus, and the *distal opening* leading into the distal colon which can be used for washing out the defunctioned colon and rectum to cleanse it for later resection of the obstructing carcinoma. If, as often happens, this lies in the sigmoid or upper rectum then, later, resection and anastomosis will be possible at a *second stage operation* and a few weeks later the colostomy can be closed at the *third stage operation*.

2. As a *protective colostomy* after a difficult anastomosis following anterior resection of a rectal carcinoma. This protects the anastomosis—which may have to be done with only one layer of sutures—during healing, the faeces emerging from the transverse colon. When the surgeon is satisfied that the rectal anastomosis is soundly healed, the loop colostomy is mobilized, closed and the colon replaced in the abdomen.

Management. In the operating theatre a colostomy is nearly always covered with a disposable adhesive bag which will receive faeces and flatus. Many patients continue to use such bags after they leave hospital and they give a feeling of confidence that there will be no 'accidents'.

In the days after operation, nursing staff will look after these bags and change them as needed. The one essential for obtaining good adhesion of the bag is that the skin around the colostomy is cleansed thoroughly and is dry—ether methylated spirit is usually best for removing old plaster and secretions. Each time this is done is an opportunity for the patient to become familiar with colostomy care, which he must increasingly take over for himself.

The patient should be told that the irregular action of the colostomy in the ward will probably settle as time goes on. Many patients find that their colostomy comes to act at predictable times and can, for example, be induced to act by taking a cup of hot tea on rising. Food has a more noticeable effect on a colostomy than when the rectum is intact. Onions, for example, cause many people to have loose colostomy actions. There is much individual variation in response to food, and patients should be encouraged to experiment with different foods and regulate what they eat by the effect on the colostomy. Some patients find it helpful to thicken the stool with cellulose (Celevac), which swells as it absorbs water in the gut. Others use codein phosphate, which is a bowel sedative.

Most surgeons are firmly of the opinion that a routine of a daily colostomy wash-out is not necessary and a needless mess and bother. A few, however, claim that this leads to colostomy evacuation at predictable times which the patient can arrange to suit his daily routine.

Views vary on what to wear over a colostomy. Some patients like the security of an adhesive bag. However, it is doubtful whether such an appliance is really necessary for a stoma which acts only a few times a day. Many patients wear some gauze and wool over the stoma and hold this in place with an ordinary 'roll-on' girdle; these are usually more comfortable than the instrument-makers' colostomy belts.

Results. The immediate mortality of operations to remove a rectal or colonic carcinoma has steadily fallen until now it is very low. Surgeons of great experience perform 100 or more such operations without a death occurring.

The long-term results depend largely on the degree of spread of the cancer at the time of operation. If there has been no spread into the glands in the meso-rectum the life-expectancy is virtually the same as in the general population.

POLYPS OF THE COLON AND RECTUM

A polyp is a localized nodular neoplasm of the colonic or rectal mucous membrane. Commonly it is an *adenoma*—and therefore benign—and it hangs on a stalk of variable length, as is well seen in Fig. 51/7. The stalk

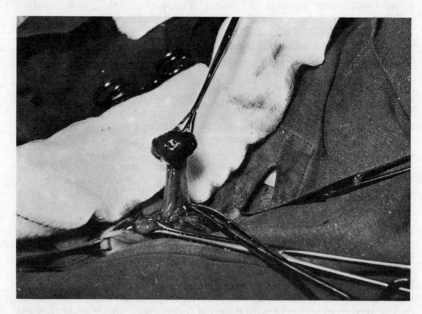

Fig. 51/7 A typical colonic polyp, exposed by colotomy. The adenoma is grasped in the forceps. The stalk is well seen; this is made up of normal mucosa which is drawn out by the pull of the adenoma. The stalk is ligated near the wall of the colon and the adenoma and the stalk removed.

may be absent and the polyp is then said to be sessile and appears as a red nodule in the mucosa. More rarely a *villous papilloma* occurs which is a more widespread nodularity of the rectal mucosa with a strong tendency to malignant change. *It is this tendency of polyps to change from benign to malignant character* that gives them special importance. If they are diagnosed and removed while still benign it is reasonable to believe that the patient may have been saved from the eventual development of a carcinoma.

Many polyps can be removed through the sigmoidoscope. If the polyp is too large, or too high in the colon, for this to be possible, then the colon is opened at laparotomy and the polyp removed (Fig. 51/7). Occasionally, resection is needed.

A special form of polyp formation—*familial polyposis*—is occasionally seen. It is a hereditary disease which is transmitted through a dominant gene to succeeding generations of a family. It is one of the outstanding examples of a pre-cancerous disease, the average age of death of polyposis patients being some 26 years younger than that of the general population.

ULCERATIVE COLITIS

This term covers a number of chronic non-specific inflammatory conditions of the colon and rectum. Their aetiology remains quite obscure in spite of much investigation.

Proctitis is the mildest form of the condition. There is a granular inflammation of the rectal mucosa which results in an excess of blood and mucus in the stools. The colon is normal and there is no general disturbance.

Procto-colitis describes a condition in which proctitis has also involved the lower colon. The inflammatory changes are not severe and do not cause general illness. Many patients continue normal lives over many years, having more or less rectal bleeding and controlling their symptoms with local steroids (given as prednisolone suppositories or retention enemata) and by taking Sulphasalazine. It is most important to recognize these conditions and one of the major reasons for performing sigmoidoscopy on every patient attending the rectal clinic is to make sure that they are not overlooked. Their symptomatology can closely resemble that of haemorrhoids but their treatment is entirely different. These mild inflammatory states are related to the more serious forms of diffuse colitis because a patient with a proctitis can quite suddenly relapse and produce the signs of true ulcerative colitis, although this is fortunately rare.

Ulcerative colitis is a term applied to chronic granulomatous inflammation of the colon which results in ulceration of the mucosa and some degree of systemic upset (Fig. 51/8). *The onset is often rather abrupt and the patient quickly becomes ill. Diarrhoea is very prominent as a symptom. General malaise, fever and rapid weight loss are usual.* The colon is often atonic and distended, sigmoidoscopy shows severe inflammation with mucosal ulceration and a barium enema usually shows that much of the colon is affected.

The behaviour of this condition is unpredictable. A few cases are rapidly and relentlessly progressive and the patient is dangerously ill within days of the onset. Perforation of the ulcerated colon is a particular hazard in these fulminant cases. More usually the patient remains seriously ill with

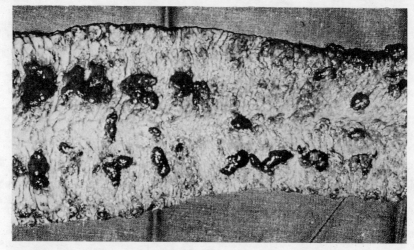

Fig. 51/8 This patient had a total colectomy for a severe relapse of chronic ulcerative colitis. The greater part of the mucosa has been shed—only a few scattered islands remain, the muscle coat of the bowel being widely exposed. Very severe diarrhoea and protein loss occurs in these circumstances.

severe diarrhoea, loss of weight, fever, progressive anaemia and hypo-proteinaemia and sometimes the complications of arthritis, pyoderma or iritis. *Intensive treatment* with systemic steroids, blood transfusions and intravenous fluids and feeding may see the patient through to remission. Relapse is, however, always a very real possibility, occurring in 75 per cent of patients.

SURGERY IN ULCERATIVE COLITIS

Total colectomy may be essential to save the patient's life or to put an end to a life of invalidism. *Emergency colectomy* may be needed for suspected or actual perforation or for severe toxic megacolon when the colon is enormously and dangerously distended. These operations may be genuinely life-saving.

Elective colectomy is done when a patient has had all possible medical treatment and is failing to improve or having repeated relapses which prevent normal life and work. An additional reason in patients who have had colitis for some years is that carcinomatous change in the diseased colon becomes increasingly likely.

The whole colon must be removed if the operation is to be effective and most surgeons advise simultaneous removal of the rectum by the abdomino-perineal approach. If this operation of procto-colectomy is done then an ileostomy is inevitable. *The prospect of a permanent stoma is a very daunting one to a young person and patience and understanding are needed when this matter is broached to the patient.* It is here that the Ileostomy Association is of the greatest help. They will arrange for a member to visit the patient. When a healthy bonny young woman looking completely normal visits a colitis patient and demonstrates that she has an ileostomy the patient can begin to believe that recovery and a normal life is possible.

There are many hints and tips which the experienced ileostomist can pass on to the patient newly operated on. *Experienced nursing and medical staff too can help the ileostomist a great deal after operation but continued advice from a fellow-ileostomist has special value.*

Pre-operative care. Considerable care is taken to put the patient in the best state for operation. Blood transfusion is used to correct any anaemia, and a high calorie and high protein diet is offered to overcome, so far as is possible, the nutritional deficiencies of these patients.

Many will have received systemic steroid treatment. If this treatment has been given for more than a few weeks then extra hydrocortisone will be ordered over the time of operation.

Bowel wash-outs are usually quite inappropriate in patients requiring colectomy for colitis on account of the profuse diarrhoea and the real risks of perforation of the diseased colon.

In *gravely ill patients* it may be decided that colectomy is more urgently needed than pre-operative treatment. *Then the mainstay is blood transfusion.*

When a patient is ambulant it is most desirable to apply the ileostomy apparatus on the day before the operation and after an hour or two to mark the place on the right iliac fossa where it rests most comfortably.

Operation. The patient is placed in lithotomy-Trendelenburg position. The minimum of ileum is removed—usually no more than two to three cm need to be taken. Most surgeons now remove the rectum at the time of colectomy through a perineal incision. The operation is concluded by constructing an **ileostomy**. A cylinder of skin, subcutaneous fat and muscle is removed at the site in the right iliac fossa indicated by wearing the ileostomy apparatus. This is equidistant from the iliac spine and the umbilicus and placed in flat skin so that the ileostomy apparatus will adhere well. The terminal ileum is brought through the hole made in the abdominal wall, its end everted and turned back and the cut edge of the bowel sutured to the skin edge around the hole (see Fig. 51/9). The ileostomy apparatus is immediately applied.

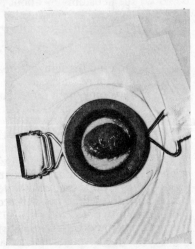

Fig. 51/9 The flange of a Chiron apparatus held in place by the double-sided adhesive square. The ileostomy protrudes exactly in the middle of the flange.

Postoperative care. The general principles of care after major abdominal surgery are followed. If steroids have been used before operation special notice is taken of the blood pressure because hypotension may indicate the need for supplementary hydrocortisone. Recovery is usually surprisingly good and it can be very striking how a gravely ill patient steadily improves from the time that the colon is excised.

CARE OF THE ILEOSTOMY

The major feature of an ileostomy is that it continuously discharges semi-fluid faeces which have a considerable enzyme content which can easily digest exposed skin. Until Koenig and Rutzen devised the adhesive rubber ileostomy bag, this tendency to skin digestion was a major deterrent to the construction of an ileostomy. Now, with care, all patients can overcome this problem.

It is important to recognize that there is not one single apparatus which suits all patients with an ileostomy. All have a bag into which ileal content is discharged, with various devices to prevent the fluid touching the skin. Each patient works out his own best method of care and should, provided it is successful, be encouraged to do it in his own way. Some believe in using an adhesive ring and bag but some find they are much better to avoid an adhesive. This can only be found by personal experiment.

Most hospitals start a patient off with an adhesive apparatus and the Chiron ring and bag, see Fig. 51/9, p. 503 (Down Bros.), is probably the most commonly used. Very many patients prefer to continue to wear this apparatus and the general principles of care apply to other types of apparatus. In application the following points must be considered:

1. No adhesive will stick on unprepared skin. Remove all traces of strapping and grease by using cotton wool and ether methylated spirit
2. Apply tinct. Benzoin Co. to the skin exposed to the adhesive
3. Cut the adhesive square so that the opening in it is larger than the ileostomy by about one-eighth inch all round
4. Remove one protective sheet from the adhesive square and apply the flange, centering it carefully.
5. Remove the other protective sheet from the double-sided plaster
6. Holding the flange, thread it and the adhesive square over the ileostomy and seat it in place, equally spaced away from the ileostomy in all directions (see Fig. 51/9)
7. Apply the bag to the flange

Most patients manage to keep the flange in position for four to seven days and become very expert at making the change of flange. Every patient needs two bags and it is wise to use a clean one twice daily if smells are to be avoided. To clean a bag effectively it needs to be turned inside out and washed in plenty of soap and water. Some like to soak it in a domestic bleach for a short time and this requires plenty of rinsing off. The bag is then hung up to drain and dry.

The number and variety of ileostomy appliances now available is considerable. Some hospitals have a trained nurse who acts as *stoma therapist*, to advise patients both in the wards and as out-patients. Experienced Ileostomy Association members can be of great assistance in this sphere.

The *complications* of an ileostomy are happily few. *Recession* of the spout is the commonest. If this causes trouble it must be corrected by operation. *Prolapses* and *stenosis* have both become very unusual since the eversion method of making an ileostomy became standardized.

Return to normal life is the rule in patients who have a procto-colectomy for ulcerative colitis. An active job and full enjoyment of sport are usual and an increasing number of women have borne children after the operation.

DIVERTICULAR DISEASE OF THE COLON

A modern translation of the Latin word 'diverticulum' would be a 'lay-by'. Diverticula are quite commonly formed in the colon, especially in the sigmoid loop, and most of the complications of this condition come from the fact that hard pieces of faeces, faecoliths, tend to be parked in these pouches. Here they may obstruct the way out, suppuration then takes place and an abscess forms in the wall of the colon. This may extend and cause a peri-colic abscess which may in turn perforate and produce a general peritonitis or make a fistulous communication with the bladder. More rarely the mucosa may be ulcerated by the faecolith, causing quite serious haemorrhage. Colonic obstruction may also occur.

This is, therefore, a disease which tends to present with its complications. Very many people have diverticula in their colons and are said to have *diverticulosis*, but they are generally unaware of this unless the complications of *diverticulitis* cause them distress. Some patients present with milder symptoms of diverticulitis—irregular bowel actions and pain in the left lower abdomen. The small quantities of blood passed so characteristically in the stools of patients with colonic or rectal neoplasms are rarely seen in diverticulitis.

The diagnosis is made by obtaining a characteristic appearance of multiple out-pouchings in the barium enema pictures of the sigmoid.

In many patients treatment is purely dietary. There is much evidence to suggest that diverticula form in races who eat a low-residue diet: this leads to localized spasm in the sigmoid colon with the build-up of high intra-luminal pressures. A high residue diet tends to produce bulky stools which prevent the high pressures building up.

If the major complications of diverticulitis occur then surgical treatment is often needed. Perforation of the colon with peritonitis is a very grave emergency requiring vigorous resuscitation of the patient and skilled surgery to close the perforation: most surgeons nowadays advise removal of the affected loop of bowel and colostomy. *A peri-colic abscess* may need incision and a *vesico-colic fistula* needs resection of the affected length of colon with restorative anastomosis and closure of the defect in the bladder. *Recurrent trouble with diverticulitis and peri-colitis is an indication for a planned resection.*

Chapter 52

Surgery of Peripheral Vascular Disease

by MICHAEL HOBSLEY

> *Introduction—obliterative arterial disease—embolism—spastic arterial disease—aneurysm—arteriovenous fistula—diseases of veins —surgical implications of arterial hypertension—surgical management of portal hypertension—diseases of lymphatics.*

INTRODUCTION

Conditions of the *arteries* and *veins* that may require surgical management are commoner than those of the *lymphatic* vessels.

Diseases of the arteries reduce the blood supply to the peripheral tissues, i.e. produce *ischaemia*, by narrowing of the lumen caused either by structural changes in the wall, *obliterative arterial disease*, or by excessive contraction of the muscular wall, *spastic arterial disease*. Sudden blockage of the lumen may also result from *embolism*. There are two types of arterial disease that may result functionally in peripheral ischaemia without a primary narrowing of the artery—*aneurysm* and *arteriovenous fistula*. Ischaemia interferes with the metabolism of the tissue cells: pain-producing substances that should be washed away by a full circulation or oxidized by a sufficiency of blood-borne oxygen accumulate in the tissues and irritate nerve-endings. If the ischaemia is sufficiently severe, tissue death occurs (*necrosis*) either in small patches (*ischaemic ulcers*) or in large areas (*gangrene*).

Diseases of the veins reduce the efficiency of the return of blood from the tissues to the heart, so that the tissues become gorged with stagnant blood. In ways we do not fully understand, this engorgement (*venous hypertension*) interferes with the nutrition of the cells and like ischaemia produces ulceration and gangrene, but with some features noticeably different from the ischaemic varieties.

A raised pressure in the arteries (*systemic hypertension*, see Chapter 22, p. 211) is an important condition because of shortened life-expectancy; occasionally it is due to a cause that can be corrected by a surgical operation. The hypertension that may occur in the portal venous system (*portal hypertension*, Chapter 22, p. 232) often requires surgical management.

Diseases of the lymphatics reduce the efficiency of the return of interstitial fluid (the fluid filling the spaces between the cells) to the great veins in the neck, and result in an accumulation of interstitial fluid, *oedema*, in the affected part.

OBLITERATIVE ARTERIAL DISEASE

Pathology

1. **Atheroma.** The most important obliterative arterial disease is *atheroma, atherosclerosis.* This is a degenerative condition of the arterial wall affecting mainly medium and large-sized arteries. It is part of the processes of ageing, since its incidence is clearly related to age, but the first signs may appear in some individuals as early as 20 years of age. Deposits of cholesterol-containing fatty material are laid down in plaques in the intima (innermost lining) of the arteries, and as they grow these plaques tend to ulcerate through the intimal layer of cells to come into contact with the bloodstream. There are no signs or symptoms of the disease itself, but the rough surfaces of the plaques encourage the deposition upon themselves of fibrin and platelets from the blood, and later red blood cells become entangled in the material. Thus a solid structure is formed from the bloodstream upon the plaque, a *mural thrombus.* Should the thrombus grow sufficiently to obstruct the lumen of the artery, thrombosis is said to have occurred.

Atheroma is a patchy process, but its presence in one set of vessels suggests that it is probably present elsewhere. For that reason, patients presenting with obliterative arterial disease of the lower limb frequently also have signs and symptoms of cerebro-vascular or cardiac ischaemic disease (strokes, angina, etc.). Involvement of the arteries of the upper limb to an extent that produces clinical disturbance is unusual, and so the clinical picture in the lower limbs only will be described. Atheroma is more common in obese subjects and in patients with diabetes mellitus.

Sites of obstruction. The common sites affecting the lower limbs are the *lower lumbar* aorta (Fig. 52/1), its *bifurcation,* and the *common iliac* arteries; the *common femoral* artery at the point high in the thigh where the profunda femoris or deep femoral artery arises, and the *superficial femoral* artery as it continues downwards towards the knee (Fig. 52/2 (A) and (B)), and the *popliteal* artery at the level of the knee-joint, where it bifurcates to form the anterior and posterior tibial arteries. Atheroma may also affect the smaller distal vessels such as the digital arteries: small vessels disease is particularly likely to be associated with diabetes.

2. **Embolism.** *An arterial embolus nearly always consists of a thrombus which has become detached from its site of origin, has travelled in the bloodstream, and has become impacted at a site of arterial narrowing.* The whole process is known as embolism. The *commonest source of an embolus* is the auricle of the left atrium of the heart in the condition of mitral stenosis complicated by atrial fibrillation (see p. 208). Alternatively, a mural thrombus may develop after a myocardial infarction with subsequent detachment of part of the thrombus. Thrombi forming in the aorta within aneurysms and on atheromatous plaques may also produce embolism. Emboli usually lodge at major arterial branches, and produce symptoms and signs of acute ischaemia in the territory normally supplied by the blocked artery.

3. **Other diseases.** Various diseases affecting the walls of arteries, such as the collagen diseases *polyarteritis nodosa* and *scleroderma,* may underlie the thrombotic process. *Buerger's disease* is an affliction of young men,

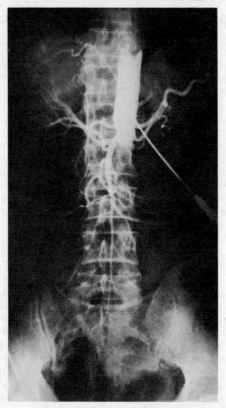

Fig. 52/1 Occlusion of the abdominal aorta by thrombus, demonstrated by lumbar aortography. The upper abdominal aorta and its branches have been opacified by injecting radio-opaque liquid via a long needle introduced from the back. Downward flow of the medium has been cut off at the upper end of the second lumbar vertebra. (There are five lumbar vertebrae: count them upwards from the sacrum.) The patient complained of intermittent claudication in both limbs.

particularly of the Jewish race, in which the smaller peripheral arteries, together with their companion veins and nerves, are involved in a fibrotic process that results primarily in distal ischaemia.

Clinical features and management

Whatever the underlying pathology, obliterative arterial disease in the lower limb presents as acute arterial insufficiency, intermittent claudication, or rest pain and gangrene.

Acute arterial insufficiency. Suddenly, the patient experiences severe pain in one or both limbs. If he is walking, he may fall. The limb feels cold and he cannot move the affected area. On examination, coldness, pallor and loss of sensation are noted, together with an absence of pulsation in those sites distal to the obstruction.

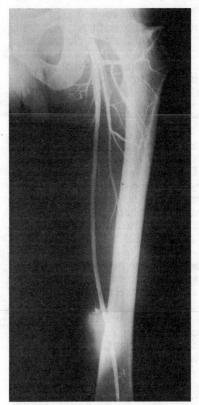 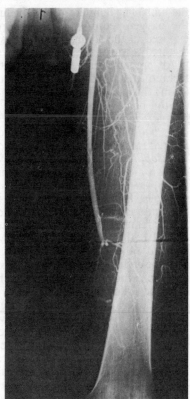

Fig. 52/2 Occlusion of the left femoral artery, demonstrated by arteriography. (*a*) A normal left femoral arteriogram for comparison. (*b*) This left femoral artery is occluded half-way down the thigh. Note the increased number of smaller arteries compared with (*a*). They are the *anastomotic* circulation, nature's attempt to circumvent the obstruction by opening vascular channels that in normal circumstances are not needed and remain empty. The arteriogram was obtained by puncturing the left femoral artery in the groin. The patient complained of intermittent claudication in the left calf.

The two causes are embolism and acute thrombosis. Embolism is suggested by the associated clinical findings of mitral stenosis, irregularity of the pulse, recent myocardial infarction or a palpable abdominal aortic, femoral or popliteal aneurysm. If these can be excluded, the likelihood is of acute thrombosis of an atherosclerotic vessel: there is frequently a previous history of intermittent claudication (see p. 510), and the acute episode is usually less dramatic than that of embolism.

Management involves care of the ischaemic limb, disobliterative surgery, and amputation. *The ischaemic limb must be handled as though it were fragile, because the least avoidable trauma may precipitate the irreversible changes of gangrene before surgery can be carried out. All examinations of the limb must be gentle, all manipulations delicate.* The head of the bed should be raised on 4-inch blocks so that gravity aids the blood supply to the limb. The temperature of the limb should be kept cool, so as to reduce the oxygen requirements of the tissues: the limb is therefore usually exposed to the room, and if necessary the breeze from an electric fan is directed towards the leg.

All pressure must be avoided: this can take some ingenuity. A useful technique is to make a collar, about 4 inches wide, of 1-inch-thick plastic foam: this is applied around the ankle and lower leg, and keeps the heel off the bed. All unnecessary movement is avoided. *The patients are in pain, often aware that they are in danger of losing a leg, so they are notoriously bad-tempered; every allowance should be made for this. Urine-testing is vital, since so many of these patients have diabetes.*

Disobliterative surgery is usually attempted if the patient is seen soon enough after the onset of ischaemia (if the time interval is as long as 48 hours, few limbs are saved), and ideally should be carried out as soon as possible. The modern operation is simple and no great strain for the patient, and may even be performed under a local anaesthetic.

The femoral artery of the affected limb is exposed in the groin, and a special catheter (Fogarty) which has an inflatable bulb near its tip is inserted either upwards or downwards, according to the site of the block. The fine catheter passes through the block, and then the balloon is inflated and the catheter withdrawn, thereby extracting the embolus. A free flow of blood following the removal of the obstruction testifies to the success of the operation. When this treatment is successful, pulses become palpable in the feet and the limb swells and the skin becomes red because the capillaries, damaged by ischaemia, passively dilate when the blood supply is restored and are more permeable than normal.

Amputation is necessary if gangrene is already present when the patient is admitted, or if disobliterative surgery fails.

Intermittent claudication. Claudication means limping. *Intermittent claudication* is a phrase used to describe the common symptom-complex in patients having a degree of ischaemia in the lower limbs compatible with perfect function at rest, but inadequate when the oxygen demands of the muscles increase during exercise.

The main symptom is *pain*, which is often described as a tight or bursting sensation, and which is most commonly situated in the calf, though it may occur anywhere in the lower limb or buttock. The pain is not present at rest, but comes on after an amount of exercise that is fairly constant for any one patient at a given stage of the disease. For example, the pain may come on after the patient has walked slowly for 200 yards on the level ('claudication distance' 200 yards), or quickly uphill for 100 yards. Although there is a tendency to deteriorate, the pattern for the patient may persist for months or years. The *pain disappears rapidly* on resting: *patients develop a technique of standing still at intervals to allow the symptoms to subside before carrying on walking.*

In most patients with intermittent claudication, the relative ischaemia of the lower limb is due to a gradual thrombosis (based on atheroma) in major vessels such as the aorta, iliac or femoral arteries. A minority of patients have more peripheral obliterative disease (diabetes, Buerger's disease, etc.) so that only the foot pulses are missing.

Management of intermittent claudication. All patients require advice on looking after the limb, because the risk of gangrene developing is always present. Minor trauma which would be of no consequence in a normal limb may precipitate massive death of tissue in the absence of an adequate blood supply. *The patient must avoid extremes of temperature (sitting too near the living-room fire, and using a hot-water bottle in bed are particularly dangerous habits); maceration by sweat must be prevented by regular washing and drying with a soft towel together with the use of foot powder,* fungus infection between the toes requires prompt treatment; and ideally toenails should be trimmed professionally to reduce the risk of trauma during this procedure. *Smoking ought to be given up completely.* Vasodilators such as Priscol are often prescribed, but there is no evidence that they help.

If the patient can do his job and reasonably enjoy his leisure within the limits imposed by his symptoms, there is no indication for surgical treatment, the results of which may be disappointing. However, if there is grave disturbance of leisure or interference with work, and if the patient's general condition is good enough to allow major surgery to be contemplated, the investigation of *arteriography* should be performed.

The aim of arteriography is to demonstrate the anatomy of the obstructive lesion or lesions so that the feasibility of *reconstructive surgery* can be assessed. The usual procedure is called *lumbar aortography*: the patient is admitted, and under a general anaesthetic a long needle is inserted from the back into the abdominal aorta at the level of the 1st lumbar vertebra. A radio-opaque liquid injected through the needle opacifies the distal arteries. Short localized blocks, particularly in the aorto-iliac rather than in the femoro-popliteal region, are the most amenable to reconstructive surgery; increasing length of the block, multiplicity of obstructions, and widespread atheroma of neighbouring segments of the arterial tree, are all factors that militate against surgical success (see Figs. 52/1 and 52/2, pp. 508, 509.)

Reconstructive surgery takes two main forms: *disobliteration* and the *construction of a by-pass.* In disobliteration or *endarterectomy* the surgeon reams out from the artery the solid mass of atherosclerotic intima and thrombus leaving the rest of the arterial wall behind. A channel to *by-pass* the blocked segment of artery may be constructed from synthetic material (e.g. Dacron) or from the patient's own long saphenous vein. If the vein is used, it is excised and reversed before re-insertion so that the valves it contains which are designed to permit blood to flow proximalwards, will not interfere with the movement of blood distally within it.

Postoperative care. Long incisions in the thigh are painful. *The surgeon usually wishes the affected limb to be kept still for several days, but the patient must be encouraged to move the rest of himself as much as possible.* A cradle keeps the pressure of the bedclothes off the limb. Deep vein thrombosis is particularly common after this sort of operation. Some surgeons use anticoagulants in the postoperative period to reduce the risk of blood clotting, both at the operation site and in the deep veins of the calf.

A successful reconstruction results in the restoration of palpable pulses in the feet, though these cannot always be felt immediately after operation, and *the nurse may be asked to chart the presence or absence of these pulses, and the condition of the limb with respect to colour, temperature and swelling.* Haematomas in the wound are common, even in the absence of anticoagulants, and infection is a dreaded complication because secondary haemorrhage from the operation site may threaten not only the limb but life itself. *Mobilization is usually commenced about the end of the first week.* The patient goes home or to a convalescence centre during the third week: the risks of smoking are emphasized before he goes, and he is advised how to modify his life to reduce the demands made on his leg.

Rest pain and gangrene. Intermittent claudication often, but not always, precedes these conditions. Pain, similar in distribution and nature to the pain of intermittent claudication, becomes a continuous manifestation and is typically worse at night because warmth induced by the bedclothes increases the tissue metabolism and oxygen demands. The patient may get relief by invoking the aid of gravity and hanging the leg out of bed.

The chief site of origin of the pain appears to be skin rather than muscle. The skin is pale and smooth, often to the point of looking glossy. Skin appendages suffer from poor nutrition: hair growth is defective, nails are deformed. Passive elevation of the limb results in severe pallor, especially noticeable in the soles of the feet; subsequent dependency causes a purple flush and swelling as a result of the stagnation of the inflow of blood in the damaged and permeable capillaries. In a leg like this, it is only a matter of time before some incident of minor trauma produces localized necrosis, which may spread with alarming rapidity to massive gangrene.

The site of the obstruction is deduced from the presence or absence of the peripheral pulses. The prognosis for the limb is so grave that aortography is mandatory, even if the chances that reconstructive surgery might be feasible appear slim. In this situation, even if peripheral areas of gangrene have become established, successful reconstructive surgery along the lines described above may save the greater part of the limb and allow amputation to be performed much more distally than would otherwise have been necessary.

Amputation. Apart from war surgery, the commonest indication for an amputation at some site in the lower limb is obliterative arterial disease. When the indication for amputation is urgent (embolism, major arterial trauma) there is usually no problem in getting the patient's permission, but the patient with rest pain and threatened gangrene is often reluctant to give his consent. *He may discuss the situation with the nurse, who can emphasize that amputation is not a destructive procedure, but an essential preliminary to the constructive procedure of supplying the patient with a useful limb in place of the useless (often painful) limb that he possesses. Demonstrations by ex-patients of their expertise with crutches and artificial limbs may be valuable.* All patients awaiting amputation should be warned that they will still be aware of the sensation of possessing the limb after it has been removed, *phantom limb*; and that although the phantom may be painful at first, the painful element always disappears in time.

Where time allows, *pre-operative physiotherapy* is most valuable. Exercises are given to strengthen the arms, which must deal with the unfamiliar task of using crutches, and the sound limb, which must bear extra weight until a satisfactory prosthesis is fitted. Practice with crutches takes the edge off one of the difficulties awaiting the patient after operation. In some cases (particularly where a through-knee amputation is contemplated), the patient can be sent to the limb-fitting centre for measurement for his *pylon* (the temporary peg-leg prosthesis which all amputees get at first) before operation. An adjustable pylon has been invented which can be fixed to the patient's bended knee for walking practice before operation while the leg is still in place.

The operation should become an incident in the total treatment of the patient, not an overwhelming climax. Techniques vary, but the two main principles include section of the bone at a point further up the limb than the cuts through muscle and skin, so that the bone-end can be well covered, and careful haemostasis to avoid haematoma formation that would invite infection and prejudice healing. The wound is often drained. The *site* of amputation is necessarily a compromise between the removal of the whole lesion and the desire to preserve as much of the limb as possible. In ischaemic problems, the performance of the amputation through an area with an adequate blood supply is essential. Until recently, the optimal sites for amputations were dictated largely by the mechanical limitations of the artificial limbs available: five inches below the knee, *below-knee amputation*, or ten inches below the greater trochanter in the thigh, *above-knee* or *mid-thigh* amputation. Nowadays, however, prostheses are mechanically so ingenious that the exact length of the stump is no longer crucial. Amputation *through* the knee-joint has become much more common.

In *postoperative management* the important features are the adequate relief of pain, the danger of reactionary haemorrhage, and the importance of avoiding contractures. The latter are due to the altered balance between flexor and extensor muscle groups as a result of the amputation. For example, after an above-knee amputation there is a marked tendency for flexion to occur at the hip. *This tendency is counteracted by nursing the patient in the supine position with the stump held flat on the bed by the pressure of a roller towel running across the front of the stump and secured on each side of the limb by sandbags.* The frequent adoption of the prone position in bed also helps to prevent contracture at rest. Meanwhile, exercises for the rest of the patient are not neglected.

When the risk of reactionary haemorrhage is past, and drains have been removed and healing appears to be progressing satisfactorily (usually about the fourth day), the stump is mobilized and later the patient is got up on his crutches to practise walking. Stitches are removed from the tenth to fourteenth day. Necrosis of the skin flaps due to an inadequate blood supply is a very serious complication diagnosed by a dark-blue discoloration. Amputation higher up the limb may eventually prove necessary. Necrosis may be followed by infection, or the latter may occur without necrosis. When the wound is well healed, the patient is sent to a limb-fitting centre for measurement for a pylon.

A good stump for the limb-fitters is conical, and this shape can be achieved by bandaging the stump twice daily to express oedema fluid, starting quite firm turns distally and letting the turns become gradually slacker as one bandages along the stump proximally. The scar should not be adherent to the deeper tissues. There must be no contracture of the joint above the amputation, because this would prevent the prosthesis from reaching the ground. The stump must have enough muscular power to control a heavy artificial limb. The definitive artificial limb is usually fitted about three months after operation, when all the natural shrinkage of the soft tissues of the stump has had time to occur.

These patients often need a great deal of social support. They may need to find a new job, new accommodation at ground level, or some sort of wheeled transport. One amputee can keep the medical social worker, as well as the physiotherapist, busy for months after the surgical work is done: but the reward of seeing a human being, well adjusted to his disability, returning to his work and leisure as a fully integrated member of society is well worth the effort.

SPASTIC ARTERIAL DISEASE

The calibre of small arteries and arterioles is determined by the degree of contraction of muscle cells lying in their walls. Calibre is influenced by a large number of factors: local stimuli such as acidity, oxygen and carbon dioxide tension, and the presence of certain chemical agents that are formed during metabolic processes; local nerve reflexes activated by external stimuli such as heat and cold; and systemic influences mediated by the *sympathetic nervous system*. The latter is the major determinant of the size of the small arteries and arterioles at rest. Acting both through the level of the hormone adrenaline circulating in the blood, and through the impulses conveyed along the sympathetic nerves to the blood vessels, the effect of sympathetic stimulation is to produce *vasoconstriction*.

Spastic arterial diseases result from excessive vasoconstriction of small arteries and arterioles. Most commonly the vasoconstriction is *intermittent*, that is it develops for short periods with remissions between each attack.

Intermittent arteriospasm

Clinical features. Since only small vessels are affected, the pulses are normal. Arteriospasm is much more common in the *upper* limb (contrast obliterative arterial disease), although severe symptoms occasionally arise in the feet. The extremities of the limb are most affected, presumably because their remoteness from the centre of the circulation makes them most susceptible to a reduction in the local blood flow: the possibility of alternative pathways is small.

In a typical attack, the fingers become cold and white and they feel numb. As the spasm continues, the stagnant blood in the capillaries loses more oxygen than usual by exchange with the tissues, and the high concentration of reduced haemoglobin results in cyanosis so that the white fingers gradually become blue. When the spasm finally passes off, the vasodilator action of the local metabolites produced by the tissues during the ischaemic phase encourages a marked arteriolar vasodilatation. *In consequence, the skin becomes pink and hot, and the tissues swell with oedema fluid that accumulates by excessive transudation across the walls of the transiently damaged capillaries.* This series of changes of colour and temperature is called *Raynaud's phenomenon*.

If the condition is of long-standing, the nutrition of the tissues may become permanently affected so that ischaemic necrosis of the tips of the fingers may occur. There is no great likelihood of the gangrene extending proximally unless organic obstruction arises in the larger vessels, or unless spasm is maintained continuously for long periods.

Causes. *Raynaud's disease* is the commonest cause of Raynaud's phenomenon. This disease mainly affects young women: the small arteries supplying the digits are particularly sensitive to cold, and respond to exposure to cold by marked spasms of vasoconstriction. Attacks may be precipitated by immersing the hands in cold water. Emotion also plays a part, presumably via the sympathetic nervous system. The best management for this condition is that the patient should live in a warm climate but in any case must take particular care to avoid exposure to cold. Wool-lined mittens should be worn in winter. If despite conservative measures the symptoms remain severe, sympathectomy is advised (see below).

Other causes of Raynaud's phenomenon. A variety of diseases can be associated with this clinical picture, including collagen diseases such as polyarteritis nodosa, and scleroderma. Workers with vibrating tools such as pneumatic drills may also suffer.

Treatment. The underlying cause of Raynaud's phenomenon must be treated if possible. Sympathectomy offers best results in Raynaud's disease, but has a place in other causes of the syndrome.

Sympathectomy produces a warm dry pink limb and prevents the attacks of Raynaud's disease. Unfortunately, its effect is not usually permanent. For the upper limb the operation performed is *cervical sympathectomy*. The incision is usually in the lower part of the neck, and the sympathetic chain—which lies deep in the neck, near the posterior end of the first rib—is approached across the summit of the pleura. Pneumothorax due to accidental damage to the pleura is a possible complication. The lower part of the *stellate* (*inferior cervical*) ganglion, the second and third thoracic ganglia, and the sympathetic chain linking these ganglia are excised. For the lower limb, the operation is *lumbar sympathectomy*. The lumbar sympathetic chain is exposed via a skin-crease incision in the anterior abdominal wall and flank at the level of the umbilicus. The chain and ganglia are excised from above the second lumbar to below the third lumbar ganglion.

Persistent arteriospasm. Severe persistent arteriospasm results in ischaemic necrosis which needs no special description. The causes are traumatic: in any major injury of a limb, the blood-supply to the periphery may be threatened by spasm of major vessels despite the fact that they are not completely occluded or transected. During the exploration of such a wound, the surgeon attempts to relieve spasm by the application of the antispastic agent papaverine to the affected vessels. If this fails, resection or by-pass grafting is necessary.

An important cause of spasm may be encountered by the nurse in a dramatic fashion, while she is assisting an anaesthetist during the induction of anaesthesia. If thiopentone is injected into an artery instead of into a vein its extremely irritant properties provoke an intense arterial spasm throughout the distal arterial tree. This is a major emergency which may cause the loss of the limb: the anaesthetist will keep the needle in the artery and attempt to flush the thiopentone through the arteries and on into the veins (where it does not cause spasm) with large quantities of saline. He may also wish to inject vasodilator drugs. The nurse must be prepared to move fast according to his instructions, as seconds matter.

ANEURYSM

An *aneurysm* is a dilatation of an artery due to weakness of the arterial wall. By far the commonest cause of the weakness is atheroma. Other causes include:

(i) Congenital weakness due to a lack of muscle in the wall.
(ii) Syphilis, which destroys the elastic tissue in the wall.
(iii) Rarely, destruction of the whole wall by the lodgement of an infected embolus in one of the small arteries supplying the vessel wall (mycotic aneurysm).

The commonest sites are the abdominal aorta, the cerebral vessels, and the popliteal artery behind the knee, but they may occur anywhere.

Clinical features. An aneurysm may be asymptomatic and found on routine clinical examination. Eventually symptoms do occur. The *size* of an enlarging aneurysm may itself constitute a symptom. *Pressure effects* on neighbouring structures may produce symptoms: for example, an abdominal aortic aneurysm produces pain in the back by eroding the lumbar vertebrae. *Rupture* of an aneurysm of a large vessel like the aorta may produce sudden death from blood loss; leaking aneurysms produce localized haematomas which themselves have pressure effects. The roughened, distorted wall of an aneurysm favours local mural thrombosis. The process of thrombosis may progress until the arterial lumen is narrowed or occluded producing *distal ischaemia*; or fragments of the thrombus may become detached and travel in the bloodstream to lodge more distally—*embolism*.

Management. The dangers of an aneurysm are so great that in general they require treatment even if not producing any symptoms. Ideally, an aneurysm is excised and replaced by a graft or prosthesis, and this procedure—particularly when a prosthesis is used—works well for the abdominal aorta. Some aneurysms are inoperable, but when the affected artery can be dispensed with, tying the artery either before or beyond the aneurysm encourages the obliteration of the aneurysm by thrombosis.

ARTERIO-VENOUS FISTULA

Normally arteries only communicate with veins via the very small-bore capillaries. An abnormal large-bore communication is called an arteriovenous fistula. Such fistulae may exist in large numbers in a localized area as a congenital abnormality, *congenital arteriovenous fistula or malformation.* Acquired arteriovenous fistulae usually result from penetrating wounds, e.g. stab- or bullet-wounds.

An arteriovenous fistula short-circuits blood away from the peripheral regions supplied by the affected artery, and so there may actually be ischaemia of these regions. Usually, however, the cardiac output increases by way of compensation (see p. 413), and the net result is an abundant supply of well-oxygenated blood. When this arises during childhood, the affected limb grows larger than the normal limb.

A large leak from the arterial circulation lowers the arterial blood pressure, and to compensate for this the heart has to work harder and pump out more blood. The arterial pressure is particularly lowered during diastole, and so the pulse pressure (difference between systolic and diastolic pressure) widens. A sphygmomanometer reading of 130/60 would be typical. In severe cases, the heart may be incapable of maintaining the arterial blood pressure and fails.

These local and systemic sequelae of a large arteriovenous fistula make it desirable to close the leak by direct attack, and where possible such an operation is carried out. This gives excellent results in acquired arteriovenous fistulae, but widespread congenital malformations may make surgery hazardous or impossible.

DISEASES OF VEINS

Deep vein thrombosis and pulmonary embolism. (See p. 467.)

Venous return from the legs. When a human stands upright, the *return of the blood from the veins of the lower limb* against the influence of gravity depends upon the efficiency of a system that has been called the 'peripheral heart', and consists of the *muscles* of the lower limbs, the *valves* in the veins, and the unyielding tough membrane that encloses the muscles, the *deep fascia*. When the muscles contract the pressure within the deep fascia rises; blood in the deep veins is squeezed by this pressure and constrained to move towards the heart because that is the only direction of movement that the valves permit.

There are also valves in the superficial veins, breaking the long column up into small segments, but the muscle-pump deep to the deep fascia cannot squeeze these superficial veins. However, the superficial veins are connected to the deep veins by communicating veins that perforate the deep fascia, and contain valves that direct flow from the superficial to the deep veins only. Hence when the muscle-pump empties the deep veins, there is an indirect effect via the communicators sucking blood from the superficial into the deep veins, and so the superficial veins are kept empty.

Disturbances of the venous return are due either to blockage of veins, i.e. *deep vein thrombosis*, or to incompetence of valves. The latter can produce two different clinical pictures according to the site of the incompetence.

1. Varicose veins

If there is an incompetence of the valve in the main vein draining the superficial tissues, the long saphenous vein, at its point of entry into the femoral vein high in the thigh, the superficial venous system distends under the high pressure relayed from the deep system and in time more distal valves lose their functions as their bases are separated. The superficial veins are visible as distended, tortuous vessels, and such veins containing incompetent valves are called *varicose veins*.

Varicose veins are unsightly, and cause aching towards the end of the day. *Because of their superficial situation, they are easily damaged, and the bleeding produced is copious and frightening, though it is easily controlled by elevating the limb.* The stagnation of the blood in these veins predisposes to inflammation, which often affects a short segment (about three inches) of a varicose vein causing it to become hard (because the blood in this segment clots), painful, and tender while the overlying skin becomes red—*superficial phlebitis*, or *thrombophlebitis*. Rarely, superficial thrombophlebitis may be the origin of a pulmonary embolus, though emboli usually come from deep veins. For all these reasons, varicose veins should be treated.

Treatment of varicose veins is by operation or by injection. Fashions change, but at the moment the vogue seems to be *injection therapy*, which can be done in the out-patient department. A short segment of vein containing an incompetent valve is entered with a hypodermic needle, and the segment is then emptied and isolated by suitable external pressure; an irritant material (e.g. ethanolamine) is injected to produce a chemical thrombophlebitis. The inflammation resolves with much fibrosis that destroys that segment of vein. The process is repeated till all the superficial varicosities are obliterated.

Operation always involves interrupting the leaks from the deep system, and especially the highest leak where the long saphenous vein empties into the femoral vein in the groin. The procedure to divide and tie off the upper end of the long saphenous vein is called *Trendelenberg's operation*. Long lengths of vein are stripped out of the superficial tissues by passing a flexible metal rod along the vein, fixing the rod to the far end of the vein, and pulling from the near end so that the vein is pulled out. After such operations the patient returns to the ward with firm crêpe bandages up to the knee or higher, and the foot of the bed is elevated to reduce the chance of venous bleeding. Pain may be considerable at first, but settles surprisingly fast, and the patient is encouraged to walk the day after operation.

2. Gravitational ulcer

A different clinical picture is produced by incompetence of communicating veins (often called *perforators*) in the region of the ankle. The upper part of the lower limb is normal, but in the region overlying the perforators the full force of the venous hypertension is sustained by superficial tissues which start with the handicap of a relatively poor arterial blood supply. The results are oedema, staining of the tissues with brown pigments formed from haemoglobin that has leaked out of the distended capillaries, and itching due to the formation of irritant metabolites in these anoxic congestive conditions. The irritation evokes scratching, which may be sufficiently active to produce an eczematous reaction of the skin (see Chapter 31, p. 315), and when the interference with local nutrition is sufficiently great any minor trauma results in necrosis of the superficial tissues and ulceration.

Such an ulcer is called a *gravitational ulcer*, because it can always be healed by reducing the venous hypertension in the superficial tissues by putting the patient to bed with the foot of the bed elevated. The ulcer tends to return when the patient gets up and about again, but this may be prevented by firm elastic bandaging from the base of the toes to just below the knee with a crêpe or (better) red-line bandage. To be effective, this bandaging must be done before rising from bed in the morning. If the condition is long-standing and therefore intractable, *Cockett's operation* is performed through a longitudinal incision behind the lower two-thirds of the calf to find and tie the incompetent perforators. In addition, an indolent ulcer may need to be excised and a split-skin graft applied (see Chapter 67, p. 700).

Gravitational ulcer is often called varicose ulcer, but this term is misleading because there may be practically no superficial varicose veins. The condition is often a sequel to deep vein thrombosis: the affected deep and perforating veins in the calf have become recanalized but their valves which have been destroyed by the thrombosis do not regenerate.

SURGICAL IMPLICATIONS OF ARTERIAL HYPERTENSION

Arterial hypertension is a serious disorder because it is associated with a reduction in life-span due to its deleterious effects upon the heart, upon atheromatous disease of arteries—particularly of the heart and the brain —and upon the kidneys. Surgery has been used in the management of severe cases in the past, because sympathectomy releases peripheral arterioles from the constrictor influence of the sympathetic nervous system and the resultant vasodilatation lowers the arterial blood pressure (see p. 36). However, the effect of sympathectomy was short-lived; there is little place for surgery in this role now that adequate hypotension-producing drugs have been discovered (see Chapter 22, p. 215).

Surgery does, however, have another role. While most cases of hypertension are of unknown aetiology, there is in some instances an underlying cause which may be amenable to surgery.

Causes of 'surgical' secondary hypertension

Coarctation of the aorta (Chapter 59, p. 599).

*Tumour of the adrenal medulla—phaeochromocytoma—*and, *tumours of the adrenal cortex*: Cushing's syndrome (Chapter 29, p. 298).

Renal causes. Reduction in renal blood flow produces arterial hypertension through a complex chain of events called the *renin-angiotensin system*. The reduction in renal blood flow stimulates a group of specialized renal cells called the *juxta-medullary apparatus* to secrete an enzyme called renin, which acts on a circulating protein to produce ultimately angiotensin II. This substance is the strongest known constrictor of arterioles, and hypertension results.

If only one kidney is ischaemic, its removal may cure the hypertension. This situation arises due to congenital stenosis of the renal artery, or some acquired cause such as atheroma that may reduce the calibre of the renal artery. Occasionally the lesion is amenable to direct arterial surgery by endarterectomy or by-pass. Unfortunately many cases of renal hypertension are due to bilateral renal diseases such as chronic pyelonephritis, chronic glomerulonephritis, etc. and surgery is not then possible. It must be emphasized that arterial hypertension from whatever cause itself damages the kidneys and produces ischaemic changes that then complete a vicious circle by producing further hypertension.

PORTAL HYPERTENSION

The *portal circulation* comprises the venous pathways between the intra-abdominal alimentary tract and the spleen on the one hand and the liver on the other. The *splenic vein* is joined by the *inferior mesenteric vein*, which brings blood from the left half of the colon, and then unites with the *superior mesenteric vein*, which drains jejunum, ileum and the right half of the colon, to form the *portal vein*. The latter receives blood from the stomach and duodenum and enters the liver, where it breaks up into small-calibre vessels only a little larger than capillaries, the *hepatic sinusoids*. The hepatic sinusoids drain into the inferior vena cava by the hepatic veins. At the periphery of the portal circulation there are potential communications with systemic veins: the chief portal-systemic anastomoses are at the junction of the stomach and oesophagus, at the umbilicus, and in the anal canal. Normally, when the portal pressure is only 10 mm Hg, the anastomoses are not patent.

Serious consequences of an increase in portal venous blood pressure, *portal hypertension*, do not usually arise until the pressure exceeds 20 mm Hg, and in some patients a level of 50 mm Hg may be exceeded. Nearly all cases are due to *resistance to outflow from the portal tract*. The possible sites are:

(1) *Pre-hepatic*, i.e. affecting the portal vein. The commonest cause is thrombosis of the portal vein, which may occur in infancy due to umbilical sepsis in association with separation of the cord, or from infective portal phlebitis following intra-abdominal sepsis in later life.

(2) *Intra-hepatic*, usually due to the various forms of cirrhosis of the liver. In these patients, the effects of the derangement of liver-function are added to those of the portal hypertension.

(3) *Post-hepatic*, i.e. an obstruction in the hepatic veins, or a rise in pressure in the inferior vena cava due to cardiac disease. These are rare causes.

Consequences of portal hypertension. (1) The *collateral circulation* is opened up: the sub-mucosal veins in the region of the gastro-oesophageal junction enlarge enormously, a pattern of radiating veins may appear at the umbilicus, '*caput Medusae*', while haemorrhoids may form in the anal canal. The high pressure in the thin-walled veins is liable to cause bleeding, particularly from the oesophageal varices. Haematemesis and melaena result.

(2) *The spleen enlarges and becomes palpable.* The normal destruction of red and white blood cells and platelets in the splenic pulp may be exaggerated in a large spleen, so that there is *anaemia* and *leucopenia, and a low platelet count with deficient coagulation* (this effect is referred to as hypersplenism).

(3) *The diversion of blood from the portal to the systemic system exposes the brain to the influence of certain toxic substances derived from ingested food.* These toxins, which include ammonia, are normally destroyed in the liver, and especially if the cause of the portal hypertension is a damaged cirrhotic liver the discharge of these toxins into the systemic circulation produces the clinical picture called *portal-systemic encephalopathy*: lack of co-ordination of movements (often tested as poor writing), a coarse ('flapping') tremor, slurring of speech, changes in behaviour and mental deterioration. Since the toxins are produced from proteins in the food by bacteria in the large intestine, it may be possible to control the symptoms by reducing oral protein-intake, washing out the large bowel to remove blood (protein) following a gastro-oesophageal bleed, and giving neomycin to reduce bacterial activity in the gut.

Surgery of portal hypertension. The dominant consideration is the dangerous bleeding from oesophageal varices. The only method of *permanently* reducing the portal pressure is to construct a large by-pass between the portal and systemic systems, accepting the risk of encephalopathy. However, in the emergency situation two *temporary* measures may be valuable: *Pituitrin* injections reduce the pressure by constricting the arterioles supplying blood to the gut, and *direct pressure* on the oesophageal varices with a *Sengstaken tube* may stop the bleeding. The Sengstaken tube is a gastric tube with an extra lumen through which two balloons near its tip can be inflated. The patient swallows the tube, the position of its tip is adjusted so that when the balloons are inflated they lie one just beyond and one just above the oesophago-gastric junction. After inflation, a small weight is fixed to the external end of the tube to maintain slight upward pressure on the bleeding veins. The stomach can be washed out and aspirated through the main lumen of the tube. This method of treatment is uncomfortable and alarming, and adequate sedation and reassurance are extremely important because adrenaline and noradrenaline increase portal pressure.

By-pass operations. The commonest is the *portal-caval shunt*, in which an anastomosis is made between the portal vein and the inferior vena cava. This is a major operation, performed through a right thoraco-abdominal incision. The after-care and complications therefore combine those following thoracotomy and those following laparotomy, together with the possibility of portal-systemic encephalopathy developing and the consequences of operations upon patients with diseased livers. It is not surprising that the mortality of these operations is high: they are contra-indicated by severe liver damage (persistent jaundice; plasma albumin less than 3 g per 100 ml), and by age (because people over 60 years are particularly liable to encephalopathy). Other possible shunts are splenic vein to renal vein (following splenectomy) and superior mesenteric vein to inferior vena cava.

Operations on the varices are less successful in the long term, but less hazardous at the time. The varices can be obliterated by sclerosing injections (as for varicose veins in the legs) through an oesophagoscope, or by sutures inserted after opening the oesophagus (a left thoracotomy incision is used in this procedure). This operation can be used as an emergency to control the bleeding before proceeding to a definitive portal-caval anastomosis at a later date.

DISEASES OF LYMPHATICS
(See also Chapter 23, p. 220)

Acute lymphangitis. This is the only common surgical disease of the lymphatic vessels. The affected vessel appears as a thin red subcutaneous streak, as a result of acute inflammatory change. The source of infection is usually a streptococcal lesion somewhere in the area drained by the lymphatics. Antibiotics cure the condition.

Lymphoedema. The lymphatic channels drain interstitial fluid from the regions surrounding the cells to make room for fresh interstitial fluid being formed by filtration through capillary walls. The lymph is returned to the great veins in the root of the neck. Obstructions in the lymphatic pathways, reduction in the number of lymphatics, or abnormalities of their valves interfere with the drainage of lymph from the periphery and result in oedema. The oedema fluid is richer in protein than is the oedema fluid produced by increased capillary transudation in venous obstruction, and the protein tends to organize and form fibrous tissue. For this reason, the oedema of lymphatic obstruction (lymphoedema) does not usually pit on digital pressure.

Causes of lymphatic obstruction. These include certain specific infections such as *filariasis*, long-standing chronic non-specific infections, and particularly neoplastic disease. Treatment is that of the cause.

Congenital lymphoedema may become manifest in childhood, adolescence or much later. One or both lower limbs becomes swollen (*elephantiasis*) and characteristically the skin desquamates in fine dry particles. No evidence of venous obstruction is found, and the oedema is non-pitting. The *diagnosis* may be confirmed if necessary by *lymphography*. A dye that is selectively taken up by lymphatics (e.g. Patent Blue Violet) is injected subcutaneously into a web-space of the affected foot. Shortly afterwards, under local anaesthesia, an incision is made over the dorsum of the foot down to the deep fascia. Any lymph channel cut across by the incision shows as a dye-stained spot on the cut surfaces. The proximal end is cannulated with a very fine cannula, and a slow injection of radio-opaque material made over the course of several hours, using a mechanically driven syringe. Subsequent X-rays of the limb show the lymphatics and confirm *hypoplasia* (less lymphatic channels than normal) or lack of valves. If there is complete *aplasia* of the lymphatic channels, no dyed spots are seen in the incision.

Management of congenital lymphoedema. Conservative measures—invoking gravity, the use of elastic stockings—may keep the patient comfortable. Operations aimed at bringing normal lymphatics into the area from elsewhere have been devised and can be successful, but are usually themselves disfiguring and so not indicated unless the disfigurement of disease is gross. In the severest cases, a useless limb that is a burden to the patient may require amputation.

Chapter 53

Operations on the Thyroid, Breast, and Adrenal Glands

by MICHAEL HOBSLEY

Thyroidectomy—the breast—adrenalectomy

THYROIDECTOMY

Indications
Thyroidectomy is performed for a variety of thyroid conditions. A *solitary nodule* is removed because it may be a neoplasm and because it may press on the trachea and cause obstruction to breathing. A generalized enlargement may be operated on because it too may cause tracheal obstruction, and to prevent gross deformity. *Thyrotoxicosis* is an indication for surgery to reduce the mass of the gland and hence limit its hypersecretion of the thyroid hormones that control the metabolic rate: other lines of treatment for thyrotoxicosis are the anti-thyroid drugs and radioactive iodine.

Preparation for operation
The recurrent laryngeal nerves lie close behind the thyroid gland, one on either side of the trachea, and control the movements of the vocal cords. They are at some risk during operations on the thyroid. The cutting of one nerve produces a varying degree of hoarseness, but this symptom usually improves with time as the opposite vocal cord increases its activity in compensation. Injury to both nerves is a catastrophe because the paralysed vocal cords fall together and obstruct the movement of air in and out of the chest: a permanent tracheostomy must be constructed and normal speech is impossible.

Because of the serious effect of damage to these nerves, and because it is not very uncommon to find patients who already have a weakness of a vocal cord before thyroidectomy, many surgeons insist that the patient is examined by an ear, nose and throat surgeon *before* operation, and the state of his vocal cords assessed as a baseline for comparison with the situation after operation.

Control of thyrotoxicosis
To perform thyroidectomy on a patient with thyrotoxicosis is dangerous: the manipulation of the gland during the operation liberates large quantities of thyroxine into the bloodstream and produces an intensification of

thyrotoxicosis, *thyroid crisis*, that can prove fatal. The thyrotoxicosis must therefore be brought under control by medical measures before the operation. Potassium iodide, 60 mg t.d.s. for 10 to 14 days before operation, may be used for this purpose.

This regime is often used even if the patient has been made *euthyroid* (normal in thyroid function) by the slow-acting drugs such as Neo-Mercazole during the preceding months, because many claim that the iodine treatment reduces the vascularity of the gland and makes the operation easier. *The nurse may be able to record objective evidence that the anti-thyroid treatment is working*; a *falling pulse rate* (especially the *sleeping pulse rate*) and a rise in *weight*.

The wound

Reactionary haemorrhage is a dreaded complication during the first 24 to 48 hours. The tissues of the neck are particularly vascular, and to make the operation easier the anaesthetist often lowers the blood pressure. If the blood pressure does not regain its normal level before the surgeon closes the wound the subsequent rise in blood pressure to normal levels may result in a haematoma if haemostasis was not perfect. The seriousness of this complication is that a large collection of blood in the neck compresses the trachea and produces acute obstruction to respiration. *The nurse may find the patient suddenly changes from his normal appearance to a choking, blue figure gasping for breath, with an obvious swelling in the neck. This is an emergency of the greatest magnitude, and while aid should be summoned immediately the nurse should not hesitate to act if no doctor or senior nurse is present.*

The life-saving procedure is to open up the skin wound so that the blood can reach the exterior instead of building up pressure in the neck. *Sterile stitch-scissors or Michel clip-removers should be kept at the bedside for 24 hours after operation.* The gush of blood from the opened wound may be an alarming sight, but the nurse may take comfort that the rate of bleeding will never be so fast as to kill the patient by loss of blood in less than an hour, whereas the same blood loss into the neck can by obstructing the trachea produce death in four minutes. Once the pressure has been relieved, arrangements can be made to return the patient to the operating theatre where the surgeon will re-explore the wound and stop the bleeding.

Wound drains. Most surgeons use drains in an effort to avoid the above complication. These can usually be removed by the second or third day.

Skin closure is by sutures or metal clips. In either case, since the wound heals very rapidly, they may be removed on the third or fourth day.

Thyrotoxic crisis. Danger signals are a rise in pulse rate, blood pressure and temperature, agitation progressing through confusion to stupor, and sweating. This complication is very rare nowadays. Treatment includes sedation and intravenous iodine and attempts to lower the temperature, e.g. ice-packs. The drug propranolol is useful in combating the toxic effects of thyroxine upon the heart.

Recurrent laryngeal nerve. The patient is often hoarse for a few days, but this does not necessarily mean that a recurrent laryngeal nerve has been damaged; the hoarseness may result from the irritation of the endo-tracheal tube used by the anaesthetist. The ear, nose and throat surgeon examines the cords again before the patient leaves hospital. *The nurse should not discuss the prognosis of hoarseness or the likely outcome of damage to the nerve: all queries from the patient should be referred to the medical staff or a senior nurse.*

THE BREAST

A lump in the breast

Women, at least in sophisticated societies, have come to realize that a *lump in the breast* must be taken seriously because it may be a *carcinoma*. Unfortunately, this does not always lead them to report the presence of a lump to their doctors at an early stage.

Carcinoma of the breast

This is the commonest form of malignant disease in women in this country. It has been calculated that one woman in 20 develops this lesion. It does not occur until puberty, and the incidence remains low in young women until about the age of 35 years. Henceforward, the incidence increases rapidly to a peak about the time of the menopause, and remains high in older women. Since other causes of a lump in the breast become very uncommon after the menopause, a lump in the breast first appearing then is very probably (but not certainly) a carcinoma.

Clinical features. The lump is frequently neither painful nor tender, and indeed the presence of the lump is usually the patient's only symptom. There may be a serous or bloodstained discharge from the nipple, but non-malignant tumours can also cause this symptom. The surgeon in his examination looks for *signs of spread*, both *local* and *at a distance*. Signs of acute inflammation usually (but not always) mean that the disease is not malignant.

Modes of spread. *Local* spread is indicated by tethering of the lump to the overlying skin, or to the underlying muscle. *Distant spread* occurs *via the lymphatic channels*, laterally to the lymph nodes in the *axilla* and then to nodes above the *clavicle* (collar bone), and medially to lymph nodes behind the medial ends of the ribs near the *sternum* (breastbone), where they lie along the internal mammary artery. These various groups are called respectively the *axillary*, *supraclavicular*, and *parasternal* or *internal mammary* lymph nodes. Distant spread also occurs *via the bloodstream*, and metastatic deposits may form anywhere, but common sites are the lungs, the bones, the liver and the brain.

Diagnosis. No features of a lump in the breast, not even the signs of local spread, are proof that the lesion is a carcinoma. They can all be simulated by various non-malignant conditions. Most surgeons therefore make it a strict rule to obtain a biopsy by operation or by techniques involving the use of a needle, so that it can be sent for microscopical examination and exact diagnosis. Only if this test has proved positive would the surgeon consider undertaking mastectomy.

Non-malignant lumps in the breast

Young women between the ages of 15 and 25 years are prone to develop a small hard mobile lump called a *fibroadenoma*. Women during the 10 years before the menopause are prone to develope breast *cysts*. These lesions may occur at any age during the reproductive period, but the common ages are as given. Other non-malignant causes of a lump in the breast are much less common.

Management of a patient with a breast lump

If the lump is a *fibroadenoma*, the surgeon can from his examination make a reasonably confident diagnosis. Nevertheless, he advises the patient to come into hospital to have the lump removed under a general anaesthetic and the diagnosis confirmed pathologically. This operation is minor: to prevent reactionary haemorrhage a pressure dressing may have been applied in the operating theatre, and this may be reduced to a small gauze dressing on the day after operation. Stitches are usually left in 7 to 10 days, but the patient can go home on the second day, or as soon as the histological report is available. Very occasionally, the lump is reported to be a carcinoma after all, and further treatment must be undertaken.

The surgeon's diagnosis of a *breast cyst* is also fairly accurate. Some surgeons advise that even a cyst should be excised. Others aspirate the fluid in the cyst with a needle and syringe as an out-patient procedure: if the lump has disappeared completely, and if the fluid obtained is typical, the patient is reassured that such cysts do not predispose towards breast cancer and that is the end of the matter.

There remain the patients in whom the surgeon fears the diagnosis is carcinoma or in whom there is no clinical evidence either way. Here the management may be exactly as that for a fibroadenoma, an excision-biopsy, followed if necessary a few days later by definitive treatment.

If special facilities are available whereby the pathologist can examine the biopsy specimen within 15 minutes of receiving it (a popular example of such techniques is the so-called 'frozen section' technique in which the tissue is frozen by exposure to solid carbon dioxide—dry ice—so that thin sections can be cut immediately to put under the microscope), the surgeon will probably seek the patient's permission to proceed immediately with the definitive treatment under the same anaesthetic. This policy requires that before the biopsy is undertaken the surgeon frankly discusses with the patient the possibility that the lump is malignant.

The *choice of treatment* depends on many factors, one of which is evidence of spread. The pre-operative evaluation of a patient with a possible carcinoma of the breast always includes a chest X-ray, and a haemoglobin estimation (looking for evidence of the anaemia that may result from metastases in the blood-forming bone marrow). In some cases evidence of bone destruction may be sought (X-rays, calcium losses in the urine—a series of 24-hour collections will be requested). If there is distant spread, any operation on the breast itself can clearly only be palliative; if there is no distant spread, the treatment advised for the breast is aiming at cure.

Radical treatment for carcinoma of the breast

Medical opinion is sharply divided on the best method of treatment, and the nurse must not be surprised to see many different regimes, possibly even in the same surgical ward. Instead of attempting to describe all these regimes, the commonly performed operation of *radical mastectomy* will be discussed. The essence of this operation is that the breast is removed with the axillary lymph nodes. Since the tissues around the carcinoma must be excised widely to prevent a local recurrence of the growth, in some patients there is not enough skin left to cover the deficiency left by the operation, and a thin graft of skin is cut (often from the front of the thigh) and applied to the defect immediately. The care of this skin graft is as described in Chapter 67, p. 702.

Suction-drainage is usually used because the chest wall is a very vascular area. Sometimes a reactionary haemorrhage occurs and requires control by re-operation. To encourage healing of the wound, the patient is advised to avoid vigorous movements of the arm on the side of the operation for three or four days: then mobilization exercises must be started to prevent the shoulder from becoming too stiff.

Some patients have a lot of trouble with the shoulder, and require much encouragement with their exercises. A clear goal should be stipulated for her endeavours at every stage—for example, to be able to brush the hair at the back of her head. Sutures are usually retained till the 10th or 12th day. It is important to inspect the wound daily because, especially if the skin flaps have been sewn together under some tension to avoid the use of a skin-graft, necrosis may occur along the edges of the wound: the appearance of any colour change, red, blue or black, in the skin should be reported immediately.

By far the most important nursing task after this operation is to treat the patient's psyche. There is no need to dwell upon the psychological consequences of this mutilating operation. Modern surgery, by judicious placing of the scar so that the patient can ultimately wear low-cut dresses with a *prosthesis* (artificial replacement), does what it can, and the attitude of the patient's husband is necessarily crucial. *In between these influences, the nurse can work steadily through her own attitude and encouragement for the patient's acceptance of the situation.*

Palliative treatment for carcinoma of the breast

The main forms of treatment are *X-rays* for localized deposits, *chemotherapy* (see Chapter 64), and *hormone therapy*.

Between one-third and one-half of breast carcinomas are sensitive, at least for a time, to the concentration of sex hormones in their environment. In such cases the progress of the disease can be arrested, at least for some weeks or months, by altering the hormonal environment. The methods used are the giving of hormones by mouth and injection, e.g. *stilboestrol*, *testosterone* (Chapter 29, and Appendix 2), or by operations to remove the sex glands (oophorectomy), the other source of sex hormones, the adrenal glands (adrenalectomy), or the pituitary gland which controls the ovarian secretion of sex hormones (*hypophysectomy*).

ADRENALECTOMY

The two adrenal glands are situated at the upper poles of the kidneys and are relatively inaccessible should surgical excision be required. Each gland consists of two components: the inner *medulla* and the outer *cortex*. Adrenaline and noradrenaline are secreted from the medulla; they are secreted in excess by the benign tumour of the medulla, *phaeochromocytoma* (Chapter 29, p. 299). Two of the many hormones secreted by the cortex are essential for life. They are *aldosterone* which conserves sodium by controlling the rate of loss in the urine, and *hydrocortisone* which has a vital function in maintaining the blood pressure. Without hydrocortisone the patient dies from hypotensive shock (Addisonian crisis, p. 297). An excess of aldosterone (Conn's syndrome) or an excess of hydrocortisone (Cushing's syndrome) may result from hyperactivity of the whole cortex, from a benign hyperfunctioning tumour of the cortex, or rarely from carcinoma. Both glands may also be removed to alter the hormonal environment in cases of advanced breast carcinoma.

Operation

Adrenalectomy may be carried out through an abdominal incision or through a loin incision. As with all loin exposures, there is a danger of pneumothorax from damage to the pleura, and a careful watch for post-operative respiratory difficulty should be kept. The choice of incision is usually one of personal surgical preference. For bilateral adrenalectomy many prefer a single abdominal incision to two loin incisions.

Replacement therapy

The essential adrenal hormones must be replaced regularly for life after bilateral adrenalectomy and replacement may be required temporarily after a unilateral operation where suppression of the remaining gland has occurred. Hydrocortisone in suitable dosage is started before operation, and maintained by intravenous injection for several days after operation until the surgeon is sure that the patient can absorb oral medication, whereupon the treatment changes to drugs with a similar action to hydrocortisone but which can be taken by mouth. Hydrocortisone possesses some of the salt-retaining properties of aldosterone, but in certain cases it is necessary to prescribe another drug with specific electrolyte functions, e.g. *fludrocortisone. The nurse should appreciate that after adrenalectomy a patient is extremely reliant upon his adrenal replacement therapy.* Patients are given cards to carry with them always, containing information about the drugs and dosage of their treatment.

In the early postoperative period the surgeon may find it difficult to diagnose whether a state of shock is hypovolaemic and due to internal reactionary haemorrhage, or else due to adrenal hormone deficiency. *Accurate fluid balance charts, especially the volume, specific gravity and chloride concentration in the urine, may be a vital factor in the assessment.*

Sepsis is predisposed to by an excess of adrenal cortical hormones, and such patients should have every possible precaution against sepsis both before (several baths with an antibacterial agent such as chlorhexidine in the water), during and after the operation. Infection of the wound is a common complication, and often rather silent in its onset.

Chapter 54

Surgical Conditions of the Genito-urinary Tract

by J. E. A. WICKHAM

*Kidney and ureter—congenital anomalies—trauma—infections—
calculus—tumours—hydronephrosis—operations on the kidney and
ureter—bladder and urethra—congenital anomalies—trauma—infections—calculus—tumours—retention of urine—operations on the
bladder and urethra—the penis—the scrotum and contents*

THE KIDNEY AND URETER

Congenital anomalies. Mistakes in development, such as the absence or
reduplication of a kidney or ureter, or the fusion of the two kidneys at their
lower poles (horseshoe kidney) are not uncommon; these conditions are
symptomless unless the malformation interferes with the drainage of
urine and predisposes to urinary tract infections. The best defence the
urinary tract has against infection is the normal flow of urine along it
which flushes any pathogenic micro-organisms to the exterior; any tendency to stagnation invites infection to become established. Occasionally
the valvular mechanism at the lower end of the ureter is defective and
allows urine to regurgitate from the bladder into the ureter and renal pelvis
during micturition. This 'ureteric reflux' may give rise to recurrent urinary
tract infections, especially in children. Surgical correction of the
abnormality may be required.

Trauma. The kidney may be contused or partially ruptured in an injury
to the back or lower chest. It is frequently difficult to distinguish renal
injury from other intra-abdominal damage but the patient is usually
shocked and evidence of haematuria confirms the renal injury.
Treatment. General resuscitation treatment for shock is carried out.
Intravenous pyelography is then performed to assess the extent of any
damage. Surgical intervention is rarely necessary; with bed rest and general
nursing care the haematuria gradually abates and the kidney ultimately
heals with surprisingly little residual abnormality in function or anatomy.
Nephrectomy may very rarely be indicated for progressive bleeding from
major renal disruption.

Acute infections (see Chapter 25).

Chronic infections. The common varieties are:

> Non-specific.
> Tuberculous.

Non-specific infections. This is the condition of chronic recurrent pyelonephritis which results from recurrent acute attacks of urinary infection leading to ultimate destruction of the renal substance. The place of surgery is usually ablative, the diseased organ being removed by nephrectomy if the contralateral kidney is normal.

Tuberculous infections. Tuberculosis of the kidney arises as a blood-borne infection leading to the development of multiple abscesses in the renal substances. Treatment is primarily the administration of the anti-tuberculous drugs: streptomycin 1·0 g daily for three months coupled with INAH (Isoniazid) 100 mg t.d.s. and PAS (para-amino-salicylic acid) 16·0 g daily for two years (see p. 206). *Surgical treatment of renal tuberculosis* is confined to removing the hopelessly destroyed kidney, drainage of localized abscesses in the renal substance, *cavernotomy*, and correcting obstruction from fibrosis and stricture which may occur in the healing stage of the disease.

CALCULOUS DISEASE OF THE KIDNEY AND URETERS

Renal calculi form in the collecting system of the kidney as concretions of substances normally present in solution in the urine. The common substances which give rise to stone formation are calcium oxalate, calcium phosphate and uric acid. Rare stones are made of cystine and xanthine. The reason why the majority of stones form is not known. A proportion occur because of poor drainage in the urinary collecting system leading to stasis and infection, whilst a small proportion form when excessive calcium is excreted into the urine in the metabolic disorder *hyperparathyroidism* (see Chapter 29, p. 296). Stone formation is also related to poor fluid intake, especially in hot climates; the urine becomes highly concentrated and the crystalloid substances in the urine become easily precipitated.

The stones form first in relation to the renal papillae in the calyces and may gradually increase in size to fill the whole renal pelvis—the so-called 'stag horn' or 'cast calculus'. Symptoms depend upon the size and mobility of the calculi. Small calculi remaining wedged in a calyx are usually symptomless, but *small calculi which become dislodged into the pelvis or ureter cause considerable pain and give rise to the condition of ureteric colic* as they pass down the ureter to the bladder. Large stones are usually symptomless unless they become wedged in the pelvic-ureteric junction, when they may cause considerable loin pain and back pressure with hydronephrotic destruction of the kidney. If such a hydronephrotic kidney becomes infected then the whole organ may be converted into a large closed abscess or *pyonephrosis*.

Medical treatment is to encourage a high fluid intake and to correct any metabolic cause for further stone formation such as hyperparathyroidism and to remove any persistent cause of infection. There is little evidence that adherence to any particular type of diet is important in the prevention of stone recurrence as long as a high fluid intake maintains a dilute urine.

Medical treatment of the acute attack of ureteric colic is to administer a high fluid load to induce diuresis and to relieve pain with strong analgesics such as pethidine at frequent intervals. Antispasmodic drugs such as Pro-Banthine or atropine are also used in an attempt to relax the smooth muscle of the ureter.

Surgical treatment. Most stones of less than 0·5 cm in diameter will be passed spontaneously down the ureter into the bladder. Ureteric colic is usually occasioned during this passage and surgical removal is only contemplated if the calculi become arrested at any point. If the stone becomes stuck within the lower two inches of the ureter it may be dislodged by passing an endoscopic stone extractor (Dormia basket) into the ureter through a cystoscope. Stones wedged higher in the ureter must be removed by open operation, *ureterolithotomy*.

Renal stones are usually removed from the kidney if they are causing obstruction, recurrent infection or renal pain. The stones may be removed from the pelvis of the kidney by pyelolithotomy or through the renal substance by nephrolithotomy.

TUMOURS OF THE KIDNEY AND URETER

Benign tumours. These are excessively rare and cause negligible symptoms.

Malignant tumours. There are three malignant tumours of the kidney.

The embryoma or Wilms' tumour is a tumour of the first seven years of life. *Symptoms* are usually haematuria or the development of an abdominal mass. Treatment is nephrectomy usually followed by radiotherapy. The prognosis is poor.

The adenocarcinoma is the common tumour of the renal substance in the adult. The usual age of presentation is the fifth decade and the symptoms are painless haematuria, occasional loin pain or palpable tumour. *Treatment is nephrectomy followed by radiotherapy*. The prognosis is determined by the histological differentiation of the tumour: poorly differentiated tumours having only a 30 per cent five-year survival; well differentiated have a 65 per cent five-year survival.

The transitional cell tumour of the renal pelvis is a carcinoma of the lining epithelium of the renal pelvis. It is a very malignant tumour and presents with haematuria. *Treatment is nephrectomy, ureterectomy and radiotherapy*. The prognosis is poor, with a five-year survival after surgery of less than 25 per cent.

Tumours of the ureter are rare and present with haematuria or loin pain. Treatment is nephro-ureterectomy as the pelvis of the kidney may be frequently involved with other tumour foci.

Hydronephrosis. This condition supervenes when the collecting system of a kidney becomes obstructed. Back pressure causes atrophy and distension of the renal substance ultimately converting the kidney into a large urine-filled sac.

The causes of obstruction are varied but probably the commonest is the so-called congenital pelvic-ureteric junction obstruction. This is a functional disturbance at the pelvi-ureteric junction of one or both kidneys which prevents the normal peristaltic advancement of urine from pelvis to ureter. Other causes of hydronephrosis are the post-tuberculous ureteric stricture, the impacted ureteric calculus and the ureteric tumour.

Bilateral hydronephrosis occurs with severe bladder neck obstruction when the persistently high intra-vesical pressure is transmitted backwards to both upper urinary tracts. The symptoms of hydronephrosis are dull pain in the kidney region, often coming on in attacks. The treatment is removal of the obstruction, be it stone, tumour or bladder neck obstruction. The treatment of congenital pelvi-ureteric junction obstruction is by pyeloplasty (see operative section, below).

OPERATIONS ON THE KIDNEY AND URETER

The surgeon approaches the kidney either through the loin or through the abdomen. The after-care of patients who have been operated on via the abdomen does not differ from that after any other laparotomy (see Chapter 49, p. 464). The loin incision is made just below the twelfth rib, or through the bed of the rib after its resection.

The upper end of the ureter is approached through the loin, but the lower half requires an incision in the lower anterior abdominal wall, either an oblique one in the iliac fossa or a vertical paramedian.

Loin incisions are painful and adequate analgesia is vital. The patient should sit well up in bed and be encouraged to take deep breathing exercises and to cough in order to prevent pulmonary segmental collapse. Early mobilization is encouraged. The stitches are removed about eight or ten days later.

Almost always the wound is drained, usually with a corrugated rubber drain. The drain can be removed after 48 hours. Any operation involving an incision with subsequent repair in the urine-conducting channels— calyces, pelvis, ureter—may result in a leak of urine. If no leak occurs, the drain may be removed in 48 hours; if there is a leak, the drainage should be maintained for at least 24 hours after it has dried up.

Nephrectomy, the removal of a kidney, is performed by mobilizing the kidney, and clamping, ligating and dividing the artery, vein and ureter. *Partial nephrectomy* may be required for the removal of a grossly destroyed or distorted segment of kidney involved in calculous disease, in order to prevent stones forming again in the diseased area. The renal pedicle is temporarily occluded with a soft clamp, the diseased portion excised, and the wound in the kidney and pelvis sutured. *Reactionary haemorrhage is a particular risk of this operation, and the blood pressure should be monitored hourly for the first 12 hours.* Other conservative operations upon the kidney are the removal of stones through an incision in the kidney, *nephrolithotomy,* or in the pelvis, *pyelolithotomy,* and a plastic reconstruction of the pelvi-ureteric junction (*pyeloplasty*) in the treatment of hydronephrosis. *Ureterolithotomy* is the removal of a stone from the ureter.

A nephrostomy, or opening into the kidney, is a drainage tube connecting the renal collecting system to the exterior in order to divert the urine flow permanently or temporarily. Indications are obstructive lesions affecting the ureter, or the necessity to protect a suture line in the collecting system (as for example after pyeloplasty) by reducing the flow of urine through the anastomosis. A nephrostomy tube inserted for the latter reason is usually removed about the eighth day, by which time the anastomosis should have healed.

All operations on the urinary tract, if the urine is infected, are liable to the infective complications of surgery—wound infection, sub-phrenic abscess, etc. Most surgeons believe in starting suitable antibiotics or chemotherapy, to which the organisms grown from a mid-stream specimen of urine are sensitive, before operation, and continuing for at least five days afterwards.

THE BLADDER AND URETHRA

Congenital anomalies. *Ectopia vesicae.* In this condition the anterior wall of the bladder and abdominal wall fail to close in the embryo and the child is born with an incomplete lower urinary tract. The base of the bladder is seen as a flattened red and bleeding area of mucosa at skin level just above the pubis, and urine drains from the ureteric orifices onto the skin surface producing considerable excoriation. The *treatment* of this condition is to excise the bladder remnant and to perform urinary diversion using an ileal conduit.

Epispadias is a lesser degree of the above condition where only the urethra remains unfused in the midline, the bladder having closed in normally. A minor degree of epispadias may be corrected by plastic surgery if the bladder sphincters are normally formed, but if the child is incontinent urinary diversion is the best treatment.

Hypospadias is the commonest congenital defect. The urethral tube does not form normally along the undersurface of the penis and the urethral orifice may be situated as far back as the peno-scrotal junction. Various plastic procedures may be undertaken to construct a normal urethra.

Urethral valves and congenital bladder neck obstruction. Occasionally folds of abnormal mucous membrane obstruct the urethra or the urethra may be abnormally narrow at the bladder neck. These conditions can cause serious back pressure on the urinary tract and the obstructions must be relieved by operation or death may ensue from gross hydronephrosis and renal failure.

Trauma. The bladder and the urethra are frequently injured in fractures of the pelvis involving the pubic bones. The bladder may be torn allowing urine to extravasate into the perivesical tissues or peritoneum and the urethra may be partially or totally avulsed from the bladder.

Symptoms. The patient is unable to void and blood may be seen coming from the external meatus.

Treatment. The patient should be instructed to hold his water lest gross extravasation occurs into the surrounding tissues from the damaged area. Immediate operation is indicated to repair any rupture in the bladder surgically and to re-align the urethra over a catheter. *On no account should an attempt be made to catheterize the patient in the ward.* Further operation at a later date may be required to correct any residual urethral stricture.

Infection. *Cystitis* is due to the introduction of pathogenic organisms into the urethra and bladder through the external meatus. The great frequency with which cystitis is seen in women is a reflection on the short-ness of the urethra and the ease with which the female introitus can be contaminated with vaginal secretions and faeces. Recurrent urinary infections in women may be avoided by scrupulous attention to local perineal hygiene. The classic symptoms are frequency and burning pain on voiding. There is little systemic disturbance unless the infection ascends to the upper tract (see Pyelonephritis, Chapter 25, p. 248).

Treatment. This is the bacteriological identification of the organisms in the urine and the administration of the appropriate antibacterial therapy. *This should be coupled with a considerably increased fluid intake of at least 3·0 litres in the 24 hours to flush out the bladder and to maintain a dilute urine to inhibit bacterial multiplication. Local perineal hygiene should be encouraged with twice-daily washing with an antiseptic soap.*

Prostatitis is a bacterial infection of the prostate gland and can be acute or chronic. Organisms are introduced by way of the urethra.

Symptoms are extreme frequency and dysuria accompanied by perineal pain.

Treatment is identification of the infecting organisms and appropriate antibiotic treatment. *Chronic prostatitis* runs a prolonged and recurrent course and if the local infection defies eradication prostatectomy may be indicated.

Urethritis. The commonest organism to give rise to acute urethritis is the gonococcus. Infection occurs by venereal contact. A profuse urethral discharge ensues accompanied by severe dysuria. *Treatment* is identification of the organism and appropriate treatment with penicillin in high dosage.

Complications of gonorrhoea. Urethral stricture may supervene many years after an attack of gonorrhoea due to healing of the urethra by fibrosis producing narrowing and obstruction.

Treatment depends on the site of the stricture. The modern trend is to treat these lesions if at all possible by plastic urethral operations (see below). Alternatively the stricture may be dilated by the use of graduated metal or gum elastic sounds until a normal calibre is achieved. This latter treatment usually requires repetition at fairly frequent intervals, and some cases may need weekly attention to maintain adequate urethral patency.

Calculous disease of the bladder. This is almost always associated with some degree of bladder outlet obstruction and urinary infection (see below). In areas where nutrition is poor bladder calculi are still seen in association with vitamin deficiency.

Treatment. Small stones may be crushed, *litholapaxy*, within the bladder by an instrument called a lithotrite passed through the urethra and the stone fragments flushed out with water. Larger stones require direct surgical removal through a suprapubic incision, *cystolithotomy*.

Tumours of the bladder and urethra. *Papilloma of the bladder* is a benign, fronded tumour which grows from the bladder lining. *Carcinoma* of the bladder is a malignant tumour of the bladder epithelium and may be papillary or solid in configuration. Poorly differentiated and invasive tumours are usually solid.

Both tumours cause similar symptoms, the principal one being painless haematuria. There may be some frequency and occasional suprapubic pain.

Treatment. The nature and site of the tumour is determined on cystoscopic examination of the bladder and a biopsy taken. Bimanual examination of the bladder under anaesthesia reveals whether the tumour is invasive or fixed to surrounding structures. Superficial well-differentiated lesions can be controlled by repeated diathermy coagulation through the cystoscope. Regular check cystoscopies are mandatory to control recurrences and treatment continues for the rest of the patient's life.

Poorly differentiated and extravesical lesions are probably best treated with radiotherapy, while a small number of tumours which are too extensive for cystodiathermy but have not yet spread beyond the bladder may be suitable for total cystectomy and urinary diversion (see below). *Survival* is again very much related to the histological grade of the initial tumour. Well-differentiated tumours may allow up to 80 per cent five-year survival, poorly differentiated tumours have a survival as low as 10 per cent.

Benign prostatic adenoma. This is the common cause of lower tract urinary obstruction in the elderly adult male. The glandular tissue of the prostate gland increases with age causing an increasing constriction of the prostatic portion of the posterior urethra.

The symptoms start with *frequency of micturition*, particularly at night (*nocturia*), and difficulty in initiating the act of micturition (*hesitancy*). Later the urinary stream loses force and calibre, and the patient complains that he cannot complete the act sharply; urine continues to dribble for some time. The frequency is due to incomplete emptying of the bladder and the constant stimulation of the voiding reflex by the pool of residual urine in the bladder.

Retention of urine is an inability to empty the bladder by micturition. It is not necessarily due to prostatic enlargement, though that is the commonest cause in the older male. The patient with *chronic retention* gradually develops an enlargement of the bladder which may be palpable in the abdomen above the level of the umbilicus. Back-pressure may be transmitted to the kidneys to produce hydronephrosis and renal failure. The bladder may become over-distended so that it loses the ability to contract, and becomes a passive reservoir from which a little urine constantly seeps down the urethra (*overflow incontinence*). *The stagnation of urine predisposes to urinary infection.*

In *acute retention* no urine is passed at all. There are two varieties:

Simple acute retention which comes out of the blue suddenly with few previous attacks.

Acute-on-chronic retention in which a definite history of past difficulty with micturition can be elicited. The precipitating factor is often alcohol, or a large fluid load.

Treatment of retention. Decompression is required urgently for the relief of pain in acute and acute-on-chronic retention, but not in patients with uncomplicated chronic retention in whom it is important not to pass a catheter (which might introduce infection) before the definitive operation to relieve the obstruction.

Decompression is by urethral catheterization (unless the catheter will not pass, for example in patients with a urethral stricture).

Treatment of benign prostatic hypertrophy is by removing the obstructing portion of the gland, either via the urethra (*transurethral resection*) or by an open operation, *retropubic prostatectomy, transvesical prostatectomy.*

Malignant prostatic obstruction. Carcinomatous change can occur in the epithelium of the prostate gland with enlargement of the gland, obstruction of the urethra and spread to other pelvic organs. The symptoms of malignant prostatic obstruction are similar to those of the benign condition but there may be associated perineal pain.

Treatment. If obstructing symptoms are severe transurethral resection of the growth is indicated. The condition can in the majority of cases be controlled by the administration of oestrogens which have an inhibitory effect on the tumour producing shrinkage and relief of obstruction. This control can be maintained for a considerable number of years with good symptomatic relief, a 65 per cent five-year survival not being uncommon.

OPERATIONS ON THE BLADDER AND URETHRA

Most suprapubic operations in this area are carried out through a small transverse suprapubic or *'Pfannenstiel incision'*. The rectus muscles are not cut but are spread apart to give access to the bladder and the prostate.

Partial cystectomy. The bladder is exposed as above, identified and opened. Any localized tumour may then be excised taking a full thickness of the bladder wall. Tumour that cannot be fully excised with the bladder wall is removed by diathermy coagulation. Some surgeons at this time implant radioactive gold grains or radon seeds into the tumour base to treat any residual tumour that may remain. *The bladder is closed in two layers with catheter drainage and a suprapubic drain to the wound. The catheter remains for 10 days and the suprapubic drain for 4 days. The patient should be encouraged to drink copiously and be mobilized early.*

Total cystectomy. This operation inevitably entails some form of urinary diversion (see below). The bladder is exposed as above. The ureters are divided and diverted. The bladder is then mobilized and excised after ligation of the vessels and transection of the urethra. The wound is closed with suprapubic drainage. *There may be considerable reactionary haemorrhage from the operation and a close watch must be kept on drains and blood pressure. Early mobilization is important.*

Methods of urinary diversion. There are two principal methods.

The uretero-colic anastomosis. Here the ureters are detached from the bladder and transplanted end-to-side into the sigmoid colon. A rectal tube is passed and the wound closed with drainage. *A close watch must be kept on the rectal drainage to ensure that an adequate urinary output is being maintained.* On removal of the rectal tube on about the eighth day the patient voids from the rectum. *Urinary voiding should be encouraged at two-hourly intervals* and faeces are usually passed as a solid motion once a day. This method of diversion is used in the elderly and the palliative type of case.

The ileal or colonic conduit. Here a segment of bowel, either ileum or colon, of about eight inches in length is isolated from the main alimentary stream and the gut reconstituted. One end of the isolated loop is closed whilst the other is brought to the skin surface as a *terminal ileostomy or colostomy*. The ureters are implanted end-to-side into the loop, and urine drains to the surface and is collected in a special type of ileostomy bag fitted with a stopcock at the lower end through which the urine may be emptied. The wound is closed in layers with the drainage. A catheter may be placed in the loop for a few days until healing has occurred. *A considerable ileus is usually seen after these operations and progress is generally slow with intravenous therapy being continued for five to seven days. Nursing care and assistance with the ileostomy apparatus in the early postoperative period is most important.*

Ileo- and colocystoplasty. This is occasionally necessary to increase the capacity of the patient's bladder when it has become contracted by chronic disease such as healed tuberculosis. This may be achieved by further use of the isolated bowel segment. A loop of ileum or colon is isolated and incised completely along the antimesenteric border and opened out to form a flat sheet of tissue. The dome of the bladder is incised transversely and the flattened sheet of gut wall, still on its mesentery, is anastomosed to the bladder thus considerably increasing its capacity. The wound is closed with a catheter in the bladder and a corrugated suprapubic drain is inserted.

Endoscopic surgery—*cystodiathermy*. Bladder tumours if restricted to the mucosal lining may be treated by diathermy fulguration using a fine electrode passed along the operating sheath of a standard viewing cystoscope.

Transurethral prostatic resection. This method of prostatectomy is used for the small benign gland or for the obstructing carcinoma. A small 1·0 cm diameter diathermy cutting loop is passed into the bladder through an instrument known as the *resectoscope*, which is similar to but slightly larger than a cystoscope. With this loop the obstructing portions of the gland are pared away from within the urethra and bleeding points are coagulated. A catheter is inserted and connected to a closed or bag drainage system. *Reactionary haemorrhage with blocking of the catheter may be a problem in the immediate postoperative period but this can be relieved by bladder irrigation (see p. 254).*

Suprapubic prostatectomy. A Pfannenstiel incision is used and the bladder and prostatic capsule exposed in the retropubic space. In the *transvesical operation* the bladder is opened and the obstructing prostatic adenoma enucleated through the bladder neck. A urethral catheter is passed and the bladder is closed with suprapubic drainage to the perivesical area. In the *retropubic* or 'Millin's' operation the prostatic capsule is incised directly and the adenoma removed followed by capsular closure over an indwelling urethral catheter. Suprapubic peri-vesical drainage is also used. *Postoperative reactionary haemorrhage* must be watched for and any tendency of the catheter to block with blood clot is corrected with gentle closed irrigation. *Early mobilization* is the rule and the drain is removed in two days and the catheter at five days.

Urethroplasty. Solitary strictures of the urethra can occasionally be excised and the ends of the divided urethra reanastomosed, Marion's operation. A number of strictures are, however, multiple and require that some form of plastic repair be done to bridge wide areas of scarring. A large number of operations have been designed for this purpose and all depend upon the utilization of suitably designed skin flaps to produce a new urethral tube which is then buried under further skin flaps. The operations are performed in the perineal area and the urine is temporarily diverted by way of a suprapubic drainage tube inserted into the bladder.

THE PENIS: THE SCROTUM AND CONTENTS

The penis. *Phimosis* is a condition where it is impossible to retract the prepuce. It can occur in children and in elderly men. Smegma accumulates beneath the foreskin and can become infected, *balanitis. Treatment* is circumcision.

Paraphimosis occurs when a tight prepuce cannot be returned to the forward position after being fully retracted. If unrelieved, oedema and ulceration of the glans will occur. *Treatment* is circumcision, or if this is not possible a dorsal slit of the constricting band will achieve relief.

Carcinoma of the penis usually involves the skin of the glans and grows as a fungating bleeding tumour. Treatment is partial amputation, or total amputation with inguinal node clearance if the growth is extensive. The prognosis is generally poor.

The scrotum. *The undescended testicle.* In some male children the testis fails to complete its descent into the scrotum from the posterior abdominal wall and may become arrested at any point from the region of the kidney to the external inguinal ring. *The testes should be in the scrotum at birth but a few may be delayed and descend in the first year of life.* If the testis has not come down by the age of six the descent path should be explored and the testis mobilized and put down in the scrotum if the spermatic cord will permit. If not the organ should be removed because of the higher risk of later malignancy in the malpositioned organ. The operation of correction is known as orchidopexy (see below).

A hydrocele is a benign collection of fluid in the tunica vaginalis of the testis which may reach considerable proportions. *Treatment* is either by repeated aspiration or radical excision of the hydrocele sac.

Spermatocele. These are small benign cysts arising from the epididymis of the testis. If causing discomfort they should be excised.

Tumours of the testis. There are two main types and both present as hard testicular swellings.

The seminoma. This is a true carcinoma of the testicular substance.

The teratoma. This is a malignant tumour arising from embryonic tissue persisting in the testis into adult life.

Treatment of both these tumours is by orchidectomy followed by radiotherapy to areas of likely glandular spread, namely the iliac and para-aortic lymph nodes.

Prognosis for the seminoma is very good with a 95 per cent five-year survival. For the teratoma the five-year survival is about 50 per cent.

OPERATIONS ON THE SCROTUM AND CONTENTS

Orchidopexy is performed when the undescended testis lies in the inguinal canal. A small inguinal incision is made and the testis mobilized. A small tunnel is made down into the scrotum and the testis passed down to lie in a normal position. Various methods have been devised for retaining the testis in this position, but the most usual is to retain it in a subcutaneous pocket made in the layers of the scrotal wall.

Orchidectomy. *For malignant disease* this is performed through an inguinal incision and the spermatic cord tied at the internal inguinal ring to prevent dissemination of cancer cells during manipulation of the testis. The testis is then withdrawn from the scrotum and excised.

Radical cure of hydrocele. The scrotum is incised and the hydrocele sac opened. The walls of the sac are excised and oversewn and the scrotum closed after suitable haemostasis.

The postoperative care of all cases of scrotal surgery involves the observation and prevention of haematoma formation. This may be avoided by closely strapping the scrotum to the thigh with 3-inch Elastoplast for the first 48 hours after operation or by wearing a suspensory bandage to produce scrotal elevation.

Scrotal stitches if unabsorbable remain for at least 10 days.

Chapter 55

Orthopaedic Surgery—Part 1

The Use of Splints—Plaster of Paris and Traction

by L. C. L. GONET

Varieties of splint: Thomas' splint, weight-relieving caliper—plaster of Paris: application, general care, bi-valving a plaster—traction: balanced, fixed, skeletal, skin, Hamilton-Russell type—nursing points

SPLINTS

Splints are rigid structures used to support a broken bone, to give protection to part of the body or to correct deformity, whether congenital or acquired. Splints may be for external or for internal use and the reader is referred to the chapter on fractures showing the several methods of internal fixation (see Chapter 56).

Wooden splints are rarely used except when applied to the anterior aspect of the forearm to prevent a young child touching his face after operation, or to restrain a confused or delirious patient or as a first-aid measure.

Metal splints. The Thomas' bed splint remains the most valuable (see below). Others include the cock-up splint for wrist drop and spring-loaded splints for fingers.

Cramer wire is malleable and is sometimes incorporated in a plaster cast.

Aluminium splints are foam-backed long strips which can be cut to the size needed and easily bent to the desired position.

Plastic splints are light in weight and include finger splints, polythene spinal jackets and cervical collars; these splints are also used for knee and other joint deformities as in rheumatoid arthritis.

Inflatable pneumatic splints are in use as first-aid measures.

The Thomas' splint is still in constant use for immobilizing the lower limb in transit. It consists of a metal ring covered with soft padded leather. From the ring two parallel bars extend for varying lengths finally meeting in a 'W' (Fig. 55/1). There are rings of different sizes, and right and left splints for the right and left lower limbs. The ring is not circular as the posterior part is bigger than the anterior.

For the splint to be correctly chosen, the ring when threaded over the limb should fit snugly *in the groin* preferably a finger's breadth away from the skin to avoid pressure. The outer side of the splint is higher up the thigh about the level of the great trochanter, the posterior part being against the ischial tuberosity. The end of the parallel bars of the splint should be about

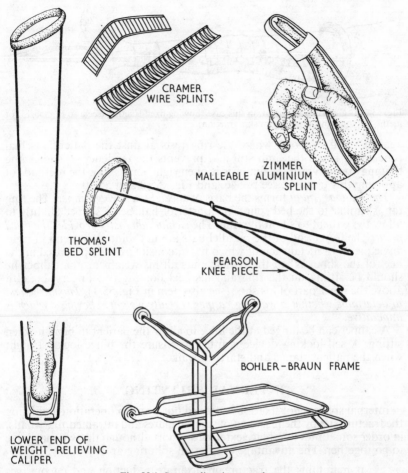

Fig. 55/1 Some splints in general use.

8 inches (20 cm) longer than the distance from groin to heel of the patient. Measurements on the sound leg will ensure the correct size of the ring and length, but some allowance should be made for swelling of the upper thigh in a case of a fractured femur.

Slings made of six-inch (15 cm) domette bandage are laid across the parallel bars and each fixed on the outer side with bull-dog clamps so that when the limb rests in the splint it is supported by these slings (Fig. 55/2). *The tension of the slings* should be such that the limb lies between the bars of the splint—a point which should be noted whenever a patient is moved. The heel should not be included; it should be free. In the elderly it is wise to place gamgee between the slings and the limb to protect the skin. Daily inspection of the sling is important. Loose slings should be tightened (see tension above) and creases removed.

The essential feature of the splinting action with this splint is the application of traction to the leg along the line of the limb. This traction, acting

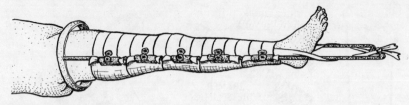

Fig. 55/2　Leg in Thomas' splint, in this case showing fixed traction (see also Fig. 55/13 for method of applying strapping in skin traction).

against the fixed point where the ring rests against the patient's ischial tuberosity, keeps the limb still and prevents the tendency to shortening that may occur when the femur is broken right across. For the methods of applying this traction, see p. 546, and Figs. 55/2 and 55/10.

The Thomas' splint forms the basis of a *weight-relieving caliper*. The ring top is similar to the bed splint, the posterior half being shaped slightly to allow the patient to sit on the ring. The *ischial tuberosity provides the fixed point*. The lower end of the parallel bars are not jointed, but end in right angle pieces of metal each of which fits into a slot already prepared in the heel of the shoe. When the patient puts all his weight on the caliper he should be sitting on the ring and his heel floating two fingers' breadth above the inner part of his shoe (see also item in Fig. 55/1). *This is the test to determine whether a walking caliper is really weight relieving—which is imperative.*

A caliper can be hinged at the knee to allow the patient to bend it when sitting. A self-locking device is fitted to ensure the hinge locks straight when the patient stands and starts to walk.

INTERNAL SPLINTING

Internal splinting or fixation is carried out by open operation and fixing the fracture site by the insertion of screws, plates and intramedullary nails, in order sometimes to replace external support although the two may have to go together. The advantage of internal splinting are:

> It maintains the fracture in accurate reduction and encourages healing.
> It makes it easier for the patient to be nursed, and move or be moved about in bed.
> It allows a patient to exercise his limb independently.

Internal fixation does not shorten the period of immobilization of the fracture, but can allow early weight bearing, as in intramedullary nailing of the femur (see Fig. 56/3).

PLASTER OF PARIS

This is the most frequently used material for external splintage as it can be made to fit the exact shape of the body and varied in thickness for strength. *The nursing staff in modern hospital practice are taking an increasing part in the application of plaster casts.* It is an art which can only be acquired by experience under skilled tuition. *Proprietary bandages* of varying widths are in general use; they are sensitive to moisture and should be stored under dry conditions. After immersion in tepid water, they are applied in slabs and rolls (bandages). A well-applied plaster should fit closely and comfortably, immobilize the joints above and below the cast, be strong and durable but not heavy.

General principles in applying plaster. *The padding* used must be carefully applied as it should fit smoothly and snugly; *a well-fitting stockinette* is first put on to keep the area of the skin smooth, free from wrinkles and to support it; over this a layer of cotton wool, orthopaedic wool or *Orthoband* is applied.

A slab the length of the intended plaster is soaked in tepid water; creases and excess moisture should be removed by smoothing on a flat surface.

A roll of plaster with the end held is then soaked until all bubbles have escaped, surplus water turned out and the roll (or bandage) applied round and round the limb smoothly but not tightly from top to bottom.

When several layers have been applied the plaster should be moulded, using the palms of the hands in firm long strokes.

Before applying the final plaster bandage (or in the case of a slab, the cotton bandage) the stockinette and padding are turned down at each end of the cast and the plaster bandage is carried up to within a quarter of an inch which gives a smooth edge and finish to the cast.

During the setting of the plaster care must be taken to see that there are no finger or thumb dents in it and no ridges, which are common causes of plaster sores.

Before the patient leaves the department his fingers or toes should be washed, dried and examined for discoloration; the plaster should be checked to ensure that no rough edges have been left and that the joints not in plaster are quite free. If there is any doubt that padding is inadequate the cast should be split from top to bottom and lightly bandaged with a crêpe bandage.

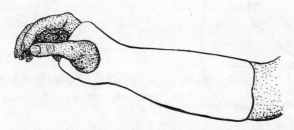

Fig. 55/3 Cast for Colles' fracture. The plaster does not extend beyond the main palmar crease, allowing full movement at the metacarpo-phalangeal joints of the fingers and full movement of the thumb.

Tight plasters lead to interference with the blood supply to the muscles of the limb which may cause fibrosis in the muscles affected with shortening and contracture.

The correct methods of applying plaster casts for certain fractures are well illustrated in Figs. 55/3, 55/4 and 55/5.

General care of plasters. They should all be exposed to the air for drying.

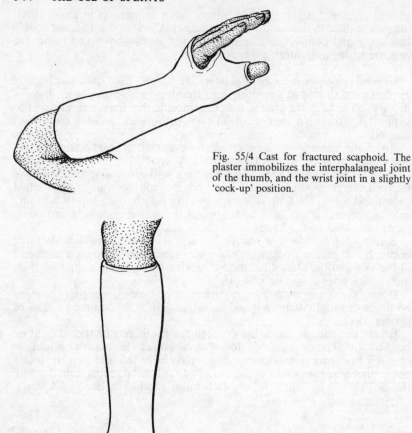

Fig. 55/4 Cast for fractured scaphoid. The plaster immobilizes the interphalangeal joint of the thumb, and the wrist joint in a slightly 'cock-up' position.

Fig. 55/5 A walking plaster extending from the tibial tubercle to the metatarsal heads, showing one type of walking piece—the wooden rocker.

Body temperature dries plasters. It is inadvisable to use artificial heat as a means of drying.

Once the plaster is dry normal behaviour should be resumed as far as possible. Using a limb in plaster will ensure a better functional result when the plaster is removed. If the injury is such that the limb must be rested the patient should be instructed in exercising the limb above and below the cast.

Circulation in the exposed parts should be noted and the patient or relative advised of the importance of returning to hospital should the fingers or toes become painful, swollen or discoloured, if the parts within the cast become painful or should the plaster become soft or cracked. A printed form is given to patients conveying these instructions. In any case the first check should be carried out next day.

Removal of plasters should be as carefully carried out as the application. Fig. 55/6 shows the instruments available. Saws can be dangerous and electric saws (which should not be used by the unskilled, or under general anaesthesia) are frightening, especially to children as they are noisy. A good pair of plaster shears does not need force to be effective; *the inner blade of the shears must be held parallel* to the patient as in Fig. 55/7.

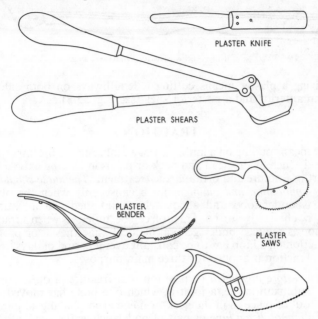

PLASTER KNIFE

PLASTER SHEARS

PLASTER BENDER

PLASTER SAWS

Fig. 55/6 Instruments used in plaster work.

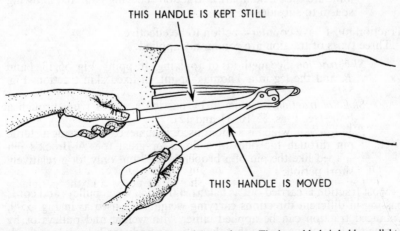

THIS HANDLE IS KEPT STILL

THIS HANDLE IS MOVED

Fig. 55/7 Method of holding shears to cut down a plaster. The inner blade is held parallel to the patient; the outer blade moved carefully along does the cutting.

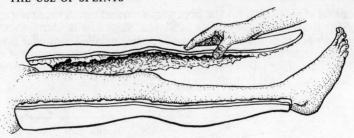

Fig. 55/8 A bi-valved plaster.

Bi-valving a plaster means cutting it lengthways on both sides, thus having an anterior and a posterior shell (see Fig. 55/8).

TRACTION

Traction means pulling on a limb, part of a limb, such as the finger, or part of the body such as the head and neck or pelvis in its long axis; it plays a large part in fracture and orthopaedic treatment. *The nurse should understand its application and maintenance* because only when the object of traction is understood and adequately maintained can a patient 'on traction' be efficiently nursed. Traction can be 'quick' as when a fracture or dislocation is reduced under general or local anaesthesia, or prolonged, when traction on a limb has to be constant over a period of days, weeks or months. Traction is applied for three main purposes:

To restore alignment or position of a fracture, a dislocation or a subluxation, i.e. a joint in which one bone has moved slightly out of place as in the neck or metacarpo-phalangeal joints.

To immobilize a limb or part of body such as the head and neck.

To overcome spasm when muscles that move an irritable joint contract and result in deformity. The inflamed bony surfaces of a joint are then held apart in traction relieving pain and allowing spasm to subside.

Traction must have counter-traction to be effective.

Three types of traction are commonly applied:

Skin traction. See methods of applying strapping, Fig. 55/13 *A* and *B*, and the leg in a Thomas' splint, in fixed skin traction, Fig. 55/2.

Skeletal traction is achieved by passing a pin or wire through a bone (see Figs. 55/10, 11 and 12).

Pulp traction, which is seldom used, is achieved by passing a sterile pin through the pulp of a finger or great toe. A Brock's pin shaped like the pin of a brooch is used but only for a relatively short period.

Most traction is carried out as **balanced traction** when pulleys and cords passing in different directions carrying weights are used as in Fig. 55/9. Balanced traction can be applied either with weight and pulleys or by raising the foot of the bed so that the patient's body tends to slide towards the head end, thus providing counter-traction.

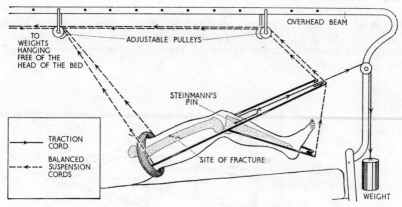

Fig. 55/9 Balanced skeletal traction using a Thomas' splint with Pearson knee piece (Fig. 55/1). Steinmann's pin is passed through the tibia (see Fig. 55/10), a cord from a stirrup running over a pulley on the upright bar carries the weight which extends the thigh. Cords from both ends of the splint, passing over pulleys on the overhead beam, enable it to be raised from the bed and easily manipulated by the patient as he moves about.

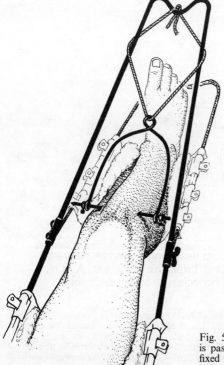

Fig. 55/10 A diagram showing how the pin is passed through the tibia. In this instance fixed traction is employed as compared with balanced skeletal traction in Fig. 55/9.

Less often **fixed traction** is employed when traction is exerted between two points. When a limb is put on skin traction on a Thomas' splint, as in Figs. 55/2 and 10, and simply tied to the lower end of the splint the counter-traction or fixed point is the ring of the Thomas' splint impinging against the ischial tuberosity.

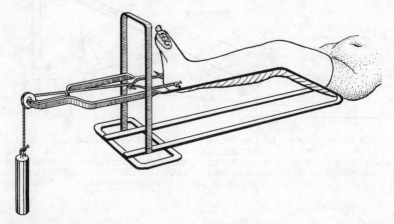

Fig. 55/11 *Skeletal traction* through the calcaneum for unstable fractures of the tibia and fibula (see text, p. 549).

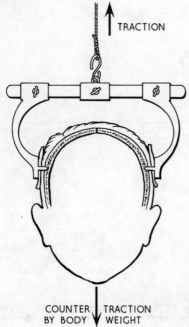

TRACTION

COUNTER TRACTION
BY BODY WEIGHT
(HEAD OF BED RAISED)

Fig. 55/12 *Skull traction.* The anchor pins penetrate only the outer cortex. This method is generally used for reduction of fracture—dislocations of the cervical spine (see text, p. 557).

Skeletal traction consists of a steel pin (usually a Steinmann's) or Kirschner's wire passed transversely through a bone. The upper end of the tibia (see Fig. 55/10) is a favourite site, the pin is introduced two fingers' breadth below and in front of the head of the fibula to avoid injuring the lateral popliteal nerve. A *stirrup* is fitted to the pin and a *cord* is attached which leads in turn *over a pulley to weights* as in Fig. 55/9 or alternatively may be fixed to the end of the splints as in Fig. 55/10.

Other sites for skeletal traction are the calcaneum (see Fig. 55/11), the olecranon and the skull, Fig. 55/12.

Skeletal traction is more efficient than skin traction (see below) provided it is properly maintained; greater pull can be exerted and with weights more traction applied. Side-to-side movement of the pin leads to loosening which may be followed by infection along the pin track and on either side at the entrance and exit wounds. *Daily inspection is essential* and the doctor should be informed of any alteration in the position of the pin. An efficient functioning skeletal traction is usually painless.

Skin traction. While skeletal traction can be applied only by a doctor as it is a surgical procedure, skin traction is more often applied by an experienced member of the nursing staff, and with modern equipment it is a speedy, safe and reliable method.

The limb is first shaved, Tinct. Benzoin Co. is then painted on both sides from thigh to ankle and extension strapping applied from the upper thigh along the outer aspect of the limb to the external malleolus, curved round a wooden spreader (Fig. 55/13a) some six inches from the sole of the foot and up the inner side of the limb to mid-thigh. Areas to be padded are the head of the fibula to protect the lateral popliteal nerve, and the medial and lateral malleoli to give protection to these bony prominences.

The extension strapping stretches sideways, not lengthwise, and is secured by crêpe bandages from just above the malleoli to mid-thigh. One or two holes in the spreader enables a cord to be fixed either to the end of a splint if *fixed traction* is required or allowed to hang over a pulley with weights in *sliding traction. The nurse must inspect the apparatus daily* to make sure that no slipping has occurred and the skin has not been abraded. Particular care must be taken in old people as the skin tends to be friable, thus skin traction is only suitable for short periods and provided not too much weight is applied.

Once traction, in whatever form, is applied it is the duty of the nursing staff to see that it is maintained. The pull must not be altered during routine nursing, such as bed bathing, attention to pressure points and toilet. Children are very persuasive and may often have their weights taken off by another child in the ward or by a visitor and especially when the child is in a room by himself. Interference with continuous traction may lead to delayed union of the fracture, to shortening and deformity of the limb.

A fractured neck of femur in the elderly provides a good case for the application of *Hamilton-Russell traction*. Skin traction is used for the longitudinal pull, and by having a sling under the knee and four pulleys an upward pull is also obtained, the final traction force being about double the weight hanging from the last pulley (Fig. 55/14).

Nursing points. *In nursing patients wearing splints, plaster or extensions* the general attitude of the patient should be watched and discomfort relieved whenever possible.

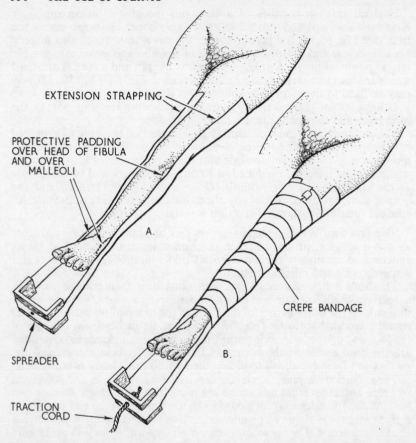

EXTENSION STRAPPING

PROTECTIVE PADDING
OVER HEAD OF FIBULA
AND OVER
MALLEOLI

A.

CREPE BANDAGE

SPREADER

B.

TRACTION
CORD

Fig. 55/13 Application of strapping to leg for skin traction (see (*a*) for first application and then (*b*)).

A small pillow under an arm or leg, in the nape of the neck or the small of the back may help.

Cradles should be employed whenever possible so that the weight of bedclothes does not rest on a splinted limb.

The *extremities should be watched* for indication of interference with the circulation to a limb. This may be overcome by elevating the limb. The toes and fingers should be warm, not blue and cold after a splint or plaster has been applied. When a patient complains of pain, this should be reported and investigated and not treated by analgesics. The splint or plaster may require adjusting or releasing.

It is important to avoid footdrop; the heel should not rest on a splint too long nor the foot hang over so that the tendon of Achilles is made sore.

The nurse should be very familiar with the effect the surgeon desires to obtain by any appliance the patient is wearing and see that this is not interfered with, the slightest alteration of the position of a splint or any movement of an extension being reported without delay.

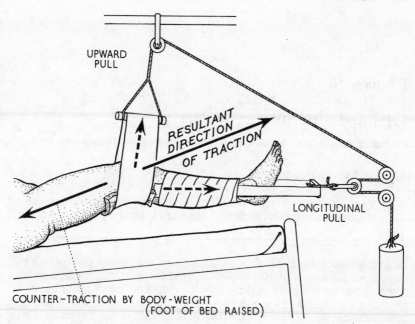

Fig. 55/14 Hamilton-Russell type traction (see text, p. 549).

Chapter 56

Orthopaedic Surgery—Part 2
Common Injuries to Bone and Joint—Outline of Treatment

by L. C. L. GONET

The incidence of road accidents—types of fracture—principles of treatment—selected fractures—injuries to joints

Statistics issued by H.M. Government show that every year over 6,000 people are killed and about 500,000 injured on the roads of Great Britain alone. The vast majority of these have fractures of one or more bones, so that at a glance one can see the enormous numbers of fractures and soft tissue trauma which have to be expertly dealt with in our hospitals. To be added to this are fractures caused in the home, the schools and playgrounds and the growing numbers of factory or industrial injuries. In some countries where hospitals are relatively few and far between, two doctors accompany the ambulance to the scene of the accident, and while one ensures that the patient has an efficient airway the other puts up a saline or blood drip and by means of electric leads (E.C.G.) monitors the rhythm and heart beat. In Great Britain the ambulance staff are highly trained and after giving any necessary first aid, transport the patient to the nearest accident and emergency centre.

A **major accident and emergency unit** is one which is staffed and equipped to deal immediately with major injuries and other emergency cases at any hour of the day or night. The major units are designed to provide service for a population of 150,000 or more, though there are smaller units which serve a correspondingly smaller community. Ideally, the staffing of a major unit consists of three teams of medical personnel each with a consultant surgeon, medical officers of intermediate and junior grade, and a similar set-up of nursing personnel so that an eight-hour shift can be undertaken by each team. In addition there must be adequate numbers of radiographers, pathology technicians, physiotherapists and clerical staff.

Fracture and orthopaedic work is essentially team work and the best results come from a team that is conscientious, devoted and above all interested.

TYPES OF FRACTURE

A *fracture* is a break in the continuity of a bone. One is often asked by an anxious patient if it is a fracture or a break. Both words mean the same thing. Fractures are usually caused by injury, either deliberately as when a surgeon divides or breaks a bone to correct deformity, or accidentally. The violence may be: direct, indirect, or by muscle action.

A *direct blow* on a limb, or a motor car running over a person's legs causes fractures by *direct violence*. A twist injury may result in a fracture usually seen in ski-ing accidents, or an elderly lady may catch her foot and fracture the neck of her femur. These are examples of fractures by *indirect violence*.

Examples of fractures which occur by muscle action are some transverse fractures of the patellae due to the pull of the quadriceps muscle during the act of rising from a squatting position. More common examples are *stress fractures* such as fractures of the ribs in the debilitated due to over-acting intercostal muscles and a large variety of *athletes' fractures* due to prolonged muscle action as in fractures of the fibula in cross-country runners.

Pathological fractures are due to disease of the bone such as carcinoma,

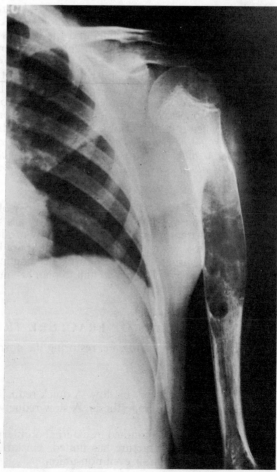

Fig. 56/1 Bone cyst in humerus which led to a pathological fracture.

Paget's disease, bone cysts; softening of the bone as in rickets, osteoporosis and osteomalacia predisposes to fractures (see Fig. 56/1). A congenital condition known as *fragilitas ossium* causes multiple bone fractures during the early years of the patient. A characteristic diagnostic feature of the condition is that the patient has blue sclerae.

There are two main *clinical types of fractures: simple and compound.* A simple fracture is one where there is no break in the skin.

A *compound fracture* is when there is loss of continuity of the skin either by a puncture wound, cut or laceration. These may occur from without but may also occur from within; because of the violence of a fracture, a piece of bone penetrates the skin. A compound fracture is more dangerous than a simple fracture because of the risk of bone infection.

Treatment is wound toilet and débridement or cutting away dirty skin edges and tissue and rapid closure of the wound, performed at the earliest opportunity so as to convert a compound fracture into a simple one. Bad handling of a simple fracture may cause it to become compound.

Varieties of fractures as seen on an X-ray film are listed as *transverse, oblique, spiral* depending on the direction of the fractures and *comminuted* when there are several fragments and the bone is splintered. Naturally combinations of all these occur. In children incomplete fractures of the long bone may occur and these are called *greenstick fractures.* If two portions of a broken bone are pushed into one another the fracture is said to be *impacted.* In the skull a *depressed fracture* is one where due to a direct blow a piece of bone is indented towards the brain; *fissured fractures* are the commonest, but occasionally a *stellate* or star-shaped fracture may occur when a flat blunt object strikes the skull.

Bone must not be regarded as the dead inanimate object seen in the classroom skeleton, but a living tissue continually responding to stress and strain, renewing its blood cells, providing marrow and growing up to the end of puberty.

Symptoms and signs of a fracture. Pain, loss of power, swelling and deformity are the general features. In long bones shortening of the limb may be seen. Attempts to move the limb may produce a grating sound at the fracture site known as crepitus, but should not be used as a method of diagnosis. The surgeon usually confirms his diagnosis by taking an X-ray in two or more views. These help him to plan his method of reduction and subsequent management.

PRINCIPLES OF FRACTURE TREATMENT

Reduction, or setting, i.e. restoring the normal position.
Immobilization.
Rehabilitation.

Reduction may be quick or slow. A quick reduction is obtained by pull under general or local anaesthesia. A slow reduction is obtained by prolonged traction.

Immobilization is maintained by external or internal splintage, and must be kept up until the fracture has united. Unstable immobilization may result in delayed union or even non-union.

Rehabilitation means to try to restore the patient's limb to its former normal function, but it is important also to rehabilitate the patient as a whole, both physically and mentally. Rehabilitation starts from the moment of reduction and the patient is encouraged to move the fingers or toes or the limb as a whole, within the limits of the method used for immobilization. Team work is required. The surgeon is aided by the nurses, physiotherapist, occupational therapist and later by the social welfare worker in order to safeguard the patient's job and ensure a return to adequate housing conditions and home help. At all times the patient must be encouraged to do things for himself, and not to consider himself an invalid as all too often broken bones lead people to think. (See also Chapter 68.)

Healing of fractures. When a fracture occurs blood is poured out around the fracture site. Soon the blood clots and a haematoma is formed, which gets invaded by blood vessels bringing cells which take away dead tissue and replace it with new material including calcium, forming what is called *callus*. At first this callus is soft and easily broken but if immobilization is firm *the callus hardens into hard callus* binding the two fragments of bone together and allowing for the formation of canals and spaces which contain bone marrow. Undue movement of the bones at the fracture site in the early stages of soft-callus formation is liable to delay union.

Complications of fractures and of fracture treatment

Shock may be due to pain or a combination of pain and loss of blood, for it is known that a pint of blood or more may be lost into the tissues in fractures of the femur. Even the slightest crack in a bone causes intense local pain, but is relieved by analgesic drugs or the injection of morphine. The haematoma may give rise to a mild fever during the stage of absorption of tissue.

Infection of bone may be due to organisms introduced from without as in compound fractures, or by germs already circulating in the patient's bloodstream. In fact this may be the cause of most cases of osteomyelitis where a minute crack in a bone forms a localized haematoma and provides a breeding ground for circulating organisms, especially *Staphylococcus aureus*.

Injury to nerves and blood vessels may occur at the time of injury or during transit or during manipulation and reduction of the fracture. Interference with the blood supply from the swelling of the limb within a plaster cast leads to a condition, *Volkmann's ischaemic contracture*, in which the blood supply to the muscles is cut off and the muscles degenerate into fibrous tissue causing contractures.

Late complications of healed fractures are wasting of muscles, stiffness of joints above and below the fracture site and osteoporosis of bone. This loss of calcium from the bones may result in the formation of kidney stones, especially if the patient has been immobilized for a prolonged period in bed.

The following are a few of the commoner fractures and their treatment. The principles of management apply similarly to all fractures in whichever bone they occur.

FRACTURES OF THE SPINE

The spine consists of several components of which the body of a vertebra is the biggest part. When we speak of a fractured spine, we usually mean a fracture of the vertebral body or bodies. The spine may be fractured by direct violence in flexion. This occurs in road accident injuries when the body is thrown forward forcibly into a bent position, or in coal-miners working in low shafts in a bent position, being pushed further into a stooping position by perhaps a fall of coal on their shoulders. Fracture of the body of a vertebra is usually called a wedge compression fracture (see Fig. 56/2) and may proceed further to a fracture dislocation of the vertebra if the ligaments are ruptured. In the latter case the cord may be damaged. *Fracture dislocations* are commonest in the cervical and lumbar vertebrae.

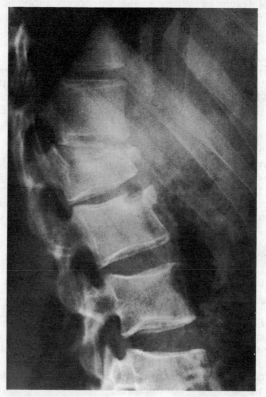

Fig. 56/2 Wedge compression fracture of the 1st lumbar vertebra with angulation and avulsion of a corner of the 2nd lumbar vertebra.

Compression fractures are often found in cases of osteoporosis of the spine and secondary carcinoma. These are examples of pathological fractures as the degree of violence is often minimal.

Signs and symptoms. As in all fractures there is pain, loss of power and possibly a deformity of the spine at the level of injury, especially with a fracture dislocation. Shock is common. Paraplegia means paralysis from the waist down; quadriplegia (or tetraplegia) means paralysis of all four limbs. Even if the spinal cord has not been actively damaged or crushed, it may be in a state of spinal concussion. There is total paralysis below the level of the injury together with loss of sensation. The sphincters may also be affected, leading to incontinence of urine and faeces and retention of urine in other cases. Recovery from spinal concussion may be from a few minutes to as much as 24 hours. In cases of injury to the spinal cord there is no recovery if the cord is completely transected or divided, but if there is a partial crush, then recovery is possible months and even years afterwards.

Treatment. Most *wedge compression fractures* are stable as ascertained by clinical and radiological examination and are treated by simple bed rest on fracture boards, with analgesics for the first few days until the initial pain has diminished, followed by graduated active back exercises. The period of recumbency is from one to three weeks, depending on the degree of wedge compression and pain.

For more severe injuries a plaster jacket is applied in extension of the spine. *In fracture dislocations of the cervical spine*, head traction (see p. 548, Fig. 55/12) is applied to reduce the dislocation. The skull is pierced by ice-tong-like calipers from which a cord passes over a pulley to which weights can be applied. X-ray examination at intervals shows when reduction has been achieved. *Later the neck may be immobilized in a plaster collar*, the most dependable being the Minerva jacket which extends down to the symphysis pubis.

Open operation may have to be carried out to reduce a severe fracture-dislocation at any level of the spine, especially if there is any hope of saving further damage to the spinal cord. Stabilization is then achieved by internal fixation by plates or screws or by spinal fusion. See Medical Care of the Paralysed Patient, p. 269, and read also Nursing the Paralysed Patient, p. 133.

FRACTURES OF THE PELVIS

These are usually caused by a crush injury resulting in a fracture dislocation of the acetabulum and head of the femur, a splitting open of the symphysis and a subluxation of the sacro-iliac joint, or in milder cases simple fractures of pubic and ischial rami of the pelvis. The severer degrees may cause partial or complete rupture of the urethra and bladder neck. In the usual fractures of the pubic and ischial rami, simple bed rest on fracture boards until the painful stage has passed is instituted, followed by graduated exercises and walking rehabilitation.

In the severer cases movement of the pelvis by injudicious handling may further damage the bladder or urethra. The patient must not be allowed to pass urine; a catheter is passed and the quantity measured. Blood may escape and if the catheter cannot be passed by the surgeon then a partial or complete rupture has occurred and this will necessitate an open operation, and suprapubic drainage. Antibiotic cover is started early. Wide separation of the symphysis pubis may be reduced under general anaesthesia by turning the patient on the side whilst fracture dislocations of the hip may require an open operation should closed manipulation fail. Prolonged skeletal traction may also be employed. Avascular necrosis of the head of the femur must be watched for and too early weight bearing avoided.

Fractures of the neck of the femur. This fracture deserves a special note for the frequency with which the nurse will be called upon to care for these usually elderly patients in the wards of most general hospitals.

The older one gets the poorer the blood supply to the head of the femur. A sudden twist or catching a foot on a mat may result in a fracture of the neck of the femur. In general the fracture occurs through the neck (subcapital) or through the base of the neck (basal or pertrochanteric). The subcapital type has a poor prognosis as regards healing of the fracture, because of the poorer blood supply than the basal type which generally has a good healing prognosis.

Treatment. For *subcapital fractures*, the usual practice is a reduction under general anaesthesia and fixation of the fragments by a Smith-Petersen type of pin or nail if the reduction is good and the patient reasonably young. In *older patients* or if it would appear that reduction would not be accurate and therefore the chances of union very slight, *an Austin Moore* (see Fig. 56/14, p. 565) *or Thompson prosthesis is employed.* This allows the patient to get up and bear weight early, thus making nursing easier; early ambulation also prevents hypostatic pneumonia. *Intertrochanteric fracture of the neck of the femur* is best treated by pin and plate fixation. For general rehabilitation see Chapter 68, p. 710.

Fractures of the shaft of the femur occur mainly in young male adults from motor-cycle accidents. Fractures may be transverse, oblique and comminuted. Pain, loss of power, deformity and shock are the usual clinical features. The loss of two pints of blood at the fracture site is not uncommon. *Skeletal traction on a Thomas' splint* (see Chapter 55, Fig. 55/9) is generally accepted as the standard treatment, but if the fracture is transverse and not too oblique or comminuted, open operation and introduction of a Kuntscher nail (see Fig. 56/3) is carried out at the first opportunity. This allows early ambulation as against 10 to 12 weeks on traction. In children under 5 years, the gallows traction method is employed, both legs being put in skin extension strapping and the limbs suspended by cords and pulleys just sufficient to keep the buttocks off the bed, as well as maintaining a pull at all times during general nursing. Four to six weeks traction is usually long enough.

Fractures of the tibia and fibula. These occur in the mid-shaft, in young adults, due to road accidents, and games such as football or rugby; ski-ing is a common cause. The fracture may be simple or compound; all varieties (see p. 552) may occur.

Treatment. Simple fractures which are stable are usually treated by manipulation under general anaesthesia and immobilized in a full-length plaster cast from mid-thigh to toes. Early weight bearing is allowed if the fracture is transverse. For very unstable and comminuted fractures skeletal traction through the calcaneum (see Fig. 55/11) is carried out until stability is ensured. Fractures difficult to get into correct alignment are best treated by open reduction and plate fixation or by the introduction of an intra-medullary nail.

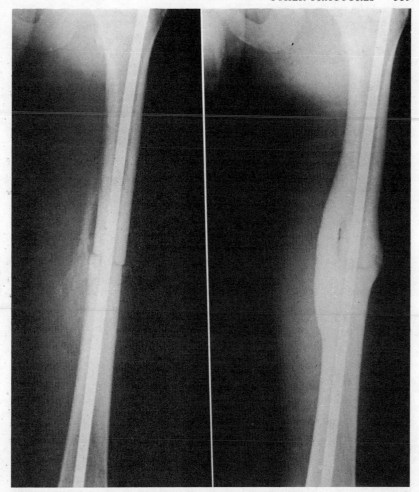

Fig. 56/3 Kuntscher nail fixation for fractured femoral shaft, and one year later, showing extensive callus formation.

OTHER FRACTURES

Colles' fracture. This is a fracture of the lower end of the radius mainly and the ulnar styloid process, with backward rotation of the lower fragment producing the typical dinner-fork deformity of the wrist, which enables one to diagnose a Colles' fracture, especially in an elderly lady who has fallen on the outstretched hand (see Fig. 56/4). Snow and ice produce large numbers of these injuries. *The treatment is to support the injured wrist bandaged to a wooden splint and when in hospital prepare for a quick reduction* under general anaesthesia and immobilization in a padded plaster cast or a plaster back slab. Should any swelling occur, splitting the padded plaster may be needed. Should the patient have eaten within

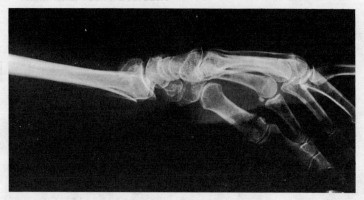

Fig. 56/4 Typical Colles' fracture showing a dinner-fork deformity.

four hours of the accident, reduction under general anaesthesia must be delayed or can be carried out under local infiltration anaesthesia. The plaster cast is usually kept on for four weeks.

Fractured ribs usually occur by falling against a solid object. In road traffic accidents the patient has fallen against the door of the car. Stress fractures of ribs occur in the debilitated during the period of deep breathing as in pneumonia and in pathological conditions already mentioned. *Complications of a fractured rib* include surgical emphysema or pneumothorax or even a haemothorax should the pleura and lung be punctured. *Multiple fractures* may produce paradoxical respiration, if the depressed bones are not elevated. Strapping of the ribs has largely been discarded in simple fractures. Deep breathing is encouraged from the start and in multiple fractures helped by local anaesthetic infiltration into the fracture sites. In the rare cases in which strapping has to be employed, it should be applied in expiration, with each strip overlapping the midline back and front.

Pott's fracture of the ankle is a fracture dislocation of the ankle-joint where a severe twist causes fractures of the medial and lateral malleoli with a dislocation of the talus backwards under the tibia. There is considerable bruising and swelling and tearing of ligaments and a lateral shift of the talus as well. Treatment is by closed reduction under general anaesthesia, and immobilization with a plaster back slab at first to allow for swelling and later in a complete plaster with the foot at right angles. A walking piece may be added later, but immobilization should be approximately eight weeks. As in most fractures, check X-rays are taken at intervals and if the position deteriorates or reduction is not satisfactory an open reduction with or without internal fixation may have to be carried out (see Figs. 56/5 and 56/6).

Supracondylar fractures of the humerus are common in children falling out of trees, and may produce severe displacement and subsequent disability and deformity. Considerable swelling may occur and the circulation must be closely watched. Reduction by skilled manipulation under general

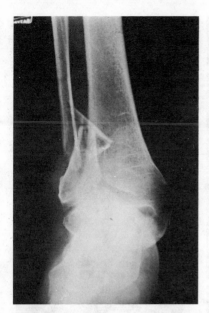

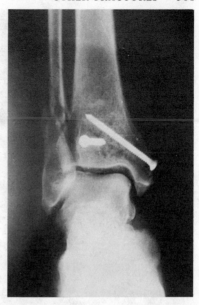

Fig. 56/5 Antero-posterior view of a comminuted Pott's fracture, i.e. a fracture of the lower third of the shaft of the fibula and of the tibial malleolus, with dislocation upwards and backwards of the ankle-joint, before treatment (see also Fig. 56/6).

Fig. 56/6 The same Pott's fracture as Fig. 56/5 after open reduction and screw fixation.

anaesthesia is attempted under X-ray control, and when satisfactory the forearm is flexed and held in a collar and cuff. Flexion should prevent the fragments from slipping. However, the degree of flexion that can be obtained may be limited because the swelling at the elbow may, combined with the flexed position, press on the brachial artery sufficiently to obliterate the radial pulse. Therefore it is important to check by X-ray the position of this fracture for two more days and repeat the manipulation if a gross slip has occurred. Plaster immobilization is not recommended for fear of further interference with the circulation.

Fractures of the shaft of the humerus are usually immobilized as a first-aid measure by bandaging the arm to the chest and supporting the forearm in a sling. Later a U-shaped plaster is applied for four to six weeks. In elderly patients fractures of the *surgical neck of the humerus* are common. The fracture is generally impacted and therefore stable. The patient is given analgesics to control the pain for the first few days and is encouraged actively to abduct the arm from the beginning to prevent stiffness of the shoulder-joint.

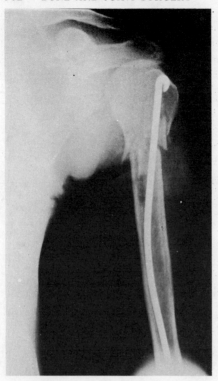

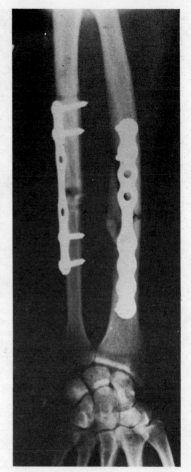

Fig. 56/7 The Rush intramedullary nail inserted for fractured humerus. It can be left in indefinitely, but if and when it should extrude, a small incision is made and the nail is taken out.

Fig. 56/8 An antero-posterior view of plate and screw fixation for mid-shaft of radius and ulna, showing correct alignment of both bones.

Fig. 56/8

Fig. 56/9 Plate fixation for fractured shaft of tibia. Note also fracture at upper end of tibia and fractured fibula.

Fig. 56/10 Capener nail plate for intertrochanteric fracture of neck of femur.

Fig. 56/11 Posterior fracture—dislocation of hip.

Fig. 56/12 Same case of fracture—dislocation of hip reduced by open reduction. Fracture secured by screw and staple.

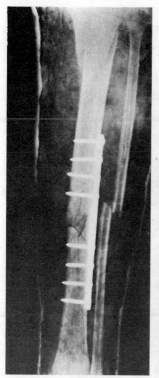

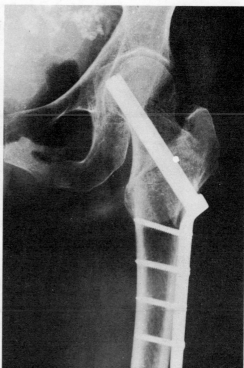

Fig. 56/9

Fig. 56/10

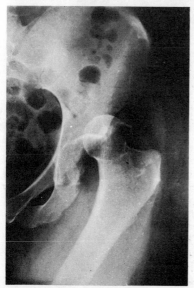

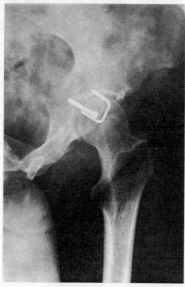

Fig. 56/11

Fig. 56/12

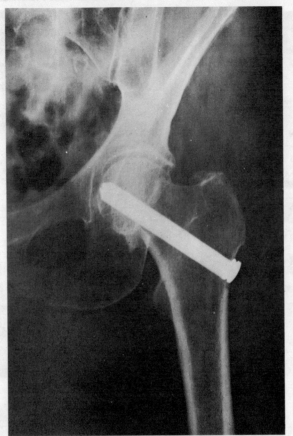

Fig. 56/13 Watson-Jones pin for subcapital fracture of neck of femur.

Fig. 56/14 Austin Moore prosthesis for bilateral fractured neck of femur.

Fig. 56/15 Moore's pins for slipped femoral epiphysis.

Recent advances in fracture treatment include the use of the *image intensifier*. This allows the surgeon to see what he is doing on a television screen, thus enabling him to position his guide wires more accurately and avoids time spent in developing the films. Smith-Petersen pinning operations are best carried out by this method. *Internal fixation* (see Figs. 56/7 to 56/15) is performed by using material which is relatively inert when implanted into human bone. These include stainless steel, titanium, vitallium, cobalt and molybdenum. They must all match up to a high standard of British specification. The theatre sister must make sure that all implants are of the same material. For instance, stainless steel plates must have steel screws, etc., otherwise a reaction may cause loosening of the plate and screws. *Acrylic cement* is in use to bond metal implants into bone.

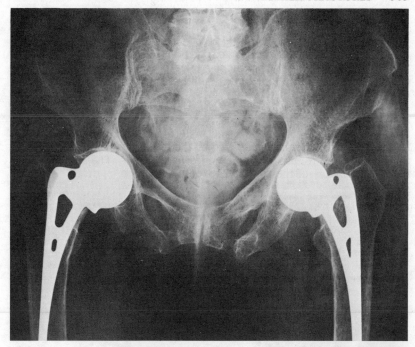

Fig. 56/14

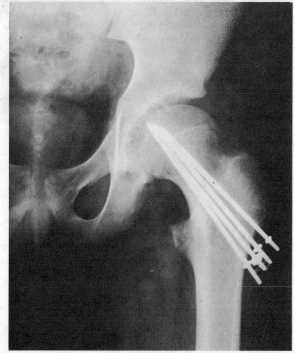

Fig. 56/15

INJURIES TO JOINTS

Dislocation of the joint occurs when by virtue of the force the capsule of the joint is torn, allowing the head of one bone to pass through or allowing the capsule to push away from the socket of the other bone. A subluxation occurs when the head of one bone is still in contact with the socket of the other, but displaced.

Common dislocations are those of the shoulder-joint (Fig. 56/16), usually easily reduced by what is known as Kocher's method, posterior dislocations of the elbow (Fig. 56/17) and dislocations of the finger-joints or knuckles, and if recurrent, stabilized by the Bankart or Putti-Platt operations. Dislocations may be accompanied by fractures. The best known is the *Pott's fracture* of the ankle (see p. 560).

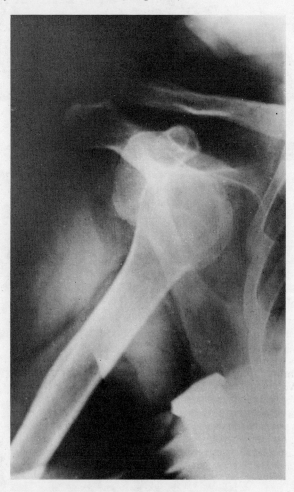

Fig. 56/16 Anterior sub-coracoid dislocation of the shoulder joint.

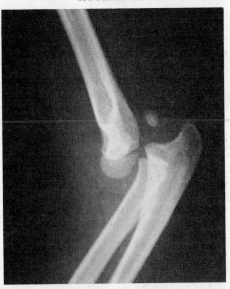

Fig. 56/17 Posterior dislocation of the elbow joint.

Sprains. This is a term given to torn or stretched ligaments around a joint. A tear of the external lateral ligament of the ankle-joint causes pain and swelling. Complete tears of ligaments may require open operation and repair, less severe cases may need plaster immobilization while minor sprains may only require Elastoplast strapping to support the affected part.

INJURIES TO THE KNEE-JOINT

Strains and tears of the medial and lateral ligaments.
Tears of the cruciate ligaments.
Tears of the medial and lateral semilunar cartilages (meniscus).
Fractures of the patella.
Dislocation or lateral subluxation of the patella.
Cysts due to trauma of the lateral and medial cartilages.

These injuries have a special place in the United Kingdom, as a nation of footballers, and on the Continent in skiers. Any one or a combination of them may occur, although in footballers a tear of either one or the other of the menisci most often happens.

The stability of the knee-joint depends primarily on the quadriceps muscles. Wasting of the muscles occurs rapidly when there is any abnormality of the joint; this cannot be fully accounted for by disuse, but must also have a reflex origin. *Pre- and postoperative quadriceps exercises are most important for the success of any operation on the knee-joint.* Strains and partial *tears of the collateral ligaments* are best treated by a course of heat, massage and quadriceps exercises; complete tears are sutured. *Tears of the cruciate ligaments* result in anterior and posterior laxity and often are part of more severe derangements of the knee-joint. In recent years several techniques for the repair of the anterior cruciate ligaments have been available.

Tears of the medial meniscus are the commonest form of injury, especially in footballers. The tear is caused by a twist which results in a split of the cartilage. If this extends the whole length of the cartilage the tear is of the 'bucket handle' type.

Signs and symptoms. Pain on the medial side of the knee, swelling, and a feeling of 'locking' of the knee when the torn portion of the cartilage becomes nipped between the femur and the tibia occur. Unlocking is often accompanied by a click.

Tears of the external meniscus produce similar signs and symptoms on the outer-side of the knee, but are less common than tears of the medial meniscus.

Treatment. Once a torn meniscus is diagnosed it is best to remove it entirely at the earliest opportunity, to prevent wasting of the quadriceps muscles and the risk of locking at inappropriate moments such as when crossing a road. This operation is known as *meniscectomy.*

Cysts of the lateral menisci are almost ten times commoner than on the medial and occur more frequently in women than in men. A small tear in the lateral meniscus may accumulate fluid and form a sac of its own which gradually pushes its way out through the lateral line of the joint, forming a cyst. The treatment consists in removal of the cyst and meniscus.

Arthroscopy is the technique of viewing the inside of a joint, such as the knee-joint, by an instrument known as an arthroscope. Almost the whole joint can be viewed, photographed, and a biopsy specimen taken for examination. Arthroscopy is very useful in the problem knee and may avoid unnecessary removal of a semilunar cartilage.

Fractures of the patella may occur by direct or indirect violence, or by muscle action. The fracture may be transverse, comminuted or a simple linear crack under the capsule and periosteum. Transverse fractures with separation are best treated by open operation and fixation of the two fragments by wire or a screw, together with repair of the capsule. Comminuted fractures are usually excised and the capsule reconstituted and a plaster cylinder applied for three weeks. Linear fractures may be treated by strapping.

Dislocation of the patella may occur as a result of severe violence, or spontaneous lateral subluxation may occur. Stabilization of a recurrent dislocation of the patella is best achieved by transplanting the insertion of the patellar ligament medially.

Notes on effusions. Injury to a joint produces a synovial reaction, *traumatic synovitis*, with outpouring of fluid, which on aspiration is usually clear straw-coloured and viscid. Injury to a blood vessel inside a joint may result in a *haemarthrosis* when aspiration must be carried out through a wide-bore needle which taps the dark altered blood. Most effusions into the knee-joint are controlled by the application of a Robert Jones' bandage. The correct way to apply this bandage is to use plenty of cotton wool and a domette or crêpe bandage with the patient's leg in as full extension as possible: the first complete layer of cotton wool is wrapped round the knee from mid-thigh to mid-calf and firmly bound with a crêpe bandage six inches wide; a second layer of cotton wool is then applied and again encircled firmly by a six-inch crêpe bandage.

PROLAPSED INTERVERTEBRAL DISC

A prolapsed intervertebral disc, sometimes described as a slipped disc or a protruded intervertebral disc (see also p. 662) may occur as a result of strain or injury and is the commonest cause of low back pain when it happens in the lumbar region. A prolapse may occur in the cervical and dorsal region as well.

The clinical symptoms are usually pain, weakness of the lower limbs or arms, tingling and numbness in the hands or feet, sciatica when roots of the sciatic nerve are pressed upon, and inability to stand erect or walk without a list to one side (sciatic scoliosis). The symptoms may become chronic, the backache coming on from time to time with acute episodes.

Treatment may be conservative or surgical. The former consists of adequate bed rest with a board underneath a thin Dunlopillo mattress or a hair mattress alone to give firm support to the back. The application of a plaster of Paris jacket often relieves acute pain, limits movement and provides support. Skilled manipulation of the spine with or without general anaesthesia can shorten the period of recovery. Additional support to the back is provided by wearing a made-to-measure lumbosacral belt.

Physiotherapy such as heat, traction, and back exercises plays an important part in conservative treatment and is prescribed from the start, and the patient taught to pick up heavy objects in the correct way with knees bent to minimize further back strain.

This conservative management provides an opportunity for natural changes to take place in the lesion, such as to allow local oedema to subside and bring about relief of pressure. Intermittent attacks of pain may occur when a return to one of the forms of rest and management advocated above is again indicated.

Surgical Treatment is undertaken only when adequate conservative measures have not proved effective. Usually a special X-ray called a **myelogram** in which an opaque dye is put into the spinal canal to localize the site of the prolapsed disc is done before operation. A laminectomy, or fenestration, i.e. excision of part of the ligamentum flavum over the appropriate intervertebral space is performed and the entire protruded disc is removed. Recumbency after operation varies from 7 to 21 days, but physiotherapy is employed from the outset.

Chapter 57

Orthopaedic Surgery—Part 3
Examples of Orthopaedic Conditions

by L. C. L. GONET

> *Acquired and congenital deformities: congenital dislocation of hip,
> congenital club foot—postural defects and deformities: scoliosis,
> torticollis, flat foot, claw foot, hallux valgus, hallux rigidus, hammer
> toe, deformities due to rickets—degenerative disease of bone and
> joint—osteomyelitis*

The word orthopaedics is derived from the Greek language, and means
'the bringing up of straight children'; but in addition to the treatment of
congenital and acquired deformities, orthopaedic surgery embraces not
only bone and joint surgery (Chapter 56) but the surgery of the entire
locomotor system including tendons, ligaments and muscles. Orthopaedic
surgery is essentially a team effort. It includes surgeons, nurses, physiotherapists, technicians for measuring, making and fitting appliances,
medical social workers and other experts in training and after-care in
school and factory. Deformity may be congenital, i.e. the child is born
with a deformity, or the condition may be acquired as a result of injury or
disease affecting the locomotor system.

ACQUIRED AND CONGENITAL DEFORMITIES
Acquired deformities
Acquired deformity may be due to injury to the skeleton as in fractures
and dislocations, and injury to soft parts such as interference with the
blood supply to muscle and tendon (Volkmann's ischaemic contracture)
and in contractures following burns. Contracture of the palmar fascia of
the hand is called Dupuytren's contracture. Diseases of bone and joint
include arthritis, tuberculosis, osteomyelitis, tumours of the bone,
primary and secondary growths, osteomalacia and rickets. Conditions of
the central nervous system, e.g. poliomyelitis and spina bifida, may also
result in deformity.

Examples of acquired deformities in growing children include flat foot,
scoliosis and kyphosis.

Congenital deformities
These may be single or multiple and are present at birth. There are

several main factors: heredity, injury or disease of the growing fetus in the uterus, and abnormal pressures in the uterus. Congenital dislocation of the hip, and osteogenesis imperfecta, known also as fragilitas ossium, and diaphyseal aclasia or multiple exostoses are good examples of hereditary bone and joint deformity.

The administration of certain drugs in early pregnancy may result in deformities, similar to those of the thalidomide disaster. If a woman has contact with a case of German measles (rubella) during the first three months of pregnancy her baby may be deformed.

Congenital dislocation of the hip (see Fig. 57/1). This condition occurs in about one in 700 births in Great Britain and is six times more common in girls than in boys.

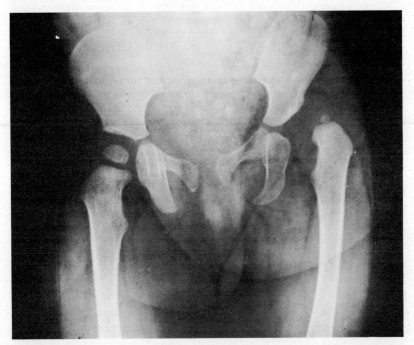

Fig. 57/1 Unilateral congenital dislocation of the hip-joint—note the shallow acetabulum on the left side.

Nurses in general hospital training may never see a child with congenital dislocation of the hip or hips, but all nurses should be aware of this condition for the earliest possible recognition of it, and the earlier treatment is commenced the better will be the result.

In a congenital dislocation the head of the femur lies above a shallow acetabulum and by employing Barlow's test, with which doctor, midwife or nurse should be familiar, the condition can be diagnosed and dealt with from birth—Barlow's sign is demonstrated as follows.

Abduct both hips at right angles with the infant's trunk, placing the fingers over the greater trochanter, and the thumb over the lesser trochanter of the femur. Pressure then applied upwards or downwards will result in a click as the head slips in or out of the acetabulum. Other useful signs are:

Unequal skin creases in unilateral cases.
Shortening of the affected leg.
Palpation of the femoral head on the back of the acetabulum.
Telescopic movement and absence of the femoral pulse on the affected side.

Treatment consists of simply abducting the legs and retaining this position in a splint or plaster of Paris. The frog position in plaster is generally used but splintage must be prolonged for approximately 12 to 18 months, or until the hip has become stable.

When the condition is not noticed until the child begins to stand and walk, which is itself later than average, she will be noticed to have an awkward gait with marked lumbar lordosis and an ungainly limp. Closed reduction is usually impossible and the following surgical measures may have to be undertaken:

Open reduction and excision of any constricting band of limbus.
Osteotomy of the femur to bring the limb into reasonably correct alignment for walking.
Pelvic osteotomy in order to rotate the acetabulum onto the head of the femur.
The shelf operation by which a piece of bone is turned down from the ilium to deepen the acetabulum.

A new type of pelvic osteotomy now brings hope to those untreated or failed cases who have developed osteoarthritis in adult life.

Congenital club foot—talipes equinovarus (see Fig. 57/2). This is the commonest type of talipes, affecting boys oftener than girls. The foot is

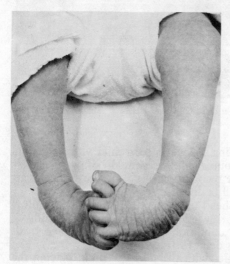

held downwards in *equinus at the ankle, the heel is inverted* or turned inwards and *the forefoot is adducted* or turned towards the other foot.

Treatment. Many mild cases respond to simple manipulation which should start at birth. Stimulation of the peroneal group of muscles by gentle massage may result in the newborn infant actively everting the foot. *More resistant cases* require planned treatment preferably in the hands of

Fig. 57/2 Talipes equinovarus—or congenital, bilateral, club foot.

one surgeon for years until full correction and mobility has been achieved. Gradual correction of the deformity by simple strapping, Denis Browne splints and serial plasters are preferable to forced manipulation under anaesthesia. Soft tissue operations are performed when full correction has not been achieved. Lengthening of the tendo Achilles and various soft tissue corrections help to restore normal gait and mobility.

In later years when the child is about 4 years old bone operations may be undertaken, and even in adult life a wedge osteotomy of the tarsal bones enables the patient to walk on the sole of his foot (plantigrade) instead of on his ankle (talipes). *The after-care of club foot must be continued until the child has grown up, since the tendency to relapse is ever present.*

Postural defects and deformities

Postural defects are variations from the accepted normal posture which can be corrected by the active effort of the patient. It is seldom that one part of the body alone is involved and usually the entire posture is at fault. Examples of the commoner postural defects are *postural scoliosis* as distinct from structural scoliosis where one or more vertebrae are at fault, knock knees and bow legs and valgus ankles. The spinal column and lower limbs support the weight of the body and are therefore subject to postural strains. Some individuals have a pelvis with an abnormal tilt forward and a more pronounced *lumbar lordosis*. Others with a less pelvic tilt have a flatter back. Patients with paralysis of the abdominal muscles as in poliomyelitis have an abnormal lumbar lordosis, and a similar situation occurs in late pregnancy.

Scoliosis of the postural type is usually a generalized lateral curvature of the spine. Bad posture, such as sitting badly at a desk at school, together with diminished muscular tone may result in shortening of ligaments on one side and convert a postural into a **structural scoliosis** (see Fig. 57/3).

Treatment. Improvement in the general state of health and nutrition and training in how to maintain correct posture are first prescribed with back and abdominal muscle exercises together with hanging exercises during the period of growth of the child. Structural scoliosis and postural scoliosis which is deteriorating are treated by a spinal brace, serial plaster jackets, of which the Risser type is most frequently employed, and finally operative surgical measures such as a wedge resection of an affected vertebra.

Torticollis. Congenital wry neck is a birth injury to the sterno-mastoid muscle either by rupture of some of its fibres or interference with the arterial blood supply. A sterno-mastoid 'tumour' soon develops which is tender and pulls the head by spasm over to the affected side, the face turning slightly to the sound side. Later the tumour becomes fibrosed and actively shortens the muscle.

Treatment is mainly by manipulation and correction of the position of the head by sandbags or in plaster of Paris. When a fibrous band can be felt, either a subcutaneous tenotomy or an open operation by division of the fibrous band is performed.

Flatfoot or pes planus. Two main groups are affected, children and young adolescents as the results of a generalized faulty posture, and the adult patient in whom the condition develops as a result of muscular fatigue

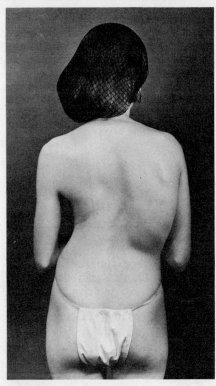

Fig. 57/3 Dorso-lumbar scoliosis of the structural type.

from long hours of standing such as in nurses, policemen and soldiers. The foot is made up of a series of arches; the inner longitudinal and the anterior transverse metatarsal arches are affected (see Figs. 57/5 and 57/6). Flat foot may be painless as in toddlers and in the majority of bare-foot walking

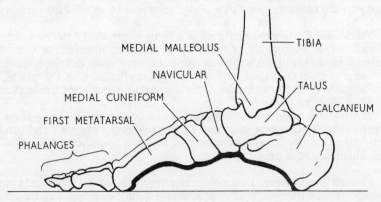

Fig. 57/4 Normal bony arches of the foot showing formation of the internal longitudinal arch.

nations. *Painful flat foot* occurs when there has not been complete collapse of the foot and the ligaments have to take the strain. *Symptoms of acute foot strain* are pain over the instep and inner side of the foot and in the calf. Nipping of a digital nerve between the metatarsal heads is a very painful manifestation of flat foot, known as Morton's metatarsalgia.

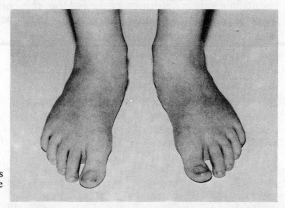

Fig. 57/5 Bilateral pes planus or flat foot—seen from the front.

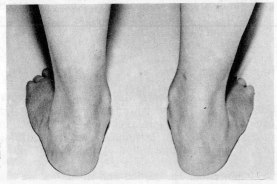

Fig. 57/6 The same patient as in Fig. 57/5, showing inward or valgus list of the ankles—from behind.

Treatment. In the acute stage rest is necessary. The ligaments may be supported by a well-fitting arch support but muscle re-education foot exercises must be instituted early. *In chronic flat foot* massage, manipulation and passive stretching are helpful. Manipulation under an anaesthetic may be necessary to mobilize stiffened joints. Patients with shortened gastrocnemius muscles, peroneal muscle spasm, fractures of the calcaneum may all result in flat foot. Morton's metatarsalgia mentioned above is treated by excision of the neuroma on the digital nerve. Plastic heel seats (Helfet) would be effective for Fig. 57/6.

Claw foot or pes cavus, also known as high arched foot, is an exaggeration of the arch of the foot. The condition may be congenital or paralytic as in poliomyelitis. *Treatment* in the early stages consists of muscle re-education, shoes without heels and later surgical shoes with cork insoles. Surgical treatment includes soft tissue division, arthrodesis of the toe joints and tendon transfers, wedge resection of the bones and a triple arthrodesis of the subtaloid and mid-tarsal joints.

Hallux valgus is a deviation of the great toe outward. Friction of the shoe over the inner part of the head of the first metatarsal causes an exostosis and a bursa, the whole being known as a *bunion* (see Fig. 57/7). Hallux valgus may be due to an out-growing first metatarsal in children, known as metatarsus primus varus. The wearing of unsuitable shoes at adolescence results in a valgus deformity of the big toe; this condition is treated by an osteotomy of the first metatarsal to allow the bone to grow straight.

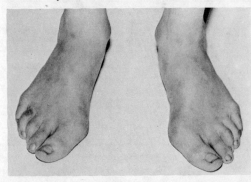

Fig. 57/7 Bilateral hallux valgus.

In adults treatment is directed by prescribing suitable footwear, toning up the intrinsic muscles of the foot, care of the bunion to prevent sepsis and finally operative treatment. Keller's operation, which consists of excision of the base of the first phalanx of the great toe, removal of the exostosis and bunion and careful repair of the capsule, is routine procedure. The bandage should not be disturbed for 10 days when the patient, on removal of the sutures, may be allowed to bear weight on the ball of the foot in proper shoes.

Hallux rigidus occurs when there is restriction of dorsiflexion of the great toe. It interferes with normal walking and constant injury leads to osteoarthritis of the joint increasing its stiffness. Pain results. Deposits of uric acid crystals in the joint lead to the same signs and symptoms and are a frequent manifestation of gout (see p. 309).

Hammer toe. The second and third toes are generally affected in association with hallux valgus or pes cavus. The proximal phalanx is dorsiflexed, the middle phalanx plantar flexed and the long extensor tendon contracted. *Treatment* consists of straightening the toe by a spike arthrodesis and tenotomy of the extensor tendon if this is tight.

Deformities due to rickets. Rickets is due to a deficiency of vitamin D, principally occurring in infancy and childhood, characterized by disturbance of normal ossification (see Fig. 57/8 *a* and *b*). Owing to softening of the bones, deformities arise particularly in the weight-bearing bones (see Figs. 57/9 and 57/10).

DEGENERATIVE AND PROLIFERATIVE DISEASE OF BONE AND JOINT

Osteoarthritis, also known as degenerative arthritis or hypertrophic arthritis, is essentially a disease affecting joints in the middle and older age group.

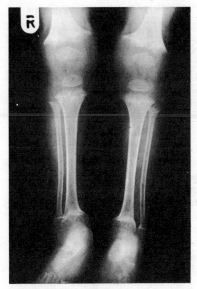
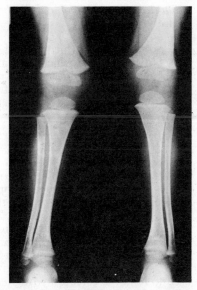

Fig. 57/8 (a) X-ray showing changes in bones of lower limbs in rickets. Note the splayed-out and widened epiphyseal plate and softened bones. (b) Six months later after vitamin D therapy. A complete contrast; note the compact epiphyseal plates and bone density.

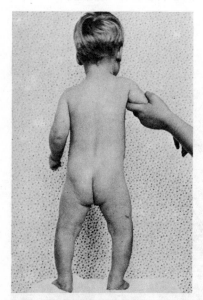
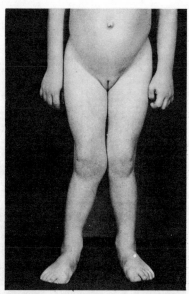

Fig. 57/9 Bilateral genu varum or bow legs.

Fig. 57/10 Bilateral genu valgum or knock knee.

Surgical treatment of osteoarthritis. There are three main forms of operative procedures:

> *Arthrodesis*—which aims at a fixed painless joint.
> *Arthroplasty*—which aims at a movable joint.
> *Osteotomy*—which aims at re-aligning bone in relation to the joint and also helps to bring a fresh blood supply so that the degenerative process may even be reversed.

In the knee-joint a *compression arthrodesis* in the manner of Charnley was most frequent. In the hip-joint an *arthroplasty* usually consists of replacing the acetabulum and the head and neck by a prosthesis which is inserted separately and fixed with cement in the case of the McKee-Farrar (Fig. 57/11) and the Charnley type of total hip replacement (Fig. 57/12), but in the Ring arthroplasty (Fig. 57/13) the acetabulum component is fixed into the pelvis by a long screw.

Replacement by an Austin Moore or Thompson prosthesis is still carried out (see Internal Splinting, p. 565, Fig. 56/14).

High femoral osteotomy is much favoured in Great Britain; McMurray, a Liverpool surgeon, first popularized this procedure. Internal fixation is used to hold the osteotomy fragments together and in recent years compression fixation (see Fig. 57/14) aids early union and allows earlier weight bearing, a considerable advance in nursing care and rehabilitation.

The nursing and after-care is one of team work. The patient should be trained to understand and practise what is expected of him *before* the operation. He sits out of bed on the third day, partially bears weight on the

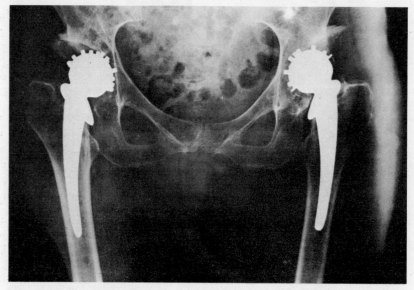

Fig. 57/11 Bilateral McKee-Farrar arthroplasty for osteo-arthritis of the hips.

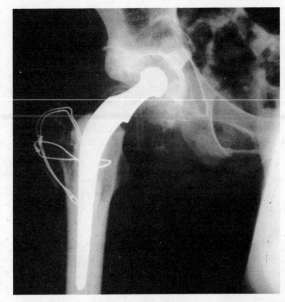

Fig. 57/12 Charnley total hip replacement.

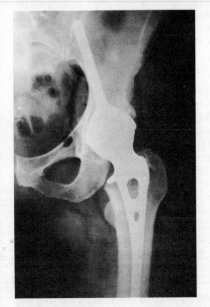

Fig. 57/13 Ring arthroplasty for osteo-arthritis of left hip.

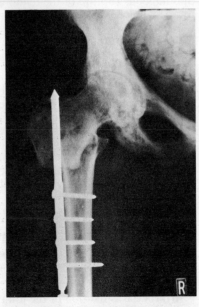

Fig. 57/14 High femoral osteotomy with Gonet's compression-plate fixation.

fifth day and rapidly progresses to full weight-bearing. Such early ambulation diminishes the risk of deep vein thrombosis in the calves and pulmonary embolism. Experimental work is still going on to reline worn-out articular cartilage, as is seen in osteoarthritis, by fresh healthy joint cartilage.

Rheumatoid or proliferative arthritis is a manifestation of a generalized disease (see Chapter 30).

Surgery is playing an increasing part in the treatment of *rheumatoid arthritis*, not only in the correction of deformity but in arresting the progress of the disease itself. Very close co-operation between surgeon and physician is essential. Minor procedures such as a release of a tendon sheath constriction may be of enormous benefit to the comfort of the patient. Major surgical procedures are synovectomy of joints and tendon sheaths, tendon repair, arthroplasty and arthrodesis.

Synovectomy. Removal of the entire synovial membrane of the knee-joint is extremely valuable. In long-standing cases the synovial membrane is thick like a pile carpet, but the best results occur when the operation is done during the synovial phase of the disease and when the X-ray appearances of the joint are nearly normal. However, even in late stages good results can be obtained. The metacarpo-phalangeal joints and the interphalangeal joints are also being subjected to synovectomy with good results, thus reducing the amount of destruction and future deformity of the hands and fingers. Proliferation of the tendon sheaths can cause considerable swelling and pain, particularly on the dorsum of the hand. Spontaneous rupture of the tendons may occur. Careful dissection of the hypertrophied tissue must be undertaken to avoid damage to the already weakened tendons. Because of the poor quality of the ruptured ends, an end-to-end suture is not often practicable and tendon transplant may be necessary.

Arthroplasty. With the introduction of the total hip-replacement procedures using high-density acrylic cement to bond the two sections into the bone, arthroplasty has become much more successful in rheumatoid joints than hitherto. Knee-joints may be made movable joints by types of hinged knee prostheses, bonded into bone by the high-density cement, such as the Shiers, McKee, Macintosh and other prostheses. Arthroplasty of the elbow is becoming increasingly successful. The knuckles and finger-joints can be replaced by highly successful malleable rubber joints. Severe clawing of the toes causing pain can be relieved by Fowler's operation which involves excision of the proximal half of the proximal phalanx of the great toe and all the other toes and excising the prominent part of the metatarsal head in order to bring the toes into the same line. The patient can then walk on the forefoot instead of the heel as is commonly seen in the flat foot of rheumatoid arthritis.

Arthrodesis is fixation of the joint which is most commonly carried out in the knee-joint and in the metacarpo-phalangeal joint of the thumb. Correction of an ulnar deformity of the wrist can be very satisfactory, allowing the patient much more function. When the active phase of rheumatoid arthritis has died out and osteoarthritis of the joint has become superimposed then surgical procedures as outlined under osteoarthritis, p. 578, may be performed.

OSTEOMYELITIS OF BONE

Acute haematogenous osteomyelitis is a disease of childhood in areas of overcrowding as a whole. The infecting organism in 90 per cent of cases is the *Staphylococcus aureus*. The organism is carried in the bloodstream from a remote boil or pimple or an infection in the nasopharynx. Minor trauma on either side of a joint may precipitate the disease. *The usual sites of infection* are the upper end of the tibia, the lower end of the femur, the radius, the lower end of the fibula and the humerus, but every other bone may be involved and not uncommonly the vertebral bodies. *Tension* develops and pus tracks towards the medullary cavity and towards the periosteum, forming a sub-periosteal abscess. *Superficial cellulitis* occurs and a full-fledged fluctuant abscess is formed. Because of the intra-medullary tension, necrosis of bone rapidly occurs.

Symptoms in the fully developed case are dominated by intense pain. The child cries out at the slightest movement (and even at the approach of the doctor for examination). Extreme tenderness and fluctuation may be elicited. Septicaemia may make the child delirious and/or comatose with a very high temperature. Milder cases do, however, occur and the physical signs are often masked by antibiotic therapy previously given.

Treatment. At the first suspicion of osteomyelitis, the patient is given an antibiotic and the limb rested in a splint or by means of skin traction. Progress depends on whether the organism is sensitive to the antibiotic, in which case the disease will be arrested, if insensitive the disease will increase in severity. Admission to hospital is essential. *The following blood tests should be instituted immediately:* blood culture, haemoglobin, white blood cell count and a blood sedimentation rate, and preparations completed for treatment of a possible septicaemia. Should the local cellulitis, that is the area of tenderness and fluctuation increase within the first 24 hours then surgical drainage with decompression of the medullary cavity by drill holes gives prompt relief, provides material for bacteriological studies to identify the organism and its sensitivity and permits the use of an effective antibiotic. Splinting or traction of a limb should be continued until all clinical evidence of infection has disappeared to prevent subluxation at an epiphysis or joint. Antibiotic therapy is continued for several weeks after quiescence of signs and symptoms.

Chronic osteomyelitis may be of two varieties: the result of incomplete resolution of an acute osteomyelitis, or a focus of infection in a bone, forming a well walled-off bone abscess (Brodie's abscess). The condition is essentially one in which infected cavities are surrounded by sclerosed bone. The cavities are filled with infected granulation tissue and loose bits of dead bone known as sequestra or, if single, a sequestrum. Sinuses lead out from the infected area of bone and the usual picture is one of recurring periods of quiescence, local abscess formation, discharging sinuses and quiescence again.

Treatment. Recurrent flares are controlled by antibiotic therapy, but local abscess formation may need incision and drainage. Persistent discharging sinuses and the obvious presence of a sequestrum or sequestra on X-ray examination may need débridement of the cavity, removal of all the loose bone and granulation tissue and saucerization of the cavity to allow free drainage.

Chapter 58

An Outline of Thoracic Surgery

by MARY P. SHEPHERD

> *The mechanics of respiration—pre-operative investigation and pre-paration—thoracic surgical procedures—postoperative care and complications—chest trauma*

The surgical treatment of diseases of the chest is designed firstly to correct or remove the abnormality in the thorax or mediastinum, then to restore the integrity of the thoracic cage and finally to restore the conditions necessary for normal respiration.

THE MECHANICS OF RESPIRATION

The lungs are the essential organs of respiration, each lying in an air-tight compartment in the thorax. The pleura is a double-layered membrane, one layer adherent to the chest wall and diaphragm—the parietal pleura—and one layer adherent to the surface of the lung—the visceral pleura. The two layers are in continuity at the hilum of the lung, that is, the point of entry of the bronchus, artery and veins into the lung. The lungs are elastic structures which, if removed from the thoracic cavity, will contract down and become airless. When in the thorax, however, the visceral and parietal layers of pleura are in contact with one another and, though the lungs are elastic and tend to contract, the pleural layers will not separate to allow this, unless an air leak occurs in the air-tight thorax. Thus, while the pleural layers are intact, the lungs will follow the normal excursions of the chest wall and diaphragm during respiration. This results in air being drawn into and expelled from the lungs.

If either pleural layer is breached, and air allowed to enter, the pleural layers will separate and the lung collapse. Air can originate from the lung itself, e.g. in spontaneous pneumothorax, or from the outside through the chest wall, e.g. at operation (see p. 584). When this happens air, blood or fluid must be removed from the pleural space and the two layers of pleura brought together again in order to restore the conditions necessary for normal respiration. The standard method by which this is achieved is by an intercostal tube with underwater seal drainage. This one-way drainage system is also known as 'intercostal drain' or 'underwater seal' (Fig. 58/1). Drainage of fluid, blood and air is assisted by coughing and the respiratory efforts of the patient. Air cannot return to the thorax via the tube because

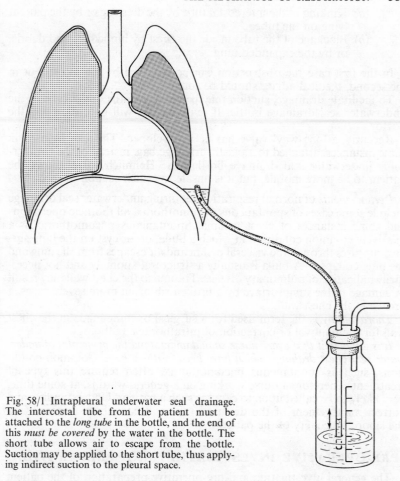

Fig. 58/1 Intrapleural underwater seal drainage. The intercostal tube from the patient must be attached to the *long tube* in the bottle, and the end of this *must be covered* by the water in the bottle. The short tube allows air to escape from the bottle. Suction may be applied to the short tube, thus applying indirect suction to the pleural space.

of the water in the bottle. During expiration, water and not air is sucked up the long glass tube. Because of this, *it is important for the nurse to ensure that the bottle is never raised up to the level of the patient, unless the tubing is first clamped*, because the contents of the bottle would then be siphoned into the pleural space. *The bottle therefore must always be kept well below the level of the patient's chest. Also, great care must be taken to keep the bottle upright at all times, otherwise the long tube will come out of the water and air will immediately enter the pleural space.* In case of any doubt as to whether the apparatus is working properly, clamp the intercostal tube and summon help.

Owing to the changes of pressure inside the pleural space with inspiration and expiration, the level of the column of fluid in the long tube in the bottle will oscillate, or 'swing'. If the drainage tube is blocked, the 'swing' will cease. This may be due to either:

(a) Kinking of the intercostal tube by the dressing or by the patient lying on the tube.

(b) Blockage of the tube inside the chest by blood clot and debris, or by the expanded lung.

In the first case the obstruction can be removed by the nurse, but in the second, medical advice should be sought.

To facilitate drainage, suction may be applied to the outlet tube of the underwater seal drainage bottle. If required this will be ordered by the doctor.

Recently, a 'one way' valve has been developed. This can be used in some instances, attached to a plastic drainage bag, instead of the cumbersome underwater seal drainage bottle. The Heimlich valve allows the patient to be more mobile, but it is unsafe to attach suction to this.

Derangements of normal respiration requiring underwater seal drainage include some cases of spontaneous pneumothorax, all thoracic operations and some instances of chest trauma. Spontaneous pneumothorax is a relatively common condition in which a bulla, or air cyst on the lung surface ruptures through the visceral pleura and air escapes from the lung and the lung collapses. A bulla is usually a structural anomaly and not necessarily indicative of pulmonary disease. Trauma to the chest wall may result in damage to the lung surface by a broken rib or, in more severe cases, a breach in the chest wall.

Thoracotomy is the term used for a surgical opening made in the chest wall for the removal or correction of intrathoracic pathology.

It is important that every nurse should understand the principles of underwater seal chest drainage which have been outlined here. Common conditions, such as spontaneous pneumothorax, often require this type of treatment. Therefore a nurse working on a general ward is, at some time, very likely to be called upon to care for such a patient. Understanding and correct management of the drainage tube will contribute materially to the smooth recovery of the patient.

PRE-OPERATIVE INVESTIGATION AND PREPARATION

The general investigation and pre-operative preparation of the patient is similar to that for any other major surgical operation (see p. 424), but special attention is paid to the heart and lungs, and dental and oral hygiene. The patient is advised not to smoke.

To confirm the clinical assessment of the patient's lung function and reserve, various *respiratory function tests* may be carried out.

Blood samples are taken for haemoglobin and serum electrolyte estimation, blood grouping and cross matching for transfusion at operation.

Radiological examination of the chest is made in various positions, and may include tomograms, bronchograms, and barium swallow or meal examinations.

Specimens of sputum are examined for pathological bacteria, including the tubercle bacillus, and for malignant cells.

Bronchoscopy or *oesophagoscopy* are carried out to examine the bronchial tree or oesophagus.

Oesophagoscopy is always, and bronchoscopy nearly always, performed under general anaesthesia. The patient is prepared for an anaesthetic in the normal way and is usually given his pre-medication in the ward, but occasionally it is given intravenously in the anaesthetic room. Following bronchoscopy oxygen administration is required and, during recovery, constant care must be taken to maintain a clear airway. The patient is not allowed food or fluids for at least four hours after either general or local anaesthesia.

Physiotherapy, consisting of breathing and shoulder exercises, instruction in coughing, and postural drainage if necessary, is important before operation to ensure that the patient is using his lungs efficiently, to remove retained secretions, and to prepare him for what will be required of him after his operation.

Antibiotics are given pre-operatively if there is definite infection of the lungs. Operation may be postponed until any infection has been eliminated.

People with oesophageal obstruction may have lost a lot of weight and be dehydrated. They will require ample nourishing fluids or semi-solid foods and vitamins until fit for surgery.

THORACIC SURGICAL PROCEDURES
(See Fig. 58/2)

Bronchoscopy. The bronchoscope is passed through the mouth, larynx and vocal cords into the trachea. The procedure is performed for the removal of an inhaled foreign body, and for the diagnosis of disease by

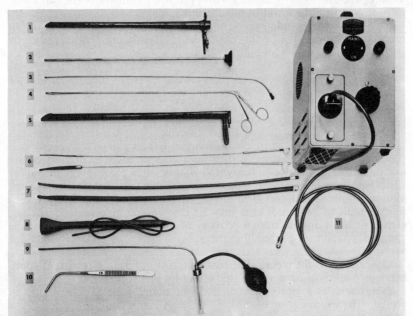

Fig. 58/2 Instruments for bronchoscopy and oesophagoscopy. 1. Bronchoscope. 2. Telescope. 3. Suction cannula. 4. Biopsy forceps. 5. Oesophagoscope. 6. Oesophageal bougies—Chevalier Jackson (supply the set). 7. Oesophageal bougies—gum elastic (supply the set). 8. Mousseau-Barbin tube. 9. Local anaesthetic spray. 10. Local anaesthetic swab-holding forceps—Kraus. 11. Fibre-optic light, source and lead.

obtaining specimens of sputum or tissue biopsy from the bronchi for examination. It is necessary for the assessment of the extent of lung resection likely to be required in cases of bronchial carcinoma. It may be required for aspiration of retained secretions if the patient is unable to cough after an operation on the chest. In this instance local anaesthesia is generally used. *Complications* include haemorrhage, anoxia, cardiac arrest and the necessity for immediate thoracotomy.

Oesophagoscopy. The oesophagoscope is passed through the mouth into the oesophagus. The procedure is performed for the removal of a swallowed, impacted foreign body, for the diagnosis of oesophagitis and assessment of its severity in cases of hiatus hernia, and the diagnosis of the cause of obstruction of the oesophagus, whether due to carcinoma or benign stricture, by tissue biopsy. It is necessary to determine the level of the obstruction so that the correct surgical procedure can be selected. A benign stricture can be dilated with oesophageal bougies through the oesophagoscope while in instances of inoperable carcinoma of the oesophagus a Mousseau-Barbin or Celestin tube is inserted in order to provide a passage for saliva, liquids and semi-solid food.

Following oesophagoscopy, clear fluids only may be given until the chest has been X-rayed the morning after the examination, and the film seen by a medical officer. There is a definite incidence of perforation of the oesophagus after oesophagoscopy even in the most experienced hands. This regime allows early detection and prompt treatment of the complication, so averting the onset of mediastinitis.

Complications include perforation of the oesophagus with resultant mediastinitis unless the perforation is detected early and treated promptly by intravenous feeding and antibiotics.

Mediastinoscopy. This is a surgical procedure performed under general anaesthesia. The investigation is designed to examine the paratracheal and hilar lymph glands. A transverse suprasternal skin incision is made and the dissection deepened in the midline until the pre-tracheal fascia is reached. This is incised and a gloved finger inserted into the mediastinum immediately in front of the trachea. Enlarged lymph glands are readily palpated. The mediastinoscope is then inserted and, after further dissection and careful identification of the lymph glands, small pieces are removed for histological examination. The deep tissues of the neck are sutured and the skin incision closed. Diseases involving the mediastinal lymph glands, such as tuberculosis or sarcoidosis may be diagnosed. Involvement of these glands with carcinoma from a primary of the bronchus indicates that the pulmonary lesion is probably inoperable.

Operations on the pleura. Patients who are suffering a recurrent spontaneous pneumothorax are treated either by pleurodesis or pleurectomy.

Pleurodesis is a procedure carried out under general anaesthesia in which, after examination of the lung through a small hole in the chest wall using a thoracoscope, iodized talcum powder is insufflated into the pleural space, care being taken to distribute the powder evenly over both visceral and parietal layers of pleura. An intercostal tube with underwater seal drainage is inserted (see p. 583). The powder irritates the pleura and causes adhesions to form between the two layers of pleura, so preventing lung collapse on a future occasion. The pleurisy caused is painful and analgesics are required postoperatively.

Fusion of the lung to the chest wall is achieved by removal of the parietal layer of pleura lining the upper part of the chest wall, or pleurectomy. This is done at thoracotomy and when the lung re-expands it adheres to the raw area of chest wall.

In conditions in which the pleura becomes enormously thickened and rigid, preventing normal rib movement and lung expansion, *decortication* may be necessary. The thickened layers of parietal and visceral pleura are carefully stripped off the chest wall and lung and removed at thoracotomy. Pleural thickening may follow a previous empyema or a haemothorax.

Operations on the lungs. The diseases requiring removal of lung tissue at thoracotomy are carcinoma of the bronchus, bronchiectasis and tuberculosis.

Lobectomy is the removal of one lobe of a lung, *pneumonectomy* the removal of one lung, *segmental resection* the removal of one or more segments of a lobe of one lung, and *wedge resection* is the removal of a wedge-shaped piece of lung tissue, as, for example, in lung biopsy.

Carcinoma of the bronchus usually requires lobectomy or pneumonectomy. *Tuberculosis* may require lobectomy or segmental resection. This may be accompanied by thoracoplasty, or thoracoplasty only may be carried out (see operation on the chest wall, p. 588).

Operations on the mediastinum. Some tumours of the mediastinum such as neurofibromas, are removed through thoracotomy incisions. Other tumours, such as thymic tumours, are removed through a median sternotomy in which the sternum is divided vertically. The pleural cavities may not be opened, but if they are, intercostal-tube underwater seal drainage is instituted, as well as draining the mediastinum. Many cardiac operations are carried out through this type of incision (see Chapter 59).

Carcinoma or benign stricture of the oesophagus may be treated by oesophagectomy. The portion of the oesophagus containing the obstruction is excised and the oesophagus anastomosed to either the stomach or small bowel, or occasionally to a segment of colon which can be brought up into the chest.

A two-stage oesophagectomy is performed for carcinoma of the middle third of the oesophagus. First the stomach is mobilized through an abdominal incision and this is immediately followed by the second stage, a right thoracotomy in which the oesophagus is excised and anastamosed to the stomach which is drawn up into the chest. *Oesophagogastrectomy* is done for carcinoma of the lower end of the oesophagus, the resection being carried out through a left thoraco-abdominal incision.

Operations on the diaphragm. The commonest condition for which the thoracic surgeon operates on the diaphragm is *hiatus hernia*. A portion of the stomach herniates through the oesophageal hiatus into the chest. The presence of *reflux oesophagitis* may result in bleeding from the inflamed oesophagus, producing anaemia, or the formation of an oesophageal stricture. At left thoracotomy, the hernia is reduced and the stretched oesophageal hiatus repaired. *Congenital hiatus hernia* also occurs in infants. Medical treatment, including weaning onto more solid food and nursing in the upright position (see p. 173, Fig. 18/2) is tried first. If it fails, surgical repair may be necessary.

Operations on the chest wall. The correction of the congenital deformity of pectus excavatum, or depressed sternum is usually carried out for cosmetic reasons, but occasionally there may be cardiac effects of the deformity. The procedure involves the removal of many of the costal cartilages of the ribs, fracturing the sternum across and lifting it forwards. The sternum is fixed in the raised position by implanting a steel bar across the front of the chest wall, underneath the sternum. The bar is removed a few months later.

Thoracoplasty is done to decrease permanently the size of one hemithorax either to produce collapse of the underlying portion of lung affected by tuberculosis, or following resection of the diseased portion of lung. The procedure involves the removal of a selected number of the upper ribs, allowing that portion of the chest wall to fall in. Thoracoplasty is not required nearly as frequently today as it was before drugs were available to treat pulmonary tuberculosis.

Rib resection is performed for drainage of a *chronic empyema*, a localized collection of pus in the pleural cavity. Under general anaesthesia, a two- to three-inch segment of the rib situated over the most dependent part of the empyema cavity is excised. The cavity is opened, emptied of pus, fibrin and debris, and a large intercostal tube inserted. *Underwater seal drainage* is maintained until maximum lung expansion has been achieved. *The drainage tube is then cut short* and allowed to drain into a surgical dressing until the cavity has completely filled in. However, the procedure may be avoided by *early treatment of an empyema* with daily aspiration of the pus and instillation of the appropriate antibiotic into the pleural space, combined with systemic antibiotic administration.

POSTOPERATIVE CARE AND COMPLICATIONS

Postoperative care of the thoracic surgical patient is basically the same as that given after any major surgical operation, and similar complications such as shock, pulmonary embolus, haemorrhage and wound breakdown can occur. However, additional complications may arise, such as pneumothorax, sputum retention, respiratory failure, cardiac arrhythmias and cardiac failure. In efforts to avoid these, several measures are taken.

Intercostal underwater seal drainage of the opened pleural space is always instituted (see p. 582). One, two, or three tubes may be inserted at the end of the operation. These are removed when fluid and air drainage has ceased and clinical and radiological examination of the chest shows that the lung has expanded and the pleural space is obliterated.

Blood pressure, pulse rate and respiratory rate are noted and recorded regularly, half-hourly or hourly during the first few hours postoperatively.

The patient may be sat up in bed as soon as he has regained consciousness and his blood pressure is satisfactory. This assists the physiotherapist who re-institutes treatment, as soon as the patient is conscious enough to co-operate, to encourage coughing and expectoration. Analgesics are given to relieve pain which also helps the patient to breathe and cough. The physiotherapist treats the patient at least twice daily if possible during the first few postoperative days, and more often if necessary. This regime reduces the incidence of postoperative sputum retention and pulmonary collapse requiring bronchoscopy for aspiration of the retained secretions which, under local anaesthesia, is an unpleasant procedure for the patient. Occasionally tracheostomy is required in the very ill postoperative patient to enable copious secretions to be aspirated regularly.

Antibiotics are given routinely for five days after operation, or longer if indicated, and anti-tuberculosis chemotherapy is continued in people with pulmonary tuberculosis.

An indwelling naso-gastric tube may be inserted in patients undergoing repair of hiatus hernia. It is always introduced at oesophagectomy to allow the stomach, or bowel, to be kept empty during the period of paralytic ileus which invariably follows the latter operation and may last several days. *Oral hygiene* is *particularly important during this period* as little or no oral feeding is allowed, the necessary fluid and calorie intake being given intravenously. When bowel sounds reappear, oral feeding is recommenced.

Whenever possible *the patient sits out of bed on the first postoperative day*. Mobilization is gradually increased so that, when the drainage tubes are removed, the patient becomes fully mobile almost at once. The increasing activity assists lung expansion and venous return in the legs.

A chest X-ray is obtained on the first postoperative day, and usually every four to five days thereafter to confirm the clinical evidence of the patient's progress. The patient usually goes home about two weeks after operation, but those with pulmonary tuberculosis may be in hospital considerably longer.

Complications of operations on the lungs. *Collapse*, or *atelectasis*, of lung tissue may result from sputum retention, and pneumonia or bronchospasm from infection of lung tissue. These conditions can lead to respiratory failure and therefore require prompt treatment. In severe cases tracheostomy may be necessary.

Cardiac arrhythmias can occur, most frequently atrial fibrillation. The patient may be treated with a digitalis preparation.

Pneumothorax may persist and surgical emphysema (or air in the tissues) may appear. If the emphysema becomes marked it usually indicates some obstruction or fault in the chest drainage system.

During a pneumonectomy for carcinoma, it is sometimes necessary to remove a portion of pericardium. In these cases there is *a risk that the heart may herniate through the defect* in the early postoperative phase and prove rapidly fatal. *It is important therefore, that these patients, whether lying down or sitting up, are inclined at all times to the side which has not been operated upon.* This can readily be achieved, and the patient kept comfortable, by the strategic positioning of pillows.

Broncho-pleural fistula arises if the bronchial suture line leaks. This can be very serious following pneumonectomy, because after removal of a whole lung the space fills with fluid and it is possible for this fluid to flood the bronchi of the remaining lung resulting in sudden respiratory failure and cardiac arrest. The development of a fistula must be suspected if the patient has a haemoptysis postoperatively or starts to cough up considerable amounts of watery bloodstained fluid. *If these symptoms are noted they should be reported immediately.*

Empyema, or infection of the pleural space, occurs less frequently after surgery today, because of the availability and use of antibiotics.

Deep-leg-vein thrombosis may arise at any time during the first 10 to 14 postoperative days. This can lead to the more serious complication of pulmonary embolus. A complaint of calf pain or ankle swelling should be reported. These symptoms may be associated with a low grade fever or this may be the initial, or only sign, of a deep vein thrombosis. If this diagnosis is made, the patient is usually treated with anticoagulants (see Chapter 22, p. 214).

If a pulmonary embolus occurs, it may be necessary to perform emergency pulmonary embolectomy, often under cardiopulmonary by-pass, or to use a streptokinase preparation administered directly into the pulmonary artery. Anticoagulants and drugs to support the heart are given.

Complications of operations on the mediastinum. *Tumours of the thymus* may be associated with myasthenia gravis (see p. 268). The treatment of this condition must be continued after the operation for removing the thymus until improvement of the myasthenia occurs. *The early postoperative period may be complicated by an exacerbation*, or *myasthenic crisis*, causing severe weakness of the muscles of respiration. Pulmonary complications are therefore very likely to arise. It may be necessary to ventilate the patient for a time. This is achieved by using a respirator and, in the first instance, an endotracheal tube. *Tracheostomy* may be done if the patient requires artificial ventilation for more than a few days.

Following oesophagectomy, a leak may occur at the site of anastamosis. This gives rise to the serious complication of *mediastinitis*, which can lead to abscess formation or death unless treatment is prompt and vigorous. Surgical drainage of an abscess in the mediastinum is usually necessary.

Complications of operations on the diaphragm. After repair of a hiatus hernia, acute dilatation of the stomach may occur unless the stomach is decompressed postoperatively by means of an indwelling naso-gastric tube. Early dysphagia usually disappears in time, as does distressing flatulent indigestion which sometimes arises. A stricture of the oesophagus at the site of repair can follow operation. This may require subsequent oesophagoscopy and dilatation with oesophageal bougies.

Any surgical procedure involving surgical incision of the diaphragm can result in the late herniation of abdominal contents into the chest, despite suture of the incision at the original operation. The symptoms and signs are related to the tissues in the hernia. Surgical repair may be necessary.

Nursing care and observation. Constant vigilance is necessary after a chest operation. Regular recordings of pulse rate and rhythm, blood pressure, respiratory rate and temperature must be made, the function of the underwater seal drainage system checked (see p. 582), intravenous and oral fluid intake and urine output noted and the general condition of the patient observed, in addition to performing the routine nursing procedures to keep the patient comfortable. Any sudden alteration in the recordings, change in general condition or fault in the intercostal drainage system should be reported immediately to the ward sister, charge nurse or doctor. In this way, the nurse makes a very valuable contribution to the smooth convalescence of the thoracic surgical patient, as any postoperative complication can be detected early and either prevented or treated promptly.

CHEST TRAUMA

In a severely injured person, the most life-threatening injuries are those to the chest or head. Such damage may not be immediately obvious, particularly in the presence of other external injuries, e.g. to the limbs. Intrathoracic trauma must be suspected if there is any evidence of respiratory insufficiency (see Chapter 43). It must be remembered that it is possible to sustain damage to the soft tissues in the thorax with no external or radiological evidence of bony thoracic injury, although this is usually found.

Injury to the bony structure of the thoracic cage

Fractured ribs are commonly found after injury to the chest and may not be associated with any intrathoracic damage. If the fractured ends are displaced, however, pneumothorax or haemopneumothorax may be found. The management of a patient with one or more ribs fractured in one place only is based on the control of pain so that the patient can move the ribs comfortably and normally to allow normal ventilation and function of the underlying lung. This may be achieved by analgesics or an intercostal nerve block by injection of the appropriate intercostal nerves with local anaesthetic. Underwater seal drainage is necessary to treat a pneumo- or haemopneumothorax. Physiotherapy is important.

Fracture of several adjacent ribs in more than one place results in instability of a segment of chest wall. The portion of mobile chest wall is sucked inwards during inspiration, instead of the normal 'upward and outward' movement of the rib cage. The abnormal movement of the mobile segment is described as paradoxical and is the basis of the terms 'flail chest' or 'stove-in chest'. If the mobile portion of chest wall is large, or the respiratory function normally poor, ventilation may become inadequate and the symptoms and signs of respiratory failure will supervene. In these cases it is necessary to perform tracheostomy and perhaps ventilate the patient using intermittent positive pressure respiration. Artificial ventilation may be required for two to three weeks until the mobile segment of chest wall has stabilized, by virtue of the healing rib fractures, with restoration of normal movements.

Fracture of the sternum with consequent instability of the chest wall may occur. These patients may need artificial ventilation to stabilize the fracture, if there is evidence of respiratory insufficiency.

Fracture or fracture-dislocation of the thoracic spine may have been sustained (see Chapter 56).

Intrathoracic soft tissue injury. *Lung contusion or bruising.* Fractured ribs may not be present and there may or may not be a pneumothorax or haemothorax for which intercostal-tube underwater seal drainage is necessary.

Lung laceration is associated with fractured ribs and is usually accompanied by a haemopneumothorax. This requires either intercostal-tube drainage or thoracotomy.

Ruptured bronchus. Surgical emphysema is found in the mediastinum or tissues of the neck. Bronchoscopy is required for diagnosis and assessment, and thoracotomy for repair or resection.

The diaphragm may be ruptured. A tear in the left hemidiaphragm results in the herniation of abdominal organs into the left chest with consequent respiratory embarrassment. Thoracotomy, with reduction of the hernia and repair of the hole in the diaphragm should be carried out at the earliest opportunity. A tear in the right hemidiaphragm is often associated with considerable liver injury, and the inferior vena cava may be torn. This type of injury frequently proves fatal.

Heart and great vessels

The myocardium may be bruised and this can result in either a haemorrhagic pericardial effusion or myocardial infarction. If the interventricular septum is affected, a traumatic ventricular septal defect can be produced. Damage to the mitral valve can occur, giving rise to the sudden onset of mitral incompetence. Urgent repair under cardiopulmonary by-pass (see p. 605) is usually necessary.

The wall of any of the great vessels may be damaged. If this affects only the inner layers of the wall of a large artery, an aneurysm may form which may require surgical repair. Complete transection of the aorta or one of its large branches, or a tear in either vena cava, often proves fatal.

Chapter 59

Surgery of Heart and Great Blood Vessels, Treatment and Nursing

by DAVID I. HAMILTON

> *Introduction—patients presenting for treatment—psychological approach—special investigations—preparation for operation—obtaining bloodless cardiac field—classification of cardiac defects, congenital, acquired—treatment of individual lesions—constrictive pericarditis—tamponade—operation using the heart-lung machine—recovery ward routine—the nurse in the team—advice on returning home*

During the past 25 years tremendous progress has been achieved. In 1945 the correction of coarctation of the aorta was performed successfully by surgery; this led to the development of special vascular clamps and instruments which enabled surgeons to operate upon blood vessels safely. As techniques improved, and the possibility of curative treatment emerged, cardiologists were stimulated to investigate congenital and acquired conditions more fully. The cardiac catheter was devised for measuring the pressures inside the heart (see p. 595).

Many conditions affecting the heart and great vessels are due to obstructions (or stenoses). Surgeons first attempted to relieve these conditions by 'blind' operations, working inside the beating heart, either with the finger or with special instruments. The most successful procedure to result from this work is the relief of mitral stenosis by 'closed valvotomy'.

Gradually it was realized that the heart is a robust muscular pump which will tolerate surgical intervention well. The development of the 'heart-lung machine' during the 1950s has made it possible to support the patient's circulation with oxygenated blood so that the heart can be excluded temporarily from the circulation, and surgery under *direct vision* performed inside it.

PATIENTS PRESENTING FOR TREATMENT

It is now possible to treat patients throughout their life-span from the neonatal period to senior citizenship. Congenital malformations of the heart and great blood vessels (see p. 598) occur in approximately 8 per 1,000 live births. These infants face a trial of 'natural selection' or 'the battle of the survival of the fittest'. Some unhappily do not survive many hours or days, others develop cardiac failure during the first weeks of life. This group should be referred from the maternity hospital to an experienced paediatric unit immediately, where investigatory and surgical management may be life-saving. The less severely afflicted will grow up through infancy or early childhood; many children, however, are slow to thrive or show diminished exercise tolerance. Some are diagnosed at school clinics. Others grow to adulthood with a 'compensated heart' defect. Their life expectancy is not normal and surgical correction is usually advised. Adults of all ages present with acquired heart conditions which may be amenable to surgical correction.

MANAGEMENT OF PATIENTS AND THEIR RELATIVES

Few conditions can be more worrying to patients and their relatives. Some patients are breathless, cyanosed, prone to fainting, and most are anxious. Serious valve lesions may affect previously fit young adults with dramatic suddenness. These patients may be breadwinners or the mothers of young families. *The investigating physician, surgeon and nursing team should deal with these families with particular consideration, care and understanding. This consideration of the psychological approach to patients is fundamental to their smooth recovery*—confidence grows up between patients, medical and nursing staff and also between the medical and nursing team itself when all become united in obtaining 'a safe passage for their patients'.

Open-heart surgery is a serious measure but success means health and mobility instead of invalidism and increasing immobility.

SPECIAL INVESTIGATIONS

A careful history and general examination form the basis of cardiac diagnosis, as in all other conditions. These are followed up with a series of special investigations, as below.

A chest radiograph taken with postero-anterior and lateral views demonstrates the size of the heart relative to the transverse diameter of the chest, termed *the cardio-thoracic ratio*. The shape of the cardiac outline reveals information about *the size of the individual heart chambers and of the great vessels. Calcification* in valve cusps, mentioned several times in the text, is revealed. All this information is considered in reaching a correct clinical diagnosis.

The lung fields are next studied, noting the changes of pulmonary collapse, over-vascularization (plethora), and under-vascularization (oligaemia).

A *full electrocardiograph* (E.C.G.) gives information about the heart rate, its rhythm and the relative size of the heart chambers and which parts are undergoing strain. It also gives important information about the coronary artery supply.

Phonocardiography records heart sounds and murmurs graphically on paper, providing a permanent record of the auscultatory findings.

Cardiac catheterization. A fine flexible catheter may be introduced into a peripheral vein or artery and advanced inside the heart under radiographic control. *The venous catheter* will normally lead into the right atrium, right ventricle and pulmonary artery; *the arterial catheter* will lead into the aorta and left ventricle. *It is thus possible to measure the pressures in all four heart chambers* by connecting the proximal end of the catheter to a pressure transducer and recording the wave produced on an oscilloscope screen (see Fig. 59/1).

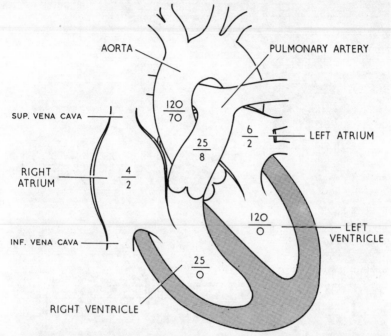

Fig. 59/1 The normal pressures within the heart and great vessels as deduced by cardiac catheterization. The right ventricular and pulmonary artery pressure is approximately one-fifth that of the left ventricular and aortic (systemic) pressure.

Blood samples withdrawn through the hollow catheter from each chamber in turn give the oxygen content at each site, thus providing basic information leading to the diagnosis of congenital and acquired conditions.

Angiocardiography is an extension of cardiac catheter technique. A special catheter is introduced into the heart from a peripheral vessel positioned by radiographic control. If contrast medium is injected through the catheter and a series of films are taken at very rapid intervals, the course of the blood through the heart will demonstrate any abnormal defect or valve deformity (see Fig. 59/2).

PREPARATION FOR OPERATION

The general principles of preparing patients for major surgery are similar (see Chapter 45). In patients for cardiac surgery a *chest radiograph and an electrocardiogram* are taken within a few days of surgery. *Pre-operative physiotherapy* with breathing exercises is commenced and *any*

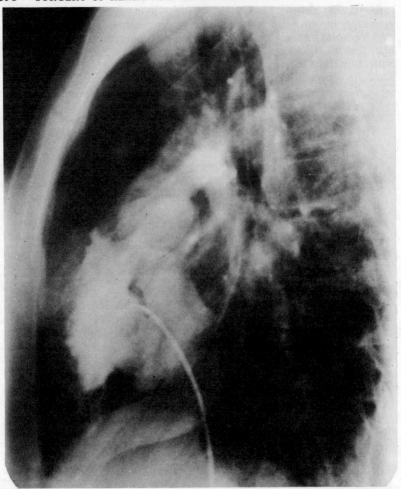

Fig. 59/2 A right ventricular angiocardiogram in a case of Fallot's tetralogy, lateral view. The catheter enters the heart from the femoral vein, inferior vena cava and right atrium, passing into the right ventricle.

sputum obtained is sent to the laboratory for culture of organisms. Estimation of antibiotic sensitivity is made. Before open-heart surgery a *dental examination* should be made, probably several months beforehand, and the necessary treatment completed. *Swabs are taken from the nose and throat* a few days before operation.

A child will usually be in hospital for several days before operation to get used to his surroundings. In patients of all ages any cold, however slight, a cough, sputum, nasal infection, defective teeth and poor oral hygiene will be investigated and dealt with. The patient may be ambulant but should be encouraged to rest as much as possible. Heart failure confines the patient to bed. As a rule he may have a normal diet. His food should be made as appetizing as possible, as these patients, particularly if children, often eat little. *Breathing exercises* and *physiotherapy* begin at once. *The haemoglobin content of the blood is estimated and the blood is grouped and cross matched with donor's fresh blood. Specimens of blood are taken for serum electrolyte and urea estimation, and special tests relating to the clotting factors in blood and to liver function* are carried out. *Blood pressure readings* are taken and the character of the pulse and respirations noted. The temperature is taken.

Skin preparation. The pubic and axillary hair is shaved three days before the day of operation. A bath containing 60 ml of 5 per cent Hibitane, using an antiseptic soap, is taken daily for three days. If the surgeon employs iodine for skin preparation in the operating theatre, then a patch skin test for *iodine sensitivity* must be performed beforehand. Serious iodine sensitivity can only be avoided in this way.

The urine will be tested. The *bowels* should have acted on the day before the operation.

The patient's *weight and height are recorded for estimation of body surface area.* This determines the flow rate through the heart-lung machine. *Antibiotics* are given the day before operation and continued for 7 to 10 days afterwards.

No fluid or food should be taken for 6 hours before operation.

Immediate preparation. A pre-medication drug is given an hour before operation and then the patient should lie quietly and not be disturbed unnecessarily.

A general anaesthetic is given and is maintained through an endotracheal tube attached to a positive-pressure pulmonary ventilator (see preparation for operation using the heart-lung machine, p. 606).

Drugs. Patients who have previously been taking digitalis derivatives should cease doing so 48 hours before operation. This is because the serum potassium level varies considerably during the use of the heart-lung machine (see p. 606) and if it falls below the normal level the effect of digoxin in slowing the heart rate may be potentiated; this can cause difficulty when the heart is beginning to take over its function again after the perfusion with the machine is discontinued.

Anticoagulants. These drugs are also discontinued 48 hours before surgery in many centres.

OBTAINING BLOODLESS CARDIAC FIELD

The *bloodless cardiac field* essential for intra-cardiac surgery is obtained in one of four ways.

1. *Inflow occlusion at normothermia* (37 °C or 98 °F). The venae cavae are clamped or snared and the heart beats itself empty. Two to three minutes only are available for a very quick surgical procedure, such as pulmonary valvotomy, to be performed.

2. *Inflow occlusion at moderate hypothermia.* The body temperature is lowered to 30 °C (86 °F) by immersing the anaesthetized patient in an ice-cold bath. When the venae cavae are occluded, 8 to 10 minutes are available to the surgeon, allowing a simple atrial septal defect to be closed.

3. *Profound hypothermia by Drew's technique.* The body temperature is lowered to 15 to 12 °C (59 to 53·6 °F). The circulation may be stopped

for 70 minutes as the tissues have a very low oxygen requirement at this temperature. The patient's lungs oxygenate his own blood, in contrast to method 4.

4. *Cardiopulmonary by-pass using the heart-lung machine.* The machine consists of an oxygenating chamber, heat exchanger and a roller pump which returns the blood to the patient. The heart-lung machine performs the work of both heart and lungs; the heart is emptied of blood, and surgery may be performed under ideal conditions lasting several hours if necessary (see Fig. 59/8, p.607).

CLASSIFICATION OF THE COMMONER DEFECTS AND CONDITIONS IN WHICH RELIEF BY OPERATION MAY BE OBTAINED

Congenital

Stenoses in the heart and great vessels
 Pulmonary valve stenosis.
 Aortic valve stenosis.
 Mitral valve stenosis.
 Coarctation of the aorta.

Left to right shunts (not cyanosed)
 Atrial septal defect.
 Ventricular septal defect.
 Persistent ductus arteriosus (P.D.A).
Right to left shunts (cyanosed)
 Tetralogy of Fallot.
 Transposition of Great Vessels (T.G.V.).

Acquired

Valve disease
 Mitral stenosis and/or regurgitation.
 Aortic stenosis and/or regurgitation.
 Constrictive pericarditis.

 Cardiac tamponade.
 Coronary artery disease (stenosis).

Congenital heart disease
 Valve stenosis. The delicate valve cusps do not always develop perfectly. The commissures dividing the cusps may be fused together leaving only a small central aperture through which the blood is forced. The heart chamber proximal to the obstructed valve must perform increased work to overcome this resistance if an adequate cardiac output is to be maintained.

 Pulmonary valve stenosis results in *right ventricular strain* and hypertrophy. Insufficient blood passes through the pulmonary circulation, causing *shortness of breath on exertion.* Operation is best performed by opening up the valve orifice, before irreversible changes of muscular fibrosis have occured in the right ventricle.

 Aortic valve stenosis is a serious condition as it affects the main outlet valve from the heart, which governs the quantity of blood reaching the coronary arteries supplying the heart itself with blood, and also the systemic circulation including the brain. These patients are liable to sudden collapse from hypotension and even to sudden death. Here the left ventricle develops signs of thickening and strain. The valve can be exposed through the root of the aorta using cardiopulmonary by-pass with the heart-lung machine (see p. 606). Incisions are made to enlarge the valve orifice. This may leave an imperfect valve, and valve replacement may be required at a later date (see p. 604).

Mitral stenosis of congenital origin is a rare condition but children or infants do present with increasing breathlessness and the signs of mitral valve obstruction. The condition is difficult to treat in children as the valve is abnormal and the valve ring is often too small to allow an artificial valve to be inserted.

Coarctation of the aorta. It is probable that the abnormality develops as early as the seventh week in fetal life. There is a narrowing in the lumen of the thoracic aorta just beyond the origin of the left subclavian artery and near the site of the ductus arteriosus (Fig. 59/3 A). The child may be born in left ventricular heart failure, and if this is resistant to medical management operation can be successfully performed in the early weeks of life.

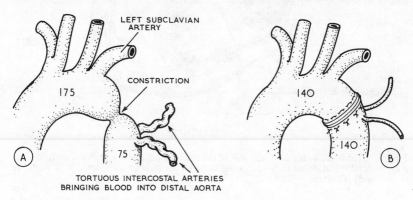

Fig. 59/3 (*a*) Co-arctation of the aorta showing the constriction beyond the left subclavian artery. This produces a high blood pressure (175 mm Hg) proximal to the constriction and a low pressure (75 mm Hg) beyond it. (*b*) After resection of the narrow segment of aorta, an end-to-end anastomosis reconstitutes the normal calibre of the vessel and equalizes the pressure differential.

Left to right shunts (not cyanosed)

The heart is a muscular pump having four chambers, two receiving reservoirs, the right and left atria, and two strong pumping chambers, the right and left ventricles. *The diagram (Fig. 59/1, p. 595) illustrates the heart chambers and the normal physiological pressures within them as deduced by cardiac catheterization.* This technique is employed in diagnosing the following conditions, as if there is a 'shunt of blood' (an abnormal passage of some of the blood passing through the heart or great vessels) from one side of the heart to the other, either left to right or right to left, then the state of equilibrium which should exist is upset and the pressures in the four chambers may be affected.

Atrial septal defect. During fetal development the *foramen ovale* is a deficiency in the septum between the right and left atria. Blood arriving in the right atrium passes via the foramen ovale to the left side of the heart. If this window does not close off soon after birth, or if there is a larger developmental deficiency in the inter-atrial septum in the same region, then an atrial septal defect results (Fig. 59/4).

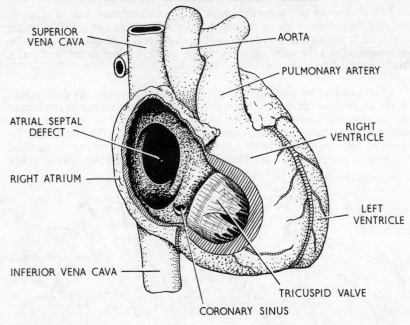

SUPERIOR VENA CAVA

AORTA

PULMONARY ARTERY

ATRIAL SEPTAL DEFECT

RIGHT VENTRICLE

RIGHT ATRIUM

LEFT VENTRICLE

INFERIOR VENA CAVA

TRICUSPID VALVE

CORONARY SINUS

Fig. 59/4 The heart with part of the wall of the right atrium and ventricle cut away to show a large atrial septal defect communicating between the right and left atria. This would be closed by direct suture.

Treatment. These defects should be closed surgically, using the heart-lung machine. This can now be performed with low mortality (1 per cent or less).

Ventricular septal defects. The interventricular septum consists of a large muscular portion and a smaller membranous upper portion. It is in the membranous portion lying just below the pulmonary and aortic valve rings that the majority of these defects are found. These communicating windows vary in size from a few millimetres to large areas perhaps 2 to 3 cm in diameter. The larger defects tend to cause symptoms early and infants may go into cardiac failure during their first few weeks of life.

Operation to close the defect is usually performed between 3 and 8 years of age. Using the heart-lung machine the right ventricle is opened and the ventricular septal defect exposed. Very small defects may be sutured with individual sutures but more commonly a patch of material is used. This condition can now be closed in infancy if indicated.

Persistent ductus arteriosus. The ductus arteriosus is a short channel, usually 5 to 8 mm in diameter, which connects the origin of the left main pulmonary artery to the descending thoracic aorta, just beyond the origin of the left subclavian artery. Before birth this provides a second mechanism for completing the circulation before the lungs expand (see Fig. 59/5).

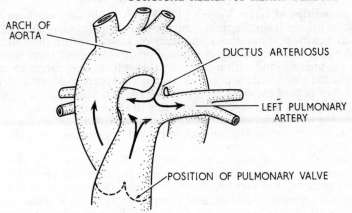

ARCH OF AORTA

DUCTUS ARTERIOSUS

LEFT PULMONARY ARTERY

POSITION OF PULMONARY VALVE

Fig. 59/5 The persistent (patent) ductus arteriosus. The arrows indicate the flow of blood after birth when the lungs have expanded. Note blood flows from aorta to pulmonary artery and to the lungs. Before birth, the unexpanded lungs provide a high resistance to blood flow which passes through the ductus and into the aorta under these circumstances.

Right to left shunts (cyanosed)

Tetralogy of Fallot. The two important elements of the tetrad are *the presence of a ventricular septal defect* and *some obstruction to the blood leaving the right ventricle*. The other less relevant, but described anomalies are an over-riding aorta (which sits astride the large ventricular septal defect), and hypertrophy of the right ventricle—the latter occurring as a result of the outflow obstruction which causes the ventricle to work harder.

The diagnosis of Fallot's tetralogy may be made when it is noted that a pink child becomes blue when he exerts himself or when he cries or strains. He may have more serious 'cyanotic attacks' which require sedation and oxygen therapy. These 'blue babies' may also present with fainting, shortness of breath on exertion and failure to grow at the normal rate. They may have *a raised haemoglobin level and red blood-cell count* which are responses to the desaturated oxygen level of the circulating blood.

On examination the right ventricle may be noticeably enlarged to palpation and there is a systolic bruit to the left of the sternum. The severity of the condition is determined from the clinical history, physical examination and special investigations.

Blalock-Taussig palliative anastomosis. If an infant or small child is suffering because insufficient blood is reaching his lungs, this can be corrected in part by anastomosing a systemic artery (usually the subclavian) to a branch of the pulmonary artery beyond the obstruction. *Total correction* performed later entails cardiopulmonary by-pass. The right ventricle is opened and the muscular or valvar obstruction removed. The ventricular septal defect is then closed. The child becomes pink as the right to left shunt has been closed and the way to the lungs opened out. Many of these children are extremely intelligent and their joy as they study their pink finger tips after operation is manifest for all to see.

Transposition of Great Vessels (T.G.V.). Some infants are born with the aorta arising from the right ventricle and the pulmonary artery from the left ventricle. Thus the aorta receives venous rather than arterial blood which leads to intense cyanosis. For survival at all, there must be some mixing of blood within the heart through either a patent foramen ovale in the inter-atrial septum, or through a ventricular septal defect. Ninety per cent of these babies die during the first year of life untreated. Recent advances have revolutionized this situation. By creating a larger hole in the inter-atrial septum using a catheter with a balloon on its end (Rashkind's septostomy technique), improved oxygenation and palliation are possible.

In specialized paediatric centres, using cardio-pulmonary by-pass and profound hypothermia a totally corrective intra-cardiac operation can now be performed in very small infants during the first year of life. The inter-atrial septum is removed and is replaced with a new spiral septum or 'baffle' of pericardium in such a way that the venous blood returning to the right atrium is directed to the mitral valve, left ventricle and pulmonary artery for oxygenation, whilst the blood returning from the lungs through the pulmonary veins flows to the right ventricle and thence to the aorta. In this way a 'physiological correction' of the condition has been achieved and the baby becomes fully pink and grows normally.

Acquired heart disease

See Chapter 22, p. 212 for rheumatic heart disease, rheumatic fever and chronic rheumatic heart disease.

The mitral valve. *Post-rheumatic mitral stenosis* develops gradually possibly over the 10 years following the rheumatic infection. The valve leaflets become thickened and stiffened with fusion of the edges of the leaflets along the line of the commissures which usually separate them. The chordae tendineae may become thick and short. The result is a diminution in the size of the central pathway through the valve which has become 'stenosed' or narrowed. The commonest symptom is shortness of breath.

On examination the patient suffering from mitral stenosis often has a malar flush and the hands and feet tend to be cold due to the poor cardiac output. This also leads to a 'small volume' pulse which may show atrial fibrillation. A *chest radiograph is taken* (see p. 594).

Pre-operative considerations. Many of these patients having developed atrial fibrillation at an earlier date are already receiving *digitalis*. To this a *diuretic* may have been added in order to increase the urine output and produce a degree of dehydration which diminishes the cardiac work load. *Pleural effusions* should be aspirated. *Physiotherapy* is begun now which will help the patient postoperatively as pain will restrict the chest movement. Good physiotherapy helps to ensure a speedy postoperative recovery and diminishes the likelihood of pulmonary complications.

Operation. Once thoracotomy has been performed and the chest wall held open in a strong retractor, the left lung becomes visible. The lung is carefully retracted and the pericardium is opened. The heart is handled as little as possible so as not to disturb any thrombus which may lie within the left atrial cavity. Fig. 59/6 illustrates how the surgeon introduces his

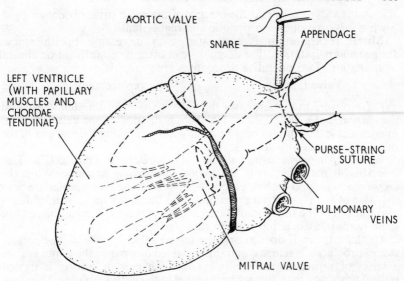

Fig. 59/6 Technique of closed mitral valvotomy. A purse-string suture placed around the neck of the left atrial appendage controls bleeding while the surgeon's index finger explores the valve.

index finger into the left atrium through its appendage. The valve is palpated and the diagnosis is confirmed. Provided the valve is suitable for valvotomy, a small incision is made in the apex of the left ventricle and the Tubb's dilator is introduced through this site. The dilator is placed across the mitral valve, its position being confirmed with the right index finger still within the atrium. The surgeon then opens the dilator with his left hand and the fused valve commissures are split open. The dilator is withdrawn and the valve function is checked with the palpating index finger as before. The finger is withdrawn from the atrium and both incisions in the heart are firmly sutured.

The results of the operation are extremely satisfactory, as the left atrial pressure is immediately lowered, pulmonary vascular congestion rapidly diminishes and dyspnoea resolves.

Mitral regurgitation may develop suddenly, or more gradually, over

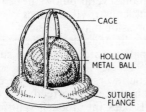

Fig. 59/7 A Starr-Edwards ball valve for mitral valve replacement. The metal ball is hollow. The metal frame is cloth-covered, allowing for tissue ingrowth.

months or years. The gradual onset of valve incompetence is often associated with mitral stenosis following rheumatic fever. The valve cusps become thickened and the commissures fused. Later calcification occurs within the valve cusps and the margin of the valve orifice becomes rigid. Such a valve may be both stenotic and regurgitant.

Mitral regurgitation is associated with increasing breathlessness, fatigue and palpitation. The diagnosis can often be established on clinical examination. Two operative procedures are available.

      1. Valve repair   2. Valve replacement

Valve repair. In certain cases the valve tissue, chordae tendineae and papillary muscles are all intact but there is dilation of the valve annulus. In such a case the annulus may be narrowed by plicating the margins of the two commissures with sutures.

Valve replacement using a ball-valve prosthesis (Fig. 59/7). This operation is performed with the aid of a heart-lung machine. When the incision is made and the heart exposed, a purse-string suture is placed about the base of the right atrial appendage and the index finger is introduced into its cavity. The function of the tricuspid valve is assessed as this may be regurgitant in association with mitral valve disease.

The left atrium is opened and the mitral valve is excised. The correct size of prosthesis is selected and this is passed down into the annulus after a series of sutures have been inserted. Each pair of sutures is ligated several times and the valve is firmly seated in the mitral annulus. The atrial incision is next sutured. As the final corner of the incision is closed great care is taken to expel any air that may have been trapped in the left side of the heart.

The aortic valve. *Aortic stenosis* may present at any age from childhood to late adult life. Although the condition is for convenience being described here among *acquired* cardiac lesions, generally speaking if serious symptoms develop during the first two decades of life, the underlying problem is likely to be that of a *congenitally malformed, usually a bicuspid valve*. Such valves may lead to symptoms during childhood, or later when the valve undergoes calcification which leads to rigidity of cusp tissue with stenosis, sometimes accompanied by regurgitation. The other main cause of aortic stenosis, like mitral stenosis, is rheumatic fever. The pathology is similar.

Paroxysmal nocturnal dyspnoea or orthopnoea are features of severe aortic stenosis. The lungs tend to be more congested when the patient lies supine and this is enough to precipitate an attack of pulmonary oedema which awakens the patient from sleep, gasping and coughing for breath. Such patients are much better propped up on several pillows in bed.

Physical signs. The pulse is normally in sinus rhythm but is of small volume with a slow upstroke. The blood pressure may be reduced but this again is not always so, many older patients having relative hypertension due to generalized atherosclerosis. These patients are in danger of sudden death and are best regarded as serious emergencies for valve replacement.

Aortic regurgitation. Following rheumatic fever, the edges of the cusps become rolled back so that they do not meet in the centre correctly. Through the deficiency so caused a jet of blood falls back into the left ventricle at each heart beat. Marked pulsation over the precordium and neck is often noticeable. *The pulse has the characteristic water-hammer action or collapsing quality* due to the sudden loss of blood back to the left ventricle through the damaged valve.

Treatment. The Starr-Edwards' ball-valve remains the most commonly used prosthesis for both mitral and aortic valve replacement and is, generally speaking, very satisfactory. The technique of replacement is similar to that employed for mitral valve replacement (see p. 604).

Coronary artery surgery. One of the debilitating symptoms of narrowing of the coronary arteries as a result of athero-sclerosis is pain, in the form of angina pectoris. This can sometimes be relieved by medical treatment. Progress has recently been made in outlining the obstructed sites in the coronary arteries by cine-angiography. In suitable cases immediate relief of anginal pain can be achieved by surgical means.

The most successful and now widely employed method is to use a length of the patient's own saphenous vein (from the thigh) as a by-pass graft from the root of the aorta (just above the aortic valve) to the affected coronary artery immediately beyond the blocked area. Two fine anastomoses are performed using delicate sutures and magnification should the surgeon find this helpful or necessary. This operation may bring dramatic relief of pain in selected patients but it is doubtful whether future 'heart-attacks' will be prevented as a result of venous by-pass grafting.

Constrictive pericarditis. Constrictive pericarditis is frequently the end result of tuberculous pericardial infection. Pus develops between the heart and the pericardial sac, which itself becomes involved in the inflammatory process. During the acute phase, if a large effusion or pyopericardium forms, cardiac tamponade (see below) may develop. Alternatively the condition may subside and its long-term sequelae may not be obvious for many years. Gradually the pericardium becomes thicker and firmer, *shrinking around the heart, which becomes encarcerated or strangled within the casing.* The patient is unwell, with the signs of right heart failure (see Chapter 22, p. 209).

The only effective treatment is surgical excision of as much of the pericardium as is possible. This can be an extremely difficult operation as the plane between the heart and the pericardium is obliterated and the thickened calcified tissue is difficult to remove without damaging the heart and coronary vessels. The results can be very satisfactory although complete relief is not always obtained.

Cardiac tamponade. This condition, although always of great importance, has assumed special significance since the advent of cardiac surgery. The patient's life may depend upon early recognition of this condition, and *it is the nurse who will be likely to observe the early changes in the patient's condition and the vital signs accompanying this.*

Tamponade arises when fluid (serum, blood or pus) increases within the inelastic pericardial sac relatively rapidly. As the sac cannot distend, being fibrous, the heart itself yields against the rising tide of incompressible fluid. The heart cavities are compressed and thus do not fill adequately in diastole and in turn put out less volume of blood at each stroke, thus the cardiac output falls, and the patient's colour becomes pale. The pulse quickens and is of low volume. The blood pressure drops and the pulse pressure narrows. The venous pressure rises and there is marked jugular venous engorgement. The patient may become restless and sweating is often a feature.

If he is under intensive care (see p. 138) and a urinary catheter is in-dwelling then a marked diminution in urine output is noticeable. *This can be the first warning sign and the patency of the urine catheter must always be ascertained to make this observation quite clear.*

The situation is urgent because, if the heart is not released by drainage of the pericardium, cardiac failure or arrest will follow quickly.

Treatment. In the case of serous effusions, these may be aspirated with immediate improvement in the patient's general and circulatory condition. Once the effusion is released, the heart is free to expand and fills properly again with a consequent improvement in its output.

Following cardiac surgery, the cause of the haemo-pericardium is likely to be leaking suture line on the heart, and in these cases it is advisable to return the patient to theatre immediately, release the tamponade and secure the bleeding point. Improvement will follow.

PREPARATION FOR OPERATION USING THE HEART-LUNG MACHINE
(For brief description of machine, see p. 598)

The patient is anaesthetized using an endotracheal tube. He is given a muscle relaxant and placed supine on the operating table. *The left radial* artery and *basilic vein* are *cannulated for monitoring the arterial and venous pressures* during and after surgery. A self-retaining urethral catheter is inserted and connected to a calibrated measuring cylinder for the assess-ment of renal function during and after the operation. *An indwelling gastric tube* is passed. Electrocardiograph leads are attached to an oscillo-scope screen to give a continuous record while the patient is in the operating theatre. *Temperature is monitored* by special probes passed into the oesophagus or the rectum. An intravenous infusion is started in a forearm vein.

A median sternotomy is made and the pericardium is opened. The patient's venous blood is taken from the heart to the machine for oxygena-tion and it is then pumped back into the arterial system beyond the heart. The patient is given intravenous heparin before the tubes are inserted into the heart. This prevents blood clotting within the circuit. Fig. 59/8 illustrates how the patient's heart is connected to the machine.

On completion of the operation the heart is allowed to take over gradually from the machine. When it is seen that the incisions are dry and the heart is able to maintain the circulation, the cannulae leading to and from the machine are removed. The heparin is neutralized by protamine sulphate given intravenously to enable blood clot to form. Care is taken to check that any major bleeding sites are controlled. If either pleural sac has been opened this is drained by underwater intercostal seal (see p. 582).

Provided the swab count is correct, the sternal and presternal tissues are closed, the wound is dressed and any chest drainage tubes are clamped during transit of the patient to the recovery ward. The monitoring pressure lines are disconnected from the equipment; the open end of each is care-fully secured either with a tap or by a syringe so that it holds pressure without leaking.

Before the patient leaves the theatre the following points will be checked:

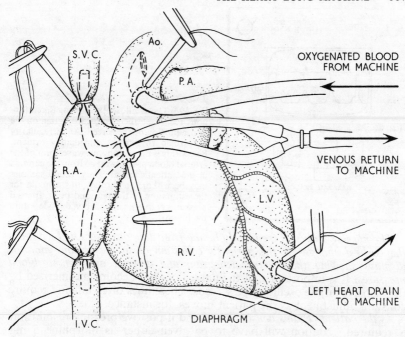

Fig. 59/8 The way in which the heart is connected to the heart-lung machine. Two venous cannulae are introduced into the right atrium via its appendage. One is passed into the superior and the other into the inferior vena cava. The arterial cannula returning oxygenated blood from the machine is placed in the ascending aorta. Once this circuit is complete perfusion is commenced and the patient's heart and lungs have been by-passed.

General condition and state of consciousness.

Rate, depth and regularity of breathing, character of pulse and its volume.

Intravenous infusions and drainage tubes are examined to see that they are accurately connected and working properly.

RECOVERY WARD ROUTINE

The patient, accompanied by anaesthetist, nurse, theatre porters and one member of the surgical team, is transferred to his own bed now in the unit. The points mentioned above are again checked.

If *positive pressure ventilation* is to be used initially, the endotracheal tube is left *in situ* connected to an oxygen source by means of an anaesthetic bag. *The intravenous fluids* are attached to drip stands. *The respirator* is connected to the endotracheal tube and set to correct pressure, rate and tidal volume. *The arterial and venous monitoring cannulae* are again connected to sterile pressure transducers which relay to an oscilloscope for visual recording. *The electrocardiograph leads are reconnected to an oscilloscope also* (see Fig. 59/9). *The urine catheter* is checked and is connected to a drainage bag or bottle, usually slung from the bed frame. *The intercostal drainage tubes* are unclamped and suction may be applied to the drainage system if desired.

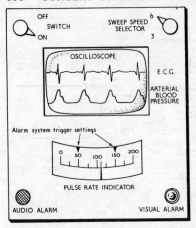

Fig. 59/9 The oscilloscope showing the continuous record of the electrocardiogram on the upper portion of the screen. Any irregularity of cardiac rhythm is immediately evident. Below this is the continuous wave-form of the arterial blood pressure taken from the cannula in the patient's radial artery. Blood samples may be withdrawn through this cannula for the estimation of the pO_2 and pCO_2 (partial pressures of oxygen and carbon dioxide within the blood).

The nursing staff will frequently be the front-line observers and will note the earliest changes in the patient's condition or in the various monitor displays showing the electrocardiogram and arterial and venous blood pressures. It is important that the nurse does not become mesmerized by the displays on the oscilloscope screens. These lines often fail and require constant adjustment as the patient moves, for instance.

As the patient regains consciousness and if positive pressure respiration is required, sedation will have to be given either as morphine 5 mg intravenously or phenoperidine 2 mg intravenously and droperidol 10 mg as required. It is essential that the patient remains sufficiently relaxed to 'accept' the positive pressure respiration from the machine, without fighting against it.

The patient's temperature may be cold at this stage, and it is essential to ascertain this early, as a cool patient tends to be vasoconstricted, with an inadequate peripheral circulation, and there is a tendency to acidosis. Blankets are usually sufficient to elevate the temperature to normality.

A rapid assessment is made of the patient's general condition and vital signs are recorded and charted.

His level of consciousness, colour, depth of breathing, chest movement for full lung expansion on both sides of the thorax, pulse volume and character.

The heart rate is obtained by counting with a stethoscope for at least 30 seconds, also noting and checking the configuration of the electrocardiograph on the oscilloscope tracing.

The arterial blood pressure is checked by 'cuff' method and compared with the tracing on the oscilloscope.

The venous pressure is obtained, making quite certain that the apparatus is working efficiently, by noting a free rise and fall of fluid in the manometer.

An *arterial blood sample* is obtained from the arterial cannula and the blood gases and acid-base balance of the patient are measured. It is best to wait for half an hour after return to the ward for this as the patient will then have settled into a state of equilibrium and a more valuable set of values will be obtained.

Any patient under treatment with positive pressure ventilation is liable to develop gastric retention and dilatation with a degree of intestinal ileus. Gastric dilatation can upset cardiac action and may cause hypotension, therefore a *naso-gastric tube* should be passed which can drain freely into a container, or be aspirated intermittently.

It is absolutely essential that the drainage tubes are kept patent by 'milking' them either by hand, or with a roller. Should these tubes become blocked with clot, in the presence of continuing cardiac bleeding, *tamponade* may develop due to cardiac compression (see p. 605).

The quantity of blood draining each 15 minutes is recorded on a cumulative chart, with the other *vital signs* mentioned above. In addition the *urine output* is also recorded as this gives an excellent measure of the state of tissue perfusion, evidence in fact of the state of the patient's cardiac output and circulatory state. *A certain volume of fluid and blood replacement* will have been ordered to be given by intravenous infusion.

Additional drugs are sometimes added to the intravenous fluids— possibly isoprenaline or potassium. *The rate at which such solutions are administered is vital.* Isoprenaline stimulates the left ventricle to contract forcibly and increases the heart rate. *If a 'drip' is inadvertently allowed to run through too quickly the patient's life can be lost as ventricular tachycardia or fibrillation may result.*

The foregoing description may cause even the 'strongest kneed' to shake a little, as the most experienced and skilled may be sorely tested during this phase of the patient's management. With proper understanding and training all this can be mastered and the work, although demanding the highest endeavour from every member of the team, is tremendously satisfying and rewarding.

THE NURSE IN THE TEAM

The patient, having been settled in bed, assisted by doctors and anaesthetist, is now in the care of his nurses. At least one and sometimes two fully trained nurses are needed for each patient in an intensive care ward. These nurses are selected for their knowledge, skill and familiarity with the apparatus in use; they must be possessed of high integrity, resource and initiative, calm and considerate and very sure, so that the patient (when he is well enough) and his relatives may always have absolute confidence in those to whose care the patient is entrusted.

An experienced doctor and an anaesthetist, stationed in the same area as the intensive care unit, are within call day and night, but the decision to summon medical aid *depends on the nurses* who must therefore be able to recognize changes in the patient's condition or in the information from the monitoring apparatus.

In no case may this patient be left unattended. *The nurse will be given instructions on the position in which he is to lie but as soon as his condition permits a patient is most comfortable when he is supported sitting up.*

The intercostal drainage tubes (there may be one to four of these) need constant observation to ensure that drainage is continuous; measurement of the amount should be noted, excessive bleeding from the tubes is observed and reported as this needs investigation. Dressings around the tubes should be watched for oozing and changed as necessary.

Blood transfusion begun in the theatre will be continued as long as is necessary and is then followed by *fluid infusion* until the patient is able to take fluid by mouth.

The stomach contents can be aspirated through the *indwelling gastric tube* until bowel sounds are normal, when the patient may begin to drink.

Urine. The *indwelling catheter*, inserted before operation, enables urine to be evacuated and the bladder kept empty. The amount should be recorded every hour, the specific gravity taken every four hours and a laboratory specimen examined for electrolyte and urea content every 24 hours. All this is essential in order to detect indication of renal failure early, as this is a serious complication.

A careful fluid balance chart is kept. It should include all fluid given as blood or fluid infusion and taken by mouth and all fluid lost by gastric aspiration, from the intercostal drainage tubes, bleeding, urinary output and from any diarrhoea.

Nursing observations which should be made without intermission from the moment the patient returns from the theatre until his condition has stabilized include: *his exact conscious state*—whether he is rational and responsive and can move his limbs when requested; his *pupils* if equal and reacting to light; any twitchings or signs of hyper-alertness and restlessness (see below). Any of these may indicate cerebral anoxia which may be due to pulmonary or circulatory factors.

Restlessness may be due to pain, to a full bladder (the indwelling catheter may be blocked), to haemorrhage, to respiratory distress, or to the patient's cerebral state just mentioned. Restlessness needs medical investigation; in the meantime, all unnecessary movement should be avoided and oxygen should always be available.

The colour and character of the skin are indications of the general condition of a patient. *The colour* should be watched for pinkness, pallor or cyanosis, and the colour of the nails noted. *The character* includes such features as whether the skin is cold and clammy, warm and clammy, dry (warm or cool), or the patient shivering.

The blood pressure is taken at regular intervals, generally every 15 minutes at first. The blood pressure should always be compared with pre-operative readings; the sounds should be distinctly audible. Drugs the patient is having may affect his blood pressure. *A raised or a low pressure and any changes in pressure should be reported.*

The pulse. The volume and regularity should be noted every 15 minutes; if the *rate* is above 120 or below 60 a minute, this should be reported. *It is important to note and record that all the peripheral pulses are of the same volume.*

Respiration. The character is a good guide to a patient's condition. *The depth of breathing* is most important after cardiac surgery. The rate, regularity, any use of the accessory muscles of respiration, whether both sides of the chest rise and fall equally, should all be noted; *a respiratory rate above 40 a minute indicates some distress which should be reported.* It may be accompanied by restlessness (see above).

When the temperature is low it is essential to prevent or stop the patient shivering, as the muscular exertion involved may result in some degree of heart failure. As a rule a sedative, e.g. morphine, is ordered and the patient may be warmed gently.

Medicines and drugs. Antibiotics first given the day before operation are continued for 7 to 10 days. Sedatives will be given if necessary. Laxatives are used as required, but fluid is carefully regulated.

Fluid intake. From the outset while given as intravenous infusion the amount is limited to 1·5 to 2 litres each 24 hours. When the patient begins to drink, this is slowly increased but he is limited to 2·5 litres each 24 hours during the time he spends in hospital both in the unit and in the general ward. When he is having light diet the fluid contained in fruit and vegetables, sauces and gravies is included in this maximum quantity. *This is a nursing point which needs the most meticulous care.*

Visitors may look at the patient for a few minutes in *the first instance* but should not be surprised if he does not appear to be aware of their presence. As the hours pass visits may be frequent but very short. *Co-operating with the nurses, visitors should be able to recognize the signs of approaching fatigue and withdraw before the patient is tired.*

Some patients are apathetic for a day or two, easily tired and should never be wearied. Some are mentally disturbed, disorientated and have hallucinations; others recover more quickly. Happily few patients remember how very ill they have been; they have forgotten the early hours of their distress. A few complain of disturbing dreams.

Time spent in the recovery ward. The patient remains in the recovery ward until it is safe to transfer him back to the general ward. This may be after 48 hours or four to five days. Occasionally a critically ill patient will require special attention with intermittent positive pressure respiration or tracheostomy for up to two weeks.

In straightforward cardiac surgery the patient may be up after a day or two. The recovery of those with valvular replacement will depend on the condition of the heart muscle at the time of operation. There is no hard and fast rule, and the patient's general condition, the length and type of illness which preceded operation, the procedures undertaken and the patient's response to postoperative measures, will all be considered.

Nursing points in the general ward. Special care is required in maintaining accurate fluid balance charts. The patient will be on a restricted fluid intake of about 2·5 litres each 24 hours and a light diet. Many patients are in some degree of cardiac failure requiring digitalis and diuretics and some valve-replacement patients may be on anticoagulant drugs.

Physiotherapy is important at this stage; many patients are remarkably well and need gradual mobilization and encouragement. Most patients leave the ward after two weeks but may need intermediate care before they are ready to return home.

Advice on returning home. Many patients feel so well within a few weeks of operation that there is a danger that they may do too much. *The heart takes many months to re-adjust fully to its new situation and this is explained to every patient.* Activity may be increased slowly and gradually. Tiredness and breathlessness are the usual warning signs that too much is being attempted. Drugs must be very clearly labelled and the regime of therapy explained fully to the patient or to relatives. He should be warned against getting tired; if he has a cold he should stay in bed and send for his doctor. The doctor will have received a detailed medical report from the hospital and a patient should never hesitate to call him in.

Chapter 60

Diseases of the Ears, Nose and Throat

Nursing Care

by L. F. W. SALMON

> *Examination of the patient—some common procedures: cleansing and syringing the ear, aural medications, ear dressings, nasal douching— diseases of the ear—diseases of the nose and paranasal sinuses— diseases of the throat—malignant disease of the ears, nose and throat*

The nursing of patients suffering from disease of the ears, nose and throat is concerned chiefly with general problems, most of which have been considered in the preceding pages. However, there are a number of nursing procedures peculiar to these patients and the description of them forms the subject of this chapter.

EXAMINATION OF THE PATIENT

Examination of the ears, nose and throat is best undertaken with the patient seated facing the surgeon, preferably in a clinical room, with the necessary instruments conveniently arranged close to the surgeon's right hand. The majority of these patients are ambulant during the greater part of their stay in hospital. A number of minor surgical procedures as well as dressing will be undertaken in the clinical room, and *the nurse should be familiar with these techniques as well as with nursing the patient in the usual sense. This aspect of her work resembles what she may be called on to do in the ears, nose and throat out-patient department.*

As well as learning to attend efficiently to the surgeon examining the patient, *the nurse should herself acquire a certain facility at examining the ears, nose and throat, since without it she will be unable to carry out properly certain of the minor procedures she may be required to undertake. These include such things as syringing the ear, inserting a gauze wick into the external meatus, removing stitches at the entrance to the ear or nose and removing a pack from the nose.* This means that she should learn to use a head mirror. The passages to be examined are usually deep and narrow and the adequate illumination of them is not possible using a torch or an Anglepoise lamp in the usual way. The source of light is placed just above and behind the patient's left shoulder and reflected from the mirror into the place to be examined. The eye is located behind the opening in the mirror so that the line of vision corresponds with the axis of the beam of light.

Fig. 60/1 illustrates the instruments in everyday use, set out as they might be in the clinical room on the ward. The manner of their use can be learned better by carefully observing the surgeon at work than by a wordy description, but a few lines about some of them may be helpful.

In many clinics the aural specula which are provided in a range of sizes are designed to fit the Siegle's otoscope. This is an instrument which, as well as providing a degree of magnification, allows the surgeon to vary the pressure in the external ear and so test, among other things, the mobility of the tympanic membrane.

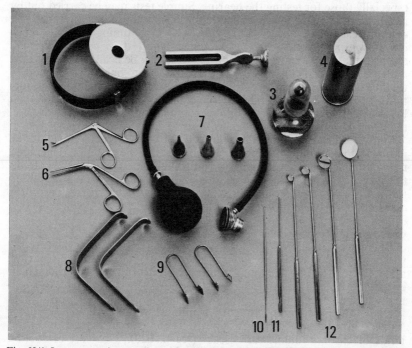

Fig. 60/1 Instruments in everyday use. 1. Head mirror. 2. Tuning fork. 3. Spirit lamp. 4. Cotton-wool dispenser. 5. Cawthorne's aural forceps. 6. Tilley's dressing forceps. 7. Modified Siegle's otoscope with specula. 8. Lack's tongue depressors. 9. Thudicum's nasal specula. 10. Jobson-Horne wool carrier. 11. Wax hook. 12. Post-nasal and laryngeal mirrors.

A range of sizes is provided, too, in the small mirrors seen on the right of Fig. 60/1. The small ones are for examining the nasopharynx or post-nasal space, the compartment at the back of the nose where, in children, the adenoids are located. The larger ones are for *indirect laryngoscopy*. If the surgeon is unable to see as much as he would like with the mirror, or if something is revealed, e.g. a growth in the larynx or deep part of the pharynx which he must remove or from which he must take a biopsy, he is likely to order *direct laryngoscopy*, usually under general anaesthesia. The throat is a sensitive place and a few patients will find that examination with the mirror produces uncontrollable retching, making adequate inspection impossible. The surgeon may then choose to spray the throat with a local anaesthetic agent such as a 2 per cent solution of cocaine. If this is done *the patient must be warned to take nothing by mouth for two hours afterwards*, or he may find it 'going the wrong way', i.e. into the larynx and air passages.

An invaluable instrument which is shown in Fig. 60/1 is the Jobson-Horne wool carrier. It is *not* used as a probe. The plain end is intended to take a *wisp* of cotton wool for ear mopping, etc., while the ring is useful for many purposes such as removing wax from the ear.

Testing the hearing

In the out-patient department many other instruments will be needed, especially those for testing the hearing. Simple tests may be carried out by requiring the patient to repeat spoken or whispered words, listening first with one ear then the other, and by using a simple tuning fork. *The nurse can demonstrate the essence of the tuning-fork test on herself.* She will discover that the sound of the vibrating fork may be heard not only when the prongs are held close to her ear (air conduction) but also if the butt of the fork is pressed on the mastoid process, behind the ear (bone conduction). Normally the sound is heard longer or louder by air conduction than by bone conduction but in middle-ear, in contrast to inner-ear, disease, the reverse holds true.

Simple tests such as these are not sufficient, however, to elucidate the nature or to determine the degree of deafness with the precision demanded today. Sophisticated electronic apparatus (audiometers) are needed to do this and the help of technicians skilled in their use. *The nurse is advised to watch an audiology technician at work and acquaint herself with the essentials of this kind of test.*

Operating microscope

Reference is made on p. 622 to the use of the operating microscope without which no ear, nose and throat operating theatre can be regarded as complete. It will not be long before such an instrument is considered an essential feature of the equipment of the out-patient department, too, and many of the larger hospitals provide this facility.

One of the procedures frequently employed with the help of the microscope is aspiration of keratin found to accumulate in the ear in certain kinds of chronic middle-ear disease (see p. 620). This sort of suction clearance is an everyday feature of the work of a busy ears, nose and throat department, in the out-patient department as much as in the operating theatre, and imposes on the nurse concerned the need to be familiar with a further technicality.

Investigating giddiness

The inner ear is concerned not only with hearing but also balance, so that the disease which interferes with the function of this part is likely to cause giddiness as well as deafness. The full investigation of giddiness is something that only a few hospitals are equipped to undertake. Most ears, nose and throat departments, however, will employ caloric testing for such cases and the doctor performing the tests will rely greatly on the nurse's help. If water considerably above or below blood heat is used to irrigate the ear (see p. 617) the patient is likely to feel giddy and develop characteristic regular jerky movements of the eyes called nystagmus. By controlling the temperature of the water and the duration of the irrigation and by measuring the duration of the resultant nystagmus, important information may be obtained about the function of the balance component of the inner ear. *The careful adjustment of the temperature of the water used and the timing of the test with a stop-watch, not to mention the sympathetic management of an apprehensive patient, is usually the responsibility of the nurse.*

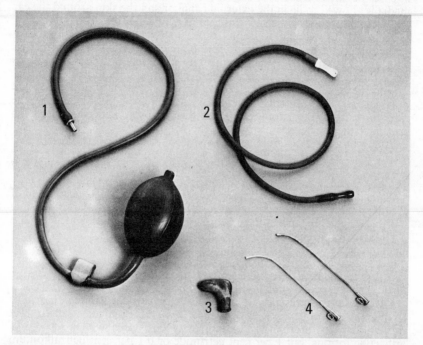

Fig. 60/2 Apparatus for inflating the middle ear. 1. The Politzer bag. 2. Auscultation tube. 3. Gardiner-Browne's nosepiece (the vulcanite mount to connect with the Luer fitting on the Politzer bag is not shown). 4. Eustachian catheters.

Finally attention must be drawn to the Eustachian catheter and related apparatus for inflating the middle ear by way of the Eustachian tube (Fig. 60/2). The Politzer bag is attached to the catheter after it has been passed through the nose and manipulated so that the tip engages the lower end of the Eustachian tube. The auscultation tube allows the surgeon to listen to the sound of air passing through the tube. The Gardiner-Browne nosepiece is suitable for inflating the ear in children or where the use of the Eustachian catheter is otherwise contra-indicated. It is used to occlude the nostril while air is forced through the nose with the Politzer bag.

SOME COMMON PROCEDURES

Cleansing the ear

The nurse must make herself expert at cleansing the ear and her skilled attention to the discharging ear may achieve a significant reduction in the duration of the patient's illness, diminish his discomfort and avert complications.

The discharge may be the result of infection of the middle ear, *otitis media*, escaping through a perforation in the drum-head, or of the skin of the external ear, *otitis externa*, or of both together. The last-named variety exemplifies why adequate attention to the toilet of the canal is imperative in cases of otitis media with discharge. If the discharge in a case of otitis media is allowed to lie in the external canal or soil the skin around the ear the probability is that the skin will become infected, too.

To avoid this sequence of events, the first step must be adequate control of the hair. If the hair is allowed to festoon the ear, it soon becomes matted with the discharge or even gummed by it to the external ear and its surroundings so that secondary infection of the skin is more than likely. To pin the hair back from the ear with clips is seldom adequate and the only sure method of control is to make a number of tight plaits. At the time of writing, the happy era when this problem applied only to the female of the species seems to be on the way out.

The canal is best cleansed with cotton wool mounted on a Jobson-Horne wool carrier or on a wooden applicator. Only a wisp of wool is necessary since if the mop is bulky it will not reach the deep part of the meatus or will abrade the skin if forced in. The nature of the discharge should be carefully noted and the number of mops necessary to obtain a dry ear. The nature of the discharge will provide valuable information about the underlying pathology. For instance, the presence of mucus means otitis media and a perforated tympanic membrane since there are no mucus-secreting elements in the external ear. *It will be necessary to cleanse the ear more or less often according to the amount of discharge. If discharge is visible at the entrance to the meatus or, worse, if it is seen to have dried at the entrance to the ear, it is a reflection on the quality of the nursing.*

Of course, the presence of dried discharge in and around the ear is frequently a problem at the outset of treatment and may call for wet rather than dry mopping. The mop may be wetted with a variety of antiseptic lotions, but 1 per cent cetrimide or 0·1 per cent benzalkonium chloride solution are among the best.

It is generally a mistake to tuck dry cotton wool into the meatus if the ear is discharging since the wool becomes soiled by the discharge which is thereby held in contact with the skin. The possible exception is overnight since it is not reasonable to wake the patient frequently at night to mop the ear. However, if cotton wool is to be tucked into the ear or a dressing of some sort applied overnight, e.g. by means of an ear 'cage' (see p. 619), it is imperative that the skin of the canal and the well of the ear (the concha) are protected with a layer of ointment, e.g. gentamicin ointment, painted on carefully with a cotton-dressed applicator after the last dry mopping before the patient is settled for the night.

Syringing the ear

Sometimes the best way to cleanse the ear is to syringe it. This applies particularly if wax is to be removed or if there is a considerable accumulation of moist keratin present. *Syringing an ear is not something that may be learned by reading about it and no nurse should attempt to syringe an ear unless she has been shown how to do it by an experienced teacher and has attempted it on a number of occasions under supervision.* She should not take it upon herself to decide that an ear should be syringed but should leave this decision to the doctor. The instruments required are shown in Fig. 60/3. The syringe must be checked for efficiency, in particular to ensure that the piston moves freely in the barrel, before being charged with tap water at a temperature of 37 °C (99 °F), i.e. just above blood heat. If it is too cold or too hot it will cause giddiness. Any air drawn into the syringe must be expelled with the syringe inverted.

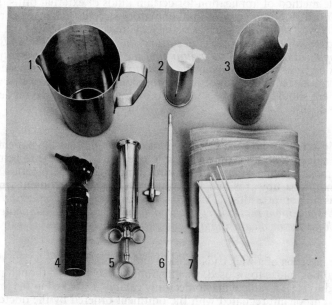

Fig. 60/3 Apparatus needed for syringing the ear. 1. Measuring jug for warm water. 2. Cotton-wool dispenser. 3. Ear trough or tank. 4. Electric otoscope. 5. Aural syringe with pipe. 6. Lotion thermometer. 7. Waterproof (plastic) cape, towel, wooden applicators for cotton-wool buds.

The patient, seated in a good light, his clothing protected by a plastic cape over the shoulders, holds a suitable receiver, a kidney dish or an ear trough, firmly beneath the ear. *The nurse pulls the pinna upwards and backwards and places the tip of the nozzle just inside the entrance to the meatus up against the postero-superior quadrant. She then ejects the water into the ear with more or less force.* Very little is needed to remove debris and discharge but impacted wax may call for considerable force. It is the question of how much force, more than anything else, that the nurse must learn under supervision. When everything seems to have been washed out, she will incline the patient's head to one side to empty the canal of fluid and dry the external ear. The ear must then be inspected with the head mirror or an electric otoscope (auriscope) to make sure that nothing abnormal remains. If anything remains, further syringing follows until the ear is seen to be quite clear and an unobstructed view of the tympanic membrane obtained. The syringing must never be regarded as completed before the external canal has been thoroughly dried, for instance with wool-dressed applicators in the way described above for cleansing the ear.

The application of medications to the ear

The nurse may be required to insert drops into the ear or apply medications on half-inch ribbon gauze, a gauze wick. The medication may be in the form of solutions or suspensions, perhaps the same as would be used on another occasion as ear drops, or as an ointment. The latter is a particularly suitable method of application for certain kinds of external otitis. Drops and ointments containing anti-inflammatory steroids like hydrocortisone together with antibiotics such as neomycin are very widely used but in this context a word of warning is necessary. *In susceptible individuals, such local applications may set up irritation of the skin and this possibility must always be borne in mind. Neomycin is particularly suspect.* The occurrence of irritation, redness and weeping of the skin in the course of this sort of treatment should always be a signal to discontinue it, pending a decision by the doctor.

To insert drops into the ear, the nurse should instruct the patient to lie on his side or hold his head well over to one side with the ear to be treated uppermost. Having drawn the required amount into the pipette she will pull the pinna upwards and backwards and expel the contents into the meatus a drop at a time. *Three drops is usually enough unless otherwise stated. The patient should keep his head in position for several minutes, long enough for the medication to apply itself thoroughly.*

The insertion of a wick calls for skill and experience. The length of half-inch ribbon gauze to be used, usually about three inches—though more is needed to treat a radical mastoidectomy cavity—is soaked in the lotion in an oil cup or impregnated with the ointment ordered by the doctor. The latter is most easily carried out by squeezing the ointment along a wooden spatula, laying the gauze on top and working in the ointment with a second spatula.

Once ready, the length of gauze must be gently inserted into the ear. If the nurse is experienced with a head mirror she will find it best to use it, otherwise the patient is seated in a good light. The ribbon gauze is gently tucked, not packed, into the meatus using an aural dressing forceps and taking care to reach the deep part of the meatus adjacent to the tympanic membrane.

Dressing the ear

It will be necessary to keep the ear covered with sterile dressings after most operations on the ear, and the nurse is usually required to change these from time to time.

There are one or two special considerations:

> Gauze loosely bunched up behind and above the ear will support it in a natural position away from the head, adding to the patient's comfort, and should be applied whether there is an incision behind the ear or not.
>
> Gauze similarly applied in the well of the ear is likely to become

soiled with discharge and adhere to the skin. It is generally desirable to protect the skin with an antibiotic ointment, e.g. gentamicin ointment (see p. 616).

For some days after many ear operations, e.g. mastoidectomy and tympanoplasty, the dressings must be held firmly in position with a suitable bandage. A loose-woven bandage, such as the Kling bandage, is very comfortable.

Within a few days it is usually possible to dispense with a bandage in favour of an ear 'cage'. This is a circular wire frame to which is sewn a fabric 'cup'. Tapes round the head apply it to the ear and maintain the dressings comfortably in place.

Nursing the deaf patient

Patients afflicted with varying degrees of deafness will be found throughout the hospital, and the more severe cases are liable to try the patience even of a nurse. Some will have hearing aids and should be encouraged to use them. The small battery may have run down and must be replaced. For those without them it may be possible to arrange for an emergency issue of a hearing aid from a hearing aid centre. Encouragement and help from the ward staff will be necessary if the patient is to overcome the difficulties inherent in learning to use the appliance. Quite apart from hearing aids, however, *there are a number of points about communicating with the deaf that the nurse should bear in mind. These include remembering to speak so that the patient can see your face, speaking slowly and distinctly and refraining from shouting.*

Inhalations

Inhalations of medicated steam are likely to be ordered for patients with such complaints as laryngitis, tracheitis and sometimes sinusitis. The details are described in Chapter 9.

Nasal drops

Nasal drops frequently do more harm than good. Nevertheless, the nurse should be familiar with the correct procedure for introducing them when ordered. The patient lies on his back with the head lower than the shoulders, the pipette is charged and the solution applied a drop at a time first into one nostril, then the other until, say, three drops have found their way high into the nose on either side. Paper tissues should be provided for the patient to mop up any excess when he sits up.

Douching the nose

Irrigating the nose with warm saline solution is indicated for such diseases as atrophic rhinitis in which the nose becomes obstructed by scabs. There are a number of ways of doing this including sniffing the solution up the nose, but the technique least open to objection entails the use of the so-called siphon nasal douche. This consists essentially of a length of rubber tubing weighted at one end to keep it at the bottom of a jug of warm saline solution and having at the other end a plastic olive. The olive is applied to the nostril and through it flows the irrigating fluid with no greater force than that represented by a head of water of some 18 inches.

First one side then the other is washed out, the patient holding his head forward over a basin situated some 18 inches (45 cm) lower than the reservoir of saline.

DISEASES OF THE EARS

The ear consists of three anatomically distinct components: the external ear, including the pinna and the external auditory meatus down to the tympanic membrane; the middle ear, including the Eustachian tube, the tympanic cavity with the three auditory ossicles, the malleus, incus and stapes and the mastoid air cells; and lastly, the inner ear locked up in the temporal bone and comprising the cochlea, vestibular apparatus and semi-circular canals. The cochlea is concerned with hearing, the other parts of the inner ear, with balance. A disturbance of the normal function of the ear may result in deafness or giddiness (vertigo). The former may result from disease of the external, middle or inner ear, whereas the latter is usually due to disease of the inner ear or its connection to or in the brain. Some of the commoner varieties of ear disease are listed below.

External ear

Wax. The skin of the external ear secretes a ceruminous substance commonly called wax. It has a protective function and constitutes a source of trouble only when it accumulates in sufficient quantity to occlude the canal and interfere with hearing. When this occurs, it may be necessary to remove the excess by syringing the ear (see p. 616).

Foreign body. Not uncommonly, a child is tempted to introduce a foreign body, e.g. a bead, into the external auditory meatus. It usually causes no trouble and may be discovered accidentally years later. *The nurse should not attempt to remove it however simple the undertaking may seem. The chances are she will push it deeper into the canal and render its subsequent removal more difficult.*

External otitis. This term is used to describe any sort of skin disease involving the pinna and external auditory meatus and is, therefore, very common indeed. It may be due to bacteria or fungi; it may be diffuse or localized; it may be primary or secondary to a discharge from the middle ear. Occasionally, it may be an outcropping in or around the ear of some generalized skin disease such as eczema or psoriasis. The treatment includes careful cleansing and the use of suitable applications as drops or gauze wicks. Less frequently systemic antibiotics are called for. From time to time, boils (furuncles) form in the external ear and, once in a while, may need incising.

The middle ear

The middle ear is particularly liable to two kinds of harmful influence, the first due to failure of the Eustachian tube to maintain atmospheric pressure in the middle ear, the second due to the onslaught of bacteria with resulting infection. Very often, particularly in childhood, the former encourages the latter.

If the middle ear is to function normally the air pressure in the tympanic cavity must be the same as that of the atmosphere outside. Most of the time, this is ensured by periodic opening of the Eustachian tube during the act of swallowing. In some individuals, for reasons not always understood, this mechanism is imperfect and a negative pressure tends to develop in the middle ear. This occurs frequently in childhood, particularly in the so-called 'catarrhal child'. It may be associated with the presence in the post-nasal space into which the Eustachian tubes open of an excess of lymphoid tissue called *adenoids*. Two common diseases may follow and, in many children, both. These are recurrent exudative otitis media and recurrent acute (suppurative) otitis media.

Exudative otitis media. Since the wide use of antibiotics has reduced the gravity and complications of acute otitis media to easily manageable proportions, more attention has been paid to a more insidious variety of ear disease in childhood. Unlike acute otitis media, it does not keep the child and the family awake with earache, it does not produce an objectionable discharge from the ear and it does not lead, in the short term, to alarming complications like mastoiditis and meningitis. It simply renders the child hard of hearing and liable to be blamed unjustly by parent and teacher alike for inattention. It is due to the pouring out of an exudate into the middle ear, displacing the air and often acquiring an intensely thick and tenacious consistency that has earned for this disease the name 'glue ear'.

Treatment includes one or more of the following measures: removal of adenoids, incision of the tympanic membrane (myringotomy) and aspiration of the exudate and, very often, the fitting of a tiny plastic self-retaining device popularly called 'a grommet'. This is insinuated into the myringotomy incision in the membrane rather like a shirt-stud in a shirt and is responsible for by-passing the malfunctioning Eustachian tube and maintaining atmospheric pressure in the middle ear, in spite of it.

Acute otitis media. Like exudative otitis media, this is characteristically a disease of childhood, but here the middle-ear cleft becomes invaded by micro-organisms from the post-nasal space. It must be regarded, therefore, as a complication of some infection involving this area. At one time, the infectious fevers of childhood, particularly measles and scarlet fever, were the commonest cause but, nowadays, the common cold leads to most of these cases. Many children have a marked predisposition to this disease and the factors considered above seem to be concerned. Frequently the infection clears up but a sterile exudate remains, or attacks of acute otitis media and 'glue ear' occur in one and the same child. Earache, fever, deafness and discharge are the distinguishing symptoms, although a mild case will resolve with or without treatment, before the drum-head ruptures and discharge appears.

Treatment is by giving the appropriate antibiotic soon enough, in adequate doses and for as long as can be relied upon to cure the individual attack. Proper care of the discharging ear (see above) is an important responsibility for the nurse, if the case finds its way into hospital.

Complications of acute otitis media. The commonest of these was mastoiditis, but this is now a rare disease. The classical picture with an abscess behind the ear pushing the ear downwards and forwards is, today, a curiosity and cortical mastoidectomy, once the accepted treatment, is now almost never performed.

Similarly, meningitis, brain abscess and venous sinus thrombosis are today extremely uncommon complications.

Chronic suppurative otitis media. The absence of pain and fever at the onset, the slow progress of the deafness, the scanty offensive nature of the discharge, the age of the patient, usually an adult, and the duration of the symptoms, often dating back many years, distinguish this disease from acute otitis media. The patient may be so little troubled by it that he regards medical advice as unnecessary although, again in contrast to acute otitis media, such complications as meningitis, brain abscess and paralysis of the face, are still encountered and a patient with chronic suppurative otitis media may, for this reason, be sitting on the edge of a volcano.

A conspicuous feature of many of these cases is the occurrence of a polyp, which may reach such a size as to present to view at the entrance to the external auditory meatus.

To complete this summary of chronic otitis media it must be recorded that many of these cases require an operation to clear them up. There forms in the recesses of the middle ear an accumulation of keratin—the horny substance produced elsewhere by the skin—and called in this location *cholesteatoma*. Its presence is associated with the risk of complications and its removal can be effected only by surgical means. The surest of these is the radical mastoidectomy in which the diseased remains of the tympanic membrane, malleus and incus are removed, sometimes with further damage to the already depleted hearing. With the arrival of the operating microscope (see p. 614) and further refinements, the surgeon of today will often attempt to conserve or improve hearing by certain reconstructive procedures called collectively *tympanoplasty*. Attempts are made to reconstruct the tympanic membrane even by the use of transplant techniques and to restore the function of the auditory ossicles.

Pre-operative nursing attention includes shaving the hair from round the ear to a distance of some two inches, and the postoperative care will include dressings and the careful cleansing of the ear as described above.

Otosclerosis is a non-suppurative condition of the middle ear which causes progressive deafness often commencing in the twenties or thirties. It is due to a change in the bone round the oval window between the middle ear and inner ear, leading to fixation of the stirrup bone (stapes), the ossicle that fits into the oval window. It is far more common than was once thought.

Treatment. The earlier operations of fenestration and stapes mobilization have now given way entirely to stapedectomy. Under the operating microscope, part of the fixed stapes is removed and replaced by a suitably shaped prosthesis made of plastic or stainless steel. The patient is giddy for a few days afterwards and may need to remain still in bed. Drugs like dimenhydrinate (Dramamine) may be ordered.

Diseases of the inner ear

The dual function of the inner ear with regard to both hearing and balance has been mentioned above, and also the place of audiometry and caloric tests in the diagnosis of the diseases affecting this part. With one exception they are rare, the exception being the deafness of old age. Patients are not admitted to hospital because of senile deafness though, as mentioned on p. 619, it will occur frequently as an intercurrent problem among those who are.

However, rare as the other diseases may be, they are important and the nurse should know of them.

Labyrinthitis. Middle-ear infection may spread to involve the inner ear, particularly in the presence of cholesteatoma (see p. 622). The resulting suppurative labyrinthitis is a dangerous disease which, at best, results in a totally deaf ear and, at worst, leads to meningitis. The patient is violently giddy and sick.

Labyrinthitis is also the term used to describe a much milder variety of giddiness unrelated to middle-ear disease and thought to be due to virus infection. It spares the hearing and complete recovery is the rule.

Ménière's disease. Usually affecting one ear only, this distressing illness results in paroxysms of disabling giddiness, noises in the head (tinnitus) and progressive perceptive deafness. It is important to differentiate it from the benign tumour of the nerve of hearing (acoustic neuroma), which may produce a remarkably similar picture.

Acoustic neuroma. Although a benign tumour, its slow but inevitable growth in the angle between the mid-brain and the cerebellum leads to increasing deafness and unsteadiness. As soon as the diagnosis is confirmed by special skull X-rays or lumbar puncture, the case must be placed in the care of a neuro-surgeon for operative treatment.

DISEASES OF THE NOSE AND PARANASAL SINUSES

Foreign body. Just as in the case of the ear, children are liable to push foreign bodies of all kinds up the nose and here, too, *the advice to the nurse is the same. Never be tempted to remove them, the danger in this case being the possibility of pushing the offending object into the post-nasal space, from which situation it may be inhaled and end up in the lung.* The foreign body in the ear generally excites no reaction. That in the nose usually does. It will produce profuse nasal discharge, sometimes bloodstained and, in many cases, a characteristically disagreeable smell.

Nose bleed (epistaxis) may be symptomatic of severe nasal disease, e.g. cancer of the nose or sinuses, or of grave generalized disease, e.g. certain blood diseases. More often it is due to direct injury, such as a blow on the nose, but far and away the majority of cases occur in the absence of any serious preceding disease or circumstance. There are two main categories.

The first is where the bleeding comes from dilated veins just inside the nose on the septum. Children and adolescents are liable to this kind of epistaxis. It is easily controlled, as a rule, by putting the head forward and pressing firmly with a finger on the side of the nose. If necessary, the veins concerned are readily cauterized, for instance by the cautious application of a caustic substance, such as trichloracetic acid.

The second category, seen characteristically in the elderly patient with arteriosclerosis, is where the bleeding may arise from anywhere in the nose, often towards the back. It may be very copious and stop as suddenly as it starts.

Treatment. The doctor is likely to want to *pack the nose* and may give instructions for preparations to be made for a blood transfusion (see p. 456). If the nose is to be packed *the nurse will be expected to prepare a tray or trolley, including a gown for the doctor, a cape or towels to protect the patient's bedclothes, a kidney dish, gauze or cotton swabs, a box of paper tissues, ribbon gauze, nasal specula, nasal dressing forceps, a Jobson-Horne wool carrier, 2 per cent cocaine solution and sterile liquid paraffin with which to impregnate the ribbon gauze.* Sometimes the doctor will indicate his intention to introduce *a pack into the post-nasal space.* In addition to what is listed above, this calls for specially prepared post-nasal gauze packs with attached tapes and a soft rubber catheter of small gauge. The catheter, introduced through the nose, is used to draw the pack through the mouth into the post-nasal space.

In the most severe cases of epistaxis, the bleeding persists or recurs in spite of all such measures and it is necessary to tie off, in the operating theatre, the artery supplying the bleeding point.

A first-aid measure of major importance should be attempted by the nurse while waiting for the doctor, or may be ordered by the doctor before he proceeds with packing. This was originally described by Wilfred Trotter and depends upon creating the best possible conditions for spontaneous clotting to occur. *The patient is sat up, preferably in a comfortable chair, and propped forward with the head over a receiver into which the blood drips from the nose. A cork is placed between his teeth to discourage him from hawking and spitting.*

Nasal obstruction is the leading symptom in very many diseases and disorders of the nose, certain of which are described below. The commonest, the common cold, is mentioned elsewhere in connection with its complications such as otitis media and sinusitis.

Deviated nasal septum. The partition dividing one side of the nose from the other is seldom entirely straight or confined to the midline. *Treatment* is required, however, only if the deviation is sufficient to cause nasal obstruction, when the operation of *submucous resection* must be considered.

It consists of removing the distorted bone and cartilage from between the mucous membrane covering it on either side. Usually the surgeon will pack the nose at the termination of the operation, for instance, by inserting a rubber glove finger packed with ribbon gauze into either side. The front of the nose is dressed with a small gauze roll held in place with strapping. It is changed as often as it becomes soiled. *The packs are removed some 12 to 24 hours after the operation, but the gauze roll may be required for some days more.*

A haematoma may collect between the layers of the septum, in spite of the pack, but will usually settle without interference.

Nasal allergy. Vaso-motor rhinitis. Nasal polypi. Sneezing, watery nasal discharge and nasal obstruction occur frequently in some individuals without anything to suggest infection. The cause may be allergy, as in hayfever, but often nothing of this kind can be identified. Sometimes a disturbance of the nerve supply to the blood vessels and mucous glands of the nasal lining is postulated (*vaso-motor rhinitis*). A number of patients with symptoms of this kind are found to be suffering from *nasal polypi*, hanging down like grapes from the ethmoidal sinuses. They are removed with the nasal snare, but are liable to recur.

Sinusitis. The bones of the skull round the nose are hollowed out by air-containing spaces called the *para-nasal or accessory air sinuses*. They communicate with the nasal cavity so that infection of the nose is liable to spread to them, when we speak of sinusitis. Most cases of sinusitis originate, therefore, from a cold in the head.

Far and away the commonest form is *maxillary sinusitis* in which infection involves the large air-containing space in the upper jaw, called the maxillary sinus or antrum of Highmore.

The disease has an acute onset with pain in the upper teeth, round the eyes or in the forehead. There is a degree of nasal obstruction on the affected side and a yellow nasal discharge, but never swelling of the cheek. *Treatment* includes antibiotics and nasal decongestants.

Chronic sinusitis may be relatively silent and X-ray examination necessary to make the diagnosis. Most cases of chronic maxillary sinusitis come to need antrum puncture and irrigation (antrum wash-out), not only to confirm the presence of pus in the sinus but also, by flushing it out, to speed up recovery.

Antral irrigation. From time to time, both in the out-patient department and in the ward, the nurse is likely to be called upon to prepare for and assist at this minor operation. Local anaesthesia is employed and the patient, appropriately draped, sits up in a chair facing the surgeon.

The following items must be available:

A suitable receiver, which the patient holds.
Two Lichtwitz pattern trochars and cannulae properly sterilized.
Two Higginson syringes, properly sterilized.
A supply of sterile normal saline solution.
Paper tissues.

Not every case of maxillary sinusitis will recover on conservative treatment however carefully judged and carried out, and operative treatment becomes necessary. The most widely practised operation is the sublabial radical antrostomy, the so-called *Caldwell-Luc operation.* Under general anaesthesia (a local anaesthetic will do if indicated or required) an incision is made under the lip in the sulcus between it and the alveolus, over the affected antrum. The antrum is opened and the diseased lining removed. An opening is then fashioned into the nose close to the floor to provide better drainage for the products of infection.

The incision is loosely sutured.

Postoperative care. During the few days spent in hospital after the operation, the patient must be encouraged to keep food to the sound side of the mouth and to take particular care with mouth-washes. If he fills his mouth and inflates his cheeks with the mouth-wash, he may force it into the antrum and out into the nose. Instead he should gently carry the mouth-wash round the mouth with the tongue.

Trans-sphenoidal hypophysectomy. It is a strange modern development that leads to the nursing in the ear, nose and throat wards of patients with advanced carcinoma of the breast. The reason is that in some of these cases a significant remission may be obtained by removing the pituitary gland (hypophysis cerebri) at the base of the brain. Originally a problem for the neuro-surgeon, this operation is now widely undertaken by the ear, nose and throat specialist working with the operating microscope through an incision between the eye and the root of the nose.

The pituitary gland has a widely varied function, but it is indispensable for its effect on the suprarenal gland which it stimulates to produce *cortisone*. Without it, the patient is obliged to take cortisone by mouth for the remainder of her life.

Starting on the morning of the operation a carefully regulated regime of medication is commenced, including hydrocortisone, penicillin and sulphonamides. The patient returns to the ward with a pack in the right side of the nose maintaining in place a muscle graft taken from the thigh and used to seal off the empty pituitary fossa. *The pack remains in place for 10 days. A careful watch must be kept on blood pressure, fluid balance and electrolytes.*

DISEASES OF THE THROAT

Foreign bodies. Foreign bodies in the pharynx, oesophagus, larynx, trachea and bronchial tree constitute an even more important problem than foreign bodies in the ear and nose and represent, along with epistaxis and respiratory obstruction, one of the few remaining ear, nose and throat emergencies.

Sharp foreign bodies, such as fish bones, may lodge in the back of the tongue, tonsil or oropharynx and a skilled doctor may remove them using a laryngeal mirror and an angled forceps. Larger foreign bodies, such as meat bones or dentures in adults or toys in children may lodge at the thoracic inlet or elsewhere in the oesophagus. They must be removed as soon as possible under a general anaesthetic in a theatre equipped with a full range of endoscopic instruments. Delay exposes the patient to the risk of mediastinitis, a grave complication.

All manner of small foreign bodies may be inhaled accidentally, usually by children, the most notorious being the peanut. If the foreign body is large enough to become impacted in the larynx, it may asphyxiate the patient at worst, or produce severe respiratory difficulty with stridor at best. Tipping the patient upside down and slapping him on the back is a desperate first-aid measure that has been known to succeed.

If the foreign body has passed into the trachea it will cause violent coughing, sometimes with shuttling of the foreign body up and down the trachea. If it lodges in a lower bronchus, as the peanut usually does, there may be wheezing and, sooner or later, partial collapse of the lung.

Foreign bodies in the air passages are major emergencies and the patient must be placed in the care of an experienced ear, nose and throat or thoracic surgeon without delay. He will proceed to remove the foreign body via the bronchoscope, not always an easy undertaking (see Chapter 58, p. 585).

Infections of the throat

These are such familiar occurrences that a general description is not necessary, but certain special sorts of infections require special consideration.

Tonsillitis. Infection in the throat is often localized to the tonsils, which may be generally inflamed and swollen, or covered with patches of exudate round the openings of the crypts (follicular tonsillitis). Occasionally, usually in adults, infection may spread outside the tonsil, where it may form an abscess between it and the subjacent muscle layer. This is called a *peritonsillar abscess or quinsy.*

Tonsillar infection is characterized by fever, difficulty and pain on swallowing, and enlargement and tenderness of the lymph nodes at the angles of the jaw. In quinsy there is also trismus, i.e. difficulty in opening the mouth.

Very many attacks of tonsillitis are due to infection with the haemolytic streptococcus and the organism is always penicillin-sensitive. Thus penicillin is to be regarded as the treatment of choice.

Once pus has formed and a quinsy is present, surgical drainage is imperative, although spontaneous rupture of the abscess may save the patient an unpleasant minor operation.

It will be seen, then, that tonsillitis is rarely a serious illness and that it can be expected to respond readily to treatment. The problem is that in many children and some adults the disease recurs frequently. A large proportion of this group comes to be treated by removal of the tonsils, tonsillectomy.

Tonsillectomy. Usually, in children, the operation is combined with removal of adenoids and, not infrequently, with attention to a middle-ear exudate (see p. 621).

The nurse need not be familiar with the steps of the operation except to know that the tonsils may either be enucleated with a guillotine or else dissected out. The latter operation is favoured by most surgeons today, although in the hands of an expert, the former is an entirely satisfactory procedure. Most surgeons remove the adenoid with a curette. The blood supply of the regions concerned is rich and bleeding is inevitable. It is the surgeon's duty to control this by means of packing, ligatures or diathermy before the patient leaves the operating table, but reactionary bleeding within hours of the operation is not uncommon, and secondary bleeding four to eight days later, an occasional complication. The former is much the more serious and its management calls, in the first place, for competent nursing care.

The postoperative care. The ideal arrangement is for the patient to be taken direct from the operating theatre to a recovery room or ward within the theatre suite. Here he can be observed by specially trained nurses during the most dangerous period before recovering from the anaesthetic. Suction is available to remove clot, which might obstruct the airway, and if bleeding is manifest he can be returned, if necessary, to the operating theatre. The patient's position during this period is very important. *He is placed on his side with the arms and the uppermost leg flexed. The head is unsupported by pillows and the face visible so that any blood will tend to run out of the nose and mouth.* The foot of the bed should be blocked. On return to the ward the patient is likely to be restless and to need an injection to settle him, for instance papaveretum injection B.P.C. (0·8 mg per year of age is a useful guide to the dose). While he remains asleep, the aim should be to maintain him in the same position as described above, but as soon as he is thoroughly awake, he should be sat up.

Regular careful observations are necessary for the 24 hours following the operation. *The pulse rate is recorded every 15 minutes in the recovery room and every 30 minutes for the first 6 hours after return to the ward. A rising pulse rate will alert the nurse to the possibility of bleeding and must be reported at once to the doctor.* Similarly, the doctor must be told of any suspicion that the patient is swallowing blood, or proof of it if the patient should vomit blood or of any suggestion of obstructed breathing. He will want to examine the patient carefully using a head mirror or head light, remove clot from the throat using a tongue depressor and Luc's forceps and perhaps apply pressure to a bleeding point with a small cotton-wool ball wrung out in 1 in 1,000 adrenaline. If the bleeding is from the post-nasal space he may wish to introduce a post-nasal pack as for the control of epistaxis (p. 624). Everything required should be put ready in advance.

Occasionally, it will be necessary to return the patient to the operating theatre and ligature the bleeding vessel, but it must not be forgotten that this is a serious decision since the patient must be re-anaesthetized while bleeding is occurring from the throat.

The throat will remain sore for 10 days or so, at first with pain referred to the ear. Some ease can be obtained at meal times by offering Disprin swallows 300 to 600 mg in water a few minutes before. Children seem to find ice cream easy to swallow.

Respiratory obstruction. *Obstruction to breathing is a terrifying experience for the patient and a most anxious one for the doctors and nurses responsible for his care.*

The causes of stridor are manifold and include such diverse pathological processes as foreign body in the larynx (see p. 626) and paralysis of the vocal cords complicating operation on the thyroid gland. It is not necessary for the nurse to be familiar with all these causes, but she should know something about the commoner ones.

Neoplasms. Malignant tumours of the larynx may obstruct the breathing and are considered in the final paragraphs of this chapter. Various innocent tumours of the larynx do so too, and among the most troublesome are the multiple papillomas (warts) of the larynx seen in children.

Infection. Simple inflammation of the larynx, *laryngitis*, rarely causes stridor, but certain special infections may do so, particularly in children. Among these are *laryngo-tracheo-bronchitis* and a rare but very important disease called *epiglottitis*.

Management. Patients with stridor demand the most careful and experienced observation since a proportion of them will need the obstruction bypassed by means of the operation of tracheostomy, and *the nurse must be on the look out for danger signals. These include a rising pulse rate, recession (sucking-in) of the soft tissues between the ribs and at the root of the neck, and the development of cyanosis.*

Tracheostomy. An incision is made in the midline of the neck exposing the upper part of the trachea. The trachea is opened at the level of the third and fourth rings and a curved tracheostomy tube introduced and tied in place with tapes round the neck. A skilled anaesthetist will usually be able to give a general anaesthetic without risk, but local anaesthesia may be necessary, or rarely in the event of a life-saving emergency, no anaesthetic at all.

Many types of tube are in use (Fig. 60/4) *and it is a first principle of the nursing management of these difficult cases that the nurse must be familiar*

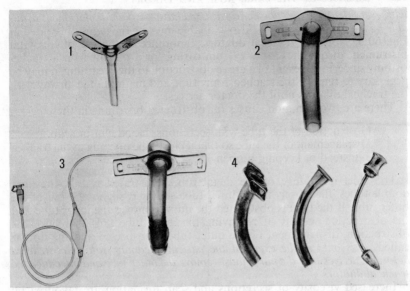

Fig. 60/4 Some tracheostomy tubes. 1. The Great Ormond Street pattern for infants. 2. Portex tracheostomy tube. 3. Cuffed tracheostomy tube. 4. Negus' tracheostomy tube with inner tube and pilot (the inner tube may be fitted with a valve to make speech possible in certain cases).

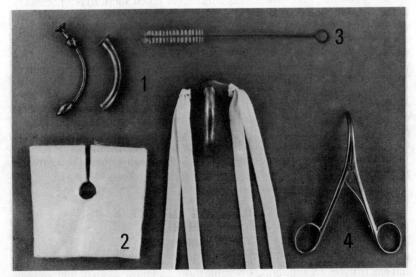

Fig. 60/5 Items needed at the bedside of the patient with a tracheostomy. 1. Spare tracheostomy tube. 2. Keyhole dressing in non-stick fabric. 3. Bottle brush. 4. Tracheal dilators. In addition to the items shown, the following will be available at the bedside of patients dependent for breathing on a tracheostomy tube: (a) A suction apparatus or piped suction with a supply of polyethylene catheters. (b) Oxygen. (c) An atomizer or other means of humidifying the air. (d) Disposal bags for soiled dressings, used catheters, etc.

with every detail of the tube concerned and have an exact replacement available by the patient's bedside. Also available must be the items illustrated in Fig. 60/5. Note the tracheal dilators. Ignorance of the use of this vital instrument disqualifies a nurse from caring for a patient with a tracheostomy since, in the event of a grave obstruction to the breathing, it may be necessary to remove the tracheostomy tube and maintain the airway with the tracheal dilators until the doctor arrives.

There are two common causes for obstructed breathing in these cases:

Obstruction of the tube with secretions, blood clot or scab.
Displacement of the tube so that it closes the opening in the trachea instead of keeping it open.

The chief advantage of the metal tubes illustrated is that they are double tubes, the closely fitting inner tube sliding easily in and out of the outer tube. If the tube is obstructed the nurse removes the inner tube and the obstruction with it. If removing the inner tube fails to relieve the obstruction, displacement of the outer tube is suspected and the doctor called. *It is only in the event of the patient becoming totally obstructed before he arrives that the nurse must remove the outer tube and introduce the tracheal dilators.*

Increased viscosity of secretions and scab formation are favoured by drying of the tracheal lining, and to avoid this the air breathed must be humidified. There are a variety of humidifying devices that attach to the tracheostomy tube, but they are designed for use with a plastic tube and these are not usually fitted with inner tubes. They must be kept clear by means of suction, and a suction apparatus (or piped suction) is a necessary item of equipment in these cases. A polyethylene tube attached to the suction apparatus is passed through the tracheostomy tube whenever the nurse's ear tells her it contains secretions. Tracheo-bronchial suction by similar means is also desirable in many cases, and very often it is to facilitate this that the tracheostomy is performed (e.g. in unconscious patients and in tracheo-bronchitis).

Those in attendance on patients treated by tracheostomy must never forget that the presence of a tube in the trachea robs the patient of the use of his voice. This should have been explained before the operation but, if not, the patient may be reassured by demonstrating that his voice is restored if the tube is momentarily blocked with a finger over the opening.

The special problem of *the end-tracheostome* is dealt with on the following page.

MALIGNANT DISEASE OF THE EARS, NOSE AND THROAT

Newer surgical techniques, antibiotics, modern anaesthesia and the application of a better understanding of the physiology of the tissue fluids and electrolytes are rendering operable more and more cases of malignancy in these regions, which previously would have been regarded as suitable for terminal nursing only. Very often such cases make heavy demands on the nursing staff and nowadays constitute the major part of the work load in the ears, nose and throat ward, particularly on the male side where this type of case is commoner. To describe the problems characteristic of each disease would require more space than is available, but certain general considerations must be mentioned.

Radiotherapy. At some stage of treatment, many of these patients will receive a course of radiotherapy (see Chapter 64). The local reaction referred to is in these instances likely to occur in the mouth and throat as well as in the skin. Secondary infection may occur, calling for antibiotic treatment.

Carcinoma of the larynx and pharynx. Removal of the diseased larynx (laryngectomy), sometimes with a large part of the pharynx (laryngo-pharyngectomy) and often with gland-metastases in the neck (block dissection of the neck), is a major undertaking, but nowadays may be dwarfed by the steps necessary to repair the regions concerned. The colon or stomach may be moved up into the neck either through the mediastinum or beneath the skin of the chest wall so that nursing care must be directed towards three major anatomical compartments, the abdomen, the thorax and the neck. Some of the problems likely to be encountered are considered in Chapters 50 and 58 and only those relative to the neck will be touched on here.

The end-tracheostome. If the larynx has been removed, the trachea will have been cut across and the lower end sewn to an opening in the skin of the neck just above the sternal notch. In many respects the nursing care will be the same as for a patient with a tracheostomy (see p. 628), but with certain important differences. A larger tube, a laryngectomy tube, will be used and the anxiety related to the displaced tube will not arise since the tube, if it is in, is bound to be in the trachea and, if it is out, will leave the patient able to breathe easily just the same. *The need for good humidification of the inspired air is of even greater importance in these cases, however, and becomes a major preoccupation of the nurse in the immediate postoperative period.*

Unlike the patient with an ordinary tracheostomy, the laryngectomized patient will be robbed of speech altogether and will never again speak in the familiar way. He will come, eventually, under the expert guidance of the speech therapist who will teach him oesophageal speech, enabling him to modify the rough sounds produced by regurgitating swallowed air into a rather gruff and staccato speech.

The pre-operative preparation of the patient must include psychological preparation, therefore, aimed at enabling him to accept this voiceless phase and the rehabilitation of the voice that must follow. It should include a meeting not only with the speech therapist, but also with a patient or patients who have recovered from similar operations and learned to speak again.

Tube-feeding. The patient will return to the ward with a naso-gastric tube in place and for some 7 to 10 days, sometimes longer, will be fed by this route. The principles of this type of feeding are described in Chapter 17.

Fistula formation. Not infrequently, and usually where radiotherapy has preceded surgery, the tissues of the neck will fail to heal by first intention and a *pharyngeal fistula* will form. Through this the patient's saliva will leak into the dressings or even, if care is not taken, into the trachea. The taking of food or drink by mouth must be prohibited, therefore, for as long as the fistula persists, sometimes until it has been repaired by plastic surgery. *It is in these cases that naso-gastric feeding needs to be persevered with for long periods though often with serious consequences so far as the morale of the patient is concerned.*

Cancer chemotherapy. A number of chemicals are now known which have a destructive effect on the rapidly dividing cells of malignant neoplasms. In recent years they have been used increasingly in an attempt to treat advanced cancer of the ear, nose and throat, for instance, carcinoma of the post-nasal space.

They are referred to as cytotoxic drugs and include such agents as methotrexate and cyclophosphamide. They may be given by mouth or by intravenous injection, but are likely to be most effective if they can be concentrated in the area of the disease. In an attempt to achieve this, surgeons now perfuse the tumour with the cytotoxic agent by injecting it directly into the blood supply, for instance by way of the superficial temporal artery. A special pump is necessary to overcome the arterial blood pressure.

The technique is not without considerable danger, since these drugs damage the bone marrow as well as the tumour cells and produce a fall in the white cell count in the blood. Regular blood counts are necessary, therefore, and the patient must be isolated and nursed with barrier precautions to reduce to a minimum the risk of cross-infection. With the number of white cells seriously depleted, it is highly likely that infection, once established, would prove fatal.

Chapter 61

The Nursing of Patients with Diseases of the Eye

by DESMOND P. GREAVES

> *Introduction—basic nursing care—examination of the eye—out-patient and casualty equipment—local treatment of the eye—affections of the eyelids and conjunctiva: trachoma—affections of the cornea and iris—affections of the lens—glaucoma—retinal detachment—strabismus—enucleation of the eye*

In recent years considerable changes have occurred in the nursing, as well as in the medical care, of patients suffering from eye complaints. Whereas not so long ago it was common to find patients after eye surgery with dressings on both eyes and confined to bed for up to 10 days or so, it is now more usual to place the dressing on the operated eye only and to allow patients to get out of bed the day after operation. This change has in part been brought about by the increasing use of sutures in cataract surgery, making for greater security of the wound.

This relaxation of a rather rigid regime which was, and still is, feared by so many patients, has led to a far greater mental calm and confidence, to say nothing of the greatly reduced incidence of general complications from prolonged bed rest such as pneumonia and thrombosis with pulmonary emboli. At the same time the results as far as the eye itself is concerned are no less satisfactory.

To be in charge of eye patients a nurse requires special training and should be highly experienced. Apart from her technical abilities, she will have developed an insight into many of the special problems and fears which afflict people threatened with failing vision and possible blindness. Many junior nurses, by virtue of the needs of general training, have little enough time to learn more than the elements of ophthalmic nursing, and newcomers naturally often worry about this inexperience. They should try not to let this lessen the patient's confidence. By talking to him and taking an interest in his affairs and condition and acting under the guidance of the sister and staff nurse, they will learn quickly to play their part in the team.

Great attention is given to detail but, though a strict ward routine and discipline is essential, it should be carried out with gentleness and relaxation. Nurses should move quietly, though the silent approach is to be

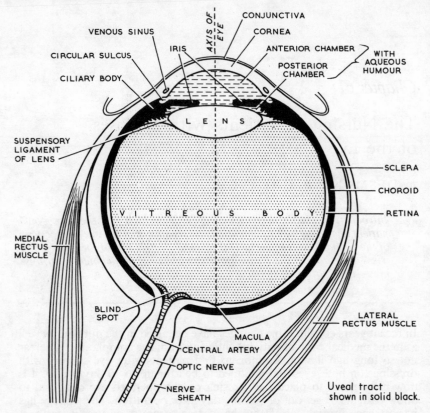

CONJUNCTIVA
CORNEA
VENOUS SINUS
ANTERIOR CHAMBER
IRIS
CIRCULAR SULCUS
POSTERIOR
CHAMBER
WITH
AQUEOUS
HUMOUR
CILIARY BODY
AXIS OF EYE

LENS

SUSPENSORY
LIGAMENT
OF LENS

SCLERA
CHOROID
RETINA

VITREOUS BODY

MEDIAL
RECTUS
MUSCLE

BLIND
SPOT
LATERAL
RECTUS MUSCLE

MACULA
CENTRAL ARTERY
OPTIC NERVE

NERVE
SHEATH
Uveal tract
shown in solid black.

Fig. 61/1 Horizontal section through the right eye, seen from above.

avoided, especially to blind patients or those with both eyes padded; by speaking quietly before she touches the bed, a nurse will thereby avoid a sudden startled response.

BASIC NURSING CARE

The patient about to undergo an eye operation generally enters hospital one or two days before. He should be received kindly and sympathetically. After the routine of admission it is helpful to explain what will happen and to relieve groundless fears, for many people still think it will be necessary for them to have both eyes covered for several days and to lie very still. Such is now not so.

General lighting in wards should be adequate to avoid any depressing effect, though not so bright as to cause discomfort since at some stage most patients are hypersensitive. *Individual lighting over each bed is also desirable. The bed should not be too high* so that, on getting out of bed, an elderly or partially sighted patient is able to feel his feet touch the floor easily.

To dispel boredom some form of occupation must be encouraged. While some patients are able to read before operation, this is generally not practicable for a few days afterwards. Freer visiting, some handicrafts and the radio all help to relieve the tedium.

The patient will already have had explained to him the nature and aim of the operation. *The side to be operated should be marked above with a skin pencil,* though this is primarily the responsibility of the surgeon.

Some surgeons insist on pre-operative conjunctival cultures being taken 48 hours before surgery to reduce the risk of postoperative infection. Others maintain that, in the absence of clinical evidence of extra-ocular infection, such a procedure is unreliable and of no value.

Particular attention should be paid to cleansing the head of the patient, with shampoo for the hair and washing the skin of the face thoroughly with soap. Many surgeons prefer the eyelashes to be cut short one or two days before operation (see p. 644) and sometimes irrigate the lacrimal sac. Antibiotic drops, such as 0·5 per cent chloramphenicol are instilled three-hourly into both eyes to reduce the risk of latent infection.

Routine urine and blood pressure examinations are made and an assessment of the patient's general condition is carried out by the doctor. If the patient is having any general medication this is usually continued but may be modified by requirements of the eye surgery and general anaesthesia. *Persistent troublesome cough can lead to serious postoperative complications and should be dealt with, any smoking discouraged,* or the operation postponed to a more suitable season. Constipation should be treated with a gentle laxative. A mild sedative is often helpful for the nervous patient.

On the morning of the operation the patient is prepared for general or local anaesthesia, and appropriate drops are instilled as ordered (see p. 642). For example, in cataract and retinal detachment surgery, it is important for the pupil to be widely dilated, whereas for glaucoma surgery a small pupil is desirable. *The patient is dressed in a jacket split at the back for ease of removal, and a cap and warm socks. Special split canvas sheets with lifting poles help a great deal in reducing the disturbance of the patient in transit to and from the operating theatre.*

On the theatre table the skin around the eye is finally cleansed with some antiseptic preparation such as Savlon and spirit, care being taken to avoid any fluid entering the eye between the lids. The surgeon arranges the drapes and proceeds with the operation. Immediately the operation has been completed drops may be instilled before the dressing is applied.

On return to his bed the patient is generally kept flat on his back until his blood pressure recovers from the effect of the anaesthetic and pre-medication, when in most instances he can be allowed to adopt a sitting position in bed. He is warned not to try to get out of bed alone and not to touch the dressing, and he should be instructed to ask for the nurse if he needs anything. Restlessness is dealt with by sedatives, and *pain* with appropriate analgesics.

For a few days the diet should be light, avoiding strong flavours. A nurse should help feed him for a day or two, especially where both eyes are covered. Some patients worry about missing a daily motion but it should be explained that on a light diet with little residue the stimulus may be absent for a few days. However, if constipation leads to discomfort, a mild aperient or glycerin suppository can be given. *Smoking should be discouraged to reduce the risk of coughing and also of fire.*

Visitors are often allowed the day after operation, the patient's wishes being carefully considered, though too many visitors should be discouraged, as should laughing and talking by the patient.

On first being allowed up (first to fifth day, according to the surgeon's wishes) the patient is helped out of bed and warned of possible temporary weakness of the legs.

The first dressing is generally carried out the day after operation and is most important; it is frequently done or attended by an experienced doctor. The patient should be encouraged to relax and asked not to squeeze the eye. He should also be warned not to expect immediate visual results. Strapping should be cut and the dressing removed gently, watching it carefully to avoid any sudden drag from its adhesions. The usual sterile precautions are adopted. Any discharge of mucus is gently swabbed away. The patient is asked to open both eyes and to look straight ahead. The eye is inspected, raising the upper eyelid gently if necessary, and avoiding any pressure on the globe. Undue redness or chemosis of the conjunctiva, or cloudiness of the cornea may indicate infection. The pupils should be round, the anterior chamber present and the wound satisfactorily closed. Drops are instilled as ordered, again warning the patient against squeezing the eye, and a pad and shield applied. Patients are washed gently in bed for two or three days. Men may be shaved on the fourth day, though a trim on the operated side may be done earlier with an electric razor to aid adhesion of strapping. Dark glasses are usually ordered about the sixth day but the eye covered at night with a pad and shield for a further week.

EXAMINATION OF THE EYE

People with eye diseases are generally first seen in a hospital out-patient or casualty department. The patient giving his history to the doctor may tell of an injury or be complaining of something obvious such as a red, painful eye or a swelling or distortion of an eyelid, or he may have noticed some disturbance of function such as a change in sight or upset of his binocular mechanism which may cause him to experience double vision. The doctor will inquire about past eye troubles and any family history of eye disease. It is also important to know of any general disease or treatment, since this may have an important bearing on the eye condition.

Subjective examination

Visual acuity. Distance vision is taken with the patient 6 metres from a Snellen's test chart (Fig. 61/2). With distance glasses worn, each eye is tested separately, first the right and then the left, care being taken to cover the other eye efficiently with a small card. Acuity is recorded according to the lowest line read correctly, the top letter being 6/60 down through 6/36, 6/24, 6/18, 6/12 (approximately equivalent to reading a car number plate at 25 yards), 6/9, 6/6 (average normal) and 6/5. For a child or illiterate person a chart with numbers or 'Es' turned in different directions can be helpful (Fig. 61/3). Should he be unable to read the top letter, the patient is taken nearer to the chart until he can see it, the numerator of the fraction 6/60 being replaced by a figure representing the distance away from the chart, e.g. 2/60 if he has to be taken up to 2 metres from the chart in order to see the top letter. With even poorer vision he is asked whether he can 'count fingers' (CF) or appreciate 'hand movements' (HM) at 1 or 0·5

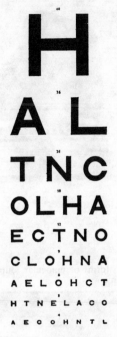

Fig. 61/2 Snellen's test chart.

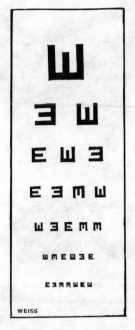

Fig. 61/3 'E' test chart.

metre. Sometimes 'perception of light' (PL) only is possible with 'accurate' or 'inaccurate' projection, according to whether he is able to say from which direction the light is coming. Lastly there is total blindness or 'no perception of light' and, with the exception of acute retrobulbar neuritis or very temporary interruption of the blood supply to the retina, this indicates damage beyond hope of recovery.

Near vision is taken with a reading card having different sizes of type. The patient is asked which is the smallest print he can read and should wear his reading glasses if he has any.

Field of vision. Visual acuity is not the only indication of how well anyone can see, for, while fixing on any small object, we are aware of a much wider 'field of vision'. This can be estimated roughly by confrontation with the examining surgeon facing the patient who, while fixing with each eye separately straight ahead (e.g. on the eyes of the examiner), is asked to say when he is aware of a small white or coloured (often red) target, such as a hat pin which is brought in slowly from different directions. More accurately the peripheral field can be recorded by a perimeter, and the central field comprising the inner 20 degrees or so by means of the Bjerrum screen. This latter method is used considerably in the diagnosis and follow-up of glaucoma.

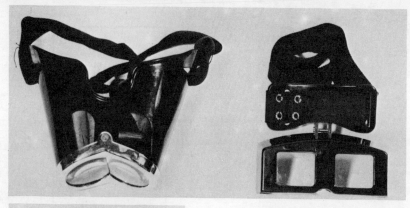

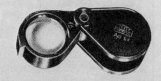

Fig. 61/4 Two forms of binocular loupe and a monocular loupe.

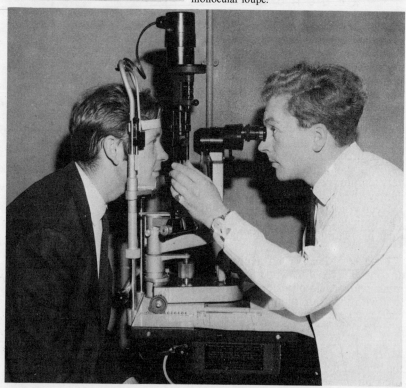

Fig. 61/5 A corneal microscope or slit lamp.

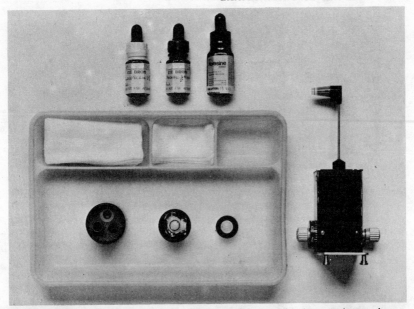

Fig. 61/6 Plastic applanation prisms and, used in conjunction with these, gonioscopy lenses, various eye drops, an applanation tonometer and swabs. A box of paper wipes should also be provided.

Objective examination

This consists of a general external inspection of the eyes, their relative position and appearance of the lids, the colour of the conjunctiva and underlying sclera, clearness of the cornea and regularity of the pupils and their reaction to light and to accommodation. Movements of the eyes are tested mainly in the six cardinal positions of gaze: to right and left, *up* to the right and left, and *down* to the right and left. In carrying out a more detailed examination of the anterior segment of the eye, the surgeon uses some form of magnification such as a binocular or monocular 8 or $10 \times$ loupe and pen torch or some other source of focal illumination (Fig. 61/4). Greater detail still is possible with the aid of a corneal microscope or slit-lamp (Fig. 61/5). The latter is expensive but has attachments for special aspects of eye examination. These include the use of plastic contact lenses to examine the angle of the anterior chamber (gonioscopy) and the fundus oculi, and plastic prisms for applanation tonometry (Fig. 61/6). *Constant care should be taken to protect these instruments from dust or rough handling, and to avoid scratching plastic lenses, they should be wiped with soft paper tissue.* Sterilization of the lenses is done by placing them in a solution of 1/5,000 chlorhexidine.

Tonometry. The assessment of the intra-ocular pressure (ocular tension) is important since any undue rise can cause permanent damage to the eye (primary and secondary glaucoma). Feeling the tension with the fingers (digital tonometry) is unreliable and various instruments have been devised to give more accurate information. The Schiotz tonometer, besides being portable, is fairly simple and relatively cheap. The plunger should

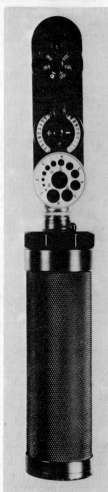

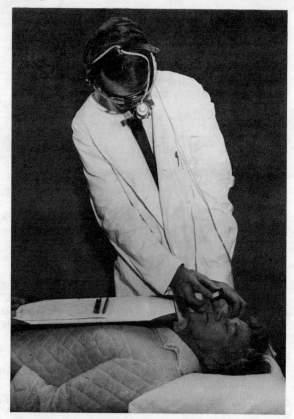

Fig. 61/8 Use of indirect ophthalmoscopy.

Fig. 61/7 A modern ophthalmoscope for direct use.

be removed for regular cleaning and be seen to move freely. Sterilization is conveniently done by holding the foot in the flame of a spirit lamp for 30 seconds. It is used by having the patient lie on his back. The cornea is anaesthetized with 1 per cent amethocaine and the instrument is then allowed to rest freely on the cornea. Displacement of the plunger is read off on the scale, the pressure being found by reference to a chart.

Owing to its weight and other factors, this instrument is much less accurate than the applanation method mentioned earlier. The latter is done with the patient sitting at the slit-lamp (see Fig. 61/5), the eyes being anaesthetized with a mild surface anaesthetic containing a small amount of fluorescein (e.g. Novesine/fluorescein) or fluorescein put in afterwards. Using a blue filter in front of the light source, the examining surgeon sees two green half-circles and adjusts the loading on the prism to produce overlap of the ends to give a ∼ shaped appearance. The pressure reading can then be read directly from the loading on the prism arm. In between examination the plastic prisms are kept in 1/5,000 chlorhexidine solution to avoid the possibility of transference of infection, particularly of virus origin, from one patient to another.

Internal examination of the eye is done with an ophthalmoscope, the pupil frequently being dilated with a mydriatic such as 2 per cent homatropine and 2 per cent cocaine, 1 per cent Mydrilate, 10 per cent phenylephrine, etc. Direct ophthalmoscopy is done usually with a battery model (Fig. 61/7) held close to the patient's eye, while indirect ophthalmoscopy is usually done with a binocular apparatus worn on the head of the surgeon with an objective lens (15 to 30 dioptres) held interposed 10 to 20 cm from the eye of the patient (Fig. 61/8).

Examination of children

This often calls for great patience and tact. Much information may be gained by simply watching the child on his mother's knee. It is often better to resist any temptation to restrain a child, though it may be necessary to wrap him securely in a blanket on a couch. The nurse can then lean over the child with her forearms alongside his body, holding his head still while the doctor carries out his examination. However, for anything except the simplest inspection or treatment, an examination under anaesthesia is the only satisfactory way of dealing with a difficult child.

OUT-PATIENT AND CASUALTY EQUIPMENT

Apart from the charts and instruments already mentioned, the clinic doctor will need a small set of drugs and dressings together with some simple surgical instruments for casualty work.

Drugs

These will be mostly in the form of drops, fresh bottles being used for each clinic to reduce the risk of contamination. There are also available various proprietary sterile single-dose preparations which eliminate all such risks. Occasionally tubes of ointment may be used. The list will vary according to the individual preference of the doctor. A useful list would be as follows:

Local anaesthetics: 1 per cent Amethocaine.
2 per cent Cocaine (tends to dilate the pupil).
2 per cent Lignocaine for injection.
Mydriatics: 2 per cent Homatropine+2 per cent Cocaine.
1 per cent Cyclopentolate.
10 per cent Phenylephrine.
Miotics: 2 per cent Pilocarpine, or 0·5 per cent Eserine.
Vasoconstrictors: 1/1,000 Adrenaline.
Antibiotics: 0·5 per cent Chloramphenicol.

Two per cent fluorescein (in small containers) is used for staining corneal ulcers and abrasions. It is particularly important that this substance be used fresh since *Pseudomonas aeruginosa* may even flourish in it and convey a serious infection to an otherwise clean abrasion. Sometimes fluorescein-impregnated paper strips are used to overcome this risk, or the fluorescein conveyed via a sterile glass rod. Normal saline can be used to wash out excess fluorescein.

There should be a tray with containers of 1/5,000 chlorhexidine for sterilizing plastic gonioscopy lenses and applanating prisms with saline for rinsing, and sterile glass rods and small swabs or paper wipes.

Treatment, including minor operations such as syringing of tear sacs and curettage of cysts, is carried out in a tilting dental chair or on a couch.

In many larger hospitals the introduction of central sterile supply units has meant the provision of sets of instruments and dressings packed and supplied already sterilized in special paper bags. *They would contain various needle holders, lid speculum, Saunders' needle (for removing foreign bodies), Meibomian clamp and curettes, lacrimal cannulae and punctum dilators, etc.* Such packs could also contain sterile paper towels, swabs and eye pads or these could be arranged as separate packs. Disposable needles and syringes, especially 2 and 5 ml, are now in almost universal use.

LOCAL TREATMENT OF THE EYE

Eversion of the eyelids

This is done with the patient looking down. The upper lashes are grasped to pull the lids downwards and each lid everted by gentle pressure on its central portion. Occasionally, in patients who cannot relax their orbicularis muscle easily, it is necessary to use a blunt glass rod to press on the central area of the lid.

Care should be taken not to abrade the cornea or cause pain or damage by undue pressure.

Removal of surface foreign bodies

These may be found in the conjunctival fornices or subtarsally under the upper eyelid after it has been everted. Removal is effected by means of a small swab stick or with a pointed piece of filter paper. Surface anaesthesia with 1 per cent amethocaine often makes this manœuvre easier for the patient and nurse or doctor, but it is essential if the foreign body is on the cornea. For the latter a good light, such as from an Anglepoise, is important and the patient should be on a couch or reclining in a dental chair. Loosely attached foreign bodies can often be removed with the tip of a small piece of filter paper. If embedded, a sterile Saunders' needle or disposable No. 1 gauge hypodermic needle is required. Great care should be taken not to damage other parts of the corneal epithelium. Antibiotic drops are instilled and the eye is padded, the patient being seen the following day and followed up as necessary until the lesion has completely healed.

To insert drops

Drop bottles are made of glass and have a screw cap with pipette incorporated, or may be of plastic with a small exit nozzle so that by squeezing the bottle a drop is expelled. The label should always be checked to ensure correct use; the word *guttae* is sometimes used to indicate *eye drops*. Two or three drops are inserted at one time into the lower conjunctival sac or fornix with the patient looking up, and a swab is used to pull the lower lid gently down and to absorb excess as it spills over the lid margin with any tears. Care should be taken to avoid touching the lashes or lid margin. Where a number of different drops have been prescribed, a minute or so should be allowed between them for absorption to take place through the conjunctiva and cornea. Placing drops in the upper fornix with the patient lying flat is sometimes helpful in conditions where disease particularly affects the upper tarsal and bulbar conjunctiva, and sometimes allows better absorption if the conjunctiva of the lower fornix is oedematous (chemosis). Ointment (Oculentum) from small tubes is sometimes used to increase the effective time a drug is present and also for conditions affecting the lid margin. Any crust or exudate should first be gently removed with a small swab moistened with saline or 2 per cent sodium bicarbonate solution.

To irrigate the eye

This may be necessary to remove chemicals splashed in an eye or mucopurulent exudates prior to other treatment (Fig. 61/9). It is done with a sterile undine containing 4 to 6 oz (120 to 180 ml) saline at body temperature (Fig. 61/10). *The nurse should check that the tip of the undine spout is smooth; if chipped it should be discarded.* The patient lies down or reclines on a chair with a headrest and the head is inclined to the same side as the eye being treated.

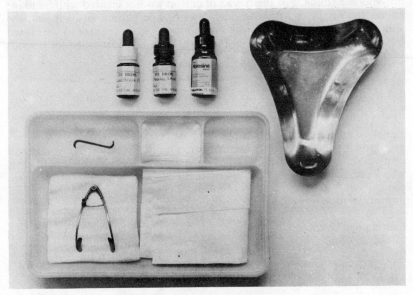

Fig. 61/9 Sterile tray containing lid speculum, wire lid retractors and paper towels; swab sticks and swabs are also needed. The appropriate drop bottles, an undine and sterile receiver should also be supplied.

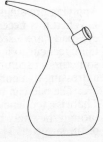

Fig. 61/10 A glass undine for use in irrigating an eye.

The nurse, usually standing behind the chair, places a receiver appropriately against the cheek, showing the patient how to hold it and herself prepares to use the undine. For the right eye the undine is held in her left hand so that she has her right hand free to open the eyelids. *The undine is held an inch or two away from the lids and, after warning the patient, a steady stream of fluid is poured first on to his cheek and then directed onto the eye, mainly at the inner canthus so that a stream flows across the eye laterally.* It often helps to move the lids a little and to ask the patient to move his eyes in different directions during the procedure. When all the fluid has been used the eye is allowed to close and dried with a swab before the receiver is removed. Where any solid caustic matter is present such as lime, it is important to remove all the particles with a swab stick or forceps prior to irrigation with double eversion of the lids. The instillation of a little local anaesthetic (1 per cent amethocaine) is very helpful in these cases.

Application of heat

This is best done with a small electric pad (Maddox heater) placed over a gauze swab. An alternative method, especially for home treatment, is hot-spoon bathing. For this a wad of cotton wool is secured with bandage round the broad end of a wooden spoon. The patient sits, dipping the spoon into a jug of boiling water and holding the spoon *near* to the closed eye so that the heat radiates onto the eye. Heat can be applied for periods of 15 minutes every three or four hours.

Application of cold

Frequent ice packs or compresses are occasionally useful to help reduce congestion or haemorrhage.

Epilation and electrolysis of lashes

Ingrowing lashes can cause irritation and risk to the cornea and immediate relief follows epilation. This is done with good epilation forceps which can grip the lash along its length. Since the lash tends to grow again, electrolysis, after the injection of a little 2 per cent lignocaine into the lid margin, gives a more permanent result.

Cutting eye lashes

This is done sometimes prior to operation. Blunt conjunctival scissors are smeared with Vaseline petroleum jelly to help catch the loose lashes which adhere to the blades. For the upper lid the eye is closed; for the lower, the patient is asked to look up.

Applying dressings

When it is necessary to apply a dressing to an eye, special oval-shaped eye pads are used made of white wool between layers of fine gauze. Gamgee, cut to a suitable size and shape, may also be used. Tulle gras is sometimes used under the pad, especially after operations. When applying a dressing to a conscious patient he should always be told first to *close the eye.* The pad can be fixed with Sellotape or other special non-irritant tape. There is a tendency now for roller bandages to be used much less frequently, though they may be employed in certain instances according to the wishes of the surgeon; $1\frac{1}{2}$ inch crêpe or woven edge are the best type. For a single eye bandage one or two turns are taken round the forehead in a direction from the operated to the unoperated eye. Several turns are then brought below the ear and up over the dressing and secured in the centre of the forehead with a safety pin or strapping.

AFFECTIONS OF THE EYELIDS

A stye (hordeolum) is a small abscess in a lash follicle and is usually due to staphylococcal infection. Hot-spoon bathing frequently gives some relief, though dry heat is better as being less liable to cause the spread of infection to other lashes. The application of antibiotic ointment to the lid margins also helps to prevent spread, and the offending eyelash should be removed as soon as it becomes loose. Recurrent styes require investigation to exclude possible systemic disease such as diabetes, and other sources of chronic infection should be excluded by taking swabs of the nose. Advice on local hygiene should be given to avoid re-contamination from cosmetics, etc.

Meibomian cysts (tarsal cysts or chalazia) are due to chronic infection of the sebaceous glands in the tarsal plates. They are generally painless and require incision and curettage from the conjunctival aspect. Occasionally they may become acutely infected and resemble styes.

Blepharitis is a mild infection of the lid margins frequently associated with dandruff. It is often due to staphylococcal infection and may ulcerate and form a sticky exudate. The lashes tend to fall out and grow irregularly.
Treatment consists of gentle removal of the exudate with a moistened swab stick after which the lid margins are dried and ointment applied generally containing an antibiotic together with a steroid. Any dandruff should be attended to with medicated shampoos. As the condition tends to recur, courses of treatment may be required from time to time.

Ectropion is eversion of the eyelid and may follow infection or injury. Epiphora and chronic conjunctivitis result and the *treatment is operative.*

Entropion is inversion of the lids and is mostly seen in old people. It is due to weakness of the subcutaneous elastic tissues giving insufficient support to the tarsal plate. Temporary relief can be given by placing a piece of strapping across the eyelid, though surgery is usually necessary to give more permanent relief. Entropion may also follow spasm of the orbicularis associated with chronic irritation.

Epiphora, or watering of the eye, may be due to excessive formation of tears, as may happen with irritation of the conjunctiva or cornea following injury. It may, however, be due to insufficient drainage from an obstructed tear duct and syringing of the duct will yield further information on this point. Sometimes lacrimal obstruction is accompanied by marked dilatation of the tear duct which becomes filled with mucopurulent material, forming a mucocele of the lacrimal sac. *This is treated by dacryocystorhinostomy*, in which a new drainage pathway into the nose is effected. *An acute dacryocystitis* occasionally develops in the tear duct and gives rise to a very painful tender swelling just below the inner canthus.

Treatment is by systemic antibiotics and no attempt at instrumentation of the lacrimal passages should be made.

Ptosis is drooping of the upper eyelids and is usually a congenital deformity requiring surgery. It can occur, however, in later life as a manifestation of myasthenia gravis.

CONJUNCTIVITIS

Conjunctivitis is inflammation of the conjunctiva and is often due to bacterial or virus infection. It may, however, be of allergic origin as a result of local drug sensitivity or reactions to cosmetics. Conjunctivitis may be acute or chronic and generally affects both eyes. As a surface phenomenon the eyes feel hot, the conjunctiva appears bright red and there is often considerable discharge, especially in the mornings on waking. Since many cases are infective in origin, advice should be given to the patient to avoid risk of transference to others in his family. *Treatment* should aim at removal of the exudate by saline irrigations with an undine or eye-bath and the frequent application of antibiotic drops during the day and ointment at night. The temporary use of dark glasses helps relieve photophobia but under no circumstances should a pad be placed on the eye.

Laboratory investigation may be necessary in the presence of resistant organisms. A particularly virulent form follows infection with the gonococcus. The condition progresses rapidly and produces large amounts of purulent secretion; the cornea is also at risk and in severe cases may perforate. Apart from its occurrence in adults it may occur in the newborn child, *ophthalmia neonatorum*, by infection during the child's passage through the birth canal. Although the risk of the latter is now much reduced it is by no means eliminated and it is probably wisest to take precautions by instilling drops of 10 per cent sulphacetamide into both eyes of the child at birth after first gently cleansing the lids with saline swabs. For many years 1 per cent silver nitrate (Credé's method) was used routinely instead.

Trachoma is a widespread infection found particularly in the Middle East, India and in some parts of Africa, but it can also occur as a primary infection in temperate zones. It is perhaps responsible for more cases of blindness in the world than any other condition. It is caused by a large virus-like body of the lymphogranuloma psittacosis group. It is particularly prevalent in communities living under conditions of poor hygiene and is spread in the first instance among the children of the family by fingers or clothing (e.g. a mother using her sari to wipe the child's eyes), and by flies which settle on the baby's eyes. It thus tends to be recurrent and chronic, eventually leading to corneal scarring and vascularization with marked scarring of the tarsal conjunctiva and inturning of the eyelashes.

Treatment is by local and systemic tetracycline preparations, though in the latter stages surgery to the eyelid and cornea may be necessary. Preventive measures of improved hygiene and large-scale local treatment of schoolchildren have helped reduce this scourge. Attempts have also been made to find a suitable vaccine.

AFFECTIONS OF THE CORNEA AND IRIS

The cornea is the transparent window of the eye. It consists of many layers of collagen fibres and is covered by fine epithelium. A little over 0·5 mm. in thickness, it is normally avascular. However, it may become scarred and vascularized with disease.

Corneal ulcer may be due to local injury or infection by a bacterial, virus or, more rarely, fungus organism. The ulcer appears to be a greyish patch which interferes with the normal bright reflex from the anterior surface of the cornea. The full extent of the ulcer can be shown by the instillation of fluorescein. The eye is usually red, particularly round the cornea (circumcorneal injection), though if the ulcer is marginal the redness may be concentrated at that point.

Since many corneal ulcers are of bacterial origin (e.g. pneumococcus), *treatment* consists of frequent instillations of local antibiotics together with dilation of the pupil with atropine. Occasionally systemic antibiotics are used. Of particular interest and difficulty nowadays is the *dendritic type of ulcer due to the herpes simplex virus*. This produces a characteristic form of ulcer with fine finger-like branching extensions. These ulcers are frequently treated by the direct application of phenol or iodine. In recent years an anti-viral substance, IDU (5 iodo-2′-deoxyuridine) has been used successfully in some cases. This is used at hourly intervals during the day and two-hourly during the night, though the ointment form reduces the frequency of such applications. It is important to avoid using local steroid preparations in the active stage of the virus.

Many different organisms can be involved in causing corneal ulcers or keratitis and extensive laboratory investigations are frequently necessary to determine which antibiotic is appropriate. In all cases it is generally better to pad the eye firmly and to give local heat and analgesics as necessary.

Corneal exposure. This may follow paralysis of the seventh cranial nerve (Bell's palsy). There is a serious risk of the cornea becoming dried and infected, especially during the night when there is no eye or lid movement. *Treatment* consists of the frequent application of antibiotic ointment to reduce drying and the risk of infection, and surgery may be necessary to give partial or complete closure of the eyelids, *tarsorrhaphy*.

It should also be remembered that patients undergoing general surgical operations, especially if prolonged, run a similar temporary risk of drying and damage to the cornea. During these procedures it is important, therefore, to see that the eyes are kept closed. The same precaution is essential in coma.

Keratoplasty. If permanent corneal scarring has resulted following inflammation or injury, opaque tissue may be removed either partially, as in lamellar keratoplasty, or its full thickness, as in perforating keratoplasty. Appropriate-sized discs, usually from 5 to 8 mm, are removed and are replaced by similar-sized discs taken from the recently enucleated eye of a living or deceased donor. While small grafts can be retained in place by indirect sutures or splints, it is generally safer to insert direct sutures. More recently continuous sutures of very fine monofilament plastic

(Perlon) have been used. With these the eye is much more comfortable postoperatively, and as the epithelium grows over the suture rapidly it can often be left in place for many months. While many surgeons have in the past covered both eyes after this operation, the greater safety of direct suturing and of the continuous suture has made it possible for the un-operated eye to be left uncovered and also for the patient to be got out of bed at a much earlier stage.

The first dressing is usually done 24 to 48 hours after operation to exclude infection, though some surgeons prefer to wait longer. The nursing care is essentially similar to that of other eye operations, though more prolonged. Drops of antibiotics and mydriatics are generally instilled at each dressing with the addition of local steroids at the end of the first week. *The time of removal of sutures* varies greatly according to the type used and also the surgeon's preference. A successful graft is a great joy to both patient and surgeon and when healed appears as a round transparent window in the centre of the cornea.

UVEITIS

Uveitis implies inflammation of the uveal tract which comprises the iris, ciliary body and choroid. *Anterior uveitis* is the modern term for what was formerly called iritis or irido-cyclitis, *posterior uveitis* being reserved primarily for affections of the choroid, though the ciliary body may be involved. Many different causes are known to be associated with these conditions which may appear in acute or chronic form.

Acute anterior uveitis (or, as it is sometimes described, non-granulomatous uveitis) may occur in Reiter's disease, ankylosing spondylitis and other acute systemic infections, though frequently the cause is never discovered. Chronic anterior uveitis (or granulomatous uveitis) is seen not infrequently associated with sarcoidosis. Local signs depend on the severity of the condition, but in general there is circumcorneal injection, the iris itself may be dull and the pupil small; owing to increased protein the aqueous reveals a flare of scattered light when a focal beam is passed through it. The patient complains of an aching pain and is photophobic.

Treatment should aim at discovering the cause, though early local treatment with atropine is important to avoid adhesions between the iris and lens. In addition local steroids are of great value and sometimes systemic antibiotics are helpful. Hot-spoon bathing and analgesics help relieve the pain, and dark glasses are more comfortable for the patient.

Posterior uveitis (choroiditis) usually gives rise to no external signs though the patient notices some mistiness of vision. In young people it is frequently due to infection with toxoplasmosis, though other endogenous or systemic causes must be considered.

AFFECTIONS OF THE LENS

The lens is a transparent lentil-shaped structure suspended behind the iris and pupil by the zonular ligament which attaches it to the ciliary muscle. By varying the amount of pull on the zonular ligament the ciliary muscle can change the shape of the lens, thus allowing the eye to alter its accommodation or focusing power.

A **cataract** is a partial or complete opacity of the lens. It can occur in congenital forms such as those of familial origin, or as a result of maternal rubella in early pregnancy. Acquired forms may be the result of injury, though most commonly it is found in old age as senile cataract. More rarely it may be found in association with disorders of metabolism such as diabetes or galactosaemia. True diabetic cataract is rare. When found in elderly diabetics a cataract is generally of the senile variety. All cataracts interfere with vision to a greater or lesser extent; most senile cataracts cause increasing, though slow, progressive loss of vision, and if this occurs in both eyes it causes the patient to be increasingly handicapped from a visual standpoint.

Treatment is surgical, but the need for it depends entirely on how much the vision is impaired. For many years the operation in young children was performed by needling the lens, the substance of which became gradually absorbed by its contact with aqueous. Repeated needlings, however, were often necessary. In more recent years the need for these repeated procedures has been largely obviated by aspirating the contents of the lens at the time of, or shortly after, the first needling.

In adults a different operation is necessary since the nucleus of the lens is too hard to be absorbed and the cataract is removed through a much larger incision which involves the upper half of the corneoscleral region. In the majority of patients the whole lens is removed with the capsule intact (*intracapsular extraction*). Where the capsule is intentionally or inadvertently ruptured, the hard nucleus is removed together with as much soft lens matter as possible, the latter being aided by washing out the anterior chamber with Ringer's solution (*extracapsular extraction*). A peripheral iridectomy is performed before removal of the lens in either case to prevent the iris being prolapsed in the postoperative period as aqueous builds up behind it.

Various forms of suture are used, both to oppose the corneoscleral wound edges and for the conjunctiva. Immediately following operation most surgeons use miotics where an intracapsular extraction has been performed, and atropine for an extracapsular extraction. Sometimes antibiotics are instilled before the dressing is applied which usually is now to the operated eye only. If an extracapsular extraction is done the capsule which is left behind may become thickened and interfere with vision, necessitating a *capsulotomy* or needling.

The operations for cataract extraction are usually done under general anaesthesia, though in adults it is perfectly feasible under local anaesthesia and may be advisable if the patient's general condition warrants the avoidance of unnecessary general anaesthesia.

The eye dressing consists of a layer of Tulle gras, an eye pad and some form of protective shield. The first dressing is done after 24 hours, the patient being allowed up a day or two after operation, or according to the surgeon's preference.

Postoperative nursing procedure is fairly standard following most forms of intra-ocular surgery. Local steroids and a mydriatic are usually used at some stage during the first postoperative week (especially for extracapsular extractions). Postoperative complications are uncommon. *In the early postoperative period the most important of these to consider are infection, prolapse of the iris, haemorrhage (hyphaema) and delayed formation of the anterior chamber*. The operated eye can be left uncovered from the 5th or 6th postoperative day, though it should have a pad and shield for protection during the night.

External sutures which need to be removed are dealt with on the 8th to 10th postoperative day, though the deeper buried sutures are left and generally cause no trouble.

Advice to patients going home. Patients can generally leave hospital 7 to 10 days after operation. They may wear their own glasses or temporary cataract spectacles during the day and continue with a pad at night for a further week or so. The patient should be told not to touch the eye except to instil the drops prescribed by the doctor and should take care when washing not to press on the eye. Care should be taken when washing the hair not to allow shampoo onto the face. He should also be warned against unnecessary stooping.

An appointment will be given to him to return for re-examination in one to two weeks' time.

GLAUCOMA

In this condition the pressure within the eye is pathologically raised above the normal (average 15 to 20 mm Hg). It is an important cause of blindness and in its chronic form, where the visual field becomes gradually contracted, is not uncommon, occurring in some 1 to 2 per cent of people over the age of 40. Glaucoma occurs in many different forms and may be congenital or acquired. In the latter it may occur secondary to other eye disease such as anterior uveitis, injury, etc., though its primary form is relatively common and not directly associated with any other ocular condition.

Congenital glaucoma is usually seen in infants. The raised pressure may cause discomfort and photophobia so that it is not unusual to find the child burying its face in the pillow. A severe rise of pressure may cause corneal oedema and loss of vision and if the rise of pressure is unrelieved, the cornea and eventually the eye becomes much larger, hence the term buphthalmos, or 'ox eye'. The condition is due to incomplete development of the angle of the anterior chamber with mesodermal remnants preventing the escape of aqueous.

Treatment is generally by goniotomy where a special knife is used to cut through this material and encourage opening of the angle.

Primary glaucoma. The classification of primary glaucoma is now related to the appearance of the angle of the anterior chamber and may be open, *simple glaucoma*, or closed. Open-angle or simple glaucoma is always chronic and is accompanied by insidious loss of visual field. It is otherwise usually symptom-free and may only be detected when the patient goes for a routine eye examination. If the condition has been present for some years characteristic cupping of the optic discs will be noted on ophthalmoscopy. However, in its early stages, the pressure may be pathologically raised without producing any ophthalmoscopic signs. For this reason many oculists now perform routine tonometry on all patients who seek their advice for whatever reason, especially those patients over the age of 40. Angle-closure glaucoma, on the other hand, may give rise to varying degrees of discomfort, mistiness of vision or haloes round street lights, according to the type and severity of the rise of pressure. In its most severe form acute angle-closure glaucoma comes on suddenly with much pain and congestion of the eye, the patient is distressed and may even vomit. The cornea may be hazy, the eye is very injected and the pupil dilated and fixed. Vision may be reduced to 'counting fingers' or even to 'hand movements'.

Treatment in the first instance is by medical means with frequent instillation of miotics (pilocarpine or eserine) at 10-minute intervals for one or two hours and the administration of Diamox (acetazolamide) 500 mg by mouth, or by injection, which has the effect of reducing the formation of aqueous. Applications of heat with an electric eye pad or hot-spoon bathing are often of great benefit. If the condition does not respond within 12 to 24 hours, surgery must be resorted to, a broad iridectomy being generally performed. Where the raised pressure is rapidly relieved by medical means, or in those eyes which have had evidence of previous attacks and where there is a considerable risk of a further attack, it is often advisable to perform a peripheral iridectomy in order to prevent this happening.

Chronic glaucoma, whether of the simple or angle-closure type, is generally treated in the first instance medically, miotics being applied in appropriate strength and frequency to control the pressure. Occasionally other forms of drops may be used and even systemic Diamox, or similar substances, may be necessary. The patient attends the out-patient clinic regularly for examination of ocular tension and visual fields, the latter being of particular importance in indicating whether the progressive nature of the condition has been halted.

Sometimes special investigations are helpful such as tonography, which aims at assessing the facility of outflow of aqueous, or provocative tests which are designed to reveal the risk of a rise of pressure in an eye (dark-room test or mydriatic test) or to indicate the capacity of an eye for coping with increased aqueous flow (water-drinking test). In some large centres these investigations are more conveniently carried out by having special glaucoma clinics.

Should follow-up show that medical treatment is inadequate, it is then necessary to operate on the patient to increase aqueous drainage, some form of filtering procedure being carried out in which a small perforation through the corneoscleral junction is made into the anterior chamber allowing the aqueous to escape sub-conjunctivally, as it were through a safety valve. There is, however, no guarantee that these operations will be entirely successful and continued follow-up of the ocular tensions and fields is vitally necessary so that further medical treatment may be instituted, or surgery performed, if indicated.

RETINAL DETACHMENT

The retina is the nervous membrane lining the eye (see Fig. 61/1, p. 634) and is developed as an outgrowth from the brain. Originally it consists of two layers of neural ectoderm, the innermost of which forms the neural elements such as the rods and cones, bipolar cells and ganglion cells, while the outer layer forms the pigment epithelium. A detachment of the retina is really a separation of these two primordial layers. It is caused by peripheral degenerative changes in the inner layer which go on to form retinal tears through which fluid enters. These degenerative changes occur most frequently in myopic eyes, also sometimes in aphakia (where a lens has been removed) but can also be the result of injury. As the fluid increases and causes further separation of the retinal layers, vision is gradually lost and is sometimes described as being like a curtain obstructing the field of vision.

Treatment aims at sealing the retinal tears by approximating the retina to the choroid in which a controlled inflammatory reaction has been produced. This is done by operation under general anaesthesia and applying a very cold probe (cryothermy), or diathermy to the sclera. Sometimes the inflammatory reaction is produced from within the eye by using photocoagulation or a laser beam. To help approximate the retina and choroid it is usually necessary to indent the sclera by sewing on an external plomb made of silastic or silicone rubber, or even burying these materials in pockets made in the sclera. In difficult cases the general diameter of the eye is reduced by encircling it with a silicone rubber strap which itself may be buried in part or combined with one of the previously mentioned methods of scleral indentation.

At operation a small puncture in the sclera allows release of subretinal fluid which thus allows more certain approximation of the retina and choroid. The success of the operation depends entirely on the satisfactory sealing of all retinal holes, and it is therefore vitally necessary that all of them are discovered and localized before operation. To do so it is often necessary to spend a considerable time carefully examining the retina with both the direct and binocular indirect ophthalmoscopes and also with a special contact lens which allows detailed examination of the peripheral part of the retina with the slit-lamp microscope.

Both before and after operation the patient may be postured in bed in such a position that the retinal tears are in the most dependent position. Whereas at one time both eyes were covered after operation for at least a week and the patient was left lying in the same position in bed, in recent years there has been much greater relaxation and now many surgeons cover only the operated eye and allow the patient out of bed in some instances as early as two or three days after operation. Postoperative dressings and nursing care are as carried out in the operations already mentioned. *The patient is generally allowed to leave hospital one or two weeks after operation and is given an appointment to attend two to three weeks later for follow-up. He should be warned to avoid unnecessary stooping and sudden jolting movements which may shake the head.*

Since retinal detachment is basically associated with degenerative changes in the periphery of the retina, it may well occur in both eyes. If a detachment has occurred in one eye, a careful search is made in the periphery of the other, and if any areas of ominous degeneration or actual retinal holes are discovered, even though the retina is in place, prophylactic treatment by photocoagulation surrounding these areas or appropriately located cryothermy to the outside of the eye is carried out so as to forestall the development of an actual retinal separation.

STRABISMUS

Strabismus or squint occurs where there is a failure of the visual axes to meet at the point being observed. Most cases are of congenital origin and represent a failure in the development of the normal binocular reflex processes. As such it may be due to an obstruction in the afferent pathways as, for example, a cataract or macular lesion, to some defect in the efferent or neuromuscular mechanisms, or even to a weakness or absence of the central co-ordinating mechanisms responsible for the fusion of the two images. If left untreated the eye may remain or become 'lazy' or amblyopic.

Early investigation is essential to exclude any organic disease and to institute treatment. This consists of correcting refractive errors ,with glasses, and occluding the sound eye to overcome amblyopia in the squinting eye. An orthoptist can help supervise this treatment, but surgery is often necessary if the squint persists and should be undertaken as soon as reasonable vision has been achieved in each eye. Most congenital squints are convergent and surgery consists of recession of the internal rectus muscle and resection of the external rectus, though for divergent squints recession of the external rectus and resection of the internal rectus are performed. In large-angle squints it is often necessary to operate on the horizontal rectus muscles of each eye, though at different times. The operation is performed under general anaesthesia and the eye covered for 24 hours. If fine catgut is used to close the conjunctiva in young children it is unnecessary to remove sutures and the postoperative toilet of the eye with instillation of antibiotic drops is all that is necessary, the child being allowed to leave hospital two or three days after operation.

Orthoptic exercises are often helpful in the postoperative period. A functional result is hoped for, though in many instances the absence of any binocular vision means that only a cosmetic result can be achieved.

ENUCLEATION OF EYE

This may be necessary but is undertaken only for the following reasons.

(a) A painful blind eye which causes the patient constant pain and loss of sleep and which has failed to be relieved by other means.

(b) A severe injury in which the eye is so disorganized and the contents so disturbed that all vision has been lost.

(c) In certain types of injury where, though vision is not lost, severe uveitis has occurred and may go on to produce a similar condition in the other eye, *sympathetic ophthalmitis*, and which could in fact lead to loss of sight in both eyes from injury to the one.

(d) In rare instances where a primary malignant growth occurs in the eye, it may be removed in the hope that this is done in time to prevent metastasis. Malignant melanoma of the choroid is the best known example.

(e) Occasionally in severely infected eyes (*panophthalmitis*), where the eye is virtually a bag of pus, the contents are eviscerated after removing the cornea but leaving the sclera in place.

Again it should be emphasized that every care is taken to mark the eye to be removed, and the patient agrees and signs the consent form correctly. The operation is almost always done under general anaesthesia; the rectus muscles are preserved so as to be attached to a plastic implant which, when the socket has healed, allows a much better movement of a moulded artificial eye. Some bleeding is generally encountered at operation and this is controlled by a small swab previously dipped in hot saline applied gently but firmly to the socket. The deeper fascial tissues are sutured with catgut and the conjunctiva closed with a black silk running suture which can be removed about the fifth postoperative day. *A gentle pressure pad is applied as dressing but should not be too firm, since this can cause considerable postoperative discomfort and may even lead to a slowing up of the patient's heart rate.*

We have just discussed what must be considered the final failure of ophthalmic surgery. Much of what has gone before, however, has concerned conditions which could all too frequently lead to blindness, but with treatment lead to recovery. There is nothing so gratifying to patient, nurse and surgeon as the restoration or preservation of sight, and those working in this speciality will be rewarded by their patients' appreciation and gratitude.

Chapter 62

A Brief Account of Some Neurosurgical Conditions

by A. E. BOOTH

Injuries to the head—mechanisms—immediate complications—late complications: haemorrhage in head injuries, infection, metabolic complications, remote complications—intracranial tumours—cerebral abscess—intracranial haemorrhage—spinal surgery—protruded intervertebral disc—hydrocephalus—spina bifida—surgery of pain—stereotactic surgery—postoperative care of neurosurgical patients—care of the unconscious patient—observations

---

The neurosurgeon may be called upon to treat the many conditions which may affect the brain, the spinal cord or their coverings and the peripheral nerves.

HEAD INJURY

As the density of road traffic mounts, head injury is becoming increasingly common. Over two people in every 1,000 are admitted to hospital each year with a head injury; of these over 60 per cent have been involved in a road traffic accident. Fortunately, the great majority of these patients are kept in hospital for only 24 or 48 hours of observation and make a full recovery.

A minority require longer stay in hospital, either because of the *severity* of brain damage or because of *complications* of their injury, or a combination of both these factors. *Few of these severely injured patients require surgical intervention* other than the immediate suture of lacerations. *The survival of the severe head injury depends nearly always on the quality of the nursing and medical care.* These patients provide some of the most difficult but rewarding problems in nursing.

MECHANISM OF DAMAGE TO THE BRAIN

Perhaps the most useful point to grasp is the importance of rapid changes in the speed of movements of the head, or more properly *acceleration and deceleration*. The brain has a consistency rather like a firm jelly

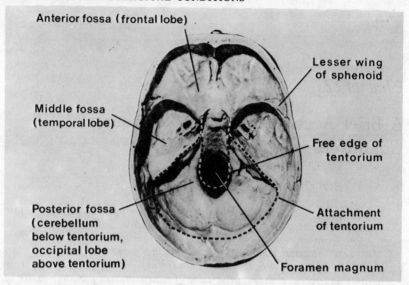

Anterior fossa (frontal lobe)

Lesser wing of sphenoid

Middle fossa (temporal lobe)

Free edge of tentorium

Posterior fossa (cerebellum below tentorium, occipital lobe above tentorium)

Attachment of tentorium

Foramen magnum

Fig. 62/1 This photograph of the skull, viewed from above, shows the many sharp edges which may injure a brain as it is shaken inside this hard bony box in a head injury.

and lies loosely inside the hard, bony skull. It is restrained but not prevented from moving by the inner foldings of the dura which form the *falx cerebri* (lying between the cerebral hemispheres in the midline), and the *tentorium cerebelli* (stretching like a tent over the cerebellum and dividing it from the cerebral hemispheres above). If the rapidly moving head is brought suddenly to a standstill, as when a motor cyclist rides into a brick wall, the soft brain is swirled and shaken inside the skull and may be bruised or torn against the sharp edges within it (see Fig. 62/1). This damage is in addition to the injury that occurs directly under the point of impact. Loss of consciousness is the direct result of the general shaking the brain receives. A man who is hit on the head by a sharp object whose mass is too low to accelerate the skull may receive a wound which penetrates deep into the brain without any loss of consciousness. The seriousness of a head injury, the length of unconsciousness, and amnesia (loss of memory) and severity of the after-effects largely depend on the amount of shaking that the brain receives and thus on the amount of change of speed which occurs in the accident.

A head injury may be classed as simple if the damage that occurs is confined to the bruising and shaking of the brain, even though this may result in prolonged unconsciousness. The *complications* of head injury can be grouped into those which occur at the time of the accident and those which arise later.

IMMEDIATE COMPLICATIONS

The severity of damage *to the scalp and skull* is a guide to the likely severity of the damage to the underlying brain. Moreover, the scalp is extremely richly supplied with blood vessels and a considerable loss of blood may occur from a scalp laceration. The bleeding can usually be controlled by pressure from a firm pad and bandage as a first-aid measure.

Fracture. A simple linear skull fracture is of itself of little importance. If such a fracture, however, runs into one of the paranasal air sinuses or into the middle ear and if the dura beneath the fracture is torn, then cerebrospinal fluid (C.S.F.) may escape from the subarachnoid space to the outside and a free route of entry for infection exists. *It is most important that these patients are not allowed to blow the nose; to do so might force infection from the nasal cavity into the subarachnoid space and cause a meningitis.* Most C.S.F. leaks stop spontaneously but it is occasionally necessary to plug the leak at operation. With more severe injuries, fragments of bone may be depressed below the contour of the skull. If the underlying dura remains intact, these depressed fractures may still interfere with brain function by pressure on the cortex. If the dura is torn and the underlying brain lacerated, there is also a considerable risk of infection.

Other injuries. The severity of the head injury must not be allowed to distract attention from injuries to other parts of the body; particularly in road traffic accidents, patients may have fractures of the long bones or of the ribs, or have injuries to abdominal or thoracic viscera.

Immediate injury to brain. Unlike cells almost anywhere else in the body, nerve cells are not replaced nor do their axons (the processes from the cell bodies) regrow within the brain or spinal cord, although they may do so in peripheral nerves. This means that brain damaged at the time of the accident cannot be replaced. Recovery of function after a head injury (or any other damage which is done to the brain, as in a cerebral haemorrhage) is a process of substitution, with other nearby cells taking over the function of those which have been destroyed. It follows that the prevention of the late complications of head injury which may lead to further brain damage gives the patient the best chance of making a useful recovery.

LATE COMPLICATIONS

The late complications of head injury are brain swelling, haemorrhage, infection and metabolic disturbances. The brain is the most sensitive of all tissues to lack of oxygen. A moderate oxygen lack greatly hinders normal cell function, and the cells so deprived respond by swelling. Complete oxygen lack for more than three minutes causes death of nerve cells. Since brain swelling (cerebral oedema) in response to oxygen lack occurs in the closed box of the skull, the result is a great increase in the pressure within the skull. This makes it yet more difficult for an adequate blood supply and thus enough oxygen to reach the brain. Hence a vicious circle is set up.

Cerebral oedema after head injury may be caused in two ways. The initial injury may have damaged the blood supply to a part of the brain; the swelling resulting is inevitable. The second probable cause is a fall in the total amount of oxygen which reaches the brain, which may be due to respiratory obstruction. As soon as an unconscious patient is seen, the adequacy of his airway must be ensured.

Treatment of cerebral oedema. Brain swelling may be temporarily reduced by sucking water out of the swollen cells into the bloodstream and thence out of the body via the kidneys. This may be achieved by giving Lasix (a diuretic) by injection. Alternatively, a concentrated solution of mannitol or urea can be given intravenously. This rapidly reduces intracranial pressure. Unfortunately, these methods only reduce brain swelling for a few hours. The more lasting control of cerebral oedema is given by the use of steroids in very high dosage, although this treatment works relatively slowly and is thus of little use in emergency.

Haemorrhage may occur either into the substance of the brain (intracerebral), into the space between the arachnoid and the dura (subdural), or between the skull and the dura (extradural). *Intracerebral haemorrhage* usually occurs at the time of the injury and is seen only in the most severe brain damage. The size of the haematoma is usually small and its operative removal of little help. In most head injuries, there is a small amount of bleeding over the surface of the brain. Occasionally, there will be enough blood clot in the subdural space to cause brain compression. *The acute subdural haematoma* large enough to warrant operative removal is always associated with severe brain damage and carries a very poor prognosis. *Extradural haematoma* is the least common of this group but it is the most dramatic. Bleeding comes from the blood supply to the dura, most commonly the middle meningeal artery which has been torn across by a fracture. The steady leak of blood forms an expanding mass between the skull and dura. The initial head injury may be relatively minor, and the patient may quite quickly regain consciousness only to sink again into deepening coma with a pupil that becomes fixed and dilated on the side of the injury, as the haematoma causes increasing pressure on the brain.

Since the associated brain damage is often slight, these patients can make a very good recovery if the clot is evacuated quickly enough. It is largely to detect this grave complication of head injury that any patient who is unconscious after an accident, even for a very short time, must be admitted to hospital for observation.

Infection of the brain following head injury is fortunately not very common. The risks of C.S.F. leak and depressed fracture have been mentioned. Careful surgical cleansing of the wound and antibiotic cover help to minimize the risk. *Chest infection,* however, frequently complicates head injury just as it may complicate the course of any patient unconscious or semi-conscious from any other cause. Such infection reduces the amount of oxygen entering the bloodstream and thus the amount of oxygen that reaches the brain. This may cause cerebral oedema (see p. 657). Prevention should be the aim and may often be achieved by repeated vigorous physiotherapy. To encourage a patient to cough and to keep the mouth and nasopharynx clear of secretions by suction should be part of the normal nursing care of these patients, and does not demand the attention of a skilled physiotherapist. Percussion of the chest to break up tenacious secretions can again be carried out by the nurse under the occasional supervision of a physiotherapist.

Metabolic complications. Brain damage in the region of the pituitary gland may interfere with the formation of the antidiuretic hormone and thus lead to an outpouring of very dilute urine (diabetes insipidus). These patients are unable to adjust their fluid output to their intake and unless a close watch is kept on their fluid balance they may become severely dehydrated. Gross electrolyte disturbances are also occasionally seen in brain damage in this area (see p. 463). *Hyperpyrexia* is another infrequent complication of head injury. Such patients may develop a fever of 41·4 °C (106 °F) or higher. The most vigorous methods may be required to reduce the temperatures (see p. 109).

Remote complications. About 10 per cent of all patients who have had a head injury will develop fits. The more severe the injury, the greater the risk of developing epilepsy. For those patients in whom the period of *amnesia* after the accident is greater than 24 hours, the risk increases to 25 per cent. *Poor concentration and slowing of the thought processes* is quite commonly seen immediately after a head injury. The large majority of patients will make a full recovery from these symptoms and return to their normal work. In a small proportion, however, this mental slowing will persist and these patients will be unable to return to their previous jobs and unfortunately must accept the drop in income that a less skilled position may imply. About 1 per cent of all patients admitted for head injury will show so severe a disability that they will be unable to return to work at all.

TYPES OF BRAIN TUMOUR

Intracranial tumour. As with any other part of the body, tumours that arise within the head may do so from nearly any of the structures within it. The single exception to this statement are the nerve cells themselves. Tumours arise when, because of an error in the normal process of cell division, a group of abnormal cells is formed which do not respond to the usual growth control mechanisms. Since adult nerve cells do not divide and no repair of nervous tissue occurs within the body, tumours of adult nerve cells do not occur.

The commonest group of tumours within the head are the *gliomas*. These arise from the brain's supporting cells—the glial tissue—which acts as the connective tissue of the brain. This group ranges from the highly malignant *glioblastoma multiforme* to the *benign cystic astrocytoma* of the cerebellum seen in children. Malignancy in intracranial tumour must be judged on other grounds than those applied to tumours elsewhere in the body. Although invasion of tissues within the brain will certainly occur, these tumours very rarely form metastases; however tumours which arise from the tissue lining the ventricular system, the *ependymomas*, may form seedlings elsewhere in the neuraxis.

Tumours of the coverings of the brain, the *meningiomas*, are as a rule relatively benign. Since they do not directly involve brain tissue, but produce their symptoms by pressure on its surface, their removal may lead to a complete cure of the patient's symptoms.

Ten per cent of intracranial tumours arise from the *pituitary gland*. These tumours may grow upwards out of the pituitary fossa to press on the optic chiasm which lies above the gland and thus cause blindness in a part of the visual field. These patients may also show some of the signs of pituitary insufficiency.

Nearly as common as the gliomas are *metastatic tumours*, seedlings from lesions elsewhere in the body. Carcinoma of the bronchus is particularly prone to give intracranial secondaries, as may tumours of the breast and kidney.

Presentation of patients with intracranial tumours. Tumours within the head call attention to themselves by their *local* effects, and by the *generalized* rise in pressure within the head that they may cause.

Local effects. Of these, *epilepsy* is perhaps the most common. Some 50 per cent of all patients who present with intracranial tumour have had one or more fits by the time of their admission. *Weakness* or *sensory change* reflects interference with the motor or sensory cortex. *Blindness* in a part of the visual field occurs in pituitary tumours which compress the optic chiasm. *Personality change*—increased irritability, forgetfulness, abnormal sleep patterns—may occur in frontal tumour. Disorders of the speech process, the *dysphasias*, are often seen in tumours arising in the temporo-parietal region within the dominant hemisphere.

The rise in intracranial pressure may reflect the size of the tumour itself. A second cause is blockage or distortion of the cerebrospinal fluid pathways giving a hydrocephalus (see p. 662), this commonly happens in cerebellar tumours since with these lesions the narrow aqueduct leading from the third to the fourth ventricle is often blocked. The third mechanism is that the more rapidly growing tumours often provoke a surrounding area of cerebral swelling.

The symptoms of rising intracranial pressure are headache, nausea and vomiting, and increasing drowsiness. Their presence lends some urgency to the investigation and treatment of the patient.

Operative treatment of tumour. The basic neurosurgical aim is the complete removal of the tumour without causing disabling damage to the surrounding brain. With the more malignant tumours, however, total excision is rarely possible and the surgeon must content himself with the removal of the centre of the mass to produce a decompression, thus reducing both the general effects of raised intracranial pressure and also diminishing the local disturbance caused by the tumour. With tumours in the frontal or temporal regions a further decompression may be obtained by performing a frontal or temporal lobectomy. *Postoperatively*, the use of radiotherapy may produce a further worthwhile reduction in tumour volume and delay its inevitable recurrence. The long-term use of steroids may help to control the cerebral swelling that the tumour has caused.

CEREBRAL ABSCESS

Abscesses in the brain may be caused by infection spreading *directly* from infection in the ear or the paranasal sinuses, or *indirectly* via the bloodstream from other heavily infected sites, such as the lung in a patient with bronchiectasis, or the heart in a patient with subacute bacterial endocarditis. Abscesses behave very much like rapidly growing tumours; they are almost always surrounded by very considerable brain swelling and these patients may deteriorate rapidly.

Treatment is by repeated aspiration of the abscess through a burr hole made in the skull and the instillation of antibiotics into the abscess cavity, together with heavy general antibiotic therapy.

INTRACRANIAL HAEMORRHAGE

Subarachnoid haemorrhage may occur from aneurysms arising from the larger cerebral vessels or from arteriovenous malformations. Here bleeding occurs into the subarachnoid space, deep to the arachnoid mater in which all the surface vessels of the brain travel before entering its substance. In this space the C.S.F. circulates after it has left the fourth ventricle, and so a subarachnoid bleed may be diagnosed by finding blood mixed with the C.S.F. at lumbar puncture. Typically the patient complains of the sudden onset of severe headache and often loses consciousness. If the haemorrhage has been massive, the blood may tear into the substance of the brain and cause hemiparesis or other localizing signs of damage.

Treatment of such subarachnoid bleeding is limited to the prevention of further bleeds. This may be achieved by clipping the neck of the aneurysm responsible, which usually sits on the wall of the parent artery like a berry on a twig, or by excising the knot of abnormal vessels which comprise the arteriovenous malformation.

Chronic subdural haematoma. Unlike the acute subdural haematoma seen after major head injury, the chronic form, although caused by minor head trauma, accumulates very slowly over a long period. The patient may not present until two to three months after the very minor injury that provoked it. Indeed, in many patients no clear history of a blow to the head is found. These patients are often elderly and give a story of recurrent headaches progressing to fluctuating episodes of drowsiness; they usually respond rapidly to the drainage of the haematoma through burr holes.

Intracerebral haemorrhage. This subject is dealt with more fully in neurology (see p. 259). Surgery has little place in the treatment of intracerebral haemorrhage, although an operation to remove a large clot may very occasionally be justified.

SPINAL SURGERY

The spinal cord and its nerve roots, like the brain, is enclosed in a bony cage. Thus a tumour within the spinal canal interferes with its function by compressing the blood vessels supplying it. *A tumour* arising within the spinal canal does not need to grow very big before severe cord compression occurs.

Patients with *compression of the cord* present with increasing weakness of the legs or, if the tumour is in the cervical region, of both arms and legs. There is a disturbance of sensation below the level of compression and often bladder control is lost. Severe pain at the site of compression is commonly seen. Tumours arising in the substance of the cord are rare and it is seldom that they can be removed. Nevertheless, a laminectomy to decompress the cord followed by radiotherapy may give a worthwhile remission. The commonest cause of cord compression is by metastatic tumour. Often the body of an invaded vertebra collapses and the tumour grows into the spinal canal to press on the dura and cord. These patients often progress very rapidly to a complete *paraplegia* (paralysis of legs) or *quadriplegia* (paralysis of arms and legs) and decompression is of little benefit. It is only when the weakness comes on slowly and there is still some power left in the legs that decompression by removing the spines and laminae which form the posterior part of the bony cage may give any worthwhile relief of symptoms.

PROTRUDED INTERVERTEBRAL DISC (slipped disc)

The normal intervertebral disc consists of a soft central *nucleus pulposus* surrounded by a thick tough capsule, the *annulus fibrosus*. These springy structures act as shock absorbers between the vertebrae. Occasionally the disc undergoes a degenerative change. A heavy strain to the back may then force the softened nucleus through the weak annulus to form a protrusion over which a nerve root may become stretched as it leaves the spinal cord. This stretching of the nerve root causes pain radiating down the leg. Since any flexion of the hip or back increases the tension on the nerve root, the patient's back is stiff and movement tends to aggravate the pain. Straight leg raising is diminished on the side of the protrusion. Sufficiently severe stretching causes numbness and weakness of the muscles within the territory supplied by that nerve root. Disc protrusions most commonly occur between the 4th and 5th lumbar vertebrae and the 5th lumbar and 1st sacral vertebra, for here the mechanical strains on the back are at their greatest.

Treatment is to excise not only the protruded part of the nucleus but also as much as possible of the degenerate material still within the disc in order to prevent a recurrence.

HYDROCEPHALUS

Some babies are born with a congenital blockage of the cerebrospinal pathways, either at the aqueduct leading from the third to the fourth ventricle or in the subarachnoid space, preventing the fluid from flowing up to be absorbed into the sagittal sinus. Since C.S.F. continues to be secreted by the choroid plexus within the lateral ventricles, the ventricles become blown up and the overlying brain squeezed and thinned. In the infant, the bones of the skull have not become fused together so that the head circumference increases rapidly. Unless the pressure inside the ventricles is relieved by draining the excess fluid away as it is formed, irreversible brain damage will be caused and may indeed already have occurred at birth.

These children are treated by draining the fluid through a *ventriculo-atrial shunt*, a tube of which one end is passed through the skull and brain into the lateral ventricle while the other end is led down under the skin into the internal jugular vein in the neck and thence down the lumen of the vein until its tip lies in the right atrium of the heart. A valve within the tube prevents the reflux of blood up the tube. These valves have the added advantage that by pressing on them as they lie on the skull under the scalp, fluid can be pumped along the tube and thus minor blocks may be cleared and the function of the system checked. The valves most frequently used are the Spitz Holter and the Pudenz. Provided that the damage to the brain *in utero* has not been too great, these children may go on to develop normally. Unfortunately, the majority will show some retardation.

SPINA BIFIDA

The brain and spinal cord form at a very early stage in the development of the embryo when it consists merely of a flat disc of cells. A groove appears in the ectoderm on the surface of the disc. The lips of the groove then meet in the midline and fuse, thus forming a tube of ectoderm buried within the disc. From this tube the central nervous system will be formed. Occasionally the burying of the tube is not completed at its lower end and at a later stage in development the laminae of the vertebrae fail to cover the back of the spinal cord, giving rise to the condition known as spina bifida.

In its mildest form, *spina bifida occulta* (meaning hidden), only the bony abnormality is present and skin and spinal cord are normal. These children usually show no neurological abnormality. In more severe forms the skin is also deficient and the cord and its coverings appear on the surface as a bulging *myelomeningocele*. In the most extreme form of the abnormality the lower spinal cord is functionless and the baby is paraplegic with no control of bladder or rectum. With lesser degrees of abnormality there may be enough power in the legs later to permit the child to walk. Myelomeningocele should be treated as soon after birth as possible (see below), for the thin sac which represents the coverings of the cord may have ruptured during birth. This open pathway into the subarachnoid space forms an easy route for infection, while the exposed spinal cord may lose yet more of its function if it is allowed to become dry.

Treatment is to excise the sac of the meningocele and to cover the defect with healthy skin. If the defect is very large, a plastic procedure may be required to swing enough skin over the defect to cover it.

Even after the defect has been closed these children demand long-continued skilled supervision. Many will require orthopaedic procedures to correct associated deformities of the hips and feet. The problem of continued incontinence may demand the formation of a new bladder from an isolated loop of ileum into which the ureters are transplanted; the other end of this loop is brought out onto the abdominal wall as a spout to which a drainage bag can more easily be attached. Nearly 50 per cent of patients with myelomeningocele go on to develop hydrocephalus, and these children will also require a ventriculo-atrial shunt.

The strain on the parents of children with this congenital deformity is enormous. It is only with the constant support, encouragement and understanding of all who have to deal with their child that they will be able to cope with the continuing burden of bringing up and caring for him.

SURGERY OF PAIN

Trigeminal neuralgia (tic douloureux). This most distressing condition usually affects the more elderly patient. Classically, he complains of lightning stabs of pain in the face involving one or more of the divisions of the trigeminal nerve. (The first, ophthalmic division supplies forehead and cornea, the second, maxillary division supplies the cheek and upper lip whilst the third, mandibular division supplies the lower cheek and lower lip.) The lightest touch may set off the pain and the patient is often afraid to eat or talk. The cause is thought to be a degenerative process affecting the sensory ganglion of the trigeminal nerve. The attacks are often controlled by the drug Tegretol, an anticonvulsant, but should medication fail to relieve the patient's symptoms the neurosurgeon may be asked to cut the trigeminal sensory root within the skull. A less certain method of control is to inject alcohol into the trigeminal ganglion. Either procedure will cure the pain but will leave the patient with a permanently numbed face.

Chordotomy. Patients with advanced malignant disease often suffer very severe pain which cannot adequately be controlled by drugs. For these patients it is justifiable to cut the spinothalamic tract. This bundle of nerve fibres runs upwards in the spinal cord to the thalamus and is responsible for carrying the sensations of pain and temperature. The procedure makes that part of the body below and on the opposite side to the cut in the spinal cord insensitive to pain and to the sensations of hot or cold. Sensation for touch is left intact.

STEREOTACTIC SURGERY

Parkinson's disease has already been discussed in the section on neurology (p. 263). If drugs fail to control the patient's symptoms surgery may be necessary. It has been found that if a tiny part of the thalamus is destroyed at surgery, the tremor and rigidity of Parkinson's disease (but not the slowness of movement or loss of balance) may be controlled. Since the thalamus is a structure deep inside the brain, an operation to expose it directly would carry a considerable risk of causing severe damage. In a stereotactic operation, an electrode held in a frame clamped rigidly to the skull can be passed with great accuracy through a burr hole until its tip lies within the thalamus. An electric current passed through the electrode destroys the tissue in the immediate vicinity of its tip. The precise direction in which the electrode is passed is calculated from a series of X-rays.

POSTOPERATIVE CARE OF NEUROSURGICAL PATIENTS

Following an intracranial operation, as soon as a patient is returned to the ward, he must be under constant observation so that the postoperative complications of secondary bleeding into the wound or brain swelling can be detected at the earliest opportunity.

Although many patients who have undergone neurosurgical procedures recover consciousness quite rapidly, some may fail to do so for many hours. The principles discussed in the section on the care of the unconscious patient (see p. 665) hold good for these cases.

Even after the immediate postoperative period, the process of recovery may be slow. The retraining of a patient recovering from a hemiparesis in the basic skills of feeding, walking and caring for himself requires the constant concern and assistance of the nurses who care for him. Often these patients are confused after their operation, they may not realize that they are in hospital or that they have had an operation. Particularly after operations on the dominant hemisphere, the normal processes of speech may be slow to return. *The nurse should realize that patients who do not speak may yet be fully aware of what is going on around them, and that their inability to communicate increases their fear and distress.* To talk to the patient and to explain what has happened and what one is about to do takes very little time but helps enormously to comfort and to reassure him.

The nurse will realize that the relatives are often more frightened and worried than the patient. They may be afraid to ask and will be thankful for a simple explanation of what has been done to the patient and how he is recovering. This is, of course, a job that must be shared by the doctors who are looking after him, but it is a role in which the nurse can play a great part. To reply to their questions with time-worn phrases would do little to ease their anxiety.

CARE OF THE UNCONSCIOUS PATIENT

Nursing care of the unconscious patient, particularly when loss of consciousness is prolonged, demands skill and constant attention. The nurse is responsible for the *support* of an individual many of whose protective mechanisms have broken down. Her accurate *observations* on the patient will be the guide to his medical or surgical management.

Airway: earlier in this chapter the paramount importance of the patient's airway has been stressed (see p. 657), and the nurse's responsibility for its maintenance does not stop until the patient has regained full consciousness. Immediately after a head injury, or other cause of any loss of consciousness (drug overdose, diabetic coma, stroke and the like), the patient's airway is threatened by two factors. The muscle tone of his tongue and jaw may be diminished, allowing the tongue to fall back and obstruct the airway. Since his protective cough reflex is diminished or absent, saliva, blood, vomit, or foreign bodies—such as broken teeth or dentures—may fill the mouth and add to this obstruction.

The immediate treatment is to clear the mouth of as much vomit or other obstructive content as possible and to turn the patient into the semiprone ('coma') position (see Fig. 8/3, p. 80). This lets the secretions drain from the mouth rather than down into the trachea and allows the tongue to fall forward. If the airway is still inadequate, it may further be improved by placing the fingers behind the angle of the jaw on each side and lifting the jaw forward so as to make the bottom teeth protrude. This manoeuvre lifts the root of the tongue forwards and upwards and again helps to maintain an adequate airway.

In the ward, where adequate suction apparatus is to hand, the semiprone position is no longer mandatory. The more deeply unconscious patient may require an oral airway while, if these measures are not sufficient, the doctor may decide that an oro-tracheal tube should be passed. The modern 'Portex' plastic tubes may safely be left *in situ* for as many as 7 to 10 days. If, however, tracheal intubation is likely to be prolonged beyond this time, then a tracheostomy may be necessary. As long as the patient breathes noisily, his airway is almost certainly unsatisfactory and every attempt must be made to improve it. Quiet, smooth respirations spell success.

Chest care. Once the anatomical airway has been ensured, constant efforts must be made to keep it clear of secretions. *Frequent oro-pharyngeal suction* is often necessary and, skilfully performed, may stimulate a good cough response and thus further help to keep the chest clear. If an endotracheal tube or tracheostomy is *in situ*, then bronchial toilet down the tube should be performed as soon as the patient sounds 'bubbly'. If the suction negative pressure is too high then the bronchial mucosa may be damaged by being sucked into the catheter. Thus the suction for endotracheal toilet should normally not exceed 100 mm Hg or 15 cm water. The suction tubes used must be soft and the suction head fitted with a side hole so that by placing or removing a finger on the hole, the suction at the catheter tip can be turned on or off as required. When bronchial suction is employed, a strict 'no-touch' technique should be used. The catheter should be handled with disposable plastic gloves and gently introduced down the endo-tracheal tube or into the tracheostomy *without* suction and then withdrawn with suction applied. A catheter should be passed once and once only.

Inspired air is normally humidified as it passes over the moist mem-branes of the nose and mouth, but if a patient has a tracheostomy or an oro-tracheal tube this humidification cannot occur. The mucosa of the bronchi and trachea become dried and the bronchial secretions thick and difficult to remove. There are several forms of *humidifier* to deal with this problem. A more simple and just as effective a method is to set up a saline drip into the trachea through a fine intravenous catheter passed down the tube. The drip should run at some six to eight drops per minute.

In all patients, whether or not a cough reflex persists, *regular chest percussion and posturing* by the physiotherapist will help to keep the bronchi clear of secretion. This is not a difficult technique and the good nurse will quite early learn to apply it.

Skin care must be meticulous (see Prevention of Pressure, p. 49).

Mouth care. The mouth of the unconscious patient quickly becomes foul and crusted with dried secretions, for the normal flow of saliva and the washing action of tongue movements are lost. Careful cleansing of the teeth and gums with swabs moistened with Glycothymoline or a similar oral antiseptic should be carried out at least every four hours (see also p. 45). In this way the risk of infection of the parotid gland may be prevented.

Eye care. Some unconscious patients lie with the eyes open or only half closed. The absence of the blink reflex allows the exposed cornea to be-come dried and may lead to abrasion or ulceration. This risk can be pre-vented by the instillation of methyl cellulose or paraffin eye drops every six hours (see Corneal Exposure, p. 647).

Control of temperature. Pyrexia above 38·3 °C (101 °F) may cause a significant deterioration in a patient's cerebral state. As the temperature of a tissue rises, so does its oxygen requirement. In the damaged brain, where blood flow may already be embarrassed by brain swelling, it may be impossible to meet such an increased demand and further hypoxia, with its consequent brain swelling, may result. The temperature can usually be sufficiently lowered by exposing the patient and playing a fan on him. The use of one to two aspirin suppositories of 600 mg each also is of value. It may occasionally be necessary to sponge the patient with tepid water in order still further to decrease his temperature. Shivering tends to drive the temperature up again and it may be necessary to control this by the use of chlorpromazine (Largactil).

Bladder. An unconscious patient may have retention of urine and then he requires catheterization and continuous bladder drainage. Intermittent drainage carries the risk of provoking an ascending urinary tract infection and should thus not be used in these circumstances. If a patient is frequently incontinent the care of his skin may become complicated by the constantly wet beds. In these circumstances, it is justifiable to catheterize females. In the male it may be possible to drain the urine away by applying a length of Paul's tubing (a Latex rubber tube which comes in a variety of sizes) over the shaft of the penis and attaching the other end to a disposable urine bag. The tube is secured to the penis with strapping or, better, by using a Latex adhesive. If this method fails then in the male, too, a catheter should be used.

Bowels. For the first four to five days of unconsciousness, no steps need be taken to empty the bowel. Thereafter, glycerin or other suppositories or a simple saline enema will usually suffice.

Feeding. The unconscious patient requires both fluid and a source of energy. A normal adult should have between 2 and 3 litres of fluid in each 24 hours to replace that lost in the urine, sweat, and as the moisture in the expired air. If unconsciousness is prolonged, gross wasting with loss of muscle bulk will result unless an adequate protein and calorie intake of between 2,500 and 3,000 calories per day is given. In the very early stages of the patient's illness intravenous fluid replacement may be required. Within 24 to 48 hours, however, the stomach and small bowel will have become normally active in most patients and nasogastric feeding can be instituted. The return of normal bowel sounds on listening to the abdomen with a stethoscope confirms that it is reasonable to start feeding by this method. A regime of 250 ml each 2 hours will give a full 3 litres in the 24 hours. Care must be taken to aspirate the tube before giving the feed to ensure that the previous feed has passed from the stomach. If the patient's fluid replacement is to be managed properly, the keeping of an accurate fluid balance chart is essential.

Restlessness in the unconscious patient may be an indication of pain or the discomfort of a full bladder. Simple analgesics or catheterization often quieten the patient satisfactorily. Codeine phosphate, 60 mg, usually relieves headache. The stronger analgesics—such as pethidine or morphine —should never be used in the unconscious patient, for these drugs may unduly depress the respiratory centre and lead to hypoxia with its attendant dangers, while their sedative effect may mask important changes in the patient's conscious level. A patient recovering consciousness after head injury may pass through a phase of irritability quite apart from that caused by discomfort. Any interference will be resented, often with violence, and the patient may become very noisy. In these special circumstances it is occasionally justifiable to use physical restraint. Hands may be wrapped in Gamgee tissue and firmly bandaged to prevent the patient from pulling out catheters or tubes, and cot sides may be used.

If possible, these patients should be nursed in a darkened side ward so that they do not disturb and are not disturbed by other patients. Sedatives may rarely be necessary but must be used with great care, for here again, a deterioration in the patient's condition that might call for urgent treatment may be masked.

OBSERVATIONS

The purpose of the repeated neurological observations made on an unconscious patient is to chart his progress. One set of observations on its own is of little value, only when it is compared with those that have been made before can the patient's improvement or deterioration be gauged.

The functions that are recorded are the patient's conscious level, pulse rate, blood pressure, temperature, respiratory rate and pupil reactions. *In assessing the conscious level* of a patient, it is important to record it in a way that is meaningful to others. The terms drowsy, stuporose, comatose, etc., are of little help unless the physical state that they describe is clearly understood by everyone. The most satisfactory method of recording a patient's conscious level is to note what responses he will give. Thus the serial observations 'unresponsive to pain'—'flexes limbs to pain'—'localizes a painful stimulus'—'responds to command but will not talk'—'will say a few words but grossly confused'—'fully alert'—will chart a patient's progress from deep coma to recovery. These records can be clearly understood by those inspecting the charts and can be reproduced by a second observer.

Pulse and blood pressure. If the pressure inside the skull rises, as when a blood clot develops or brain swelling occurs, there is a reflex rise in the blood pressure and a fall in the pulse rate. Conversely, a low blood pressure with a rapid pulse may be a sign of blood loss and an indication for transfusion.

The temperature must be monitored so that cooling may be instituted if it rises too high.

The respiratory rate and pattern should be recorded. A rapid respiration may mean that a chest infection is present and call for its treatment, while irregular respirations may be a sign of grossly raised intracranial pressure with embarrassment of the respiratory centre.

The pupils should be carefully observed. The constrictor muscle of the pupil is supplied by the third cranial oculomotor nerve. This nerve arises from the brainstem in the posterior fossa and then passes forward and upward along the free edge of the tentorium to reach the back of the eye. If the cerebral hemisphere swells, or is compressed by blood clot, the nerve may be squeezed against the free edge of the tentorium and the constrictor of the pupil paralysed. Thus a pupil that becomes fixed and dilated is a most sinister sign and may call for the institution of urgent surgical or medical means to reduce the pressure inside the head.

Frequency. In the early stages of unconsciousness or postoperative period when the patient's condition may change rapidly, frequent observations should be made, usually each 15 minutes. Later on, however, when the rate of change is likely to be slower, the frequency can be decreased gradually to four-hourly intervals.

Chapter 63

Neurological and Neurosurgical Investigation

by A. E. BOOTH

*Electroencephalography (E.E.G.)—electromyography (E.M.G.)—
brain scan, gamma scan—echoencephalography, ultra sound—radiological investigations—cerebral angiography—air encephalography—
ventriculography—myelography*

As with many specialities, diagnosis in neurology and neurosurgery relies
quite heavily on a variety of sophisticated tests. The basic principles behind
them are usually quite simple.

Electroencephalography (E.E.G.). If wire electrodes are attached to the
skull and connected to very sensitive recording equipment, it can be shown
that the normal brain has a constant electrical activity and that this activity
varies both with the site from which records are made and also with the
state of awareness of the subject. Careful recording of this electrical
activity may reveal abnormalities which help to localize a lesion within
the brain and to give some clue as to its nature.

Electromyography (E.M.G.). By recording the passage of electrical impulses along a nerve it is possible to show whether the nerve has been
damaged by local trauma or by compression, or is affected by a specific
disease of nerves (a neuropathy). Similarly, the electrical activity of a
muscle can be recorded and a weakness due to interruption of nerve fibres
to that muscle differentiated from one due to a primary disease of muscle
(a myopathy).

Brain scan, gamma scan. It has been shown that some brain tumours (but
by no means all) actively take up radioactive substances from the bloodstream. These tumours thus become more radioactive than the surrounding brain, and their increased activity can be recorded by a special 'gamma
scanner'. The resulting picture shows the lesion as a 'hot spot' (see Fig.
63/1). Brain abscesses and intracerebral haematomas are also sometimes
shown in this way. The enormous advantage of this technique is that there
is no risk or discomfort for the patient. It can be performed as an out-
patient procedure and patients who show a positive scan can then be
selected for more sophisticated neuro-radiological procedures.

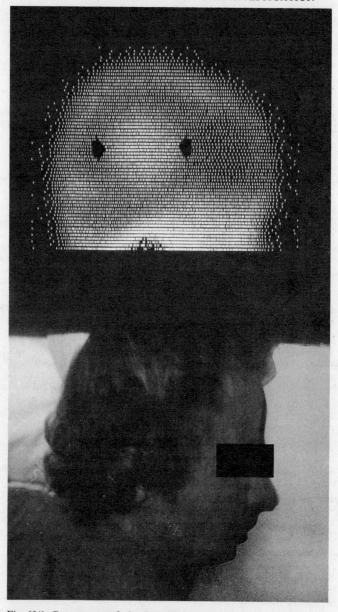

Fig. 63/1 Gamma scan of a large parietal tumour. The area of high uptake shows pale against the darker area of normal brain where the uptake is normal. The photograph below indicates the position of the patient's head when the scan was performed.

Echoencephalography, ultra-sound. This is another rapid, safe and pain-less procedure which can be of great help in selecting patients who require a more specialized investigation. By placing a special probe against the surface of the skull, it is possible to bounce very high frequency sound waves from the midline structures of the brain. By measuring the time taken for the echo to return to the probe the distance of the midline from the skull surface can be calculated. In a normal individual when recordings are taken from both sides of the skull, the midline structures should be shown the same distance away from the probe on each side. If, however, a patient has a tumour pushing the midline towards the opposite side of the head, the two recorded distances will not be the same.

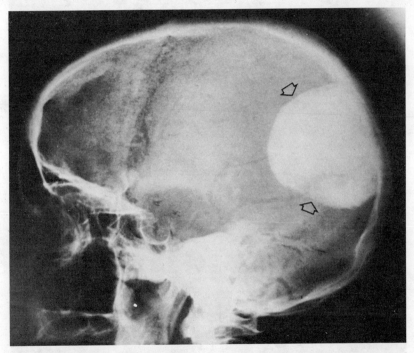

Fig. 63/2 This straight X-ray of the skull shows a very large calcified tumour at the back of the head.

Radiological investigation. Two forms of X-ray pictures may help the neurologist or neuro-surgeon. The first of these, straight X-ray (see Fig. 63/2), gives information about the bony structure surrounding the brain and spinal cord and also displays any calcification within them. Not only may fractures be shown in patients with head injury but tumours may declare themselves in a variety of ways. In a patient whose tumour is on the surface of the brain, there may be a local thinning of the skull, while the rise in intracranial pressure which may accompany a tumour anywhere within the brain causes an erosion of the pituitary fossa. In many people over 40 years old the pineal gland is calcified. This little gland is situated in the midline just behind the third ventricle. If a tumour is present in one hemisphere, then the pineal will be pushed over to the other side and this shift may be seen on plain X-rays. In the more slowly growing tumours calcification sometimes occurs within the tumour itself.

The other type of X-ray frequently used is the contrast study (see Figs. 63/3 and 63/4). Here the soft radiolucent structures within the bony

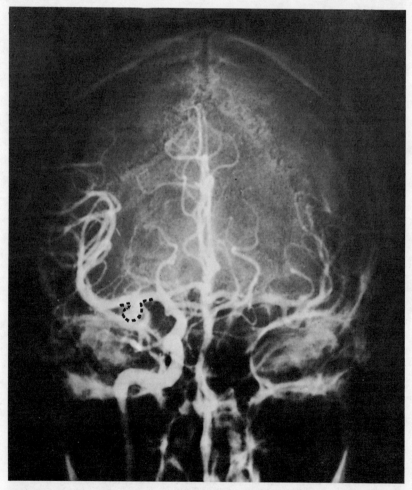

Fig. 63/3 In this carotid angiogram, in the antero-posterior projection, the right carotid artery has been injected while the left carotid has been compressed. The middle and anterior cerebral arteries on both sides of the head have been filled. The dotted outline is of a large aneurysm projecting downwards from the right middle cerebral artery.

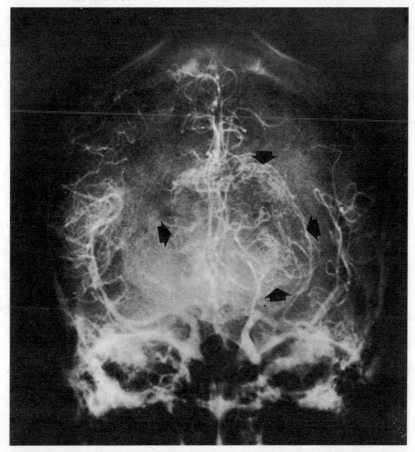

Fig. 63/4 A second carotid angiogram with a left-sided injection and right-sided compression. The arrows point to a mass of abnormal vessels within a very large metastatic sarcoma.

cage of the skull are studied. The principle behind all contrast radiography, whether it be a barium meal or an air encephalogram, is that an existing but radiolucent cavity is filled with a substance that will show on X-ray. The pictures are then studied to see how they differ from the normal and the cause of this abnormality can be deduced. Such pictures may show that normal structures are being displaced by a mass (which will itself not be shown), that normal filling is obstructed, or that abnormal spaces have formed.

Cerebral angiography. Here a contrast material is injected into the carotid or vertebral arteries, either by direct puncture in the neck or by passing a catheter into them from the femoral or brachial artery. The investigation may be done under local anaesthesia in a well-sedated patient but in children or confused patients a general anaesthetic is usually given. Angiograms may show displacement of blood vessels by tumour,

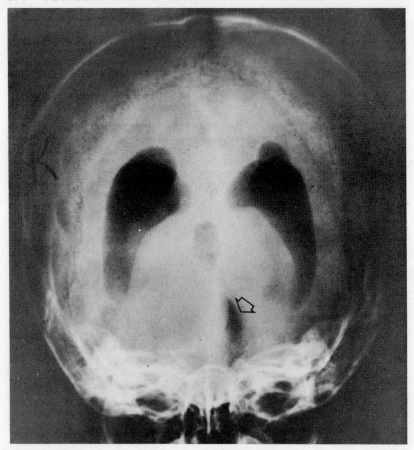

Fig. 63/5 A ventriculogram of a four-year-old boy. He is lying on his face, so that the air has risen to the posterior part of the lateral ventricles (the large comma-shaped shadows) and has filled the fourth ventricle (arrowed). The fourth ventricle has been pushed over to the left by an abscess in the right cerebellar hemisphere.

abscess or other lump within the brain. They may show the abnormal blood vessels supplying a tumour or the blockage of normal blood vessels by thrombosis or embolus, the bulging sac of an aneurysm or the tortuous vessels of an angioma.

Air encephalography. Here air is injected into the subarachnoid space at lumbar puncture or cisternal puncture. Not only does the air outline the cisterns—the pools of fluid around the brain—but with careful positioning of the patient's head the air may be made to pass into the ventricular system through the openings from the fourth ventricle.

Ventriculography. If the air will not pass from the subarachnoid space into the ventricular system, or if the presence of high pressure within the head makes encephalography dangerous, the system may be filled directly

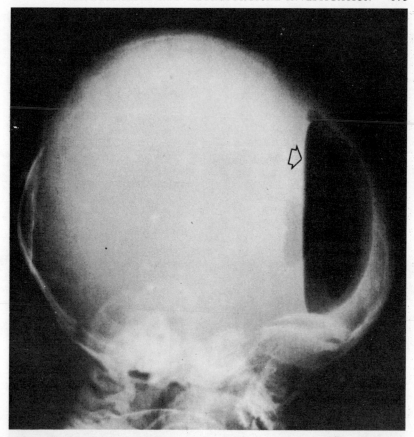

Fig. 63/6 A ventriculogram of a three-week-old infant with gross hydrocephalus. The baby is lying on her back and a lateral view has been taken. The enormous dilatation of the lateral ventricles can be seen. The arrow points to the fluid level below the bubble of air.

by making burr holes through the patient's skull and passing a thin cannula, down which air may be injected through the brain into the lateral ventricles. With suitable local anaesthesia this is a painless procedure and is usually performed on the conscious patient. Air encephalography or ventriculography may show displacement of the ventricular system by a mass or obstruction to the flow of C.S.F. causing a hydrocephalus. It may sometimes prove necessary to inject a small amount of the radio-opaque material, Myodil, into the lateral ventricles and allow it to run down into the third ventricle, aqueduct and fourth ventricle, so that these smaller spaces may be more clearly seen.

Myelography. The spinal subarachnoid space may be filled with Myodil via a lumbar or cisternal puncture; distortion of the space reveals masses arising either within the spinal cord or pressing onto it from without.

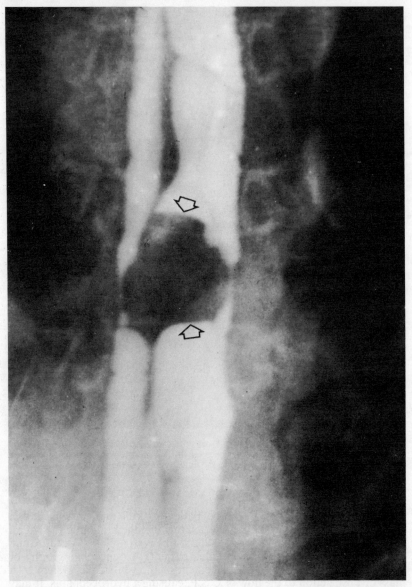

Fig. 63/7 This myelogram shows well the rounded filling defect in the Myodil column made by a small meningioma (arrowed).

Chapter 64

The Treatment of Cancer

by N. M. BLEEHEN

Types of radiotherapy—radiotherapy methods—effects of radiation—treatment of individual diseases—unsealed radioactive isotopes—cancer chemotherapy

---

Cancer may be treated by a variety of methods used either individually or in combination. Surgery, radiotherapy or drug therapy may be available. The choice of the most suitable method for the disease in an individual patient must be the subject of careful consultation between the various specialists. Methods of surgical treatment have been considered elsewhere. Other methods of treatment are discussed in this chapter. Treatments may be intended to be *curative*. In patients with the most advanced stages of disease it may only be possible to consider *palliative* measures.

Radiotherapy is the treatment of disease by ionizing radiations. These radiations are so called because they achieve their biological effect by producing ions in the irradiated tissues. There are several different types of radiation which are principally used in the treatment of malignant disease. A few non-malignant conditions are also treated.

TYPES OF RADIOTHERAPY

The type most commonly used is **X-radiation** or gamma-radiation. When the rays are produced from generators operated at very high electrical voltages they are known as X-rays. Such machines are known as superficial or deep X-ray machines and linear accelerators. The *superficial X-ray* machines produce X-rays of low energy at a voltage of from 10,000 to 100,000 volts. These will only penetrate tissue for a short distance and are therefore very useful for skin conditions. The *deep X-ray machines* produce X-rays at higher energies of 200,000 to 500,000 volts with much better penetration depth and are therefore used in the treatment of deep-seated tumours.

Supervoltage therapy has recently been introduced in which the X-rays are generated at millions of volts energy. These have considerable advantages over the lower voltage X-rays in the treatment of deep tumours. They produce much less reaction in normal tissues such as skin and bone and less general effect on the patient.

When radiation is produced by the decay of substances called radioactive isotopes the rays are known as **gamma rays**. Radium was the first naturally occurring isotope used clinically for this purpose. Artificially produced radioactive isotopes of cobalt and caesium are now commonly used to produce high-intensity beams of radiation with similar effects to that of supervoltage irradiation. Other isotopes, of iridium, tantalum and gold have also been prepared for implantation into tumours. Radioactive substances are referred to as *sources* (of ionizing radiations) and are used in two ways—as *sealed* or *unsealed* sources. Sources of radiation used for external beam therapy or implantation are isotopes which have been sealed into leak-proof containers. Unsealed radioactive isotopes are usually in a solution which is administered to the patient either orally or by injection.

Electrons are charged particles which are part of the atom. These may be produced in electrical generators such as linear accelerators or betatrons. They may be used to treat skin and other tumours close to the surface. They have the advantage of only treating a very limited depth of tissue and therefore sparing the normal tissue beyond. For this reason electron therapy is used in malignant infiltrations of the skin where it is desired to treat the whole skin surface. **Beta-rays** are electrons produced from radioactive isotopes. Beta-ray applicators are sealed sources which are used for the treatment of superficial areas of skin or the cornea of the eye. A strontium isotope is commonly used for this purpose. Another sealed beta-ray source which may be used for implantation into the pituitary gland is radio-yttrium in small pellets. Many unsealed isotopes produce their effect by the beta-rays they emit, such as radioactive phosphorus (^{32}P). Others, such as iodine (^{131}I) will also emit gamma rays.

RADIOTHERAPY METHODS

Units of radiation dosage are important to define the amount of treatment given. The dose of radiation to which a patient is exposed is known as the Roentgen after the discoverer of X-rays. The dose which is absorbed by the tissues, which is of more importance, may be very slightly different. This is given in rads.

Detection and calibration of radiation is carried out by trained physicists. Specialized detectors known as ionizing chambers, scintillation and Geiger counters are used to calibrate the radiation emitted by the various types of source, and received by the patient. A *film-badge* containing a small X-ray film is worn on the clothing of all persons working with radiation, including nurses. It is changed every two weeks, developed and measured for the radiation received. A careful check can thus be made on the radiation received by staff.

Planning of treatment is carried out by the medically qualified radiotherapist with the assistance of a radiographer and physicist. The tissue volume for treatment is defined and a dose of radiation prescribed. The optimum treatment with respect to the type of radiation source and the number of individual treatments is specified. Many external radiation schedules are fractionated so that the total dose is split into daily or less frequent exposures, spread over a few days to several weeks.

Radiation beam therapy is carried out with the patient positioned as comfortably as possible on the treatment couch. The centre of the *radiation field* is indicated with marker ink on the skin so that the treatments may be reproduced each day. The outline of the radiation field may also be indicated on the patient in special circumstances. These marks are preserved during the treatment course.

Ancillary treatments to increase the efficacy of the radiotherapy may be given as part of a planned pre-operative or postoperative management. The treatment may also be combined with drug therapy. These drugs may be used to sensitize the tumour to the irradiation or they may be cancerocidal in their own right. In this case the additive effect of the two treatments is advantageous.

Hyperbaric oxygen is a special form of radiosensitization (see Chapter 47). Patients may receive radiation while breathing pure oxygen under pressure in a special sealed tank which completely contains them. The sensitivity of cells to radiation may depend on their oxygen content and it is hoped that better clinical results will be obtained.

EFFECTS OF RADIATION

The biological effect of radiation is achieved by its destructive action on the genetic material in the nucleus of cells. This effect will be seen with both normal and malignant tissues. However, the malignant tissues will usually have a greater response, thus explaining the value of radiotherapy.

The *radiosensitivity* of tumours varies considerably. Thus tumours of the lymph glands (e.g. lymphosarcoma) may disappear with small doses of radiation. Squamous-cell skin cancers may need much larger doses. The *curability* of a disease will, however, depend also on its capacity to spread from its site of origin. A patient with skin cancer may be more certain of cure because of the lower likelihood of spread than one with lymphosarcoma.

TREATMENT OF INDIVIDUAL DISEASES

The best results of radiotherapy are obtained in the treatment of malignancies in the head and neck region and cancer of the uterine cervix. In these situations it is usually the treatment of choice.

The treatment of cancer of the *mouth* and *tongue* may be carried out by external irradiation. If the disease is localized to a small volume, a radium needle implant may be used. The needles are inserted into the tumour under general anaesthesia and stitched to retain them in position. They are left in the tissue for about six to seven days, the exact time being calculated by physicists on the basis of check X-rays of the position of the needles. Lymph nodes involved with tumour are best treated by surgery, but if this is not possible external irradiation may be given. Cancer of the *larynx* is usually treated by irradiation as the initial method. The advantage is preservation of normal function. Should the treatment fail then surgery is always possible later.

Cancer of the *cervix* is usually treated by a combination of internal and external irradiation, sometimes combined with surgical removal. The local disease in the cervix is given a high dose of radiation by insertion under anaesthesia of radium into the uterus and upper part of the vagina. One or more of these insertions may be carried out. The lymph nodes in the pelvis which may be invaded by tumour are then irradiated by external treatment. Alternatively the uterus, ovaries and lymph nodes may then be removed surgically. Cancer of the *body of the uterus* is usually treated surgically, but pre-operative insertion of radium helps to reduce the likelihood of local recurrence of the disease.

Cancers of the *ovary* should be removed for histological diagnosis and this is also the best method of treatment. Residual local tumour in the pelvis may be treated by external irradiation. Widespread disease throughout the peritoneal cavity is usually treated by chemotherapy.

Cancer of the *lung* is frequently treated by irradiation, although rarely cured. The treatments are very useful in controlling local disease for palliative purposes, but death is usually caused by the distant spread of the disease.

Cancer of the *breast* is usually treated surgically when in its early stages. However, spread to the local lymph nodes is common and these are frequently irradiated as a precaution against later recurrence. More advanced inoperable local disease and distant spread, usually to bone and brain, may be treated by irradiation with excellent palliative response of pain and other symptoms.

Painful bone deposits from many other tumours may be treated to reduce pain and the risk of fracture. *Some tumours of children* are sensitive to irradiation and are often so treated either alone, or in combination with surgery and chemotherapy. These include Wilm's tumour, retinoblastoma and medulloblastoma. *Bone tumours* are usually treated surgically where possible, but it is often desirable to give pre-operative irradiation. Tumours at many other sites are also treated by radiation with useful curative and palliative results.

UNSEALED RADIOACTIVE ISOTOPES

Many radioactive isotopes of elements can now be produced artificially in nuclear reactors and other generators. Some, as has been mentioned, are used as sealed sources for the external irradiation of patients. Others, to be considered here, are generally prepared in liquid or suspension form and are for internal administration. These isotopes are given orally or by injection intravenously or into body cavities. They may be used either for *diagnostic* or *therapeutic* purposes.

Dosage. The dosage of radioactivity present in an isotope is measured in *curies* (Ci), thousandths or millionths of a curie (mCi and μCi). This unit is named after the discoverers of radium. The radioactivity of a substance does not remain constant with time as atoms need to disintegrate to produce the radiations. The period during which half the atoms do this is known as the *half-life* of the material and is a constant for that isotope. This period varies for different substances, e.g. that for radium is 1,600 years, for radiocobalt 5·3 years and radiogold 8 days.

Radioisotopes in diagnosis. The *diagnostic* uses of isotopes are becoming increasingly important as more new techniques are developed. The commonest use is that of radioiodine to test the function of the thyroid gland. A small dose of a few microcuries is given by mouth and the quantity retained in the thyroid measured. Reduced or increased activity of the gland can then be determined. Other techniques measure the distribution of the administered isotope, such as technetium in brain and liver or radiostrontium in bone. These *scans* may then demonstrate the presence of primary or secondary tumours in those tissues.

Radioisotopes in treatment. The therapeutic uses of isotopes take advantage of the high local dosage of radiation possible with locally absorbed isotopes. Radioactive iodine may be given in millicurie doses in the treatment of polycythaemia. Other isotopes, like colloidal gold and yttrium, are produced in minute particles. These can be injected into the pleural or peritoneal cavities in the treatment of malignant effusions.

CANCER CHEMOTHERAPY

Drug therapy of cancer is usually only palliative. This may be carried out with one or more of the many *cytotoxic* agents such as nitrogen mustard, cyclophosphamide or chlorambucil. It is used for advanced malignant disease such as metastases of carcinoma of the lung, breast and ovary. A variety of these agents and others like vinblastine, procarbazine and methotrexate are also used in the combinations of treatment for leukaemias, Hodgkin's disease and other reticuloses. In these conditions, long-term remissions have been obtained in some patients and there are hopes for many more with newer combinations of drugs.

A few cancers have been cured by chemotherapy. The principal type is chorioncarcinoma occurring in women, where high-intensity drug treatment with careful sterile reverse-barrier nursing will eliminate the disease from the majority of patients.

The *complications of cytotoxic therapy* can be very severe, and include depression of the blood count, infections, haemorrhage and bowel disturbances. Careful use of the drugs will usually reduce the risks to an acceptable level.

Hormones are frequently used in the management of cancer of the breast and prostate. Prednisone, or a similar steroid, is frequently used where there are blood disorders associated with the disease or its treatment.

Chapter 65

The Nursing of Patients Receiving Radiotherapy

by MARY CRAIG

> *General considerations—examples of local reactions—care of patients being treated with small sealed radioactive sources in the wards—care of patients undergoing treatment with unsealed radioactive isotopes—protection of nursing and other staff from radiation hazards*

The majority of patients attend daily as out-patients for external radiation therapy. They are admitted to hospital if this is impractical for medical, geographical or social reasons. In either case they usually require no specific preparation (such as might precede a diagnostic X-ray examination).

They should be told the probable details of treatment procedure before the first attendance to allay their natural anxiety. This will have been discussed at the time of medical examination and decision but it should be recapitulated by the ward staff. (Radiotherapy staff will attend to the needs of out-patients.)

Nurses should visit the treatment department and be able to speak with confidence about the procedure. Patients lie on a treatment couch in a prescribed position for a certain length of time, e.g. 1 to 10 minutes in a room by themselves. They are in the care of qualified staff (radiographers) who watch them through an observation window or by closed circuit television all the time. Patients and staff can communicate with each other by microphone during the treatment if they wish.

The radiation is invisible and has no apparent effect at the time of treatment, e.g. no pain or other sensation is experienced. The patient does not become radioactive and no radioactivity remains in the treatment room, patient's clothing, etc.

When the prescribed dosage has been given the apparatus automatically shuts off the beam. This safety device is incorporated in all radiation units.

Diet. All patients should have as good and nourishing a diet as possible.

Fluid intake is important and should be adequate to enable the kidneys to excrete the waste-products of tissue breakdown—say four pints, about two litres, daily.

Bowel action. This should be normal unless the bowels are directly concerned and receiving special consideration, but patients requiring regular analgesics are likely to become constipated and require advice.

Pain from disease (usually in more advanced conditions) must be alleviated. Frequently the regular administration of mild analgesics will achieve good results.

Anxiety and depression. Anxiety may be present in many forms such as a basic fear of hospitals and any kind of disease—these are usually people who have not required hospital treatment before. There is fear of cancer. The advancement in treatment for many forms of this disease is not yet well known. Almost all forms of cancer are amenable to some form of curative or palliative measures. In advanced disease the palliative results may be short-term but helpful—reduction of pain, discharge, etc. Regular opportunities to speak to the medical staff are greatly appreciated. Anxiety may also be due to social and economic factors—should the bread-winner be off work for some months or an even longer time or how young children are to be looked after while mother attends daily for treatment or is warded.

Daily encouragement from nurses and radiographers provides essential support to all patients. We are all individuals and require individual attention, not personal involvement but a sympathetic general under-standing of the position. Medical social workers are immensely helpful to all our patients and we should work closely with them and the district nurses and health visitors who may look after our patients while they are attending hospital or after they have been discharged.

EXAMPLES OF LOCAL REACTIONS

Skin. If *supervoltage* apparatus is used changes in the skin will be minimal. Patients can usually wash and bathe normally, though being careful not to remove any skin marks connected with the treatment. Warm water, soft flannels and towels and super-fatted, non-irritating soaps—patting rather than rubbing dry.

If *superficial X-rays* or *deep X-rays* are used the skin will gradually become red, dry, flaky and probably break (moist desquamation). Washing is not usually recommended but the skin may be dabbed with surgical spirit and dusted with non-metallic dusting powder. When the skin is inflamed the spirit is discontinued and the areas may be dabbed with a solution of bicarbonate of soda (a 5 ml teaspoon to 600 ml of warm water) gently dried and dusted with the powder. Each department has its own instructions for skin care especially if moist desquamation occurs. These should be strictly adhered to.

Important points. Friction should always be avoided, e.g. from clothing such as collars, corsets, tight-fitting dresses, woollen vests or jerseys.

Heat should be avoided, e.g. direct hot sunshine, sitting close to fires, hot-water bottles or electric pads. Sunbathing is never advisable for skin areas that have been irradiated.

Mucous membranes of the mouth, nasal and pharyngeal passages. There will be dryness, loss of taste, soreness. Such saliva as there is may be thick and viscid. Increase daily fluid intake to 4 to 6 pints, approximately 2 to 3 litres, according to the total diet. Avoid very hot drinks, spices, curries. Give frequent mouth washes, nose sniffs or gargles of sodium bicarbonate solution, half a teaspoonful to a tumbler of warm water to loosen thick saliva or discharge especially before meals. This may be followed if the mouth or throat is sore, by a mildly anaesthetic emulsion, 1 to 2 teaspoon-fuls (5 to 10 ml). Undiluted spirits and smoking are likely to irritate the throat and should be discouraged. Monilia is a fungus infection which may occur in devitalized mouth and throat tissues. Signs and symptoms are severe inflammation, pain and a whitish appearance in the area. Treatment is usually suspended for a day or two and the condition responds quickly to suitable doses of nystatin.

Epigastric region. There is likely to be nausea and perhaps vomiting and consequent loss of appetite. Drugs may be given to reduce nausea and general discomfort. Rest and encouragement will help.

Pelvis. There may be diarrhoea or cystitis. Courses of treatment in this area will produce sterility unless the gonads can be shielded and this depends on the site and extent of the disease. Low residue diet, good fluid intake and suitable drugs can minimize the discomfort.

The blood-forming areas of the bone marrow. Regular haemoglobin, leucocyte and platelet counts will be made throughout the treatment. Drugs may be given to increase the efficiency of the bone marrow.

Scalp and underlying structures. Irradiation will cause the hair to come out, though usually it will grow again after some months.

Follow-up clinics. Patients attend these clinics at regular intervals after receiving radiotherapy. Progress can be assessed, queries can be answered, further help given if necessary. At first the intervals are fairly close, one, two or three monthly. Later they may be extended to six months or one year.

CARE OF PATIENTS BEING TREATED WITH SMALL SEALED RADIOACTIVE SOURCES IN THE WARDS

Gynaecological applicators. These may take the form of a nylon tube containing radium or caesium placed in the uterine cavity and two Perspex ovoids containing radium or caesium placed in the lateral fornices of the vagina held in position with non-radioactive spacers and packing. The applicators and spacers are threaded for later ease of removal. They are applied for a specified period of time, e.g. 36 hours. There may be three such applications at weekly intervals.

While the applicators are in position special precautions must be taken by the staff for the patient's care and for their own protection. Detailed instructions for these precautions are issued to every ward where such patients are nursed. They include the correct use of *time, distance* and *shielding.*

Time. Essential nursing procedures only are carried out as efficiently and speedily as possible. Duties are shared between the staff.

Distance. Beds should be spaced so that they are not near the nurses' station, ward doors or next to another patient requiring maximum attention. Long-handled forceps should be used when manipulating the sources, i.e. when they are being removed or if one should become displaced (although applied in the operating theatre they are often removed in the ward).

Shielding. Lead containers must be available at the bedside in which to put the applicators when removed and carry them back to the hospital radioactive storage room. A mobile heavy lead screen will be used when the applicators are removed.

Note. The lead gloves and aprons used in diagnostic X-ray departments are not suitable and are not used in radiotherapy.

Label. A special label with the patient's name and treatment details is attached to the bed and must be returned with the sources.

Checking. Regular checks must be made that the packing has not shifted during treatment. The number of sources must be checked on removal and signed as correct in a special book when returned to the storage room.

After loading techniques. Non-radioactive applicators are inserted in the theatre, the usual diagnostic X-rays are taken to ensure correct position and the sources are quickly introduced afterwards in the ward by a member of the medical staff. Ward care and precautions are then the same as above. These techniques eliminate the need for special precautions in the theatre and the X-ray department.

Cathetrons. These treatment units are a comparatively new development and have been installed in certain Centres. Suitably adapted, non-radioactive catheter-applicators are inserted into the uterus and vagina with or without full anaesthesia in the treatment/theatre suite. The catheters are then attached to the Cathetron. All staff leave the room and the sources are introduced and the treatment controlled by medical or radiographic staff outside the room. Such patients, of course, require no special precautions when they return to the ward; some, in fact, may be treated as out-patients.

Radium or caesium needles or iridium wires may be threaded and implanted in a specific volume of tissue. They may remain in position for five to seven days. The threads will be visible on the skin gathered together with adhesive tape. They must be regularly counted to make sure that no source has become loose.

Gold. Gold grains are minute radioactive sources. They may be implanted in surface tissues and covered by an adhesive dressing which must be checked for position as a whole. The entire dressing must be placed in the lead container and returned to the storage room at the end of treatment. Gold grains may also be implanted in small lesions in the bladder, they are intended to remain indefinitely *in situ*. Should any grain be passed in the urine during the first three days of treatment it must be removed with the long-handled forceps, put in the lead container and returned to the storage room. No further precautions need be taken after this time. *Precise details of procedure in all these situations will be in the special instructions.*

CARE OF PATIENTS BEING TREATED WITH UNSEALED RADIOACTIVE ISOTOPES

Precautions are necessary in the care of these patients because:

1. These isotopes are sources of radiation
2. They are in liquid form and there is risk of spilling and so contaminating clothing, linen, floor, hands, which could lead to ingestion or inhalation of radioactive material
3. An appreciable amount of the radioactive element may be present in the patient's urine, faeces, sweat and any vomited material

Detailed instructions for these precautions are issued to every ward where such patients are nursed.

Unsealed isotopes differ from the small sealed sources (except for the gold grains) in that they all have a short half-life, otherwise they could not be introduced into patients in a form which cannot be totally withdrawn after a stated period of treatment. Check most carefully the name of any patient who is to receive a therapeutic dose.

General points. Patients receiving an initial 'tracer' dose are nursed in the general ward. No special precautions are required. Patients receiving a *therapeutic dose* are nursed in a single room (or specially designated ward) with separate bathroom and W.C. The room should have a hand basin and be as clear of all unnecessary objects as possible. The patient wears hospital clothing and uses disposable toilet articles, paper handkerchiefs, that can be destroyed.

Gowns and *gloves* must be worn by nursing staff, who carry out their essential duties as speedily as possible. The gloved hands must be washed in the hand basin, dried on the towel provided and left ready for use. The nurse must wash her hands again after leaving the room.

Bed linen is changed daily and kept in labelled bins in the bathroom until monitored by the isotope (nuclear medicine) staff and either removed for storage or declared free from contamination.

Visitors are allowed but they must not come in contact with the patient or bedclothes. It must be emphasized that no books, magazines, sweets, fruit, etc., must be shared with the visitors—or nursing staff. Everything used for the patient, e.g. crockery, is kept in the room and everything removed, including waste food and rubbish, must be monitored before disposal.

The room is *labelled* and the precautions must be maintained until the ward is notified that the patient is clear of contamination. The room itself must be thoroughly checked before another patient is admitted.

Explanation. The precautions must be fully explained to the patient before the dose is administered so that he can co-operate fully without anxiety.

PROTECTION OF NURSING AND OTHER STAFF FROM RADIATION HAZARDS

A *Code of Practice for the Protection of Persons Exposed to Ionizing Radiations* is issued by the Department of Health and Social Security and is published by H.M. Stationery Office. A specific *Handbook for Nurses* on the subject is published by the same office.

Points covered by the *Code of Practice* include the construction of buildings, the levels of permissible dosage, techniques to be employed, details of the nature of the hazards and the methods to be used for the protection of personnel.

A radiological safety committee controls the use of all ionizing radiations in each hospital group. Safety officers are appointed to give advice on new or routine procedures—in the case of the wards they are usually the superintendent of the radiotherapy department or a radiotherapy physicist.

The *Code* lays down that detailed instructions (local rules) for the use of small sealed or unsealed radioactive isotopes must be available for the nursing staff. These rules include emergency procedures and the names and means of contacting persons whose advice may be urgently needed. Nurses may be assured that, provided this *Code of Practice* is properly applied, no one will come to any harm.

Chapter 66

Nursing Duties in the Preparation of Patients for X-ray Examination

by MARION FRANK

> *General considerations—handling films—communications between wards and X-ray department—contrast media—preparation of patient —barium examinations—cholecystography—bronchography—angiography—cardiac catheterization—lymphography—pyelography— hystero-salpingography*

X-rays are similar to light, but of shorter wave-length. Unlike light, they do not excite the sensation of vision when they fall on the retina, but like light, they affect a sensitized photographic film. Because an X-ray beam has a shorter wave-length than a beam of visible light, it is capable of penetrating to a greater or lesser extent objects that are opaque to light. The picture produced on a photographic film by a beam of X-rays after passing through an object is called a radiograph, or very often (colloquially but incorrectly) an X-ray.

The *degree of penetration* depends on the density of the object. Bones, due to their calcium content, are of considerable density and absorb the X-ray beam. Soft tissues, such as muscle, fat and most of the internal organs absorb less radiation and therefore produce blackening of the film.

A further effect of X-radiation is to produce fluorescence of certain substances, e.g. calcium tungstate. This is made use of in 'screening' or *fluoroscopy* which allows continuous observation to be made of movements of the parts being examined.

HANDLING OF FILMS

Wet films. In modern departments few wet films need to be handled. This is a major advantage of automatic processing. Dental films, or those taken in the operating theatre may have to be handled in the wet state. Wet films on hangers must be allowed to hang freely so that they do not stick together or cling to viewing boxes or other adjacent surfaces; they must be returned to the X-ray department as soon as possible.

Dry films. It is of the greatest importance to avoid getting films confused; this can occur at ward rounds and in clinics when one patient's films may be put into an envelope bearing another patient's name. It is essential always to check the name on the film with the name on the envelope. Once a film is misplaced in the wrong envelope it is practically impossible to correct the error, and repeat X-ray examinations may have to be carried out.

Any film damaged by water or in any other way must be returned to the X-ray department in order to prevent damage to the image. Damp films must not be put back in the envelope.

COMMUNICATIONS BETWEEN THE WARDS AND X-RAY DEPARTMENT

It must be realized that in the beginning the only information the staff of the X-ray department has about a patient is contained on the request form. Nurses can help the department materially and help to ensure that the patient receives maximum benefit from the X-ray examination by attention to the following details:

Request forms. Ensure that the name, age, registration number and date of previous examination are accurately recorded. Previous films must be returned to the X-ray department when the patient attends for further examination.

The condition of the patient has an influence on his transport to the X-ray department. Sick patients or those who have had some form of pre-medication must be conveyed on a canvas stretcher with poles, while others may need only a trolley or chair or may walk accompanied.

It is important to indicate on the form whether an examination *is to be carried out in the ward*.

The patient should be informed as clearly as possible, what is to be done and the help expected from him. He will have to lie very still, and great pains should be taken to see that he is comfortably placed on the table or other piece of apparatus on which he is to lie, or rest.

A nurse who is familiar with the methods of X-ray examination is a valuable ally in placing a patient at his ease.

The radiographer should be told whenever it has been impossible to carry out any or all of the preparation ordered. Information about the general condition of the patient's physical health and emotional reaction to the examination should be made known to the radiographer and any disability, including blindness, deafness, dumbness, restriction in movement, pyrexia, pregnancy or unknown allergies, noted.

CONTRAST MEDIA

The media employed in demonstrating relations and functions of certain organs include:

>   *Non-opaque*—the introduction of oxygen or air in certain situations, as in ventriculography, encephalography and in double contrast enemas.
>
>   *Opaque media* include *barium* for barium meals and enemas, and *iodine compounds* for bronchography, cholecystography, pyelography, hystero-salpingography and angiography.

Note that opaque in this context means opaque to X-rays.

Precautions. When an iodine compound is used the history of any previous allergic reaction should be investigated—asthma, food allergies, hay fever, etc. should be noted; when an allergic history is present the patient is usually desensitized to the compound before the full dose is given: otherwise a skin reaction, oedema or anaphylaxis may arise.

PREPARATION OF PATIENT

The patient should be suitably clothed, all garments should be easily removable or re-arranged without exposure of the patient. A shawl or small blanket or shoulder wrap should be at hand to cover the patient's shoulders in case for any reason he may have to wait while a cassette is re-loaded or a film developed. Slippers should be worn. The clothing should be free from all articles known to be opaque to X-rays, such as metal buttons, keys or watch. *A clean cotton dressing gown is ideal.* If the skull is to be X-rayed all hairpins, slides, combs and ribbons should be removed. Dentures should be taken out at the last moment, and kept safely. Bandages should not contain safety pins and strapping ought not to be employed.

BARIUM EXAMINATIONS OF THE ALIMENTARY TRACT

These examinations may be necessary in all gastric disorders such as hiatus hernia, suspected peptic ulcer or carcinoma (see also examination of the colon, below).

All barium examinations are carried out by *fluoroscopy* (screening) as well as by the use of films. As fluoroscopy is conducted in a darkened room the patient should be warned beforehand (modern apparatus for fluoroscopy allows dim room lighting). The examination is entirely without discomfort to the patient.

The contrast medium commonly employed is a suspension of *barium sulphate* which enables study of both the anatomy and dynamics of the organs undergoing examination to be made.

Barium swallow (see p. 473). No preparation is required for examination of the upper part of the oesophagus. For examination of the lower part, preparation is as for a barium meal.

Barium meal. In preparation an aperient should be given the day before. No medicine of any kind should be taken during the previous 24 hours lest it contain something to confuse the issue, such as an anti-spasmodic, stimulant or any opaque substance, e.g. bismuth. After examination, a further aperient is desirable as barium is constipating.

As this examination must be carried out on an empty stomach no food or drink may be taken during the preceding six hours.

A barium meal may necessitate repeated visits to the X-ray department and *the nurse should ask for clear instructions regarding the giving or withholding of food, fluids, and medicines which must be most meticulously carried out.*

Barium enema. A suspected organic lesion is the principal indication for X-ray examination of the colon (Figs. 66/1 and 66/2).

Complete clearance of the colon by cleansing enemas or colonic lavage

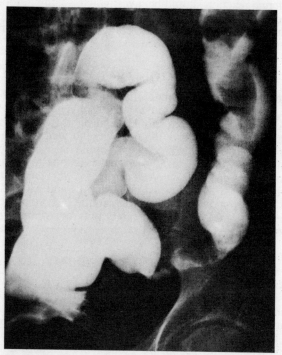

Fig. 66/1 Barium enema. A stricture is shown in the proximal part of the sigmoid colon. The persistence of this appearance in subsequent films strongly suggested a real stricture (as distinct from spasm) at this site. The lesion proved to be a carcinoma.

is essential. Films are taken at the time the barium enema is given. Movements of the colon are observed by fluoroscopy and the anatomy is demonstrated on films. The patient is asked to evacuate the barium which will take 15 to 20 minutes and films are taken after this evacuation. This examination may necessitate the patient re-visiting the X-ray department some hours later.

A double contrast enema is achieved by partially evacuating the barium and thereafter injecting air using Higginson's syringe.

CHOLECYSTOGRAPHY

Areas of the gall bladder, cystic duct and common bile duct are radiographically investigated when a calculus or chronic inflammatory condition is suspected. *Adequate bowel preparation is essential.* The oral method, *cholecystography* is usually undertaken in the first instance. Studies of the duct system are carried out by the intravenous route, *intravenous cholangiography* (also called choledochography).

A preliminary film is taken to assure complete absence of gas and faecal

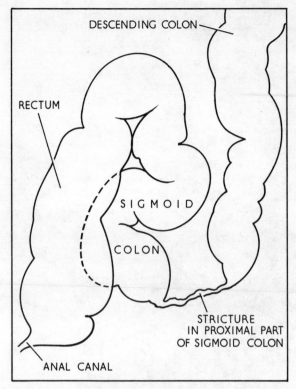

DESCENDING COLON

RECTUM

SIGMOID

COLON

STRICTURE
IN PROXIMAL PART
OF SIGMOID COLON

ANAL CANAL

Fig. 66/2 A line drawing of the colon.

matter in the right hypochondrium and the possible presence of opaque gallstones.

The medium, with a high iodine content, is excreted by the liver in the bile and reaches the gall bladder, where it is concentrated. *Once the medium has been given, the patient must abstain from the taste, sight and smell of all food and fluids*, except that sips of water may be taken. Instructions are given by the X-ray department regarding the time of administration of the contrast medium and the taking of films.

Once the anatomy of the gall bladder, and whether it contains gallstones has been demonstrated (see Fig. 66/3), a meal containing a considerable amount of fat, or some proprietary substance with a high fat content is given. Fat in the duodenum stimulates the gall bladder to contract. Films are taken after half an hour, and if necessary one hour later to show the contraction of the gall bladder.

At the operation of *cholecystectomy* a surgeon frequently requires an opaque iodine compound to be injected into the ducts using a fine tube or catheter. This will ensure that no calculi in the common bile duct will be overlooked.

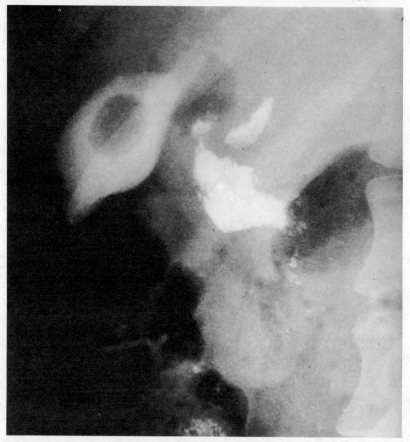

Fig. 66/3 Cholecystogram. Twelve hours after the oral administration of an opaque medium showing non-opaque stone as a large filling defect. Note residual contrast in bowel.

BRONCHOGRAPHY

This examination gives reliable information of the condition of the lungs in many chest diseases and abnormalities as it reveals conditions like bronchiectasis (see p. 199).

The contrast medium is an iodine-containing compound which may be passed into the trachea either over the tongue, or by means of a nasal tube passed into the oro-pharynx, or by puncture of the crico-thyroid membrane.

The whole procedure must be carefully explained to the patient beforehand. In particular it must be impressed on him that it is essential that he should not cough during the examination, and that he must follow exactly any instructions he is given about breathing.

No food or drink should be taken for three hours beforehand as pharyngeal irritation may stimulate vomiting. Nothing should be taken by mouth for three hours after the examination in case persistence of the local anaesthesia employed during induction should destroy the cough reflex and result in food and drink being inhaled.

Postural drainage under the supervision of a physiotherapist is ordered to follow immediately after the examination.

ANGIOGRAPHY AND LYMPHOGRAPHY

Angiography is a collective term used to describe injection into the blood vessels of a contrast medium for the purpose of X-ray examination. When an artery is injected the term *arteriography* is used, and when a vein is injected the procedure is known as *phlebography* or *venography*. Administration can be percutaneous, that is by needle-puncture through the skin, or by open operation and catheterization of a vessel.

In *preparation* sensitivity tests are carried out. The skin surface is cleansed and shaved if necessary. The patient is advised whether he may or may not have food; in many cases there is no need to fast and a light meal may be taken two hours before the injection is given. If a patient is apprehensive he is given a mild sedative.

After the examination, if a needle or catheter has been inserted percutaneously, a pressure pad is applied over the site of the injection. In order to avoid any possible haematoma or bleeding, *manual pressure should be maintained for at least five minutes. If a vessel in the arm or leg is injected the colour and degree of warmth or coldness of the limb should be noted.*

Cardiac catheterization is the passing of a radio-opaque catheter into the heart in order to measure pressure in the heart and great vessels and to calculate the size of any intracardiac shunt and for the injection of contrast medium into the great vessels or cardiac chambers for angiocardiography (see p. 595). This procedure calls for great caution and is an examination in which very serious responsibility rests on the radiologist and the cardiologist.

It is employed to diagnose and assess the extent of the cardiac lesion in congenital and acquired heart disease.

Lymphography is the X-ray examination of lymphatic vessels and lymph nodes after injecting a radio-opaque medium into a lymphatic vessel (Fig. 66/4). This examination is carried out to investigate possible causes of oedema of the arms, legs or pelvis. In order to identify lymphatic vessels, which are small and difficult to locate, preliminary injection of 2 ml of an 11 per cent aqueous solution of 'Patent Blue' is injected into the fine web between the fingers and toes and is taken up by the lymphatics which show up as thin blue vessels.

For the purpose of lymphography lymphatic vessels are injected slowly with the contrast medium, either at the dorsum of the foot, in the inguinal region, or at the elbow, depending on the area to be examined; the contrast media then flow with the lymph along its normal drainage course, when X-ray films of the lymphatics are taken. The skin may need shaving and the patient should pass urine before the injection is given because the examination *takes several hours.* It is advisable to warn patients and their relatives that the skin will appear green and that urine will be green for about 48 hours after the injection but this will pass off.

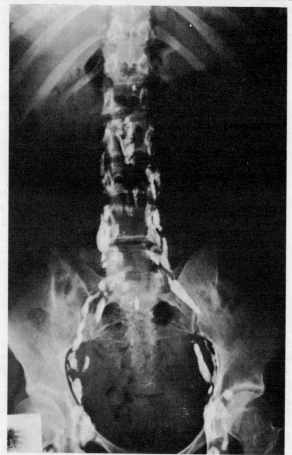

Fig. 66/4 Lymphogram. This demonstrates the peri-aortic, external and common iliac lymph nodes.

Special polythene tubes with syringe attachments and No. 32 needles are available ready sterilized, and the procedure is carried out by a doctor.

UROGRAPHY OR PYELOGRAPHY

Urography or *pyelography* is the radiological examination of the urinary tract after the injection of a fluid containing a high percentage of organic iodine. *In preparation the alimentary tract should be free of faeces and gas. Light dry diet may be given up to the time of the examination. Fluids should be withheld for eight hours to ensure concentration of the iodine compound in the urine.*

In *intravenous pyelography* the iodine compound is injected into the circulation. X-ray examination is made at intervals of 5, 10, 15 and 20 minutes when shadows of the kidneys and ureters may be seen, as in

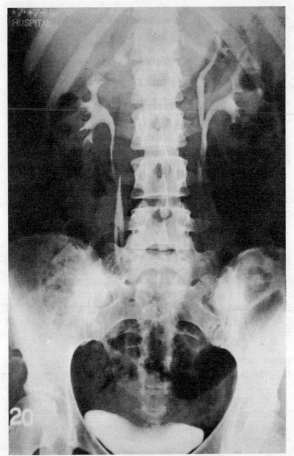

Fig. 66/5 Intravenous pyelogram. Twenty minutes after injection of an iodine compound, this shows a bilateral renal system. Note the abnormal double ureters.

Fig. 66/5. In severe hydronephrosis or diminished kidney function, later films may be necessary.

In the *retrograde method*, a cystoscope is passed and by means of ureteric catheters a similar fluid is injected into the pelvis of the kidneys.

HYSTERO-SALPINGOGRAPHY

Hystero-salpingography is the radiological demonstration of the uterus and uterine (Fallopian) tubes, using a radio-opaque compound. By this means occlusion of the tubes can be shown and the shape of the uterus determined. The medium is injected into the cervix, and films are taken on injection and after a short interval. The later film will show spill-over of the medium into the peritoneal cavity, thus proving the patency of one or both tubes.

Chapter 67

Plastic and Reconstructive Surgery

by I. F. K. MUIR

Introduction—plastic and reconstructive surgery—cleft lip and palate —repair of skin and soft tissue defects—pedicled skin flaps—burns and scalds—maxillo-facial injuries—reduction operations

The term *plastic surgery* seems to have first been used in the middle of the nineteenth century, and was used to describe the moulding and re-arrangement of tissues by operation in order to correct a deformity, or to make good a loss of tissue. The scope of the surgery of repair was much increased by the introduction of free skin grafts towards the end of the nineteenth century, and later by the introduction of the use of pedicle flaps early in this century. The original idea of plastic surgery therefore represents only a small proportion of a modern plastic surgeon's work, and the branch is now properly called plastic and reconstructive surgery. The demands of the two World Wars, with the necessity of treating many patients with severe injuries of the face and hands and burns of all parts of the body, caused rapid advances in techniques, and were also responsible for the development of special units.

PLASTIC AND RECONSTRUCTIVE SURGERY

Plastic and reconstructive surgery is concerned with the treatment of deformities, injuries and diseases of the soft tissues in general, as a result of:

Congenital deformities, such as cleft lip and palate and other deformities of the face; haemangiomata, and naevi.

Injuries with destruction of soft tissue, particularly those of the face and hands.

Deformities occurring from the treatment of diseases such as rodent ulcer, cancer of the mouth and jaws.

In addition to these groups, plastic surgery may also be used for the improvement of appearance or comfort in a person who is distressed by some unusually prominent or ugly feature, e.g. correction of outstanding ears, reduction of a large nose, reduction of excessively large breasts, reduction of excess lax skin of the face (face-lift operation). This aspect is sometimes known as aesthetic or cosmetic surgery.

General care of patients undergoing reconstructive procedures

Wounds heal badly and grafts fail to take if the patient's general condition is poor. If the repair procedure involves a series of operations it is important that the patient has a good intake of food to provide the necessary materials for the healing process, and also that a watch is kept on the haemoglobin level of the blood. This is particularly important in the case of patients with extensive burns. The final result also depends to a great extent on the local care of the wound and this requires particular attention.

Wounds and incisions on the face as a rule heal well and quickly because of the excellent blood supply. The presence of the orifices of the nose and mouth makes coverage of wounds of the face by dressings difficult and it is often much more satisfactory to leave the wounds completely uncovered. If this is done it is important that the suture line should be kept clean of discharge and crusts. It is also possible to observe the wound easily for the development of haematoma. Stitches from facial wounds should be removed early to avoid leaving stitch marks, and unless there is any tension, it is usual to remove facial stitches by four days. Any stitches which appear to be cutting in should be removed even earlier than this.

Plastic operations on limbs are often followed by the application of a pressure dressing. It is then important that the limb should be elevated to reduce the likelihood of oedema and a careful watch should be kept that there is no obstruction to the circulation. Should there be any anxiety about this the surgeon will almost certainly wish to remove and re-apply the bandage himself, and on no account should the pressure bandage applied at operation be removed without the consent of the surgeon. Some account of the special problems of the management of the different conditions will now be given.

CLEFT LIP AND PALATE

The cleft lip was often called 'hare-lip' because the deformity was supposed to resemble the lip of a hare. However, a hare's lip is cleft in the midline whereas a child's cleft lip is invariably to one side or other of the midline and this inaccurate term should therefore be dropped. Cleft lip and palate are among the more common of the severe congenital deformities and some degree of this deformity occurs in approximately 1 in 800 newborn babies. There is some hereditary tendency in this condition and the parents of a child who has been born with a cleft lip or palate often ask what the chances of further children having a similar deformity are. The precise figures have been worked out by the study of a large series of patients. If the parents themselves are normal, and if there is no recent history in the family then the chances of further children having the deformity are still fairly small. If, however, one or other of the parents or a close relative also has a cleft lip and palate then the chances of further children having the deformity are high. *The deformity is due to incomplete fusion of the parts of the face during the development of the embryo.*

Types of deformity. The deformity may involve the lip only, palate only, or the lip and palate together. In the complete form a continuous cleft exists right through the lip and hard palate and to the back of the soft palate. The deformity may be unilateral or in the most severe type of all may be bilateral (see Figs. 67/1, 67/2, 67/3 and 67/4). The condition causes the following disabilities:

Deformity of appearance.

Distortion of the dental arch; when the teeth erupt these may be displaced, causing difficulty in chewing.

Owing to the communication between the cavities of the nose and mouth, fluid which is drunk tends to come down through the nose. The nose may become infected and this may lead to infection of the middle ear.

If the soft palate is not corrected the child will be unable to speak clearly. Contrary to popular belief the deformity does not lead to difficulties in swallowing, although these babies sometimes have some additional condition which is responsible for difficulty in swallowing.

Treatment. The definitive treatment is by operation. It is usual to operate on a cleft lip at three months, the repair of the palate being performed at the age of one year so that the palatal repair is complete before the child speaks.

Feeding. Because of the deformity these babies are unable to suck, and because of this they are often very slow feeders. With only a very minor degree of deformity breast feeding may be possible but in cases with severe deformity this is impossible. In order to facilitate feeding it is necessary either to use a bottle with a large hole in the teat, or to feed the baby by spoon. An ordinary teaspoon may be satisfactory, but in cases of difficulty a spoon which is narrow but deep should be used. This may either be a special spoon, or it can be modified from an ordinary spoon by squashing it from side to side.

Dental plate. If there is difficulty in feeding then this can sometimes be helped by the use of a small dental plate which is made by the dental surgeon after taking an impression. In some cases also when there is great distortion of the segments of the jaw a special type of plate may be used to bring the segments into better position before undertaking operation— pre-surgical orthodontic correction.

Pre-operative assessment. In order that the dangers of operation may be minimized the following points are of importance:

The baby should be well, feeding well and putting on weight. It should be at least 4·5 kg (10 lb.) in weight.

It should be free of coughs and colds.

A throat swab should be taken some days before operation to make sure there are no haemolytic streptococci in the throat.

The haemoglobin content of the blood should be checked, and this should be at least 75 per cent.

If these criteria are insisted on and if the postoperative care is skilled then these babies stand operation very well.

Operation for cleft lip. This is performed under general anaesthesia at the age of three months. The technique requires a wide mobilization of the sides of the cleft so that the parts of the lip can be brought together without tension. Most modern operations involve the use of some kind of local flap and the lack of tension is usually well achieved. However, occasion-

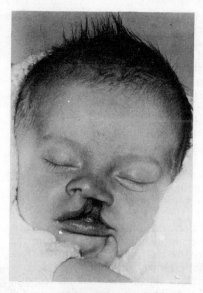

Fig. 67/1 Complete unilateral cleft lip and palate.

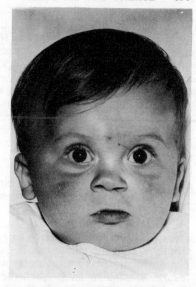

Fig. 67/2 The same child as in Fig. 67/1 after repair.

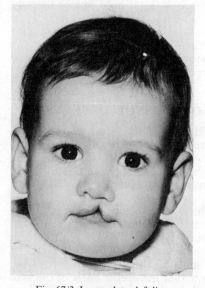

Fig. 67/3 Incomplete cleft lip.

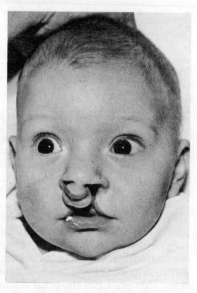

Fig. 67/4 Bilateral cleft lip and palate.

ally there is still undesirable tension and a Logan's bow can be applied to relieve the tension at the suture line.

Postoperative care. The great danger in the immediate postoperative period is obstruction of the airway due either to blood running down into the pharynx or to falling back of the tongue. In order to overcome the latter difficulty the surgeon will insert a tongue stitch with which the tongue can be pulled forward and this is left in place until the child is fully conscious. In case any blood is present the child should be nursed on his side with the head down and a sucker should be immediately available. A feed of water should be given as soon as the child is conscious, a half-strength feed can be given soon after, and if the operation has been performed in the morning it should be possible to give normal feeds by the evening. A drink of water should be given at the end of each feed but there should not be any need to clean inside the mouth. The baby's arms should be restrained by splints for the first week in order to avoid him putting his fingers into his mouth. It is important that the suture line should be kept clean and free from crusts, and stitches should be removed at 4 days or earlier if they look as if they are cutting in.

Chemotherapy. Penicillin is often given for five days.

Operation for cleft palate is usually performed at the age of one year. The operation again involves extensive mobilization of flaps within the mouth so that the palate can be sutured in the midline without tension. The postoperative care is similar to that after cleft-lip repair.

Later treatment. Even when the primary repair has been carried out, these children often need further treatment when they are older.

> By the time the child is ready to go to school, it should be possible to assess the quality of the speech. If this is poor, speech therapy will be necessary.
>
> When the teeth erupt there may be irregularities which require specialized orthodontic treatment.
>
> When the child is older some deformity may persist, particularly of the nose, and this can be corrected by treatment at a later date.

REPAIR OF SKIN AND SOFT TISSUE DEFECTS

Repair by local plastic operation. The skin of the face is of very good vascularity and relatively lax. For these reasons various types of local flaps (e.g. rotation flaps, transposition flaps) are particularly suitable for the repair of small and medium-size defects of the face and these correspond with the original use of the term plastic surgery.

Free skin grafts. These are grafts which when they have been taken are entirely separated from the body and are then applied to the recipient area.

Split skin graft. This is the commonest type of free skin graft used in reconstructive work. As the name implies it is a graft which is taken by some form of flat sharp knife which splits off the superficial part of the skin. This graft has the great advantage that the deeper parts of the skin structures remain in the donor area and the donor area can therefore heal spontaneously with little or no deformity. *A thin split skin graft* taken in this way is often called *a Thiersch graft* after the surgeon who first popularized its use. A Thiersch graft is usually taken with some simple form of skin grafting knife, e.g. Blair or Humby knife or one of its modifications. This graft has the advantage that it takes well and it is resistant to infection and for this reason is most often used in the repair of extensive defects such

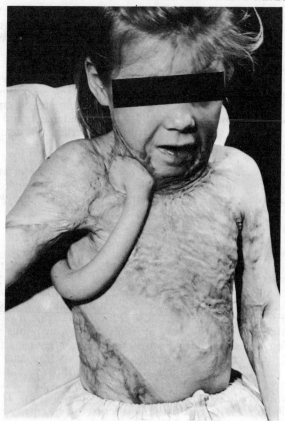

Fig. 67/5 A girl with severe contraction of the neck following a
burn, being treated by a tubed pedicle flap.

as those caused by burns. This graft, however, has the disadvantage that
it shrinks over the course of 6 to 12 weeks and where lack of contracture is
important a thicker split skin graft is used. This is often taken by a special
instrument known as a dermatome.

A full thickness free skin graft or *Wolfe graft* shows the least tendency of
all to contract. This, however, has the disadvantage that since the full
thickness of skin has been removed from the donor site this cannot heal
spontaneously and it must somehow be closed. The size of Wolfe graft
which can be used therefore is limited but it is particularly useful for
relatively small defects in the region of the eyes when the graft is taken from
the back of the ear, so called *post-auricular Wolfe graft*. The donor area
can usually be closed by simple suture leaving the sulcus behind the ear
rather more shallow than before but causing no obvious deformity.

Preparation of the recipient site for skin grafting. If the area exposed by
the loss of skin is healthy and clean then a skin graft can be applied immediately and no special preparation of the recipient area is necessary.

However, many instances will occur when it may not be possible to achieve this state of affairs in the first instance, when the area to be grafted is unhealthy and probably contains more or less dead tissue. We are then concerned with the preparation of this area so that it is in a fit state to take a skin graft.

In order to have a chance for the graft to take the area must be free of dead tissue, clean, of good vascularity, and with minimal infection. It is possible to get grafts to take satisfactorily even when bacteriological cultures show the presence of pathogenic organisms, but if the wound is dirty and there is profuse discharge of pus then the grafts will almost certainly be lost. *The haemolytic streptococcus is particularly lethal to grafts and if pre-operative swabs show the presence of this organism then it must be cleared by the appropriate chemotherapy before grafting is undertaken.* The most important feature of the pre-operative preparation of the wound is frequent and careful dressings. If any dead tissue is present then frequent dressings with eusol or Milton, e.g. two to three times a day, combined with snipping away of any obviously dead and loosening tissue, are most likely to be successful. The newer enzymatic agents which have been suggested for the removal of dead tissue have not yet proved their value.

When all dead tissue has been removed the aim is to get the raw area covered with healthy flat red granulations. If haemolytic streptococci are present then the appropriate chemotherapy should be employed to clear this. *Pseudomonas* infection produces a characteristic blue-green pus which stains the dressings and was responsible for its old name, *pyocyaneus*. This organism was previously very resistant to treatment but dressings of Sulfamylon are now usually effective. With other organisms, however, the results of treatment by chemotherapy are disappointing, and the mainstay of treatment is the frequent application of some form of wet dressing. When all the slough has been removed and if all has gone well, the surface will be covered with bright red, flat, healthy looking granulations. These granulations will take grafts readily. If, however, the granulations are pale, oedematous or hypertrophic further treatment is necessary. *A traditional treatment which is often successful is the use of dressings soaked in hypertonic sodium sulphate. In addition careful firm pressure bandaging will help to reduce oedema*, and if the raw area is on a limb then this should be elevated, and the joints exercised.

Operation of skin grafting. The donor site usually chosen is the thigh, although the upper arm may also be used for relatively small grafts. If the donor area is hairy it should be shaved before operation. If the thighs or arms are not available as may be the case in an extensive burn it may be necessary to cut grafts from the trunk and for this the electric dermatome is most generally used. The donor area is dressed with Tulle gras, gauze, wool and pressure bandage. The grafts are then applied to the raw area either in large sheets which are stitched on or in smaller strips or patches (postage stamp) grafts which are particularly useful when covering a large irregular area. It used to be thought it was always necessary to apply pressure to a graft in order for it to take but it is now known that this is not necessary, and in fact some grafts are most conveniently treated by exposure.

Treatment of grafts by exposure. The grafts are laid on the raw area and

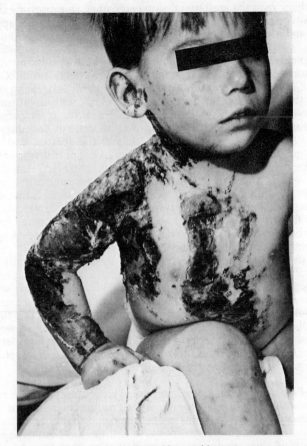

Fig. 67/6 An extensive scald treated by exposure.

no other dressing is applied. *If this is to be successful it is essential that the graft should not be rubbed or touched until it is firmly adherent, and much ingenuity may have to be exercised in splinting and protecting the area so this does not occur.* Once the graft has become adherent in four to seven days it may be more convenient to change over to treatment by dressing.

Treatment of grafts by dressing. In the simplest form of dressing a further layer of Tulle gras is applied over the grafts and then gauze, wool and a pressure bandage in the usual way. When, however, there is danger of the graft being displaced, it is usual to apply a few stitches around the edge, and then to apply the pressure bandage. When the recipient site is a fresh cut area, there is a danger of the graft being separated from its bed by bleeding or oozing of serum, and further measures are taken to prevent this occurring. A number of stitches are applied around the graft, and a pad of wool, soaked usually in acriflavine and paraffin, is built up over the graft. The long ends of the stitches which have been inserted are then brought back over the graft and tied to each other, thus pressing the pad of wool down onto the bed. The dressing is then completed by the application of wool and a pressure bandage in the usual way.

Further care. If the danger of haematoma has been avoided by the correct application of pressure, then the main danger to the graft is infection. The more risk there is of infection then the earlier the first dressing should be done. If the chances of an infection, particularly with organisms of the Gram-negative group, e.g. Pseudomonas, or Proteus, is present then the dressing must be done earlier and even as early as two days. At this time it is very easy to pull the graft off and the greatest care must be taken to get down to the level of the graft and support it while the upper layers are being removed. It is more likely, however, that it will be possible to leave the graft undisturbed until the fourth day by which time a fair amount of adhesion should have occurred. If the area is clean when the graft is applied then it can safely be left till the seventh day. By this time the stitches can be removed, and excess overlapping bits of graft edge can be trimmed away and a new dressing can be applied. Any blisters should be pricked and evacuated.

By 10 to 14 days after operation the graft should be firmly adherent and at each subsequent dressing it is important that all loose debris and crusts should be removed so that the edges of the graft and any areas where two grafts are close together can heal completely. Until the fourteenth day the area should be covered by a layer of Tulle gras, but after this time when the graft has become adherent it is useful to change back to a wet type of dressing such as eusol applied directly to the grafted area in order to assist the separation of small dead bits of tissue, excess graft, crust, etc., whose presence will delay the final epithelialization of the area.

Care of the donor area. *The patient usually complains of much more pain at the donor site than the area to which the graft has been applied and analgesics will usually be given.* This is not surprising when one thinks what a large raw area containing sensitive nerve endings has been exposed. If the dressings soak through during the first day or so, then the area should be repacked and rebandaged. If the wool becomes heavily saturated with blood this may be extremely uncomfortable, and after two days when the oozing has ceased it is best to remove the wool and apply clean wool and a new bandage. *The inner dressings are very adherent at this time and should not be disturbed.* The donor area will normally take at least ten days to heal, longer if the graft has been cut very thick. Ten to fourteen days after operation, therefore, the donor site dressing should be removed, preferably by putting the patient in the bath and letting him soak it off gently. If the donor area is healed then it can be exposed, but if some areas are still raw then further Tulle gras dressings should be applied.

PEDICLED SKIN FLAPS

When a skin defect has to be repaired free skin grafting is preferred if this is possible, because this is a relatively simple procedure and does not involve the immobilization of parts in abnormal positions. However, there are circumstances when a free skin graft is not suitable, usually because the vascularity of the recipient area is poor and not sufficient for a

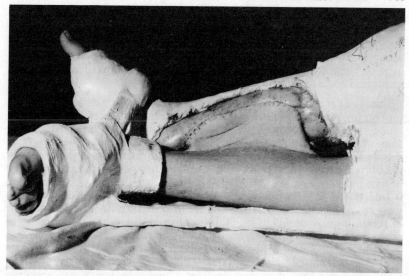

Fig. 67/7 Cross-leg flap for severe wound of leg. The injured (right) leg is receiving a flap of skin from the sound leg.

free skin graft to 'take'. This may occur, for example, when the tendons in the palms of the hand are exposed, or when there is extensive exposure of the tibia in a compound fracture of the leg. Under these circumstances the repair must be made by a flap of skin which remains partially attached to its original site so that it is always nourished by a blood supply.

This attachment through which the blood supply is maintained is known as *the pedicle of the flap.* Thus a severe injury of the hand may be treated by raising a flap of skin on the abdomen along three sides but leaving it attached on a fourth side and stitching it in place on the hand. The hand is then immobilized to the trunk by strapping and after three weeks a sufficient blood supply has grown in from the hand to make it possible to divide the fourth side of the skin from the abdomen. In a similar fashion a defect of the front of the tibia may be covered by a flap of skin from the opposite calf—*cross leg flap. During the period of healing the two legs are immobilized side by side with plaster of Paris, until after three weeks the flap can be divided from the donor leg.* These two types of flap are known as *direct flaps.*

Sometimes, however, it is not possible to provide skin from a site which can be brought into direct approximation with the site to be repaired. *The problem can still be solved, however, by using an intermediate carrier site.* Skin from the abdomen is sewn into a tube, *tubed pedicle flap,* and when healing is complete one end of the tube is transferred to the wrist which then becomes the intermediate carrier site. When the tube has healed soundly to the wrist the remaining attachment to the abdomen can be divided and, nourished by the attachment to the wrist, the tube of skin can then be transferred to the face (see Fig. 67/5, p. 701) or to the leg.

BURNS AND SCALDS

A burn is due to the action of dry heat, such as flame or contact with a hot object, e.g. a hot iron, and a scald is due to moist heat, e.g. boiling water, hot tea, steam. Burns may also be caused by electricity, ultraviolet light or chemicals, particularly strong acids and alkalis. The dangers of burns and scalds are:

Shock. This occurs during the first few hours, and the danger continues for two to three days. The shock is due to loss of fluid from the circulating blood at the site of the burn. Some of this fluid exudes from the surface and some passes into the tissues, which become oedematous. The danger of shock is dependent upon the total size of the burn and not on the depth of the burn. Therefore a superficial burn may cause just as much shock as a deeper burn.

Infection. The large raw surface of a burn is in continuous danger of infection, and this danger persists until the area of the burn is healed. In spite of recent improvements in techniques infection is still the major cause of death in burns.

If the full thickness of the skin has been destroyed by the burn, a raw area will be created. This raw area is likely to become infected, which results in great loss of protein and red blood cells which will seriously affect the general health of the patient until the raw area is closed by skin grafting. In addition the scarring associated with the healing of such raw areas is responsible for contractures and deformities.

Healing of burns. Healing is dependent upon the depth of the burn, and an important distinction to be made is between partial thickness burning of the skin and full thickness burning. If the burn is of **partial thickness depth** and infection is prevented, spontaneous healing will take place from the deeper layers of the skin, and there will be little or no deformity. When the **full thickness of the skin** has been destroyed the dead skin will form a slough which ultimately becomes black and is cast off, leaving a raw red area of granulation tissue. This area can only heal very slowly from the edge and the scarring associated with this slow healing is the cause of contraction and deformity. In this type of full thickness burn, therefore, it is important that the raw area should be healed by a skin graft to minimize the contraction.

First aid. With relatively small burns in which there is not a great danger of shock it is now generally agreed that plunging the affected part in cold water or applying a cold compress is the best treatment. The cold-water treatment should be continued until the pain has been relieved. *However, a note of warning should be sounded in the case of extensive burns. For if cold treatment were applied to a patient with an extensive burn and if for any reason the treatment of shock was delayed, then the shock might be greatly aggravated.* For extensive burns, therefore, the correct treatment is to cover the area by smooth clean towels or sheets and transfer the patient to hospital.

Treatment of shock. In minor burns the patient can make up loss of fluid by drinking extra fluid by mouth. In larger burns, however, this is not possible and intravenous transfusion is necessary. Blood plasma is the fluid most usually used for transfusion, although saline fluids may also be used, and artificial plasma substitutes such as Dextran. In patients with extensive deep burns, red blood cells are also destroyed and a blood transfusion will be necessary. Sedation, and relief of pain by morphine or Omnopon is necessary, and if the patient is being transfused this should be given intravenously into the drip. *It is necessary to continue the transfusion for 36 to 72 hours. The most important indication that the transfusion is adequate is a good flow of urine.* All urine should therefore be saved and tested, and in patients with severe burns a catheter should be passed so that the hourly urine output can be accurately measured and compared with the input. In addition, haemoglobin or haematocrit estimations of the blood will help to determine the extent of the plasma deficit.

Local treatment of the burn wound. Prevention of infection is of the first importance. Infection is most likely to be caused by particles transferred on the hands and clothing of nursing and surgical staff, and great care in the treatment of the burn wound and in the technique of dressings is therefore necessary.

Treatment by dressings. Some form of antiseptic dressing is necessary. No ideal preparation has yet been discovered but antibiotics such as neomycin, bacitracin and polymyxin, and synthetic antibacterial agents such as nitrofurazone (Furacin), chlorhexidine (Hibitane), Sulfamylon and silver sulphadiazine have been of value. Commercial products of Tulle gras impregnated with one or other of the antiseptics, e.g. Sofra Tulle, which is impregnated with 1 per cent Soframycin, are available. Alternatively, the antiseptic cream can be made up in the dispensary and spread with a spatula on large sheets of gauze which are then applied to the wound. *With relatively small burns it is convenient to add a layer of cotton wool over the inner gauze dressing and to bandage this in place. The dressing can then be left for three to four days before being changed. With extensive burns, however, it has been found that more frequent changes of dressings, at least every two days, are necessary.* The burn is covered with a single layer of gauze dressing impregnated with the antiseptic, omitting an absorbent layer. This dressing can then be changed every other day or even every day if necessary.

Treatment by exposure. This is suitable for very extensive burns which are difficult to dress satisfactorily, also for burns of the face and those involving the perineum. For the method to be satisfactory the whole burnt area must be exposed to the air, and much ingenuity may be needed to ensure that this is possible. It may be possible to do this by using various types of splints or sectional mattresses. If the burn is circumferential it is difficult, but may be helped by the use of a special frame such as a Striker frame or the Zimmer circ-electric bed. Recent developments have been a special type of air-conditioning apparatus which encloses the patient in an atmosphere of clean filtered air, and the Hover-bed, which actually supports the body on filtered air and is ideal for extensive circumferential burns.

In partial thickness burns, whichever of the above methods is chosen should be continued until the burn is completely healed.

In full thickness burns the treatment will be continued until surrounding areas of partial thickness burns have healed. Areas in which there is full thickness burning will then be covered by a black slough of dead skin. It is necessary that this should be removed before skin grafting can be performed. In some cases it may be possible to expedite matters by performing an actual surgical excision of the burn slough. In other cases, however, further treatment by dressings will be necessary to assist in the conservative removal of the slough, see page 702 (preparation of the recipient site for skin grafting).

GENERAL NURSING CARE

Fluids and diet. In severe burns vomiting may occur during the shock period and oral fluids must be restricted until this tendency has passed. As the shock comes under control oral fluid should be increased, and by the end of the shock period the patient should be on a mixed diet. After this time the patient should be encouraged to eat a full diet and he should have supplements of milk, eggs or concentrated preparations such as Casilan, so that extra protein and carbohydrates are available for the healing process. Iron and vitamin preparations should also be given.

Later treatment. The healing of an extensive burn is long and tedious for the patient and there is a great tendency for joints to become stiff. *Physiotherapy and occupational therapy are therefore important as soon as the patient is fit enough. In the case of a child it is very helpful if the mother can visit every day and help with the feeding and general management of the child.*

MAXILLO-FACIAL INJURIES

Severe injuries of the face are now common in road traffic accidents. Less severe injuries occur in sports such as football and boxing. For descriptive purposes the face is considered in thirds.

> *The upper third* is the forehead.
> *The middle third* is between the eyebrows and the line of occlusion of the teeth; this includes the nose, the malar (cheek) bones, and the maxilla (upper jaw).
> *The lower third* is the mandible (lower jaw).

The immediate danger in such injuries is *respiratory obstruction* due either to blood running down into the air passages, or falling back of the tongue in association with unstable fractures of the mandible. The first-aid treatment is to turn the patient into the coma position (see Fig. 8/3, p. 80) or right over on the face, and if apparatus is available any blood which has gone down into the throat is sucked out.

The treatment of the fractures of the upper and lower jaws involves skilled dental treatment, and if teeth are present stabilization of the fractures is usually obtained by fixing the teeth of the upper and lower jaw together either by wires or by specially constructed cast silver dental splints. In patients who are edentulous it may often be possible to use the dentures as splints, but if this is not possible then either internal wiring or external pin fixation must be used (see Fig. 67/8).

The immediate postoperative treatment of these patients is mainly concerned with ensuring that an adequate airway is maintained. *Later when the patient is conscious it is necessary to ensure that an adequate intake of*

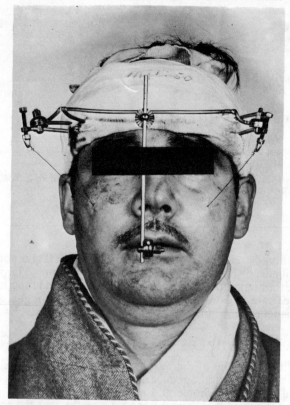

Fig. 67/8 Patient with fracture of the maxilla showing fixation with plaster of Paris headcap.

food is obtained and that teeth or splints are kept scrupulously clean to avoid any infection of the fracture sites.

REDUCTION OPERATION

Some operations in plastic surgery are performed mainly or entirely for the sake of appearance, because the appearance of an unusually ugly feature may have a serious effect on the happiness of a patient. One of the commonest operations in this group is the correction of outstanding ears, 'bat ears', which often cause great unhappiness in boys who are teased at school. In older persons a large and ugly nose is often a source of embarrassment, and a nasal reduction or *cosmetic rhinoplasty* can be performed in which the size of the nose is reduced through incisions entirely on the inside of the nose so that no visible scars remain at the end of the operation. *Grossly enlarged breasts* are also a source of embarrassment to the patient, and in addition the actual weight of the breasts may be so great as to cause severe discomfort and aching of the shoulders. The operation of breast reduction or *mammaplasty* as practised nowadays causes much less shock than the operation previously performed and gives excellent results.

Chapter 68

Medical Rehabilitation

by JAMES G. SOMMERVILLE

Definition—principles of rehabilitation—function of a rehabilitation centre

---

Rehabilitation or reablement means restoration to full and normal function after illness or injury. In some patients this will prove impossible, in which case the highest possible level of independence and function become the goal (see note on Convalescence, p. 21). To achieve the goal it is vital to treat the patient as a whole and not merely the disability.

PRINCIPLES OF REHABILITATION

Rehabilitation begins at the outset of illness or injury; when a person becomes ill his mind must be at once directed to being well again and taking his normal place in his home and at work. Similarly, when a multiple injuries unit is alerted that an accident case is on the way, the preparations made by the staff are directed to the same end whatever may be the condition of the patient when he arrives.

Doctors and nurses in hospital should have this end in view also. A period in hospital is only one stage in treatment, but it can be an educative one enabling a patient to understand, as well as his condition permits, the processes he will pass through during recovery and the ultimate result he may expect. A nurse should always be aware of this. When a patient has been very ill, in an intensive care or resuscitation unit, for example, the withdrawal of the machines by which his vital functions have been kept acting is a preliminary; this is followed by the nurse withdrawing all her work which may have relieved him of the strain of performing his own body functions and handing back to him gradually his own care of his body. His first steps out of bed will be guided, but the donning of his normal walking clothes can raise his morale. However much he may feel that he cannot manage, the fact that the nurse expects this of him will show how essential it is that he should do so. All this is rehabilitation.

These principles can be applied to every situation, a coronary heart attack for example. Reassurance must be positive; a man's family, friends and work colleagues can all be enlisted as useful collaborators. Advice given on his progress should be encouraging rather than restrictive: do's and don'ts should be studiously avoided. His own experiments may be watched and applauded. So much depends on the qualities of mind, heart and will of the patient and on the warm companionship of family and friends and the encouragement of his surgeon or physician in hospital and family doctor at home, who know so well the health-giving value of being normally active and eventually busily occupied.

The nurse, always guided by the doctors, can apply similar principles to all her patients, no matter to which team they belong. Further to what can be done in hospital or at home, a medical rehabilitation centre will deal with a number of people who need treatment, care and cure, constructive advice in the management of their lives and encouragement to persevere. Such a centre, staffed by a team consisting of physiotherapists, occupational therapists, speech therapists, nurses, remedial gymnasts and social workers working under medical direction, provides the best possible treatment for many patients. In most instances a man can return to his former work or similar work; in others this may be considered too strenuous and, after consideration of his desires and aptitude, education or training for some other sphere is advised and arranged. The aim is to provide occupation comparable to his previous work and carrying the same status and income if possible, though the attainment of this level may have to be modified.

The establishment of motivation is all important—the desire to get better; and any organization which tries to get people better must have as one of its aims the need to stimulate this motivation. One thing is certain, people who are disabled and unemployed become unemployable purely and simply by the passage of time. This is a very important fact to recognize, because whereas it is possible to do something positive for people who are disabled, it is often extremely difficult to do anything useful about those who have become set in a pattern of incapacity—that is, those who are the disabled unemployables.

In this respect it is worth noting that there are dangers inherent in providing inadequate treatment. If we lead patients to believe that they are discharging their social obligations to the community by going to the hospital two or three times a week and having some physiotherapy for half an hour and returning home, we should not be surprised if they take a long time to get better, and indeed such treatment, if it is not carefully controlled, can of itself provide a socially acceptable reason for not working.

FUNCTION OF A REHABILITATION CENTRE

A government report commonly known as the Piercy Report, which was published as long ago as November 1956, stated that the treatment of the individual patient should be planned, should be intensive and should have a background of discipline.

It was in an attempt to achieve this that medical rehabilitation centres were originally conceived and developed, and indeed were running successfully long before the publication of this Report. The only significant statistic in relation to the disabled in this respect concerns the total disability period, that is, not the time that is spent in hospital, not the time that is spent as an out-patient, but the total time that the patient is off work.

All effort should be directed towards shortening this total disability period. The best way to achieve this for the appropriate patients is by transferring them from the atmosphere of the hospital to the atmosphere of a medical rehabilitation centre as soon as possible. The Medical Rehabilitation Centre, Camden Road, London provides an example of intensive medical rehabilitation.

Patients attend daily, Monday to Friday, from 9.15 a.m. to 4.30 p.m. Lunch is provided at the Centre. A few patients attend on a half-day basis if this is desirable. Each patient is provided with appropriate clothing and a locker for keeping personal possessions and outdoor clothes.

On the first day at the Centre, normally a Monday, a full medical and social history is obtained and the patient is medically examined. From a master programme the doctor selects an individual programme for the particular patient, which is geared to the patient's needs. Thirteen major disability exercise groups are available, together with a number of specialized groups, and little difficulty is experienced in finding the right level of treatment for the patient. The approach to the problem is three-fold: directly, by means of remedial exercises, physiotherapy and specific occupational therapy; indirectly, by means of games, exercises and occupational therapy; and obliquely, by the assessment of the patient as a whole by the entire staff and by trying to solve related problems, social, legal, industrial and financial, which are militating against as rapid a recovery as possible.

There is a shift in emphasis from individual to group treatment and from passive to active therapy as the patient progresses. As far as possible patients are treated in groups and, as the staff have a full knowledge of each patient, it is possible to give appropriate attention to the individual needs of each patient.

Treating patients in groups is preferable to treating patients individually. First of all it helps the patient to get his disability, permanent or temporary, into perspective. Secondly, it subjects him to the discipline of the group and this provides a valuable filter, which rejects or shows up the patient who is not making the expected rate of progress. Thirdly, an element of competition comes into the work of the groups and this helps to stimulate positive motivation in patients where it may be lacking. The morning and afternoon periods begin with a half-hour period of exercise to music.

Special provision is made for the severely disabled. A Functional Activities Group is of great help to such patients by providing the training, encouragement and example to overcome the large proportion of the disability which is due to lack of knowledge, lack of confidence and disuse.

Severely handicapped patients have time set aside each day to allow them to be taught the basic elements of the activities of daily living. Aids and devices are provided or made in the workshops when necessary. It is significant that over 80 per cent of the patients admitted to the Centre who were dependent, i.e. unable to dress, wash and feed themselves without assistance, were able to do so after less than two weeks' treatment.

Public transport. Every effort is made to encourage patients to use public transport, and progress is made from the use of a static model of a bus to supervised journeys on buses and trains.

Invalid tricycles. These are sometimes necessary for the more severely handicapped patients and, after assessment, arrangements are made for suitable patients to be provided with these through the Department of Health and Social Security.

Resettlement. It is essential that no patient is discharged into a vacuum.

The normal practice is for patients returning to work to be discharged from a rehabilitation centre on a Friday, with a certificate which enables them to commence work the following Monday.

Those who are unable to return to their previous work can often return to modified work with the same employer, and direct negotiations are made with employers to try to achieve this.

A number require training or alternative employment, and this is achieved either directly or with the help of the Disablement Resettlement Officer. Other patients may be provided with sheltered employment or other occupation at a work group or social centre.

The nurse is, or should be, deeply involved in medical rehabilitation. Her attitude to each patient during the acute stage can have far-reaching effects upon the ultimate outcome. The nurse must look upon the patient as a whole, and not merely as a diagnosis. She must recognize the dangers as well as the advantages of bed rest and she must foster the re-establishment of independence with every means at her command.

Notes on rehabilitation in particular situations will be found throughout this book; see, for example:

The care of paralysed patients, p. 269.
Psychiatric nursing, p. 279.
The care of the elderly, p. 343.
The treatment of bone and joint injuries, p. 554.

Section 7

A. A Brief Introduction to Obstetrical Nursing

Chapter 69

An Outline of the Physiology of the Female Organs of Reproduction

by RUTH McKAY

> *Puberty—the menarche—menstruation—ovulation—fertilization—tests of pregnancy*

Puberty describes the age when the *reproductive organs develop* and make it possible for a girl to conceive. This is brought about by the pituitary gland stimulating the production of oestrogen, a follicular hormone in the ovary. In many girls at about 12 years, mental and emotional and certain physical changes take place, the curves of the body are revealed, deposits of fatty tissue round off the angularities, the breasts become fuller and the pelvis widens.

Menstruation. During the *menstrual life* of a woman oestrogen is increased; it maintains her womanly characteristics, and stimulates the preparation of the uterus for the reception of a fertilized ovum. The correct term for the *onset* of menstruation is the *menarche*. Thereafter there is a discharge of blood and cast-off endometrial cells from the uterus occurring in a rhythmical cycle every 28 days, but there are individual variations. Thus menstruation is the shedding of the old, and the preparation of a new endometrium which is peculiarly soft at this stage as it is intended to become a resting place for a fertilized ovum.

The *ovaries* are the female sex glands and the centre of the whole sex mechanism. If an ovary is cut across it is seen to contain holes, like Gruyère cheese; these are the Graafian follicles; minute cells line the walls of these follicles and a group of granulosa cells develops to surround an ovum. The follicles are filled with fluid and it is here that in the developing girl the hormones controlling puberty and also controlling the reproductive cycle and menstruation are produced.

The reproductive or menstrual cycle. The anterior lobe of the pituitary gland produces two *gonadotrophic hormones*, so called as they stimulate the gonads or reproductive organs (in this instance the ovaries).

Ovulation. (1) *A follicle stimulating hormone* (F.S.H.), controls the ripening of a Graafian follicle in the ovary and the production of oestrogen and the discharge of an ovum when the follicle ruptures. Prior to ovulation one follicle ripens and approximates to the surface of the ovary. The follicle ruptures and the ovum is swept out with the fluid, to be drawn into the uterine (Fallopian) tube. Ovulation occurs usually 14 days *before the onset* of the next menstrual period.

(2) *A luteinizing hormone* (L.H.) stimulates the growth of the corpus luteum or yellow body from the cells where a Graafian follicle has ruptured. This produces progesterone which causes increase in the preparation of the uterus and the preservation of the condition of the endometrium required in pregnancy. After about two months the chorionic villi (see below), surrounding the developing fetus, take over the production of progesterone.

If no ovum is fertilized, the corpus luteum disintegrates after 12 days, the production of progesterone is diminished and the endometrium breaks down and discharges the menses. The reproductive cycle begins once again; a Graafian follicle matures, the endometrium is renewed and is ready to respond again to the actions of oestrogen and progesterone.

Fertilization is the fusing of the male element of reproduction, the *spermatozoon*, with the *ovum* or egg cell. This usually takes place in the uterine (Fallopian) tube; the ovum which is non-motile and is a round cell is being transmitted through the tube by the action of the ciliated epithelium which passes it from the external to the internal ostium, through which it reaches the uterus.

The spermatozoon is a motile cell, shaped like a tadpole with a head and a tail; it passes up through the uterus and fights its way along the uterine tube against the stream of activity of the cilia which is bringing the ovum along, down the tube. On meeting, the head of one of the spermatozoa penetrates the ovum and the tail drops off. The two cells fuse, at this moment 23 chromosomes—which carry the hereditary factors (genes)—of the spermatozoon unite with 23 chromosomes of the ovum; at the time of fusion the sex is also determined, depending upon the type of spermatozoon—since it is the male which carries the decisive sex cell.

Cell division commences and the fertilized ovum passes along the uterine (Fallopian) tube into the uterus, which is prepared with its soft lining to receive it. Various changes now take place and different cells are formed, some going to the construction of the fetus and others to the formation of the placenta and membranes. As growth continues, small finger-like projections (villi) grow in all directions surrounding the fertilized ovum, some become embedded like roots into the inner lining of the uterus and develop into the placenta; these are known as the *chorionic villi*, the remainder eventually atrophy.

Tests of pregnancy. The first indication of pregnancy is that a period is missed. *Diagnosis* may be established, or alternatively excluded, by one of the biological pregnancy tests which depend on the gonadotrophic hormones produced by the chorionic villi being found in the urine of the patient.

Tests are undertaken to determine pregnancy as early as possible. At the present time an *immunological test* for the detection of human chorionic gonadotrophin in pregnancy urine is employed. It is a complicated laboratory procedure; several proprietary tests have been developed and are in use. One of these is Prepuerin, known as *haemagglutination inhibition test*.

Put simply, an anti-serum is prepared and added to human chorionic gonadotrophin with which it combines, some specially treated sheep's red blood cells are added, an agglutinated mass forms; then some of the suspected urine is added when, if the test is positive, the blood cells will begin to disagglutinate and this is why it is named 'the haemagglutination inhibition test'. Dilutions are put up in test-tubes at room temperature for several hours and the result is read. This test is considered to be accurate and inexpensive, providing a diagnosis of pregnancy within a few days after human chorionic gonadotrophin (H.C.G.) is excreted in the urine, which is about six weeks following establishment of pregnancy.

Biological tests for pregnancy have been used for many years but a biological test is unlikely to be positive until about the eighth week of pregnancy and the result takes several weeks to establish. Two of these tests are mentioned.

Aschheim-Zondek. Some of the pregnancy urine is injected into immature white mice, when, if positive, developmental changes take place in the generative organs of the mice. In the *Hogben test* female toads are used, and if the toads ovulate within 12 hours the test is considered positive.

Chapter 70

Pregnancy and Prenatal Care

by RUTH McKAY

Probable signs and symptoms of pregnancy—prenatal care—parentcraft—complications of pregnancy

---

The probable signs and symptoms of pregnancy. A woman is said to be pregnant when she is with child; the uterus will retain the growing fetus for 10 lunar months or 280 days, which is the duration of pregnancy. The expected date of confinement may be calculated by adding 9 calendar months and 7 days to the first day of the last menstrual period. This reckoning is correct within 2 or 3 weeks. The *symptoms and signs* by which pregnancy may be determined are divided for convenience into those which appear during the first 3 months, and those seen later.

During the first 12 weeks, amenorrhoea is considered to be a sign of pregnancy provided the woman has previously menstruated regularly and that there is no other cause of amenorrhoea, such as the onset of the menopause, anaemia or other illness. There is *frequency of micturition* during this period.

Morning sickness. This usually occurs from the sixth to the sixteenth weeks, and is thought to be due to chemical changes in the maternal blood. It may be relieved by taking a cup of tea and a biscuit before rising in the morning. The movements made when getting up should be gradual, giving time for the body to accommodate to standing up.

Skin changes are useful but not definite signs of pregnancy. *Chloasma* are pigmentary changes in the face. *Striae gravidarum* are the marks due to overstretching of the skin of the abdomen and/or the breasts. There is darkening of the linea alba, now known as the *linea nigra*. For colour changes in the areola of the nipple see below.

Breast changes commence about the *sixth week*, when the breasts are full and tender. By the *twelfth week* the breasts are firmer and some mucous secretion is present; visible veins appear beneath the surface of the skin. The nipples become erect and the areola dark in tint.

By the *sixteenth week*, little nodules, called Montgomery's follicles, appear around the area of the nipple and by the *twentieth week* the secondary areola appears. Colostrum can now be expressed from the breasts.

Progressive enlargement of the uterus. The enlargement of the uterus varies with the size of the fetus, the presence of twins or hydramnios. A full bladder or bowel can also influence the height of the uterine fundus. The height of the fundus at certain weeks of pregnancy (but no two women are alike) is generally:

At the *twelfth week* the fundus can just be felt above the level of the symphysis pubis.

By the *twenty-fourth week* it can be felt at the level of the umbilicus.

By the *thirty-sixth week* the fundus can be felt at the level of the xiphisternum. The uterus sinks to a slightly lower level in the pelvis in the last few weeks of pregnancy.

Intermittent painless contractions may be felt by the mother after the sixteenth week of pregnancy. *Quickening* is the term used to describe the sensations the mother experiences after the eighteenth or twentieth week when the fetus moves his position in the uterus.

Positive signs of pregnancy may be distinguished by:

Touch—the fetal parts can be felt.

Sound—the fetal heart sounds can be heard.

Sight—what the midwife observes.

An X-ray examination of the abdomen provides a further sign.

PRENATAL CARE

Environmental factors are of importance in successful child bearing. Prenatal care is undertaken in order to assist a woman through pregnancy and to avoid and treat any diseases or abnormal conditions which may arise, so as to ensure a normal uncomplicated labour and puerperium. Every woman should be advised either to consult her own doctor or to attend a prenatal clinic as soon as she knows she is pregnant. The date of her first attendance will be recorded, the date of her last menstrual period and the possible date of the expected confinement estimated.

The history will be taken at the woman's first visit. It is divided for convenience of making a record into:

The *medical history* which includes whether she has had any illnesses such as scarlet fever, diphtheria, rheumatism or chorea which may affect the heart. Poliomyelitis and tuberculosis may result in alteration in the size and shape of the pelvis.

Any recurring infections or disorders—colds, tonsillitis, headache, biliousness, or constipation; whether she has had any virus infections such as German measles.

Any operations undergone or accidents sustained.

The history of previous blood transfusions with dates is important because of the possible existence of the Rh (rhesus) antibodies in the patient's blood.

The obstetrical history. The following particulars are important: the length of time the patient has been married; duration of previous pregnancies, whether these were normal or complicated, and whether conducted at home or in hospital; the birth weight, method of delivery and birth conditions of her previous babies and whether they were breast or bottle fed and the present state of their health.

The family history. The following points will be considered: any diseases in the family such as diabetes, hypertension, tuberculosis or mental breakdown, any family history of twins, whether her parents are living and in good health.

Examination

At the first examination, which is fairly extensive, the woman's general condition will be closely observed, the condition of the heart and lungs investigated.

The condition of the *mouth, teeth* and *tonsils* will be noted.
The *blood pressure* and *pulse rate* taken and recorded.
The *urine* will be tested for albumin and sugar.
The patient will be weighed and her *weight recorded.*
The *pelvis* will be assessed.

At every visit *the signs of pre-eclamptic toxaemia* are looked for. These are:

Rising blood pressure.
The presence of albumin in the urine.
Oedema—swelling of the feet and ankles.
Increase in weight beyond what is expected. This may be due to oedema.

Visits will be made *every 4 weeks* during the first 28 weeks, *every fortnight* until the thirty-sixth week and then *every week*. But it is essential that the mother should clearly realize that the clinic is there to help and advise her and that if she has the slightest doubt about her condition or is in the least worried she should attend immediately, or she may telephone.

During the later visits the abdomen will be palpated to determine the position in which the fetus is lying, and the part of the baby lowest in the uterus and its level in relation to the pelvis is noted. All these points and the condition of the fetal heart sounds will be recorded, in addition to all the other points mentioned in the first examination (see above).

A number of tests which will be made at the initial examination include:

Estimation of the haemoglobin blood content which will be carried out at regular intervals throughout the prenatal period. In pregnancy there is a physiological lowering of the haemoglobin content of the red blood cells which in some instances may require treatment in order to prevent anaemia.

Blood tests. The blood is typed and grouped in case blood transfusion should be necessary. The presence or the absence of the rhesus factor so important in pregnancy is also determined (see Chapter 48, p. 459).

Serological tests are carried out for the presence of any venereal disease.

Cervical smears are taken in all pregnant women to exclude the possibility of the early development of cancer of the cervix (see p. 738).

Prenatal advice. The main points on which it is essential that a woman should be clearly advised either at a prenatal clinic or at *mothercraft* sessions are as follows:

The diet should be well balanced and nourishing, plenty of fish and meat should be taken, and all dairy produce, including two pints of milk a day. Highly spiced foods, sauces and stimulants, and strong tea and coffee are inadvisable. Plenty of green vegetables and fruit should be taken, and orange juice and vitamin tablets supplied as accessory articles of diet. The carbohydrate intake should be cut down.

Smoking in pregnancy. If the expectant mother is a heavy smoker she will be advised to cut down, or if possible stop this habit since it predisposes to alteration to the size of the fetus and even in some cases slower development at school level.

Medication in pregnancy. Self-medication during the first months of pregnancy should never be practised and only prescription as ordered by the doctor should be accepted.

Action of bowels. There should be a good action daily, only vegetable products such as Senokot are allowed as a laxative. Any lubricant containing paraffin is contra-indicated as these hinder the absorption of vitamins from the intestine.

Rest and sleep. Fatigue should be avoided and from eight to nine hours in bed is recommended. An hour or two on the bed after the midday meal should be taken if possible. Relaxation is taught during the prenatal period because of its importance during labour, and it should be practised.

Exercise. Moderate exercise is valuable but fatigue, sudden strains and violent jerky movements should be avoided. Open-air exercise is to be recommended, but every woman will have to consider this question for herself—for example, a woman who does most of her own housework, and walks about doing the shopping, does not need a three-mile walk every day as well.

Clothing should be sensible. Many women find that shoes with a moderate heel give better support than very high-heeled shoes which may increase the tendency to backache and accidents.

Care of breasts. A daily bath is advisable, and the patient should wash her breasts and nipples thoroughly whilst in the bath and train her nipples to be erect if they are at all inclined to retraction, though her handling of them should never be painful. Woolwich shells which encourage projection of the nipples may be worn under a well-fitting brassière if advised. The woman may be taught to express 'colostrum' from her breasts very gently twice a day from the thirty-fourth to the thirty-sixth week onwards in order to prevent engorgement.

It should always be impressed on a pregnant woman that if she feels unwell, gets a bad headache, has swollen feet or hands, feels sick and disinclined for food or has any other symptoms of malaise, or any loss of blood, she should call her doctor at once.

Parentcraft. A young mother who is expecting her first baby is embarking on entirely new and unknown changes within her body which run parallel with the altered emotional state of her mind; she needs guidance, understanding and help.

The expectant father will be grateful since the conception of his baby proves to him his maturity and his capacity for fatherhood and the opening of a new responsibility in providing for this additional unit to his family. He should be encouraged to take an active part in helping his wife throughout her pregnancy, and he may attend some of the classes listed below. He may desire to stay with her and encourage her during labour and to stay on after delivery to share the joys and responsibility in caring for his baby. In this way both parents make the necessary psychological and social adjustments.

The mother's emotional reaction to conception, pregnancy and labour will be influenced to some extent by her own childhood (she may have loved playing with dolls or caring for children outside her own family), her relationship with her parents, especially with her mother, and her present happiness with her husband.

At mothercraft and relaxation classes the following talks and aids will be given which will answer some of the problems which may be troubling the pregnant woman.

The nutritional values and the functions of various foods.
The fashionable wear available for the expectant mother.
The way in which a new baby grows.
The preparation for labour and the stages of childbirth.
The use of analgesics during childbirth (see below).
The equipment needed for the baby, and the preparation of his layette.
Feeding the baby.
What happens during the lying-in period.

She will also be instructed on her care of the breasts and nipples, and she will be shown how to bath and handle a newly born baby.

Inhalation anaesthesia. The Entonox machine for inhalation analgesia, is available for all mothers; the cylinder contains a mixture of 50 per cent nitrous oxide and 50 per cent oxygen.

COMPLICATIONS OF PREGNANCY

These may be divided into minor and major disorders.

Minor complications include *morning sickness* during the first two months, which may be relieved by lying for half an hour before sitting up and having a cup of tea and a biscuit before getting up.

Fainting may result from any sudden change of posture or standing for long periods as in a bus queue or being in a stuffy atmosphere.

Constipation and *haemorrhoids* may occur and in some there may be *pruritus vulvae*. A controlled diet and mild laxatives may relieve constipation but liquid paraffin or any emulsion is not recommended. *Insomnia* and *muscular cramp* may be troublesome.

Pyelonephritis due to urinary infection by the *Escherichia coli* may be severe or less severe. It may occur during the second trimester, usually from the sixteenth to the twenty-eighth weeks and may *recur* during the puerperium. As a rule the prognosis is good in pregnancy. For symptoms and treatment see p. 248.

Major complications. *Hyperemesis gravidarum* (persistent excessive vomiting) leads to a condition of acidosis. There is serious metabolic disturbance and unless treated this condition may lead to involvement of the liver. Treatment in hospital is usually necessary.

Pre-eclampsia or *pre-eclamptic toxaemia* occurs any time after the twenty-eighth week and more probably nearer term. The blood pressure rises, the urine is diminished and contains protein, oedema (see below) is generally present, headache, spots before the eyes, vomiting and other symptoms met with in eclampsia (see p. 722) may occur.

Oedema may be occult or clinical. In *occult oedema* the only manifestation is a marked increase in body weight which would be noted during prenatal examination. Any unexplained weight increase should be regarded with suspicion. The average total weight gain during a normal pregnancy is 28 lb (13 kg). *Clinical oedema* is seen first in the ankles and hands. A woman may say that her wedding ring is tight. Then the face, sacral region, abdominal wall and vulva become swollen.

Treatment includes observation and rest in hospital where she will be delivered.

> Sedatives and in some instances the use of hypotensive drugs may be prescribed.
> Diuretics may be necessary.
> A high protein diet is advocated to replace the loss of protein in the urine.
> When oedema is present salt is often restricted.
> Fluids also are sometimes restricted to two pints a day.
> The urine must be tested daily for proteinuria, and the quantity of protein is also estimated daily by means of Esbach's reagent, p. 61.
> A careful fluid balance record should be kept. The weight should be checked daily.

Complications which may occur during the pre-eclamptic state are accidental ante-partum haemorrhage, *placenta abruptio* (see p. 724), placental insufficiency, which means the baby is deprived of necessary oxygen and, the most dreaded of all—the onset of eclampsia.

Eclampsia may occur before, during and after delivery. *It is characterized by one or more fits* and usually, though not invariably, preceded by pre-eclamptic toxaemia.

> There may be severe headaches, vomiting, oliguria, diplopia, dimness of vision, flashes of light before the eyes, and epigastric pain.
> This collection of symptoms indicates the imminent onset of eclampsia.
> There is also a fulminating type of eclampsia with sudden onset without warning, which is most serious.

Treatment of eclampsia is urgent in order to prevent the patient having more fits or to avoid the recurrence of them. Heavy sedation is necessary. Hypotensive drugs may alternatively be used. The patient must be kept quiet and should not be disturbed. The blood pressure should be recorded frequently, the temperature and pulse rate four-hourly, and the respiration rate every quarter of an hour. Avoidance of all stimulation by sudden noise, light or touch is of first importance. Gentle swabbing of the mouth may be possible, but, as touching the patient may stimulate a fit, all nursing attentions must be carefully assessed.

A self-retaining catheter is inserted and released every four hours; the amount of urine is measured and charted; the urine should be tested and the quantity of albumin present estimated twice a day. A careful record of all fluids administered and of the urinary output should be kept.

An *eclamptic fit* is epileptiform in character, passing through the same stages as in epilepsy (see p. 261).

A short *premonitory* state.

A *tonic* stage when there is rigidity and cyanosis.

A *clonic* stage when convulsive movements occur.

A stage of *coma* which may last a few minutes or some hours.

During coma an epileptic would pass urine involuntarily; not so the eclamptic in whom urine is diminished and the bladder probably empty. There may be further convulsions before consciousness is regained, and cerebral haemorrhage may occur. During an eclamptic fit the woman should be turned on her side to avoid the inhalation of saliva or any gastric contents which might be regurgitated as this would be serious.

Medical aid should be summoned and oxygen, if available, should be given.

A rubber ring inserted between the teeth *during the clonic stage* may prevent the tongue from being bitten.

Labour may commence spontaneously during eclampsia, or an obstetrician may consider the advisability of inducing labour and in selected instances he may recommend Caesarean section. The fetal mortality is high in eclampsia.

Bleeding as a complication in pregnancy may occur early or later, and it may be slight or severe enough to be regarded as an obstetrical emergency.

Miscarriage or *abortion* is the premature termination of pregnancy occurring before the twenty-eighth week of gestation and generally before the middle of the third month. It is a not uncommon complication—a woman with four or five children may perhaps have had one or two miscarriages.

Causes. An *abnormal fetus* or disease of a fertilized ovum is regarded as one of the commonest causes. *Congenital abnormalities* including an underdeveloped uterus, a bi-cornuate uterus or an incompetent cervix; retroversion of the uterus and lacerations of the cervix may also cause miscarriage. Any *foreign body* or irritating material in the uterus will cause it to contract and expel the fetus, such as the occasional fibroid tumour; an induced abortion or an attempt at abortion will have the same result.

Disease in the mother has also to be considered. Chronic nephritis and any pyrexial condition or acute illness and endocrine dysfunction may result in miscarriage. Other causes of early bleeding include 'cervical erosion', carcinoma of the cervix, mucous polypus, ectopic gestation and hydatidiform mole which is rare.

In cases of habitual abortion the cause may be unknown.

Symptoms of miscarriage. A miscarriage is really a miniature labour and it may occur a few days, some weeks or several months after pregnancy began. A very usual history is that the woman has missed menstruation for two or three months; she then begins to bleed from the uterus; this is accompanied by abdominal pain, followed by a stronger flow of blood and the products of pregnancy are expelled.

Treatment depends on whether the miscarriage is complicated by continued bleeding or not. If it is not the patient should remain quiet, lying down or resting in bed. Her pads should be inspected and any products of pregnancy should be saved for the inspection of the midwife or obstetrician. The *after-care* includes observation of vaginal discharge and of the temperature and the pulse rate, as sepsis may complicate miscarriage. In all cases medical aid should be sent for and the condition will be dealt with as in any other complication of pregnancy characterized by bleeding.

Complications in which there is bleeding from the uterus after the twenty-eighth week of pregnancy and when the child is viable:

Antepartum haemorrhage is bleeding from the genital tract after the twenty-eighth week of pregnancy before complete expulsion of the fetus.

Accidental antepartum haemorrhage or *placenta abruptio* is bleeding from the site of a normally situated placenta, i.e. in the upper uterine segment, also after the twenty-eighth week of pregnancy up to the complete expulsion of the fetus.

Unavoidable antepartum haemorrhage is bleeding from a placental site which is partly or wholly situated in the lower uterine segment, commonly known as *placenta praevia*.

Treatment of any bleeding met with in pregnancy is directed to the relief of the cause. Medical aid should be summoned at once. In the meantime, the patient should be kept at rest and be reassured.

All food should be withheld in case a general anaesthetic has to be given. All sanitary pads and soaked linen should be saved for inspection so that the amount of blood loss can be estimated. A frequent record of the blood pressure and pulse rate should be kept. A falling blood pressure and a steadily rising pulse rate indicate that the bleeding is continuing. It is an important nursing point that patients who are bleeding should be disturbed as little as possible, as any movement will tend to increase the prostration and exhaustion from which a patient who is bleeding seriously already suffers. Any products of pregnancy passed should be saved for inspection.

An emergency obstetrical unit, colloquially known as 'the flying squad', which can be sent out when the need is urgent, is attached to most large maternity departments. This unit is staffed by an obstetrician, a doctor who can give an anaesthetic if required, and a midwife.

The call usually comes when a woman needs blood transfusion because antepartum or postpartum haemorrhage has occurred. This unit can perform resuscitation on the spot and give blood transfusion; later when the mother has recovered sufficiently to be moved, she would be brought into hospital if obstetrical measures were necessary.

Alternatively an emergency call may be made for resuscitation of the baby, when a paediatrician and a senior member of the nursing staff will go out.

Chapter 71

Labour and the Puerperium

by RUTH McKAY

> *The patient—delivery room—stages of labour—complications—care of the woman in labour—care of the baby—the puerperium—complications—postnatal care*

The patient. It may be presumed that the patient has had instruction in mothercraft during the prenatal period (see p. 720).

Delivery or *labour room.* The labour or delivery room is similar to an operating theatre. Obstetrician and nurse are masked, 'scrubbed up', gowned and gloved. The birth of a baby is conducted as aseptically as any major operation. All the apparatus required should be ready, in good order and clean or sterile as the case may be. The skin of the vulva, perineal area and of the patient's buttocks and thighs is carefully prepared.

The first indication of labour may be pain in the back, associated with hardening of the uterus under the anterior abdominal wall; or there may be:

> Intermittent painful contractions which tend to become stronger and more frequent.
> Or a blood-stained mucoid discharge from the vagina known as 'the show'.
> Or there may be an escape of fluid from the vagina if the membranes have ruptured.

The first stage of labour begins with the onset of rhythmic contractions and lasts until the cervix is fully dilated. The pains are due to the contractions and retractions of the uterus resulting in the gradual and complete dilatation of the cervix.

The second stage of labour lasts from the time the cervix is fully dilated, to the complete expulsion of the baby.

The third stage is from the birth of the baby, until the placenta and membranes are expelled from the vagina.

Care of a woman in labour. Those in attendance on a mother should radiate kindliness. When a nurse goes calmly about her duties this, in itself, will inspire a patient with the confidence and contentment she needs, so that she may look forward to the birth of her baby without apprehension.

The bowel and bladder should be empty so that the patient is not worried by this during the uterine contractions.

> A careful record of the amount of urine passed should be kept.
>
> Any staining or vaginal discharge should be observed and noted.
>
> The maternal pulse and fetal heart sounds should be recorded more frequently as labour progresses.
>
> The blood pressure and temperature should be taken every four hours.
>
> The urine should be tested for protein and acetone.

A woman in labour may at times have to be anaesthetized and therefore should not have food. But most women are allowed fluids fairly liberally.

The woman should not be left unattended or suffer discomfort, Entonox inhalation anaesthesia will be offered to the mother and analgesics for the relief of pain should be given sufficiently freely though they ought to be used with discretion. A warm cot in a warm room should be prepared for the baby and labels for affixing the name of the mother.

General care of the baby at birth. *The eyes* are swabbed as the head is born, using two separate sterile wool swabs to remove any organisms which may have contaminated the eyes as the baby passed through the birth canal. The action of swabbing should be from the inner to the outer canthus. The midwife should look and feel if there is any tight cord round the neck which may have to be clamped in two places and divided in between and removed; if the cord is loose enough it may be slipped up over the baby's head. By this time the baby is born.

The inhalation of mucus must be most carefully avoided by clearing the air passages, otherwise as the baby takes his first gasping breath he will inhale this mucus and any fluid which may be in his mouth or pharynx, thus blocking passage to the lungs. In hospital an air suction apparatus is often used; alternatively, a mucus extractor with a mouthpiece is employed with great care. Suspending him upside-down for a few seconds by the feet, helps to drain out any fluid. A newborn baby can only breathe through free air passages and when he cries lustily he is considered to be all right.

The cord is then safely clamped. Alternatively, a sterile linen thread ligature is passed round and *very tightly tied* two inches (5 cm) from the umbilicus; a second ligature is similarly tied two inches or 5 cm further away; by cutting between these two ligatures or clamps the baby is separated from his mother. A second umbilical clamp and a sterile dressing is then applied and the infant is wrapped in a sterile towel and warm cellular blanket and placed with head low in the prepared cot to rest and recover. *The wrist name-tapes* should now be put on.

Meanwhile the *third stage of labour* is in progress, now the placenta and membranes become separated from the uterine wall by the contractions of the uterus. This generally happens within 5 to 20 minutes of the birth of the baby. The midwife in attendance watches and may place her hand on the uterus. Syntometrine 1 ml (0·5 mg ergometrine and 5 units of oxytocin) is given as a routine measure, either with the crowning of the head or alternatively with the birth of the anterior shoulder, to accelerate the contractions of the uterus and minimize the amount of blood which will be lost during this process.

After delivery the placenta and membranes are most carefully examined as any products of conception which may have been retained in the uterus could cause severe postpartum haemorrhage (see below), or give rise to puerperal sepsis. The empty uterus should now be firmly contracted; the vaginal wall and perineum are inspected for any possible lacerations, any necessary sutures inserted, the vulva is swabbed, the mother is made comfortable and any wet linen removed from the bed. The blood loss is estimated or measured.

A cup of tea should be given as soon as possible because labour is a strenuous and exhausting physical experience.

The newly born baby may now be taken to his mother to hold, admire, kiss and fondle. She should be shown the attached name-tapes and the sex of the baby should be verified with her.

The fundal height and the consistence of the uterus should be noted and observations made of the extent to which the patient is losing from the vagina; this should not be excessive. The blood pressure, temperature, pulse and respiration rate should be taken. The mother should pass urine as the bladder ought to be emptied; a full bladder inhibits uterine drainage. She may be sponged down. Some nourishment is given provided her general condition is satisfactory. When settled comfortably she should be allowed to rest and sleep if she can.

Dangers and complications of labour. *Postpartum haemorrhage* usually occurs during or immediately after the third stage of labour, within six hours of delivery. The uterus fails to contract either before or after the expulsion of the placenta. The resultant haemorrhage is alarming and unless quickly controlled it may be fatal. This is one of the most dramatic and dangerous conditions in obstetrics. No time should be lost in summoning medical aid, including the emergency unit (see p. 724). In the meantime every effort should be directed to arresting the bleeding by encouraging contraction of the uterus. This is done by massage of the uterus through the abdominal wall, and by giving ergometrine 0·5 mg by injection.

Prolonged labour may be due to poor uterine action. Sometimes the pelvis is small or there may be a large malplaced baby, which in extreme cases causes obstructed labour.

An asphyxiated baby who does not breathe at birth may follow a difficult labour, either as the result of the use of forceps in a prolonged labour, or a breech presentation.

The main treatment is to clear the airway so that the baby can breathe and to give oxygen. If there is no response in a *severely asphyxiated baby* the trachea is intubated by means of an endotracheal catheter, any mucus is sucked out followed by intermittent positive pressure of oxygen, up to 35 cm of water, with the help of a manually operated rubber bag.

THE PUERPERIUM

The puerperium is the period of six weeks after the birth of a baby and during this period the uterus returns to its normal pre-pregnant state and lactation is well established. Sleep is essential to the mother and the amount of sleep she gets should be noted; her diet should be full, well balanced and nourishing; unless contra-indicated for any reason she may get up on the second day.

Supervision of lactation. Preparation for lactation is part of the pre-natal care. The mother washes her hands and her breasts and dries them before putting her baby to the breast. Her position during nursing should be comfortable, she may cuddle her baby to her, but should see that he has the clear airway he needs in order to be able to suck; he should have her full and undivided attention. The length of time a baby is at the breast is gradually increased and the needs of every nursing mother and baby need individual consideration.

Involution of the uterus. Measurement of the fundal height of the uterus should be made once a day, at the same time, and after the bladder has been emptied. On the first day the fundus is generally one inch (2·5 cm) below the umbilicus. Then there is a reduction of half an inch a day and the fundus should reach the level of the symphysis pubis by the end of a week.

The *lochia* is the debris discharged from the uterus; the amount and character should be noted; it should not be offensive.

The toilet of the vulva described on p. 748 should be carried out twice a day for the first two or three days and always after defaecation. The nurse performing this treatment should wear a mask; after the first day or two the patient will herself carry out the toilet of the vulva. If the perineum was torn and has been sutured the condition of healing should be noted and the stitches removed as necessary.

The placenta has covered about one-third of the uterine wall so that quite apart from any lacerations of the birth canal and perineum there is already a large wound surface to heal. This is vulnerable to micro-organisms which could be introduced either by one of the attendants or from some infection, such as a sore throat, in the mother.

Postnatal exercises directed to toning up the abdominal muscles and pelvic floor, and *breathing exercises* are aids to general recovery.

Prevention of emotional crises. A mother tends to have some emotional disturbance, and tolerance, understanding sympathy, moral support and wise guidance are essential. She has undergone extreme physical exertion and has experienced fear and anxiety and has probably suffered from loss of sleep. A great deal has depended on her. There is now time for her to think of her problems at home and she may wonder how her husband and family are getting on. At this time anything, however small and unprovoked, even unreasonable, can upset her. She needs reassurance, encouragement and help.

Complications of the puerperium. *Insomnia* and *emotional disturbances* have been mentioned. *Puerperal sepsis* is rare; it follows the course of any general surgical infection (see p. 416).

Puerperal pyrexia is defined as a rise of temperature to 38 °C (100·4 °F) even once, during the first 14 days. *Pyrexia* may also be due to some intercurrent infection; routine investigations include the taking of vaginal, cervical and throat swabs and the examination of a mid-stream specimen of urine.

Pyelonephritis which may have occurred during pregnancy may recur during the puerperium. Complete retention of urine is common and retention of residual urine with overflow and stress incontinence may occur.

Breast complications should generally be considered preventable.

Cracked nipples require rest from feeding the baby; the milk is then hand-expressed for his feeding.

An engorged breast from which no milk can be expressed may be treated by single doses of stilboestrol; or by alternate hot and cold bathings to dilate the milk ducts. The breasts should be supported by a good suitable brassière. *A full breast* can be relieved by expressing the milk from it.

A flushed breast indicates sepsis and is generally treated by giving an antibiotic in order to prevent *a breast abscess* which may follow.

Sub-involution of the uterus may be due to a distended bladder or overloaded bowel or to some uterine infection.

Venous thrombosis, if it should occur, may be slight or more severe; it may be due to infection or arise as the result of slowing of the blood in the veins because of immobility. For treatment of this condition, see p. 469. As far as a nurse is concerned every complaint of pain should be investigated. A slight cramp-like pain in the leg with a mild degree only of pyrexia, may be the prelude to the possible detachment of a clot from a thrombus in one of the veins, which might result in *pulmonary embolism*.

Puerperal psychosis may occur in patients who are very emotional or who may have a family history of mental disorder. The earliest sign of this complication is usually insomnia.

POSTNATAL CARE

In order to complete the care of the mother and her baby, a postnatal examination is held the day before her medical care ceases, normally on the ninth or tenth day after delivery.

The perineum and vaginal wall are inspected to see that they are healing well; *the lochia* should be normal. The patient's general condition is noted in order to ensure that she is fit to go home, and family planning is considered when necessary.

Six weeks after the birth of a baby all mothers should be examined in order to ensure that the uterus has returned to its pre-pregnant state. She will be questioned about her health and whether she is able to have adequate rest, her *blood-pressure is taken, haemoglobin checked, the urine is examined*, particularly if there has been any toxaemia during pregnancy, *the breasts are inspected* to see that they are normal, and inquiries are made concerning the progress of breast-feeding.

The abdominal muscles are examined by palpation and note is taken of the condition of the muscles of the pelvic floor in order to ascertain that normal strength and elasticity has been regained.

The perineum is inspected and the patient is asked to strain so that any possible tendency to prolapse of the anterior vaginal wall can be detected.

A careful pelvic examination is also carried out to note whether the uterus is normally anteverted and that the cervix appears healthy. Vaginal discharge, if present, should be only slight.

If the mother has brought her baby with her, any feeding problems, or other small worries should be discussed and alleviated; the infant welfare clinic is always ready to give any help required concerning the feeding and management of the infant.

Chapter 72

Care of a Newly Born Baby

by RUTH McKAY

Care of the baby—care of a premature baby

The newly born baby who has been lying on his side in a warm cot, snugly wrapped up with the head of the cot tilted slightly downwards in case there should be any regurgitation of fluid from the stomach which might be inhaled, is now taken up by the nurse. She wears a plastic apron and a cotton gown and has washed her hands. She takes the baby on her lap and seats herself comfortably on a low chair or stool. The room should be warm, as the heat-regulating mechanism of tiny babies is delicately balanced; they are easily chilled which must be avoided.

The baby is first carefully inspected to exclude any abnormalities:

The head, to note the size and shape, the width of the sutures and the size of the two fontanelles.

The eyes, as to whether they appear normal in size, position and appearance, and the presence of any discharge from them.

The mouth, particularly the palate to see that there is complete fusion; the tongue to see that it is freely movable.

The nose, in regard to its normal relation to the upper lip and that the nasal orifices appear clear.

The ears, that they appear normal.

The hands and *feet*, fingers and toes for any deformity.

The back is inspected for signs of deformity of the spine.

Congenital dislocation of the hip might be recognized by *broadening of the perineum*; *shortening of one leg* in unilateral cases. Barlow's test is now carried out as a routine measure at the birth of every infant in a maternity hospital. If there is any doubt of the normality of the hip joint, the baby is splinted forthwith. No child thus treated should ever have to be admitted to hospital later for reduction of congenital dislocation of the hip. Barlow's sign is an invaluable advance in preventive treatment (see p. 571). Most general practitioners and district midwives are also practising it.

As the temperature is taken in the rectum the nurse also inspects the condition of the *external genital organs*.

The first bath is given on the day of birth and the baby is weighed. He

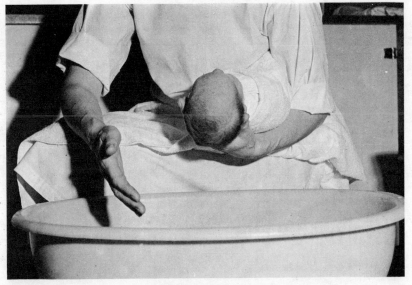

Fig. 72/1 Method of holding the baby when washing the head.

may then be bathed again on the third day, and thereafter on alternate days. This varies and some bath babies at longer intervals. The articles required for the bathing will have been placed ready; these include:

A baby bath of warm water, at 37·2 °C (99 °F).
A very mild soap.
No flannel is needed as the nurse uses her hands.
Moist cotton wool swabs (the cotton wool has been sterilized, but is no longer sterile).
Soft towels, one for the nurse's knee and one with which to dab the baby dry.
A little lubricant (petroleum jelly).

Wrapping the baby in one of the towels so that his arms are gently restrained, the nurse swabs his eyes using a moist wool swab for each eye from the inner to the outer canthus; she then washes the baby's face with moistened swabs, drying it gently. The ears, nostrils and mouth do not need attention except to remove any dried maternal blood. She then turns the baby so that his head lies over the bath of water (see Fig. 72/1), and placing her left hand on the back of the shoulders, supports the occiput and soaps the top and back of the head with her right hand, and rinses the soap off with the same hand, lifts the baby back on to her lap, and dries the head gently but thoroughly with a soft towel.

She then uncovers the baby's body, and using both hands soaps the body all over, back, front and sides, arms and legs, passing her hands well into all the crevices. She now places her left hand at the back of the shoulders supporting the occiput as before, and with her right hand under the buttocks lifts the baby over the bath and lowers him into the water (see Fig. 72/2). She puts the infant in the bath and continues to support his head and shoulders with her left hand in order to keep his head out of

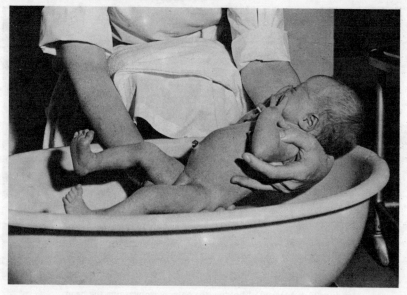

Fig. 72/2 Position of nurse's hands when lowering the baby into the bath.

the water (see Fig. 72/3). She swills water over his body to remove all soap, and lifts him back with the same movements that were used when putting him in the water, placing him on his face, on one of the bath towels. She folds the towel up over his back and dabs him dry, paying special attention to see that all creases and crevices are thoroughly dry. A little lubricant applied to the buttocks will prevent meconium sticking to the skin.

Meconium is a black tarry substance present in the intestine of a baby at birth. As a rule it is evacuated gradually; it is sterile and is considered protective against infection of the bowel. In premature babies it is evacuated more slowly.

Baby clothing. As a rule this consists of a woolly vest and gown and little bootees to prevent the baby being chilled.

Treatment of the cord. At first the stump should be looked at frequently as loosening of the clamp or ligature could result in bleeding. The cord is generally left free; it may be dried with a spirit solution, lightly sprinkled with special sterile powder and left exposed, or it may be covered with a dry sterile dressing. Alternatively it is sometimes cut quite short and sprayed with an aerosol plastic dressing. The cord will usually dry off and become detached in a few days.

THE PREMATURE BABY

Prematurity is often associated with poor environmental conditions and is therefore commonest in countries where the nutritional standards are low. In this country in about 50 per cent of cases the cause of prematurity is not known. In other instances it appears to be associated with some of the possible complications of pregnancy which organized prenatal care aims at preventing.

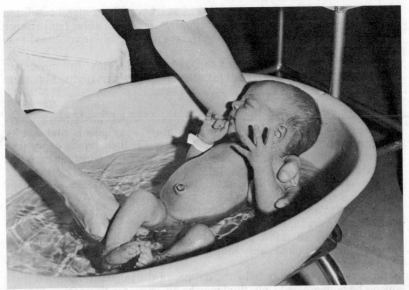

Fig. 72/3 Position of the nurse's left hand and forearm during bathing procedure.

A premature infant is defined by international standards as one weighing 2,500 g (5½ lb) or less, irrespective of the period of gestation. The baby looks like a wizened old man, the skin is wrinkled and red, the circulation is defective, there is little subcutaneous fat. He is drowsy, his cry is weak, breathing is irregular in both rhythm and depth, his movements tend to be uncontrolled.

A premature baby is seriously handicapped by his underdeveloped organs. Infections, disorders of the respiratory system, cerebral haemorrhage, jaundice and severe anaemia are amongst the conditions to be feared. Moreover, the respiratory control, the sucking and swallowing reflexes and the heat-regulating mechanism are poorly developed and the care this infant needs is based on this knowledge of his hazardous condition.

The care of a premature infant requires the skill of an experienced nurse and infinite patience. But it is most rewarding to see this tiny baby, weighing perhaps as little as about 1,135 to 1,365 g (2½ to 3 lb), grow under her care, and develop later into a lovely child.

The air passages must be kept clear, oxygen may have to be administered to relieve cyanosis and respiratory distress; it will be carefully ordered as it is not without danger; prolonged administration or too high a concentration of the gas is considered to be related to blindness in these babies.

Warmth is essential because of the sluggish circulation. The size and condition of the baby will be assessed and he will be nursed either in a warm incubator in high humidity, or in a warm cot in a heated humid or air-conditioned room.

The *temperature of a premature baby* is usually stabilized at 35 to

35·6 °C (95 to 96 °F), and as he gains in weight and his general condition grows more satisfactory this level gradually rises. Then as his temperature improves, the heat and humidity of the room in which he is nursed may reasonably be decreased.

Clothing. Preferably the infant should be naked so that full movement of his body and limbs is possible; otherwise only very light, but warm clothing may be provided.

Prevention of infection must be stressed as these delicate babies are very vulnerable. All those who handle him must wear gowns and masks, which have been sterilized, and they must wash their hands every time before attending to him. The baby should be under constant care and supervision. He should be handled as little as possible and very gently. His skin is tender, it is easily irritated; he is not bathed but may be swabbed over with sterilized olive oil.

The *vernix caseosa*, a greasy substance which covers the fetus *in utero*, is present in varying degrees at birth and is a protection to the skin of a premature baby, therefore it should not be disturbed. His body temperature should be checked every four hours.

In **feeding a premature baby** the danger of the inhalation of food must always be remembered since fluid may be diverted into the trachea because of the immaturity of the digestive system and of the cough reflex. A gastric or oesophageal feeding tube is generally employed, then when sucking becomes possible a feeding bottle, using either expressed breast milk, or half-skimmed evaporated milk may be given. The strength of the feeds is increased rapidly as improvement takes place.

Although a premature baby is not anaemic when born, the fall in the haemoglobin is dramatically rapid after birth and sometimes prolonged. Therefore the infant becomes anaemic and needs iron after the first few weeks of life. Vitamins A, D and C are also added to the feedings. In addition to the disadvantages mentioned on the previous page severe jaundice may arise because of the immaturity of the liver and should the serum-bilirubin exceed the level of 18 to 20 mg, replacement blood transfusion may be needed (see Chapter 48).

After-care. At the special postnatal clinic where premature babies are seen, both the physical health and the mental progress of the infant are carefully checked and every care is taken to help him develop into a normal child. By the age of two years he will usually have attained the progress normal at this age and unless told no one would know that he had been a premature baby. A number of well-known people were premature babies who with careful attention developed normally and became famous men and women. Every nurse and midwife should regard the care of a premature baby as a challenge to her initiative, observation and wisdom.

'The light-for-dates baby.' Although this type of baby is delivered just before or actually 'at term' he is an extremely scraggy, sickly looking infant with poor subcutaneous fat. He has suffered fetal growth retardation due either to disease of the mother or of the placenta. Because these babies have been starved during their intra-uterine lives they require immediate attention to make up for their loss of glycogen.

Section 7 (cont.)

B. Gynaecological Conditions, Their Treatment and Nursing Care

by P. A. M. WHITE

INTRODUCTION

Some of the conditions dealt with in this sub-section are brought about by hormonal imbalance and deficiency, others arise as the result of an obstetrical incident; only a few are congenital anomalies.

A number of patients will be wives and mothers who may have suffered considerable discomfort, even illness, before they could be persuaded to seek the advice and help needed. Apprehensive as a woman may be about her own condition, she is even more worried about the care of her family and home during her absence. Kindness, understanding and encouragement are essential to help these patients face whatever the future may hold.

It is assumed that nurses will revise their knowledge of the anatomy and physiology of the female genital tract before considering some of its abnormalities. It would also be helpful to read Chapter 69 in the section on obstetrical nursing.

Chapter 73

Inflammatory Conditions, Diseases and Disorders of the Female Generative Organs

by P. A. M. WHITE

Ascending infection—vulvitis—vaginitis—vaginal discharges—cervix uteri, cervicitis, cervical erosion, carcinoma, cervical smears—uterus, disorders, displacements, inflammatory conditions—ectopic gestation —ovaries, cysts and tumours

The first part of this section describes some gynaecological disorders and diseases arranged according to the organs affected. One of the most important points to remember is that *ascending infection* may affect any part of the tract as the Fallopian tubes open into the pelvic cavity. The organs affected therefore include the vulva, vagina, cervix, uterus, Fallopian tubes and ovaries. *A second part* is devoted to some of the more common gynaecological operations including the pre- and postoperative care.

VULVA AND VAGINA

Vulvitis is usually a simple inflammation due to an abrasion which may have been infected with staphylococci. In some instances streptococci may be the causative organism when the condition is more severe, the vulva becoming red, dry and swollen and possibly ulcerated. Treatment is by frequent baths and the application of antiseptic creams. The urine should be tested for sugar and ketones as vulvitis is sometimes a symptom of diabetes.

Menopausal vulvitis occurs during or after the menopause and is treated with hormones, either locally or orally.

Bartholin's cyst and *Bartholin's abscess.* A cyst is formed in the duct of Bartholin's gland situated beneath the posterior part of the *labium majus* due to blockage of the duct or to trauma (see p. 744).

Leukoplakia is a condition affecting the vulva, most commonly found in the post-menopausal patient. The patient complains of severe irritation, and on examination, white patches are seen on the labia minora and majora, sometimes spreading around the anal area. A biopsy is taken to confirm the diagnosis and to exclude carcinoma. A simple vulvectomy is performed.

Carcinoma of vulva is a malignant growth which presents as a swelling or as an ulcer giving rise to pain and a bloodstained discharge. *A biopsy is taken and if the result is positive a radical vulvectomy (see p. 745) undertaken.*

The vagina

Vaginal discharges. The vagina is always moist but its secretion should not be sufficient to stain or stiffen clothing.

Leucorrhoea is the term used to describe any excessive secretion; if at all profuse it may set up a mild *vaginitis*. Trichomoniasis and moniliasis are also mentioned below. Discharge due to gonorrhoea is mentioned in Chapter 32, p. 330.

Foreign bodies such as forgotten tampons may cause profuse discharge. *Cervical* cancers may cause discharge, but fortunately, through taking advantage of routine cervical smears (see p. 738), these conditions are being discovered early enough to treat and in most instances to cure.

Vaginitis is inflammation of the vaginal mucosa caused by various organisms.

Trichomoniasis is an infection due to the *Trichomonas vaginalis*, a flagellated organism, which gives rise to *an irritant and offensive yellowish discharge* with soreness around the vaginal introitus. It can be conveyed by sexual intercourse and consequently both the man and the woman should be treated at the same time by giving metronidazole (Flagyl) orally for seven days.

Moniliasis is an infection caused by a fungus, the *Candida albicans*; it often occurs during pregnancy and is also seen after prolonged treatment for infective conditions with broad-spectrum antibiotics. *The vaginal discharge* is white, profuse and thick; the symptoms produced are pruritus, soreness and oedema of the vulva. Treatment is by the insertion of *nystatin pessaries* twice daily for at least 10 days and external applications of nystatin cream. Alternatively the vagina may be painted with gentian violet, but this has the disadvantage of staining the skin and the patient's clothing.

Atrophic or senile vaginitis. Owing to the lowered oestrogen blood level, following the menopause, the vaginal epithelium becomes thin and easily excoriated. *There may be a yellowish or blood-stained discharge* with soreness and burning of the vulva. It is essential that these patients have a diagnostic curettage and cervical smear to exclude carcinoma of the uterus or cervix and, if relevant, a biopsy of cervix. Having excluded neoplasm this condition is treated with local or oral oestrogen therapy. It should be remembered that oestrogens given to post-menopausal patients may give rise to 'withdrawal bleeding'.

CERVIX UTERI

Cervicitis is an infection of the neck of the uterus which can be chronic or it may be caused by *cervical erosion*. It is characterized by a discharge, usually bloodstained, which is heavy before menstruation. *The treatment* consists either in cauterizing or coning the cervix. *A biopsy* should be taken to exclude neoplasm. The term *endocervicitis* is also used to indicate inflammation of the cervical canal.

Cervical erosion. The mucus-secreting cells of the cervical canal replace the normal covering of the cervix, giving it a red velvety appearance. It is seen in pregnant women sometimes associated with tears and lacerations of the cervix in childbirth. In the absence of symptoms treatment is not generally considered. It is commonly seen in patients who are taking oral contraceptives.

Carcinoma in situ. This diagnosis is made when the cervical epithelium shows features of carcinoma without invasion of the basement membrane. The treatment is usually a cone biopsy with a careful check on cervical smears performed approximately at six-monthly intervals.

Carcinoma of cervix. If a patient has a lesion suspicious of a carcinoma, a biopsy should be taken. In patients who have suspicious cells in cervical smears, cone biopsy of the cervix should always be performed. Carcinoma of the cervix should not be diagnosed by cervical cytology alone. Depending on the stage of the carcinoma, treatment is either by radiotherapy, surgery or a combination of the two. In early lesions, radium insertion followed by a Wertheim's hysterectomy (see p. 745) is often the treatment of choice.

Cervical smears. *Cytology* is the study of the origin, structure and function of the cells which has made it possible to detect pre-malignant conditions in certain tissues of the body. The taking of smears from the cervix is recommended for all women over 25 years.

By gently scraping the surface of the cervix with a wooden spatula, cells are obtained, which are then examined thus enabling a diagnosis to be made, so that the condition can be detected long before the patient develops symptoms.

UTERUS

The uterine disorders and diseases for which medical advice may be sought include:

Disorders of menstruation.
Displacement of the uterus.
Inflammatory conditions.
New growths.

Disorders of menstruation

These are frequently met with in abnormal conditions of the uterus. *Amenorrhoea*, or absence of menstruation, is normal before puberty and after the menopause; its absence during the menstruating period is *most usually due to pregnancy*, though absence may also occur as a result of general ill health, particularly associated with constitutional disease of the heart, lungs and kidneys; it also occurs as a result of emotional disturbance, disease of the endocrine organs, and is an inevitable result of hysterectomy and bilateral oophorectomy.

A rare condition described as *cryptomenorrhoea* is due to an abnormality of the hymen, when the latter is not perforated (*imperforate hymen*). In these cases menstruation occurs, but the discharge cannot escape and remains pent up in the vaginal cavity until the hymen is excised, *hymenectomy* (see p. 744).

Dysmenorrhoea is the term used to describe any difficult or painful menstruation. A number of types are described.

Spasmodic dysmenorrhoea is the type which occurs in young women two to three years after the onset of menstruation; the pain, which coincides with the onset of the period, is in the lower part of the abdomen and in the middle line, and lasts from five to six hours and in some cases for a whole day and may be very disabling. As the subject grows older it may improve —if not, it may have to be treated by dilatation of the cervix.

Congestive dysmenorrhoea occurs in older women, and is more common in those who have had children. The pain in these cases precedes menstruation for a day or two and is accompanied by severe backache.

Obstructive dysmenorrhoea is the type in which the pain is colicky. It is also described as 'clot' dysmenorrhoea, because it is thought to be due to the forcible contraction of the uterus on a clot in an endeavour to remove it—after a clot is passed the pain seems to be relieved.

Menorrhagia is excessive loss at the menstrual period, and *metrorrhagia* is irregular, acyclic bleeding.

Dysfunctional uterine bleeding is a term used to include all types of irregular and heavy bleeding for which there is no obvious cause. One exception, however, is the case of *metropathia haemorrhagica* which is diagnosed from the histological examination of curettings from the uterus. Treatment varies according to the age of the patient. Hormone therapy is given to young adults and a hysterectomy is often necessary for older women if a dilatation and curettage has not proved efficacious.

Displacements of the uterus

The commonest displacements of the uterus are retroversion and prolapse.

In *retroversion* the uterus is lying backwards instead of forwards. This is due to weakness of the ligaments which normally hold the uterus in the correct position of anteversion. This weakness is most commonly brought about by childbearing, but any laxity of muscle tone indicates laxity of ligaments and may also be accompanied by backache, excessive menstruation, leucorrhoea and dyspareunia, or the condition may be symptomless, being accidentally discovered during a routine examination.

Uterine prolapse. In this condition there is relaxation of the pelvic floor, frequently accompanied by cystocele or rectocele. Three degrees of prolapse are described:

> *First degree*, the cervix is below its normal level.
> *Second*, the cervix lies below the opening of the vagina.
> *Third*, it lies outside the vagina.
> *Procidentia* is a complete prolapse when the uterus drops outside the vulva, thus inverting the vaginal walls by dragging them down with it.

The prolapsed structures are liable to ulceration from pressure, irritation and urine contamination and become infected; prolapse may be complicated by cystocele or rectocele (see below).

Treatment. By the time a patient sees a gynaecologist, operative treatment is usually necessary, though treatment by posture, and/or the insertion of a ring pessary (see p. 740) may give relief for a time. In cases of first-degree utero-vaginal prolapse, the Fothergill operation (Manchester repair) is best performed. In cases of second- and third-degree utero-vaginal prolapse, vaginal hysterectomy and an associated repair gives the most satisfactory overall result.

Cystocele is due to herniation of the urinary bladder into the relaxed anterior vaginal wall. This condition is rectified by anterior colporrhaphy.

Rectocele is a prolapse of the posterior vaginal wall, a herniation of the rectum into the relaxed wall. In repair of this condition posterior colporrhaphy often combined with perineorrhaphy is performed.

Supportive pessaries, generally plastic ones, are sometimes used in the treatment of uterine displacement and prolapse but a repair operation is the better treatment and in most cases quite possible. *Hodge's pessary* may be inserted to correct retroversion of the uterus but if, after a few months, the correction is not maintained ventrosuspension is undertaken.

A ring pessary which can be polythene or rubber is inserted as a temporary measure for relief of vaginal prolapse in patients who wish to have further pregnancies. These rings should be changed every three months and the patient advised to douche at regular intervals.

It is inadvisable to use a ring pessary for patients of post-menopausal age owing to the danger of ulceration and the possibility of the development of carcinoma.

Inflammatory conditions of the uterus

Conditions of the uterus which are due to the ascending inflammation permeating the genital tract (see note on p. 736) include *endometritis*, an inflammation of the lining membrane of the uterus; the condition may be acute or chronic. It can occur following an abortion. The symptoms are menorrhagia, suprapubic pain, general malaise and slight pyrexia. The treatment is a course of antibiotics.

Endometriosis is a condition in which endometrial tissue may penetrate the ovaries and uterus and may be found in the pouch of Douglas. During menstruation this tissue bleeds causing cysts (chocolate cysts) to form; menorrhagia, dysmenorrhoea and pelvic adhesions may occur. The treatment varies according to the severity of the condition. Surgery, including ovarian cystectomy, oophorectomy and hysterectomy may be required if hormone therapy fails.

New growths of uterus

Uterine fibroids are benign tumours; the cause is unknown. The symptoms depend on where the tumours are situated:

> *Submucous fibroids* cause menorrhagia.
> *Intramural fibroids* cause menorrhagia and intermenstrual bleeding.
> *Subperitoneal fibroids* do not cause bleeding but may give rise to enlargement of the abdomen and pressure symptoms.

The treatment is myomectomy if the patient is under 40 years and desires to have a family, otherwise hysterectomy is performed.

Carcinoma of the body of the uterus often presents at or after the menopause, the commonest symptoms being irregular or post-menopausal bleeding. A dilatation and curettage is performed. If the neoplasm is limited to the cavity, the patient should have pre-operative radium prior to hysterectomy. This diminishes the chance of recurrence of the tumour in the vaginal vault.

FALLOPIAN TUBES AND OVARIES

Fallopian tubes

Acute salpingitis is inflammation of the Fallopian tubes due to an ascending infection. The symptoms are acute lower abdominal pain, pyrexia, general malaise and vaginal discharge. The patient is given complete bed rest, vaginal and cervical swabs are taken and the appropriate antibiotics given. It may often be difficult to differentiate between an attack of acute salpingitis and an acute-or-chronic salpingitis. The term 'pelvic inflammatory disease' is often used to cover these conditions.

Chronic salpingitis often follows an attack of acute salpingitis. The symptoms are not easily recognized but most patients complain of dull lower abdominal pain. The condition is treated with prolonged periods of bed rest and sometimes a course of short-wave diathermy is given.

Tuberculous salpingitis. Tuberculous lesions may occur in any part of the genital tract but most commonly in the Fallopian tubes. Some of the symptoms include debility, anaemia, irregular pyrexia and constant abdominal pain. This condition is treated by chemotherapy.

Pyosalpinx. The fimbrial and uterine ends of the Fallopian tubes become blocked and a purulent exudate collects in the tube. *Hydrosalpinx* may follow a long-standing pyosalpinx where the purulent exudate becomes thin and watery and is usually sterile to culture. Operative treatment consists in removal of the infected tube.

Ectopic gestation is an extra-uterine pregnancy which may occur in the Fallopian tube, *tubal pregnancy*, in the ovary and in the abdominal cavity and cervix. If undiagnosed when in the Fallopian tube the developing ovum will usually rupture the tube, causing severe internal bleeding often needing immediate emergency surgical measures. This is described as a *ruptured ectopic gestation.* Treatment is the removal of the affected tube. A *tubal abortion* occurs when the fetus is expelled from the fimbrial end of the tube into the peritoneal cavity.

Ovaries. Ovarian tumours may be cystic or solid, unilocular or multi-locular; they can become very large in size.

> A *simple cyst* contains clear fluid.
> A *pseudomucinous cyst* contains mucoid viscous fluid.
> A *papillomatous cyst* contains warty growths and serous fluid.
> A *chocolate cyst* is due to an effusion of blood into the ovary.
> A *dermoid cyst* has a thick wall and is filled with a yellow fatty-like substance and can contain hair, teeth, skin, cartilage and even bone.

Ovarian cysts are often symptomless; however, their presence is revealed either when they have grown to a very large size or some other complication has developed. A cyst may undergo torsion of the pedicle giving rise to acute abdominal pain, nausea and vomiting often necessitating immediate surgery, when either ovarian cystectomy or oophorectomy is performed.

Malignant tumours of the ovary may be cystic or solid, primary or secondary. *Sarcoma* is one of the primary type and one of the few malignant tumours of the ovary which are common in young people.

Carcinoma. The majority of these tumours arise from papillary cystadenomas and are usually cystic, but when growth is rapid they become solid. The Krukenberg tumour is a solid ovarian tumour which is always secondary to malignancy in the gastro-intestinal tract.

The onset and progress of ovarian tumours are often symptomless, therefore by the time they are diagnosed they are frequently found to be incurable; at a later stage ascites may develop.

Treatment. If the patient is operable a total hysterectomy and bilateral salpingo-oophorectomy is performed, sometimes followed by a course of cytotoxic drugs or by radiotherapy.

Chapter 74

Some Common Gynaecological Operations, Pre- and Postoperative Care

by P. A. M. WHITE

Examination—minor and major vaginal and abdominal operations—pre- and postoperative care—nursing measures used in gynaecology—abortion—the use of endocrine products

In this specialized field the most common symptoms which cause a woman to consult her doctor include bleeding from the vagina, heavy or scanty periods, low abdominal pain, backache, vaginal discharge, prolapse and stress incontinence of urine.

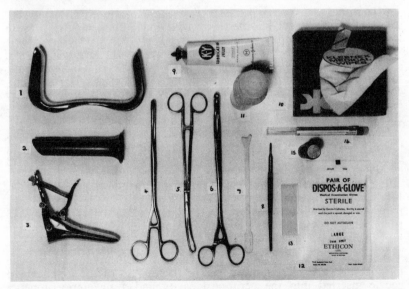

Fig. 74/1 Articles for a gynaecological examination. 1. Sims's vaginal speculum. 2. Fergusson's speculum. 3. Cusco's speculum. 4–6. Volsellum forceps. 7. Ayre's cervical spatula. 8. Diamard pen. 9. Lubrication jelly. 10. Medical wipes. 11. Cytology jar. 12. Disposable gloves. 13. Glass slide. 14. Specimen tube. 15. Specimen jar. In addition supply a covered bowl for the reception of soiled instruments and a disposal bag for used tissues and the disposable gloves.

Examination of the patient. A nurse assists a doctor during a gynaecological examination. The articles he may need are shown in Fig. 74/1. The nature of the examination is explained to the patient, as this is one a patient dislikes; the presence of a calm efficient nurse can allay much apprehension. The bed curtains are drawn or the bed screened; the patient is asked to pass urine; the nightdress is removed and a light warm covering placed over the chest; the bedclothing is folded back, leaving a sheet to cover the thighs. The doctor palpates the abdomen and the genito-vaginal examination is then carried out.

The patient is asked to lie in the left lateral, dorsal recumbent or Sims's semiprone position. Using gloves the labia are separated and one or two fingers, previously lubricated, are inserted into the vagina. The cervix can then be felt.

In a *bi-manual examination* one hand is placed on the abdomen while a vaginal examination is carried out. In this way the uterus is palpated between the two hands, thus enabling the size and position to be determined. The cervix is seen by passing a vaginal speculum; a rectal examination is also often performed. In the case of *virgo intacta* a rectal examination only is carried out.

It is usual for every patient to have a cervical smear taken for cytology (see p. 738) unless carried out within the past year. *Vaginal swabs* may be taken for bacteriological examination when there is a vaginal discharge or infection is suspected.

MINOR AND MAJOR OPERATIONS

Minor operations. *Examination under anaesthesia* to estimate the size, shape and mobility of the uterus, ovaries and Fallopian tubes, and to investigate any abnormal swellings.

Dilatation of the cervix for the treatment of dysmenorrhoea. *Uterine dilatation and curettage*, either for diagnostic purposes or as a therapeutic measure. *Coning biopsy of cervix* to examine the extent of the squamocolumnar junction. *Cauterization of cervix* by electro- or chemical cautery in the treatment of cervical erosion. *Amputation of the cervix* (see Manchester repair). *Trachelorraphy*, repair of a lacerated cervix.

Hymenectomy, excision of the hymen when rigid or intact (digital dilatation is often more satisfactory). *Perineotomy* is a plastic enlargement of the vaginal introitus. *Excision of a urethral caruncle* is usually performed by diathermy.

Bartholin's cyst is due to blockage of the duct of Bartholin's gland. The best treatment is marsupialization. An incision is made into the cyst allowing the fluid contents to escape. Fine catgut stitches are inserted round the edge of the incision which unite the wall of the cyst to the skin thus forming a pouch.

Laparoscopy. The laparoscope is used for both operative and diagnostic purposes. A small incision is made at the margin of the umbilicus, a needle inserted into the peritoneal cavity and a pneumoperitoneum induced with carbon dioxide. The laparoscope can then be passed through the abdominal wall and the contents of the abdomen inspected. This procedure is particularly useful when investigating infertility, as the Fallopian tubes and ovaries may be examined, and the latter biopsied, and in establishing diagnoses, such as ectopic pregnancy, when these are in doubt.

This may save the patient a laparotomy and a much longer stay in hospital.

Laparoscopic sterilization. Both Fallopian tubes are diathermized through the laparoscope. The patient is admitted 24 hours prior to the operation and is usually discharged home 48 hours afterwards.

Major vaginal operations. *Anterior colporrhaphy*, repair of a cystocele. *Posterior colporrhaphy*, repair of a rectocele and enterocele.

Perineorrhaphy, repair of the perineum.

Colpoperineorrhaphy, repair of a rectocele and of the perineum.

Manchester or *Fothergill's* repair consists of an anterior colporrhaphy with amputation of the cervix in order to tighten the cardinal ligaments.

Vaginal hysterectomy is removal of the uterus by the vaginal route. This is sometimes performed as a routine operation in preference to an abdominal hysterectomy (see below), when in cases of utero-vaginal prolapse it is combined with an anterior and posterior colpoperineorrhaphy.

Simple vulvectomy or excision of the vulva, excluding the vestibule, is performed in leukoplakia (see p. 736). *Radical vulvectomy* is an extensive excision of the vulva including a block dissection of the lymphatic glands of both groins generally performed in carcinoma of the vulva.

Major abdominal operations. *Hysterectomy* may be performed as follows.

Sub-total hysterectomy when the body of the uterus is removed leaving the cervix *in situ* (this is rarely done at the present time).

Total hysterectomy, the uterus including the cervix is removed.

Total hysterectomy and *bilateral salpingo-oophorectomy*, the uterus, Fallopian tubes and ovaries are removed.

Wertheim's hysterectomy consists of removing the uterus, Fallopian tubes, ovaries and the major part of the vagina and the lymphatic glands in the pelvis.

The term *pan-hysterectomy* is best avoided as it is given various meanings by different authorities.

Myomectomy is enucleation of fibroid tumours from the uterine wall thus avoiding hysterectomy, so that the uterus retains its normal function.

Ventro-suspension. In this operation the round ligaments are shortened by various means, so that the uterus which is retroverted is drawn forwards and becomes anteverted.

Sterilization implies the cutting and tying of the Fallopian tubes.

Ovarian cystectomy is the enucleation of a cyst from an ovary, and *oophorectomy* the removal of an ovary. *Salpingectomy* is removal of a Fallopian tube, and *salpingostomy* an opening made into one of the Fallopian tubes as in cases of infertility due to a blockage in the tubes. An opening is made at the fimbrial end of the tube to restore patency, or alternatively a reimplantation of the tube or tubes is sometimes carried out when the blockage occurs at the uterine end. *Salpingo-oophorectomy* is a combination of salpingectomy and oophorectomy when both Fallopian tubes and ovaries are affected.

Marshall-Marchetti operation is performed to relieve stress incontinence when a vaginal operation has proved unsuccessful. The neck of the bladder is elevated and stitched to the back of the pubis.

PREPARATION AND POSTOPERATIVE CARE

It is advisable that all patients should be admitted one or two days before operation except in the case of very minor procedures.

The doctor explains the nature of the operation to his patient, obtains a written consent and witnesses her signature. Everyone of 16 years and over may legally sign their own consent form. It is not necessary to obtain the husband's written consent for his wife's hysterectomy, but when sterilization is being considered a special form has to be signed both by the husband and wife and by an independent witness.

The patient is weighed, a routine urine test carried out; a mid-stream specimen may be needed for bacteriological examination. If the bowels have not acted a suppository or laxative will be given. An X-ray of chest is taken, if this has not recently been done. The haemoglobin is estimated and, in the case of a major operation, the blood group and rhesus factor also are determined. The patient's blood should be cross matched if she is anaemic or bleeding as in a ruptured ectopic gestation and whenever heavy blood loss is anticipated during operation. Prior to Wertheim's hysterectomy an intravenous pyelogram is carried out.

A physiotherapist instructs the patient in breathing exercises to avoid possible postoperative chest complications. In the case of vaginal operations some gynaecologists like the patient to have a preoperative douche. A sedative is often necessary the night before operation to ensure a good night's sleep.

Shaving a gynaecological patient. The ordinary articles required for shaving are prepared. The vulva and perineum cannot be properly shaved unless a good light is provided.

The order of procedure is rather important. When a 'through' shave is carried out, the hairs on the abdominal wall should first be removed, then those on the mons veneris and vulva; and after this the patient should be turned on her side and the perineum, buttocks and lower part of the back should be shaved. The patient may generally have a bath immediately after shaving to remove all the short-cut hair.

It is not always necessary to do such an extensive shaving; in some cases a 'pubic shave' or a 'vulval shave' would be adequate.

The day of operation. No food or drink is allowed for four to six hours, a bath is taken, hair clips and any artificial hair pieces removed, long hair should be plaited (in some hospitals paper caps are provided to cover the hair). Coloured nail varnish should be removed, dentures are placed in a special container, clothing is removed and replaced by an operation gown; the patient is asked to pass urine. Her name and hospital registration number are attached to her wrist. If the wedding ring is left on it must be covered with adhesive plaster as a protection against the possibility of a burn should diathermy be used. If removed, this ring with any other jewellery is listed and put into safe-keeping.

The *pre-medication* ordered by the anaesthetist is given by intramuscular injection one to one and a half hours before operation.

Postoperative care. On return from the theatre most patients will have an airway *in situ* (unless they are taken to a recovery ward), which is removed when the swallowing reflex returns and the patient regains consciousness. The *pulse rate* is recorded every 15 minutes and the character of the respirations noted until the patient's condition is satisfactory. After major operations the *blood pressure* is recorded every four hours for approximately 12 hours. If the patient is suffering from shock the foot of the bed is elevated and the blood pressure recorded every 15 minutes. Intravenous infusion may be ordered. Any abnormal bleeding or unusual signs should be reported to the ward sister. Sedatives or anti-emetics are prescribed as necessary, four- to six-hourly for the first 24 to 48 hours.

After *vaginal operations* it is essential to inspect the vaginal loss regularly for the first few hours. When a vaginal pack and self-retaining catheter have been inserted continuous bladder drainage will immediately be established. Fluids may be taken when the patient's condition warrants it; *the fluid intake and output is carefully measured and recorded.*

On the following day the patient is bed bathed and should sit up to facilitate vaginal drainage; she is given an air or Sorbo ring when necessary. The physiotherapist visits her daily to give postoperative exercises. *The vaginal pack is removed after 24 hours*; the patient has a vulval wash-down or swabbing (see below) two to three times a day until she is able to go to the bath. When fit enough a daily bath is taken.

The indwelling catheter is removed, usually after five days and the patient is encouraged to pass urine; she may be taken to the lavatory. If the patient is unable to pass urine, she is recatheterized. Even if micturition is established, the patient should be catheterized once daily after micturition until the residual volume is within normal limits. The haemoglobin estimation is checked to verify that the patient is not anaemic.

Absorbable sutures are widely used, but if any non-absorbable ones have been inserted they are removed after 10 days. When the patient is fit, usually after two weeks, she is discharged from hospital to her home or a convalescent home. The doctor will carry out a vaginal examination before discharge to make sure that no vaginal adhesions or packs are present.

After abdominal operations. When a drainage tube has been inserted into the abdominal wound the amount of blood loss from it should be noted and if necessary the wound repacked. The drain is normally removed after 24 hours. Analgesics may be required for the first few days. These patients tend to suffer from flatulence, which can be very painful; it can often be relieved by passing a flatus tube.

Movement is encouraged and the patient is allowed out of bed on the first or second day, this is helpful if she has difficulty in passing urine. *Normal diet* and fluids are given as soon as possible; the fluid intake and output being measured for a few days. A laxative or suppository may be given on the third day after operation. *Clips* are removed on the fourth or fifth day and *sutures* from the seventh to the tenth day. The patient has a daily bath from the fifth day onwards.

As with any major operation *the haemoglobin estimation* is checked on the fourth day and if the patient is anaemic a course of iron may be prescribed.

Possible complications. *Primary haemorrhage* may occur soon after the patient returns to the ward. Any excessive vaginal bleeding may necessitate the insertion of a vaginal pack. If the bleeding is internal the patient will probably have to be taken back to the theatre for laparotomy. *Secondary haemorrhage* could occur about the ninth or tenth day after operation. Retention of *urine* and *cystitis* occur occasionally after a hysterectomy but more commonly after a vaginal repair. *Excessive* and *persistent vomiting* may be a symptom of paralytic ileus (see p. 480).

Discharge from hospital. Patients are discharged approximately 12 to 14 days after operation and if the doctor advises convalescence this is arranged by the social welfare worker. After minor operations the patients may be discharged in one or two days.

On discharge from hospital each patient should be informed of the nature of her operation and given advice as to her mode of living and when she may resume her normal duties. She should also be told when sexual intercourse may be resumed as patients are usually reluctant to ask about this.

SOME NURSING MEASURES USED IN GYNAECOLOGY

Toilet of the vulva includes either a vulval wash-down or a vulval swabbing. The sterile articles contained in *a vaginal examination pack* include

> 10 swabs.
> 1 sanitary towel.
> 1 paper towel.
> 1 gallipot.
> 1 jug in pack.

One pint of normal saline (at body temperature), a pair of pack scissors, a disposable bag and a bed pan with cover will be required.

The pack is opened at the bedside and the paper wrap spread out to form a clean working field. The patient supported with pillows and having a light warm covering, is placed on the bed pan. The soiled sanitary towel is removed, the nurse washes her hands and swabs the vulval area using the same technique as before catheterization (see below).

Holding the labia apart warm saline is gently poured over the vulval area which is dried with swabs, the bed pan is removed and the patient turned on to her side to complete drying the perineum. The paper towel may be used to dry the buttocks. A clean sanitary towel is placed in position.

When *a vulval swabbing only is required* the jug of lotion and the bed pan will not be needed, otherwise the procedure is the same. The perineal and anal areas are carefully swabbed before being dried.

Female catheterization (for male catheterization see p. 253)

Catheterization carried out by means of a urethral catheter taps the urinary bladder.

The *articles* required generally placed on a bedside trolley are:

Top shelf	*Bottom shelf*
Sterile pack containing:	Normal saline, warm.
A large receiver.	Lubricant, e.g. KY jelly.
Gallipot, swabs.	Measure jug.
1 dissecting forceps.	2 prepacked sterile disposable
1 paper towel.	(Nelaton) catheters.
1 piece of gauze.	Disposable bag.
	Jar of antiseptic in customary use.

Other articles which may be required include:

> Specimen bottle, pathological forms and label.
> Syringe, needle and distilled water if a Foley catheter is used.
> Strapping and strapping scissors.
> Spigot in pack.

Disposable drainage bag, tubing in pack and carrier if continuous drainage is required.

Pack scissors.

Procedure. The patient lies on her back semi-recumbent with thighs flexed and abducted. This position is comfortable and steady if the feet are placed flat on the bed. A good light must be provided and the patient should be covered by something warm and light. The nurse now washes her hands.

At the bedside the pack is opened and serves as a sterile field. Using the dissecting forceps, wool swabs, gallipot, the piece of gauze with a small amount of lubricant on it and the paper towel are placed on this sterile field.

The towel is placed between the patient's thighs; an assistant opens the catheter pack; the nurse withdraws a catheter, lubricates it and puts it with the forceps into the large receiver now placed on the towel between the patient's thighs.

The vulval toilet is performed, first swabbing each *labium majus* after separating them with the fingers of the free hand. *The labia minora* are similarly treated and held apart by the first and second fingers during the entire procedure; the vestibule and urethral orifice are swabbed noting its size and character.

All swabbing must be done from front to the back; each swab being used once only and discarded into the disposal bag; about 12 swabs will be needed. Taking the lubricated catheter with the forceps two inches from its head it is gently introduced into the urethral orifice, urine begins to flow into the receiver, the catheter should be held steady; when the flow ceases, withdrawing the catheter slightly may tap urine at a lower level; when the bladder is empty the catheter is withdrawn and if disposable placed into the disposal bag. The receiver of urine is put on the bottom shelf of the trolley.

After *catheterization* the patient is swabbed dry; she turns on her side (back towards nurse) and the perineum is dried with swabs, and the fold between the buttocks with the paper towel which is then placed in the disposal bag. She is made comfortable in bed and given a drink if she wishes.

Report and record should include the time of catheterization, the amount of urine obtained, its appearance and character. Any problems met, rigidity or pain noted. A specimen of the urine is either put up for routine examination by the nurse or alternatively one is sent to the laboratory.

Vaginal douching

Irrigation of the vaginal canal is described as douching. It may be carried out by means of funnel and catheter or by douching as described below. It is performed:

> To cleanse the vagina when a woman is wearing a pessary and as treatment in some cases of discharge and before certain operations on the lower part of the genital tract.
>
> In the treatment of inflammatory conditions of the vagina, cervix, ovaries and tubes.
>
> In the emergency treatment of severe uterine bleeding.

The solution used varies—many mild antiseptics may be employed, but on average normal saline or a solution of sodium bicarbonate is preferred.

For cleansing purposes the lotion should be warm, in the treatment of inflammatory conditions it should be hot, 40 °C (104 °F) and for the treatment of bleeding when given by a surgeon it is used very hot, up to 43·3 °C (110 °F).

The condition of the external genitalia should be inspected carefully before a hot douche is given; it may be necessary to smear the parts with a lubricant in order to protect them from injury by a hot solution.

The articles required include a douche can, a length of tubing, clip and douche nozzle, lotion thermometer and a litre of selected solution, lotion and swabs for cleansing, paper bag for discarded swabs, disposable waterproof material and towels to protect the bed, warmed douche pan and cover, receiver for used douche nozzle unless disposable.

Procedure. As a rule the patient lies on her back with the legs drawn up and knees separated (but a douche can equally well be given with the woman lying on her side).

The bedclothes are divided and separated so that the patient and her legs are covered and only the vulval region is exposed. This region is covered by a disposable towel. The patient is placed on the douche pan.

The nurse washes her arms and hands, removes the towel over the vulva with forceps to avoid soiling her hands, discards these forceps which may be contaminated. She then separates the labia and cleanses the vulva with swabs and lotion, inspects the glass nozzle to see that it is intact, allows some lotion to flow through from the irrigation can and inserts the nozzle into the vaginal canal in an upward and backward direction. She should move the nozzle about in order to irrigate the walls and vault of the vagina.

Precautions. The temperature of the lotion should be carefully tested, all movements must be gentle; the douche can should only be raised 10 to 12 inches (25 to 30 cm) above the bed to ensure a gentle even flow, otherwise fluid may be jerked against the cervix which is undesirable. Using the tubing clip with discretion the flow into the vagina is regulated, and as the douche nozzle is moved about all parts of the vagina are irrigated.

When the treatment is over, the glass nozzle is removed and inspected carefully to see that it has not been broken during the treatment. If the patient can sit up, she may do so for a few minutes as the erect position facilitates drainage. The contents of the douche pan should be inspected and any abnormalities noted and reported.

Insertion of medical pessaries

Soluble pessaries are often used in treatment of the vagina and sometimes also before operation. Antibiotic preparations may be included and stilboestrol after menopausal age when the normally protective action of lactic acid is lessened. Alternatively lactic acid pessaries may be ordered.

When pessaries are prescribed for self-administration *the patient should be advised to introduce them as high as possible, usually when she goes to bed at night, so that the entire vagina will be in contact with the drug.*

If the nurse inserts the pessary she must check it with the prescription. She will need:

A disposable glove or caped finger stall.
Swabs for cleansing and a paper bag for their disposal.
The pessary and, usually, a sanitary pad.

With the patient preferably lying on her back, knees drawn up and feet flat on the bed, the pessary is introduced over the perineum and pushed well up into the vagina.

Packing the vagina

1. A vaginal pack may be ordered before operation to reduce oedema when the vagina may be packed daily for a week with glycerin gauze (when a complete procidentia, p. 739, is contemplated).
2. A vaginal pack may be inserted by the doctor in order to check severe bleeding either reactionary or secondary after operation.
3. A pack may be inserted in the theatre after operation, which is generally removed 48 hours later. This should be witnessed by a second person and the date and time of removal recorded.

When in an emergency a vaginal pack is inserted in the ward by a doctor the nurse will prepare the following articles:

Preparation for catheterization, see p. 748.
Preparation for packing the vagina.

A trolley is brought to the bedside containing:

On the top shelf a sterile pack from the Central Sterile Supplies Department, containing
A large receiver, large gallipot and swabs.
2 rolls of sterile gauze 2 inches wide.
1 pair disposable gloves.
1 paper towel.
1 pair of dissecting forceps.

On the bottom shelf
Sims's speculum, sponge-holding forceps, which may be sterilized or alternatively pre-packed and sterile.
Disposal bag.
Jar of antiseptic, in customary use.
Normal saline.

Position of patient. She may be lying either in the left lateral or the dorsal, recumbent position. The doctor will insert the speculum, remove any clots with the sponge-holding forceps and then pack the vagina with as much gauze as necessary.

As the patient will find it difficult or impossible to pass urine while the vagina is packed, a Foley's self-retaining catheter is inserted to drain the bladder.

Vaginal packing is almost always an emergency procedure and the patient will be taken to the operating theatre later to have the bleeding point ligatured and the vagina temporarily repacked.

Vaginal painting

Painting the vagina is generally performed by a doctor; it may be ordered pre-operatively and sometimes in the treatment of vaginal infections.

The articles required include:

A good light such as an Anglepoise lamp.
A vaginal speculum usually Sims's or Cusco's and a lubricant.
Sponge-holding forceps and suitable wool (gauze covered) swabs.

A gallipot containing the paint ordered.
Disposable mackintosh and towel to protect the bed.
Disposal paper bag.
A vaginal pad.

With the patient in the left lateral or Sims's position (see Figs. 8/1 and 8/2, p. 79–80) a swab is dipped in the paint, passed over the speculum (now in place) and the whole vagina painted thoroughly. The posterior wall of the vagina is painted on withdrawing the speculum.

ABORTION

Although abortion is more properly an obstetrical complication it is thought useful to include the various types here, and some of the abnormalities which may give rise to this emergency.

An abortion or miscarriage is the premature termination of pregnancy before the twenty-eighth week of gestation, that is, before the fetus is viable. The causes may be:

Maternal. Pre-existing conditions such as chronic nephritis, diabetes, hypertension, malnutrition and chronic heart disease.

Maternal coincidental conditions—include acute febrile illness during the early months of pregnancy, severe shock, strong purgatives, or an accident such as a fall, acute toxaemia, pernicious vomiting, or acute yellow atrophy of the liver.

Fetal—abnormal formation of the fetus, low implantation of the ovum which would lead to a placenta praevia, or a hydatidiform mole.

Parental—syphilis.

Types of abortion. In *threatened abortion* the first sign is irregular vaginal bleeding, usually slight to moderate. The treatment consists of bed rest; sedatives are often prescribed to allay the patient's fears. There is no specific treatment. The patient will be mobilized after all bleeding has ceased, and is discharged to her home having been advised to take life easy for a few weeks.

Inevitable abortion. An abortion is said to be inevitable when there is vaginal bleeding, uterine contractions, and on examination the cervix is found to be dilated. Conservative treatment is not given. The patient is put to bed and given analgesics. The end result is either a complete or incomplete abortion.

Complete abortion. The fetus and placenta are expelled spontaneously from the uterus. If vaginal bleeding persists, ergometrine may be given. The placenta must be carefully examined to see that it is complete.

Incomplete abortion. Part of the products of conception are retained, preventing the uterus from contracting and therefore causing continuous bleeding which may be severe. The patient should be admitted to hospital where her general condition is assessed and a blood transfusion given if indicated. A dilatation and curettage will be performed when her condition is satisfactory. Ergometrine may be given to control haemorrhage.

Septic abortion. The cause is almost always due to criminal interference. The patient is admitted to hospital with pyrexia, abdominal pain and vaginal discharge or bleeding. The infection spreads very rapidly. Salpingitis and pelvic peritonitis may occur and septicaemia may result. This type of abortion goes through the stages of threatened, inevitable and complete or incomplete, and the haemorrhage may cause death, which can also result from infection. To prevent infection, vaginal and cervical swabs are cultured, and the patient treated with broad spectrum antibiotics.

When the infection has been controlled, and the blood loss replaced, a curettage may be performed. The patient then improves rapidly. A complication that may arise is anuria; this may be due to hypotension owing to excessive blood loss and toxaemia. *The patient's fluid intake and output should be accurately recorded*, so that oliguria is at once noted as early treatment ensures a good prognosis.

Missed abortion. The fetus dies in the uterus, but is not expelled immediately; this is called a *carneous or fleshy mole.* There may be a slight vaginal loss or bloodstained discharge. The signs of pregnancy disappear, and after four weeks it is possible to establish that the uterus has not enlarged to its expected size. Pregnancy tests will prove to be negative. It is better to wait, and allow the uterus to expel its contents spontaneously. If after several weeks this has not occurred, a dilatation and curettage may be necessary. A blood transfusion is occasionally required.

Habitual abortion. If a patient has several consecutive abortions, she will need investigation. A hysterosalpingogram may be carried out (see p. 695) and a vaginal smear taken for cytology. If the cervix is found to be incompetent, a Shirodkar suture may be inserted at the third month of pregnancy and left *in situ* until full term. The patient will be advised as regards the need of rest.

Hydatidiform mole is an abnormal development of the placenta, giving rise to a mucoid and cystic degeneration of the stroma of the chorionic villi, thus giving the characteristic appearance of a bunch of grapes. The increased size of the placenta gives rise to a uterus which is larger than the period of amenorrhoea would suggest. Vesicles may be passed *per vaginam*, and it is necessary to empty the uterus completely. It is sometimes possible to remove the contents with sponge forceps and a curette, but occasionally a hysterectomy may be necessary. If the evacuation is not complete haemorrhage may occur. This condition may also give rise to malignant disease.

The patient is followed up for approximately two years. A pregnancy test is carried out at regular intervals, and providing the patient is not pregnant, a positive test suggests trophoblastic activity, and a dilatation and curettage is indicated to exclude chorion-epithelioma.

THE USE OF ENDOCRINE PRODUCTS

The therapeutic use of endocrines occupies a wide field in the treatment of abnormalities, hormone imbalance and deficiency in women.

Some of the gynaecological conditions treated include vulvitis, pruritus vulvae, atrophic vaginitis, amenorrhoea, primary and secondary, cyclical control of menstrual disorders and irregularities, dysfunctional uterine bleeding, habitual abortion and symptoms of sex-hormone deficiency following the climacteric, and endometriosis.

Recognition of toxic effect. It is essential that nurses make themselves conversant with any side-effects likely to occur (see Appendix ii), so that their appearance may be discovered without delay, when an alternative preparation will usually be prescribed.

Appendix i

Metric Measurements and Milliequivalents

METRIC MEASUREMENTS

Unit of weight = 1 gram

The abbreviation for gram is internationally recognized as being 'g'.

1,000 micrograms (μg) = 1 milligram (mg)
1,000 milligrams = 1 gram (g)
1,000 grams = 1 kilogram (kg)

Note: When drugs are prescribed in micrograms, it is recommended that no abbreviation should be used and that the word should be written in full. In writing prescriptions, quantities of solids less than one gram should be given in milligrams, e.g. 500 mg NOT 0·5 g.

Unit of volume = 1 millilitre   *Unit of length* = 1 metre
1,000 millilitres (ml) = 1 litre (l)   100 centimetres (cm) = 1 metre

APPROXIMATE METRIC AND IMPERIAL EQUIVALENTS

1 milligram (mg) = $\frac{1}{60}$ grain (gr.)
60 milligrams = 1 grain
1 gram (g) = 15 grains
30 grams = 1 ounce (oz.)
1 kilogram (kg) = $2\frac{1}{4}$ pounds (lb.)
6·5 kilograms = 1 stone

1 millilitre (ml) = 15 minims (m.)
30 millilitres = 1 fluid ounce (fl. oz.)
600 millilitres = 1 pint (pt.)
1 litre (l) = 35 fluid ounces

1 millimetre (mm) = 0·0394 inch ($\frac{1}{25}$, nearly)
1 centimetre (cm) = 0·394 inch ($\frac{2}{5}$, nearly)
1 metre (100 cm) = 39·37 inches (1 yard $3\frac{1}{4}$ inches, nearly)

1 inch = 25·4 mm   1 foot = 30·5 cm
1 yard = 91·5 cm

(These measures will be useful for the widths and lengths of bandages etc. when this scale comes in.)

MILLIEQUIVALENTS

The concentrations of electrolytes (such as sodium, potassium, and chloride) in the plasma or urine, and in fluids used for intravenous infusions, are routinely expressed as milliequivalents per litre (mEq/1). This system is based on the fact that when chemical reactions take place between two substances, the substances react by one or a few particles (molecules, atoms or ions) combining with one or a few particles of the other. The lightest particle which undergoes chemical reactions is the hydrogen atom. The weight in grams of any substance which reacts with 1 g of hydrogen is called the *equivalent weight* or *gram-equivalent* of the substance. A *milli-equivalent* is one-thousandth part of an equivalent. This system of expressing concentrations is simpler than the usual method which states the actual weight of the material in solution. For example, sodium chloride (saline) solution can be produced by the chemical reaction between an alkali, sodium bicarbonate, and an acid, hydrochloric acid. The *normal* or *physiological* saline frequently used in intravenous therapy contains about 4 g of sodium, 5 g of chloride, and 9 g of sodium chloride in 1 l. These differing figures quite obscure the fact that the sodium and the chloride are present in *chemically* equivalent concentration, so that the resulting solution is neither acidic nor alkaline, but neutral. This fact is much more easily understood when the saline is described as containing sodium chloride, sodium and chloride, all in a concentration of 154 mEq/1.

Appendix ii

Some Side-Effects of Endocrinological Preparations

Androgens (testicular hormones)

> Testosterone propionate.
> Methyltestosterone.
> Anabolic steroids.

Excessive dosage or prolonged administration can cause oedema through sodium and water retention, and in early puberty linear growth can be halted through closure of the epiphyses in the male. In the female, they can cause masculinization, clitoral enlargement and decrease in breast size and diminished lactation in the puerperium. Hair growth on face and chest may also be produced.

Corticosteroids

> Hydrocortisone.
> Cortisone.
> Synthetic corticosteroids, fluorinated or not.

Retention of sodium and water with loss of potassium, with inhibition of corticotrophin secretion may occur. Sudden withdrawal of corticosteroids can precipitate adrenal insufficiency, muscle weakness, hypotension, hypoglycaemia, headache, nausea and vomiting. In diabetics, the insulin requirements may be increased by corticosteroids and they may also cause rounding of the face (so-called 'moon-face').

These symptoms may result from oral or injection treatment. *Topical application* can cause similar symptoms, but this is less likely.

Insulin

Adverse symptoms may arise if the dose of insulin is excessive or if the patient fails to receive an adequate amount of carbohydrate in relation to the prescribed dose of insulin. Such symptoms include weakness, a sinking feeling in the stomach, palpitation, irritability, tremor, giddiness, pallor, sweating and salivation. Later, the higher centres may be affected as shown by depression or euphoria, lack of judgement and self-control, amnesia, hemiplegia, ataxia, diplopia and paraesthesia. The pupils are often dilated but later may become contracted and cease to respond to light. Respiration may be shallow and rapid and, in severe cases, hypoglycaemic (insulin) coma may follow. This must be differentiated from hyperglycaemic (diabetic) coma in which the breath probably will smell of acetone.

Non-specific local reactions may occur such as skin rash, urticaria, pruritus or angioneurotic oedema. In chronic diabetics prolonged insulin treatment can cause atrophy of fatty tissue at the site of injection. (See also Chapter 29, p. 303.)

Oestrogens

> Natural steroid oestrogens.

Synthetic steroid oestrogens and their esters.
Synthetic non-steroid oestrogens (stilboestrol, hexoestrol, etc.).

If given in excessive doses or over unduly long periods, oestrogens can induce premature sexual development in young females or inhibit such development in young males. They promote retention of fluid, producing oedema, premature enlargement of the breasts, over-proliferation of the endometrium and in severe cases endometrial polyps which can result in uterine haemorrhage.

An early side-effect may be the production of nausea and possibly vomiting in patients of all ages. Such an effect is more marked with synthetic oestrogens, such as stilboestrol, than with steroid oestrogens. An early indication of oestrogenic action is an increase in pigmentation of the areolae of the nipples. In males, these effects are also produced and in the high doses used in the treatment of prostatic carcinoma there is a possibility of gynaecomastia (breast enlargement) (see p. 300) with tenderness developing.

Suppression of ovulation is a common effect of oestrogen treatment which has long been used for the prevention of dysmenorrhoea (*anovulatory* menstruation is painless) and in association with progestogens, the oestrogens are used as contraceptives, usually by the oral route. When given, in combination, therapeutically, oestrogens and progestogens are usually ordered only for limited periods and their side-effects are not of such significance as when they are given as contraceptives over a number of years in the life of an individual. As contraceptives, oestrogens and progestogens combined may give rise to nausea and headaches in the first two or three months of administration but they tend thereafter to diminish and frequently disappear.

Vascular disorders, particularly of the legs, such as varicose veins, may be worsened by oral contraceptives and thrombotic tendencies are considered to be contraindications to their use. An appreciably increased rise of thrombosis is thought to be associated with doses of ethinyloestradiol or mestranol of more than 0.05 mg ($=50$ micrograms).

There appears to be no conclusive evidence that steroidal drugs or oral contraceptives can induce malignancy and there is some evidence that they may in some cases reduce the possibility of malignancy arising. In cases with a history of malignant tendencies in the genito-urinary system or breasts, however, steroidal oral contraceptives are best avoided except under specialist medical advice.

Progestogens

Progesterone.
Synthetic progestogens.

(*a*) 19-nor derivatives—ethynodiol, lynoestrenol, norethisterone, norethynodrel.
(*b*) Acetoxy derivatives—chlormadinone, megestrol acetate, medroxyprogesterone.
(*c*) Ethisterone, dydrogesterone, dimethisterone.

Progesterone is unlikely to produce untoward effects in any dosage likely to be prescribed.

The 19-norprogestogens (*a*) appear to be metabolized in part to oestrogens and possibly androgens and may therefore produce in some patients unwanted masculinizing or feminizing effects, and hepatotoxic effects could possibly arise.

The acetoxy derivatives (*b*) are virtually purely progestogenic in their effects and, except in large doses, are unlikely to produce any untoward effects, though some resembling those produced by norethisterone may be produced by large doses, possible nausea, lethargy and weight gain.

Of those in group (*c*) ethisterone may cause masculinization in female fetuses. Dydrogesterone has been reported to cause mild nausea and leucocytosis and dimethisterone in large doses may cause pain, resembling dysmenorrhoea and breast turgidity.

Pituitary (posterior lobe) hormones

> Oxytocin ('Pitocin', 'Syntocinon').
> Vasopressin ('Pitressin').

Overdosage or excessively rapid intravenous infusion of diluted injection of oxytocin may cause violent uterine contractions and rupture of the uterus or fetal asphyxia. It can also cause rise in blood pressure and tetany. The action of oxytocin is intensified by oestrogens and diminished by progestogens.

Vasopressin can give rise to marked pallor, nausea, eructation, cramp and desire to defaecate. Most dangerously it can cause angina and myocardial ischaemia.

Parathyroid

> 'Para-thor-mone'.

Overdosage with parathyroid causes abnormally high blood calcium levels, symptoms of which are weakness, apathy, vomiting and diarrhoea. With continuation of administration there may be extreme lassitude, muscular atony, lethargy and possibly coma.

Pituitary, anterior lobe

> Gonadotrophins (FSH and LH).
> ACTH.

Oversecretion of follicle-stimulating gonadotrophin (FSH) has been suggested as the cause of some menopausal symptoms (flushing, raised temperature, etc.) but clinical overdosage is unlikely. Temporary water retention and excessive corticosteroid secretion may result and allergy is a possibility, particularly to serum (pregnant mares) gonadotrophin.

ACTH (adrenocorticotrophic hormone) may in excessive dosage cause symptoms attributable to oversecretion of corticosteroid hormones. Hypertension and acne may be more marked, however, than from corticosteroids and diabetes mellitus can be exacerbated and insulin requirements may be increased.

Thyroid

> Thyroxine.
> Tri-iodothyronine (liothyronine).

Occasionally, ordinary doses of thyroid substance may cause some anginal pain, palpitation and muscle cramp at the beginning of treatment. Thyroxine is less likely to have this effect because of the delay in the onset of its action (about 10 days from starting administration). Liothyronine quickly begins to act and early onset of untoward effects is more likely. After larger doses, particularly of liothyronine and to some extent of thyroid gland substance, there may be tachycardia, diarrhoea, restlessness, cardiac arrhythmia, headache, flushing and excessive loss of weight. Thyroid hormones may increase the effect of anticoagulant drugs and upset the stability of patients receiving hypoglycaemic drugs.

Code of Ethics (Nursing)

Code of ethics as applied to nursing adopted by the Grand Council of the International Council of Nurses, July 1953 and revised June 1965

Nurses minister to the sick, assume responsibility for creating a physical, social and spiritual environment which will be conducive to recovery, and stress the prevention of illness and promotion of health by teaching and example. They render health-service to the individual, the family, and the community and co-ordinate their services with members of other health professions.

Service to mankind is the primary function of nurses and the reason for the existence of the nursing profession. Need for nursing service is universal. Professional nursing service is based on human need and is therefore unrestricted by considerations of nationality, race, creed, colour, politics or social status.

Inherent in the code is the fundamental concept that the nurse believes in the essential freedoms of mankind and in the preservation of human life. It is important that all nurses be aware of the Red Cross Principles and of their rights and obligations under the terms of the Geneva Conventions of 1949.

The profession recognizes that an international code cannot cover in detail all the activities and relationships of nurses, some of which are conditioned by personal philosophies and beliefs.

1. The fundamental responsibility of the nurse is threefold: to conserve life, to alleviate suffering and to promote health

2. The nurse shall maintain at all times the highest standards of nursing care and of professional conduct

3. The nurse must not only be well prepared to practise, but shall maintain knowledge and skill at a consistently high level

4. The religious beliefs of a patient shall be respected

5. Nurses hold in confidence all personal information entrusted to them

6. Nurses recognize not only the responsibilities but the limitations of their professional functions; do not recommend or give medical treatment without medical orders except in emergencies and report such action to a physician as soon as possible

7. The nurse is under an obligation to carry out the physician's orders intelligently and loyally and to refuse to participate in unethical procedures

8. The nurse sustains confidence in the physician and other members of the health team; incompetence or unethical conduct of associates should be exposed but only to the proper authority

9. The nurse is entitled to just remuneration and accepts only such compensation as the contract, actual or implied, provides

10. Nurses do not permit their names to be used in connection with the advertisement of products or with any other forms of self advertisement

11. The nurse co-operates with and maintains harmonious relationships with members of other professions and with nursing colleagues

12. The nurse adheres to standards of personal ethics which reflect credit upon the profession

13. In personal conduct nurses should not knowingly disregard the accepted pattern of behaviour of the community in which they live and work

14. The nurse participates and shares responsibility with other citizens and other health professions in promoting efforts to meet the health needs of the public—local, state, national and international

Commentary

The introduction points to the purpose and responsibilities of nursing and its universality—based on human need and unrestricted by circumstances of nationality, politics, social status, race and creed, belief in the essential freedoms of mankind—in other words in human rights.

(1) stresses the responsibility to protect life, lessen suffering, promote health and wherever possible cure the sick.

(2) stresses the high standard of care the public should (and will) receive if the Code is followed.

(8, 11 and 12) refer to the nurse's relationship and responsibilities to the medical profession and to others.

RED CROSS BASIC PRINCIPLES

Humanity. The Red Cross, born of a desire to bring assistance without discrimination to the wounded on the battlefield, endeavours—in its international and national capacity—to prevent and alleviate human suffering wherever it may be found. Its purpose is to protect life and health and to ensure respect for the human being. It promotes mutual understanding, friendship, co-operation and lasting peace amongst all peoples.

Impartiality. It makes no discrimination as to nationality, race, religious beliefs, class or political opinions. It endeavours only to relieve suffering, giving priority to the most urgent cases of distress.

Neutrality. In order to continue to enjoy the confidence of all, the Red Cross may not take sides in hostilities or engage at any time in controversies of a political, racial, religious or ideological nature.

Independence. The Red Cross is independent. The National Societies while auxiliaries in the humanitarian services of their governments and subject to the laws of their respective countries, must always maintain their autonomy so that they may be able at all times to act in accordance with Red Cross principles.

Voluntary Service. The Red Cross is a voluntary relief organisation not prompted in any manner by desire for gain.

Unity. There can be only one Red Cross Society in any one country. It must be open to all. It must carry on its humanitarian work throughout its territory.

Universality. The Red Cross is a world-wide institution in which all Societies have equal status and share responsibilities and duties in helping each other.

With regard to the **Geneva Conventions of 1949**, nurses are advised to approach either the local Red Cross authorities or the International Red Cross Society for advice when in any situation they may need their rights and responsibilities defined.

Appendix iv

Question Papers Set in the Final State Examination for the General Part of the Register During Recent Years

Examples of questions from papers set in the **Final State Examination** (General) recently, which indicate the standard of knowledge expected of candidates. *The percentages at the side act as a guide to the value of each part of a question and enable a candidate to judge the length of time which should be allocated to it.*

ALL ASPECTS OF NURSING CARE AND TREATMENT OF PATIENTS

October 1973
Morning Paper (3 hours and 5 questions)

1. A 35-year-old bus driver has just been admitted to your ward with a myocardial infarction.
   - (a) Give an account of the immediate treatment he will require.   30%
   - (b) What further treatment and nursing care should be given during the first 24 hours after admission?   40%
   - (c) What advice may be given to the patient on discharge regarding his future health and well-being?   30%

2. A patient is admitted to hospital to undergo partial thyroidectomy for thyrotoxicosis.
   - (a) What special pre-operative care may this patient need?   20%
   - (b) Describe in detail the postoperative care this patient will require. 50%
   - (c) With reference to anatomy and physiology how would you describe to a junior nurse the possible postoperative complications which may occur?   30%

3. A man aged 20 has been admitted to your ward in status asthmaticus.
   - (a) With reference to anatomy and physiology explain this condition to your junior nurse.   20%
   - (b) Describe the treatment and nursing care of this patient.   40%
   - (c) Discuss his long-term management.   40%

4. An eight-year-old child has acute myeloid leukaemia.
   - (a) What is meant by acute myeloid leukaemia?   20%
   - (b) How would you try to make this child happy and comfortable? 40%
   - (c) How may the child's parents be helped and supported by the hospital team?   40%

5. Discuss the role of the nurse in ONE of the following:

(A) the Theatre Recovery Room;   100%

or

(B) the initial booking of a primigravida in an antenatal clinic;   100%

or

(C) the care of a patient with senile dementia in a psycho-geriatric ward; 100%

or

(D) the first domiciliary visit by the district nurse to a patient with diabetes mellitus who has recently been discharged from hospital.   100%

6. A patient is admitted with severe crush injuries to the lower abdomen following a road traffic accident.

    (*a*) What structures may have been damaged?   10%

    (*b*) What observations would you make of this patient on admission? 30%

    (*c*) Discuss the management of this patient during the first few hours following admission.   60%

7. (*a*) What do you understand by the term 'colic'?   10%

    (*b*) Where may it occur in the body?   20%

    (*c*) Describe the signs, symptoms, treatment and nursing care of any ONE patient you have nursed during an attack of colic.
What further treatment was required for this patient?   70%

8. You may answer EITHER A or B.

(A) A teenager has meningococcal meningitis.

    (*a*) Describe the signs and symptoms of this condition.   20%

    (*b*) What treatment may the doctor prescribe?   20%

    (*c*) Give an account of the nursing care which should be given to this patient.   40%

    (*d*) Draw a diagram to illustrate the position of the meninges.   20%

or

(B) Discuss the total care of a patient admitted with carcinoma of the bronchus for a pneumonectomy.   100%

ALL ASPECTS OF NURSING CARE AND TREATMENT OF PATIENTS

October 1973

Afternoon Paper (3 hours and 5 questions)

1. (*a*) Compare and contrast the structure of arteries and veins.   20%

    (*b*) What factors predispose to the formation of varicose veins in the leg? 10%

    (*c*) What surgical treatment may be carried out for this condition?   10%

    (*d*) Describe the total care required by a patient undergoing any ONE treatment you have mentioned.   60%

2. A schoolteacher aged 30 years has been admitted to a medical ward with the provisional diagnosis of a duodenal ulcer.

    (*a*) How would you prepare this patient for a barium meal?   30%

    (*b*) Describe the procedure for obtaining specimens of stool for detection of occult blood.   20%

    (*c*) Describe the care he may be given during this period of investigations.
                                                                          50%

3. (a) With the aid of a diagram describe the hip-joint. 20%
   (b) What conditions and diseases may cause this joint to be painful? 10%
   (c) Describe in detail the total care of a patient suffering from any ONE condition you have mentioned. 70%

4. (a) Give an account of how a person may gain immunity to an infectious disease. 40%
   (b) Describe the facilities available in the community for the immunization of children and adults. 40%
   (c) Against which diseases may protection be given? 20%

5. (a) What do you understand by diverticulitis? Illustrate your answer with a diagram. 20%
   (b) A man aged 55 years is admitted to your ward with diverticulitis. He is to undergo surgery which will include a temporary colostomy. Describe in detail the pre-operative treatment and nursing care this patient may require. 80%

6. What first-aid should be given in the following situations:
   (a) a woman receives a severe electric shock whilst ironing; 50%
   (b) an elderly man has an epistaxis whilst sitting in the park; 25%
   (c) a man working in his tool shed splashes acid in one eye? 25%

7. Discuss the advantages and disadvantages of bed rest. 100%

8. If you answer this question you may answer EITHER A or B.
   (A) (a) List the possible causes of vaginal discharge. 20%
       (b) Describe the care and treatment of a patient suffering from any ONE of the causes you have mentioned. 80%
   or
   (B) (a) List the possible causes of retention of urine. 20%
       (b) Describe the total care of a patient suffering from any ONE of the causes you have mentioned. 80%

ALL ASPECTS OF NURSING CARE AND TREATMENT OF PATIENTS

June 1973

Morning Paper (3 hours and 5 questions)

1. An elderly man has broncho-pneumonia.
   (a) With reference to anatomy and physiology describe how normal respiratory function is impaired in this patient. 25%
   (b) Give an account of the treatment and nursing care he will require in hospital. 75%

2. (a) What do you understand by the term 'haemorrhoids'? 10%
   (b) What factors predispose to this condition? 10%
   (c) How may this condition be treated? 10%
   A man of 40 years is admitted for haemorrhoidectomy.
   (d) Describe in detail the nursing management of this patient. 70%

3. (a) With reference to anatomy and physiology describe how jaundice may occur. 25%
   (b) Discuss the observations which may be made about a jaundiced patient and explain why they are important. 25%
   (c) Describe the nursing care of a patient with infective hepatitis. 50%

4. Describe the facilities that are available in this country for the care of EITHER
   (A) a mentally handicapped child;   100%
   or
   (B) a physically handicapped child.   100%

5. Write an essay on EITHER
   (A) disorders of the menstrual cycle;   100%
   or
   (B) vasectomy.   100%

6. Describe the oesophagus.   20%
   A middle-aged patient has dysphagia (difficulty in swallowing).
   (*a*) List the possible reasons for this.   20%
   (*b*) Give an account of the total care of a patient you have nursed with
         ONE of these conditions.   60%

7. You are in charge of the ward for the weekend.
   What are your responsibilities for ensuring that all patients, including any who
   have been newly admitted, receive the drugs that have been prescribed?   100%

8. (*a*) List the possible postoperative complications which may occur following
        major abdominal surgery.   25%
   (*b*) Discuss the role of the nurse in the early detection or prevention of FIVE of
        the complications you have listed.   75%

ALL ASPECTS OF NURSING CARE AND TREATMENT OF PATIENTS

June 1973

Afternoon Paper (3 hours and 5 questions)

1. A school child aged 13 years is admitted to your ward with a perforated appendix.
   Describe in detail the pre- and postoperative care this child will require.   100%

2. (*a*) Draw a diagram of the heart to indicate the direction of the flow of blood
        through this organ.   20%
   A patient aged 72 years has just been admitted to your ward suffering from
   congestive cardiac failure.
   (*b*) What observations should be made about this patient on admission?   30%
   (*c*) What immediate treatment and nursing care will he require?   50%

3. If you select this question answer ONLY A or B.
   (A) A woman aged 40 years is admitted to your ward with carcinoma of breast for
       surgery.
       (*a*) What may have led this woman to seek medical advice?   20%
       (*b*) How may the nurse help in the pre-operative preparation of this
             patient?   40%
       (*c*) Describe the special postoperative care she will require. 40%
   or
   (B) (*a*) Describe the mechanism of micturition.   20%
        (*b*) List the disorders of micturition which may occur in male patients.
                                                                       20%
        (*c*) Describe in detail the total care of a patient suffering with ONE
              disorder you have mentioned.   60%

4. (*a*) Give an account of the causes of diarrhoea.   40%
   A patient in a geriatric ward develops severe diarrhoea.
   (*b*) Describe the management and nursing care of this patient.   60%

5. An elderly man is admitted to hospital having fallen and struck his head. He is conscious but dazed.

> (a) Describe the procedure for admission of this patient.   30%
> (b) What observations would you make about this patient and why are they important?   40%
> (c) Discuss the care he will require during the first night in hospital. 30%

6. What are the nurse's responsibilities regarding the following:

> (a) the support and reassurance of the patient's relatives;   50%
> (b) the preservation of confidentiality concerning the patient and his condition?   50%

7. A mother with four young children is admitted to your ward with a disc protrusion (prolapsed intravertebral disc).

> (a) How would you describe this condition to a junior nurse?   20%
> (b) Give an account of the treatment and nursing care this patient may require.   50%
> (c) Discuss the social problems which may arise from this patient's illness.   30%

8. If you select this question answer ONLY A or B.

> (A). (a) Describe the structure and relations of the tonsils.   10%
>
> A child aged five years is admitted for tonsillectomy.
>
> (b) Describe the admission procedure of this child.   20%
> (c) Give a detailed account of his postoperative care.   50%
> (d) How may the effects of hospitalization on this child be reduced? 20%

or

> (B) (a) Describe the structure and functions of the skin.   30%
> (b) Give an account of the treatment and management of a patient with psoriasis.   70%

ALL ASPECTS OF NURSING CARE AND TREATMENT OF PATIENTS

January 1973

Morning Paper (3 hours and 5 questions)

1. Give an account of the functions of the pancreas.   25%

A woman aged 20 years is admitted to hospital in hyperglycaemic (diabetic) coma. Discuss the specific medical and nursing care she will require on admission, and for the subsequent 24 hours.   75%

2. A patient is admitted to hospital with a compound fracture of the tibia.

> (a) What first-aid treatment should this patient have received before admission to hospital?   20%
> (b) What treatment and care will the patient receive in the first 24 hours after admission?   40%
> (c) What possible complications may arise from this condition and how may these complications be prevented?   40%

3. You are in charge of a ward on night duty and there is one junior nurse with you when a patient has a cardiac arrest.

> (a) How would you recognize this state?   20%
> (b) How would you deal with this situation giving reasons for your actions?   80%

4. How may a malignant growth be treated?   20%

Describe in detail the total care of any one patient you have nursed suffering from a malignant condition.   80%

5. As nurse in charge of the ward how would you deal with the following situations:
   (a) fire breaks out in the ward kitchen;   40%
   (b) during a storm at night a window is blown in above a patient's bed;
                                                                                30%
   (c) a patient's dentures are missing?   30%

6. Discuss the dangers and complications associated with the giving of intravenous fluids.   60%
   How can the nurse help to minimize these dangers and complications?   40%

7. How can the nurse's observations of a patient's vomit, sputum, urine and faeces help the doctor in reaching a diagnosis?   100%

8. If you select this question answer ONLY A or B or C.
   (A) A young man is admitted with phimosis for circumcision.
       (a) With reference to anatomy how would you describe this condition to a junior nurse?   20%
       (b) Discuss the management of this patient.   80%
   or
   (B) A woman aged 20 has been admitted with a ruptured ectopic gestation (tubal pregnancy).
       (a) Describe in detail the pre-operative preparation this patient will receive.   60%
       (b) What special complications may arise from this condition?   20%
       (c) With reference to anatomy and physiology how would you describe this condition to a junior nurse?   20%
   or
   (C) Describe the care which should be given to a mother in the week following the birth of her first child.   100%

ALL ASPECTS OF NURSING CARE AND TREATMENT OF PATIENTS

January 1973
Afternoon Paper (3 hours and 5 questions)

1. A bus driver aged 40 is admitted to a surgical ward with a confirmed diagnosis of a gastric ulcer.
   (a) How may this condition have affected the patient and his family?
                                                                                20%
   (b) Describe in detail the pre-operative preparation and care he will require.   60%
   (c) If surgery is not performed what complications may arise from a gastric ulcer?   20%

2. With reference to anatomy and physiology what do you understand by the term 'cerebral vascular accident'?   20%
   An elderly man is recovering from this condition in your ward.
   How can the nurse help to prepare this patient for discharge?   50%
   What are the various services available to enable him to return home and live within the family?   30%

3. A gentleman has had an emergency colostomy performed for intestinal obstruction.
   (a) What care should be given to this patient during the first 24 hours following surgery?   60%

(b) How should he be prepared prior to the first dressing of the colostomy? 20%

(c) Describe the structure and function of the colon. 20%

4. You may answer EITHER A or B.

(A) (a) Describe the mechanism of respiration. 30%

(b) Give an account of the special nursing care required by a patient who has had a thoracotomy. 70%

or

(B) (a) Describe the trachea. 15%

(b) For what reasons may tracheostomy be performed? 15%

(c) Give an account of the postoperative care required by a patient who has undergone tracheostomy. 70%

5. Two patients in your ward have had an above-knee amputation of leg. One is an old age pensioner of 70 years admitted from the waiting list, the other a young man of 28 years admitted as a result of industrial injury. Discuss the postoperative care and rehabilitation services required by ONE of these patients. 100%

6. Discuss the uses and side-effects of the following drugs:

(a) digoxin; 25%

(b) streptomycin; 25%

(c) aspirin; 25%

(d) cortico-steroids. 25%

7. Give an account of the formation, structure and function of the erythrocyte (red blood corpuscle). 20%

A patient is admitted with iron deficiency anaemia.

(a) List the possible causes. 20%

(b) Describe the signs and symptoms of this condition. 30%

(c) How may it be treated? 30%

8. Patients in hospital often have difficulty in sleeping.

Discuss the reasons for this and suggest how the nurse can help in the prevention of insomnia. 100%

ALL ASPECTS OF NURSING CARE AND TREATMENT OF PATIENTS

October 1972

Morning Paper (3 hours and 5 questions)

1. (a) Describe the gall bladder and its functions. 30%

An obese middle-aged patient is admitted for cholecystectomy and exploration of the common bile duct.

(b) Describe in detail the special postoperative treatment and care this patient will require. 60%

(c) What advice would you give this patient on discharge? 10%

2. A patient in your ward has a major epileptic attack.

(a) Describe in detail how you would deal with this situation. 30%

(b) What observations should be made and recorded? 30%

(c) Discuss the treatment of epilepsy. 20%

(d) What are the social implications of the condition? 20%

3. (a) What would lead you to suspect that a patient has a wound infection? 30%

(b) How does the body attempt to overcome this infection? 20%

(c) Discuss the role of the nurse in the prevention of wound infection in a surgical ward.   50%

4. You may answer EITHER A or B.

   (A) A two-year-old child is to be admitted to the Paediatric Unit from the waiting list for surgery.
       What can be done by the nursing staff to ensure the welfare and well-being of this child and his parents during his stay in hospital?   100%
   or
   (B) How can a nurse preserve the dignity, individuality and independence of the elderly in hospital?   100%

5. A 40-year-old male patient has been admitted for a nephrectomy.

   (a) Describe the kidney, including the microscopic structure.   30%
   (b) List the possible investigations which may be carried out.   20%
   (c) Discuss in detail the postoperative treatment and care this patient may require.   50%

6. (a) Give an account of the essential constituents of a normal diet.   30%
   (b) Discuss the possible causes of malutrition in the United Kingdom.   40%
   (c) What may be the effect of malnutrition on the individual?   30%

7. (a) With the aid of a diagram describe the structure of the knee-joint.   30%

   A young footballer is admitted for a miniscectomy.

   (b) Discuss the nursing management of this patient in the ward.   70%

8. If you select this question answer ONLY A or B or C.

   (A)   (a) What is meant by the term 'venereal disease'? Give examples. 20%
         (b) Discuss the prevention and control of these diseases.   40%
         (c) Give an account of the diagnosis and treatment of any one venereal disease.   40%
   or
   (B)   (a) Why is antenatal care necessary?   20%
         (b) Give an account of the care required by a young mother whilst expecting her first baby.   50%
         (c) What discomforts and complications may occur in the early months of pregnancy?   30%
   or
   (C)   (a) What do you understand by the term 'uterine prolapse'?   20%
         (b) What are the symptoms of uterine prolapse?   30%
         (c) Describe how you would prepare a woman for the surgical treatment of this condition.   50%

ALL ASPECTS OF NURSING CARE AND TREATMENT OF PATIENTS

October 1972

Afternoon Paper (3 hours and 5 questions)

1. A man aged 50 is admitted to hospital with severe chest pain following myocardial infarction.

   (a) Describe the immediate treatment and care he will require.   50%
   (b) What are the factors that predispose to coronary artery disease?   20%
   (c) With reference to the anatomy and physiology, explain what occurs in this condition.   30%

2. (a) With reference to the structures involved, how would you describe an inguinal hernia to a junior nurse? 20%
   (b) List the other possible sites of hernia. 10%

   A middle-aged man who is a heavy smoker is admitted for repair of right inguinal hernia.

   (c) What observations should be made on this patient the morning after operation? 40%
   (d) What are the advantages to this patient of early ambulation? 30%

3. (a) How may a patient's mouth become dry? 30%
   (b) List the possible complications arising from poor oral hygiene. 20%
   (c) Describe the oral care required for:
      (i) a patient who has had a dental extraction under general anaesthesia;
   or
      (ii) a patient with advanced leukaemia. 50%

4. (a) Compare and contrast the structure of arteries and veins. 20%
   (b) How would you explain varicose veins to a junior nurse? 15%
   (c) What treatments may be given for this condition? 15%
   (d) Describe in detail the postoperative care a patient may receive after any one surgical treatment you have mentioned. 50%

5. A student of 19 years is admitted to the ward with severe bronchial asthma.

   (a) With reference to the relevant anatomy and physiology of the lung how would you explain this condition to a junior nurse? 30%
   (b) Describe the treatment and nursing care of this patient. 50%
   (c) Discuss the possible causes of this condition. 20%

6. A patient is admitted with a severe crush injury of the upper abdomen.

   (a) List the structures which may have been damaged. 20%
   (b) What observations should the nurse make and how may these observations help the doctor? 40%
   (c) Describe in detail the immediate treatment and care this patient will require. 40%

7. A woman aged 40 years has rheumatoid arthritis.

   Describe the part in her care that may be played by the nurse, the physiotherapist, the occupational therapist and the medical social worker. 100%

8' If you select this question answer ONLY A or B or C.

   (A)   (a) With reference to anatomy and physiology how would you describe a cataract to a junior nurse? 20%

      An elderly patient is admitted to your ward for lens extraction.

      (b) Describe in detail the special pre- and postoperative care of this patient. 80%
   or
   (B) A child of ten is admitted to your ward with acute otitis media.
      (a) With reference to anatomy and physiology how would you describe to a junior nurse the possible complications of this condition? 40%
      (b) Describe in detail the treatment and nursing care this child will require. 60%
   or
   (C) A middle-aged man is admitted to your ward with a rodent ulcer of his face. What do you understand by 'rodent ulcer'? 10%
      Describe in detail the possible treatment and nursing care this patient will require. 90%

ALL ASPECTS OF NURSING CARE AND TREATMENT OF PATIENTS

June 1972 (Experimental Syllabus)

Morning Paper (3 hours and 5 questions)

1. A patient is admitted to your ward to undergo partial thyroidectomy for thyrotoxicosis.

  (a) Describe in detail the pre-operative care this patient will require.
  40%

  (b) What postoperative observations should be made on this patient?
  20%

  (c) With reference to anatomy and physiology how would you describe to a junior nurse the possible postoperative complications which may occur?
  40%

2. A man aged 60 years with a history of chronic bronchitis has been admitted in an acute phase.

  (a) Describe the changes which have taken place in the respiratory system of this patient.
  20%

  (b) Give an account of the treatment and nursing care.
  60%

  (c) What factors predispose to the development of chronic bronchitis?
  20%

3. What would lead you to suspect that a patient in your ward is developing:

  (a) deep vein thrombosis of the leg;
  20%

  (b) paralytic ileus;
  20%

  (c) reaction to streptomycin;
  20%

  (d) an anxiety state;
  20%

  (e) postoperative chest infection?
  20%

4. A married woman of 40 years has advanced multiple (disseminated) sclerosis, and is going home from hospital.

  (a) What problems are likely to arise at home?
  30%

  (b) Give an account of the services available for the care and welfare of this patient in her own home.
  70%

5. A man aged 50 years is admitted to your ward with carcinoma of stomach for surgery.

  (a) What are the normal functions of the stomach?
  20%

  (b) Describe the postoperative care this patient will require.
  50%

  (c) List the possible postoperative complications which may arise.
  30%

6. Discuss the factors you consider to be important in creating a ward environment conducive to the recovery of the patient, taking into consideration his physical and psychological needs.
  100%

7. A child aged 10 years has been involved in a road traffic accident and sustained multiple lacerations.

  (a) What first-aid measures should be taken at the scene of the accident?
  20%

  (b) Describe in detail the procedure for admitting this child to hospital.
  30%

  (c) What observations would you make on this patient?
  30%

  (d) What immediate hospital treatment would be necessary?
  20%

8. (a) What do you understand by the term 'hypothermia'?
  5%

(b) What measures should be taken in the home to prevent hypothermia occurring in EITHER:
  (i) an elderly person;
or
  (ii) a baby?   25%
(c) Describe the care required by a patient admitted with hypothermia.   40%
(d) Describe how the normal body temperature is maintained.   30%

ALL ASPECTS OF NURSING CARE AND TREATMENT OF PATIENTS

June 1972 (Experimental Syllabus)
Afternoon Paper (3 hours and 5 questions)

1. A middle-aged man in your ward has severe hypertension.
    (a) Give an account of the investigations which may be ordered.   30%
    (b) What treatment may be given for severe hypertension?   30%
    (c) List the complications which may occur in this condition.   20%
    (d) Describe how you would measure this patient's blood pressure.   20%

2. A sales representative, aged 25 years, is admitted to your ward with severe ulcerative colitis and is to undergo surgery resulting in a permanent ileostomy.
    (a) Discuss the role of the nurse in the pre-operative preparation of this patient.   40%
    (b) Describe the specific postoperative care.   30%
    (c) What advice would you give this patient before discharge?   30%

3. A youth of 18 is unconscious after taking an overdose of aspirin, and has just been admitted to hospital.
    (a) Give an account of the immediate treatment and nursing care he will require.   50%
    (b) On returning to consciousness what further treatment and care may be given?   50%

4. An elderly patient is admitted to hospital with a fractured neck of femur following a fall at home.
    (a) With reference to anatomy outline the surgical treatment which may be carried out.   20%
    (b) How can the nurse help in the rehabilitation of this patient in hospital?   40%
    (c) How may accidents to the elderly in the home be prevented?   40%

5. A man aged 36 years is dying from an inoperable carcinoma of larynx.
    (a) Give an account of the total care of this patient.   70%
    (b) How could you, as a senior nurse, support the junior nurses in the care of this patient?   30%

6. What are the nurse's responsibilities with regard to:
    (a) the custody;
    (b) the administration;
of drugs in a hospital ward?   100%

7. A patient is to have a transfusion of three units of Group O, Rhesus Positive blood.
    (a) What do you understand by 'Group O Rhesus Positive blood'?   20%
    (b) How would you prepare this patient for the transfusion?   20%

    (c) What are the nurse's responsibilities for this blood prior to and during the transfusion?   20%
    (d) What complications may arise during the transfusion and how may the nurse recognize them?   40%

8. If you select this question answer ONLY A or B or C.

(A)   (a) Describe the position and structure of the uterus.   30%
    A young married woman is admitted to hospital with uterine fibroids.
    (b) Discuss the pre- and postoperative care she would require.   70%
or
(B) Describe in detail the observations carried out on a newborn baby.   100%
or
(C)   (a) List the causes of acute retention of urine.   15%
    (b) What dangers are associated with catheterization in the male?   10%
    (c) Discuss the investigations that may be undertaken prior to prostatectomy.   35%
    (d) Describe the immediate postoperative care of this patient.   40%

ALL ASPECTS OF NURSING CARE AND TREATMENT OF PATIENTS

January 1972 (Experimental Syllabus)
Morning Paper (3 hours and 5 questions)

1. A middle-aged man is admitted to hospital following severe haematemesis.
    (a) What are the causes and aggravating factors of haematemesis?   20%
    (b) Discuss the nursing care and treatment of this patient.   60%
    (c) What changes occur in the body as a result of severe bleeding?   20%

2. A patient is admitted to hospital with acute appendicitis.
    (a) Describe the appendix and its relations.   20%
    (b) What are the symptoms of acute appendicitis?   30%
    (c) Discuss the nursing care and treatment this patient will receive.   50%

3. Discuss the uses and side-effects of the following drugs:
    (a) digitalis;   25%
    (b) cortico-steroids;   25%
    (c) penicillin;   25%
    (d) chlorpromazine (largactil).   25%

4. What can a nurse do to minimize the discomfort and complications of the following procedures:
    (a) lumbar puncture;   20%
    (b) a naso-gastric feed to an unconscious patient;   20%
    (c) an intramuscular injection;   20%
    (d) intravenous therapy to a baby;   20%
    (e) a surgical dressing?   20%

5. (a) Describe the formation of urine.   40%
    (b) What are the characteristics of normal urine?   20%
    (c) In what conditions do the following substances occur in abnormal amounts in urine:
      (i) ketones;
      (ii) protein;
      (iii) blood;
      (iv) bilirubin?   20%
    (d) What would cause you to suspect a patient has a urinary infection?   20%

6. Describe the rectum and its functions. 30%

   An elderly man is admitted to hospital with carcinoma of the rectum. How may the nurse help in the pre- and postoperative management of this patient? 70%

7. Discuss the problems associated with obesity. 60%
   Describe in detail a reducing diet. 40%

8. Describe the structure and function of the skin. 30%
   Describe the nursing care and treatment of a child admitted to hospital with severe burns of the trunk. 70%

ALL ASPECTS OF NURSING CARE AND TREATMENT OF PATIENTS

January 1972 (Experimental Syllabus)
Afternoon Paper (3 hours and 5 questions)

1. A patient with a haemoglobin of 40% (5·9 g per 100 ml) is admitted to hospital.

   (a) Describe haemoglobin and discuss its function. 20%
   (b) List the causes of anaemia. 30%
   (c) Describe the treatment and nursing care of only ONE cause you mention. 50%

2. A patient is admitted to hospital with acute intestinal obstruction.

   (a) List the causes of this condition. 20%
   (b) Discuss the observations and records the nurse should make of this patient. 50%
   (c) Describe the changes which occur in the body as the result of intestinal obstruction. 30%

3. If you were a staff nurse in charge of a ward for the weekend, describe how you would:

   (a) prepare a patient for a barium meal on the Monday morning; 20%
   (b) ensure the collection of a 24-hour specimen of urine; 20%
   (c) deal with a patient who wishes to leave hospital against medical advice; 30%
   (d) care for a patient who has collapsed in the toilet. 30%

4. Describe the first-aid treatment that YOU would give for the following:

   (a) an abrasion on the knee due to gravel; 20%
   (b) a splinter in the finger; 20%
   (c) a fractured clavicle; 20%
   (d) a bleeding nose; 20%
   (e) a 'black eye'. 20%

5. What are the illnesses to which the elderly are prone? 60%
   How may these conditions be prevented or minimized? 40%

6. You may answer EITHER A or B.

   (A) (a) Describe the cervix uteri and give its relations. 20%
   (b) What are the symtoms of carcinoma of the cervix? 20%
   (c) What methods are available for the early diagnosis of carcinoma of the cervix? 20%
   (d) Discuss the postoperative nursing care following hysterectomy. 40%

   or
   (B) (a) Describe the urinary bladder and its anatomical relations. 20%
   (b) What are the symptoms of bladder cancer? 20%
   (c) Describe the postoperative nursing care of a patient after partial cystectomy. 60%

7. Describe the heart.   40%
   Give an account of the special nursing care of a patient with left ventricular failure
   (cardiac asthma).   60%

8. Describe the trachea.   20%
   List the causes of tracheal obstruction.   20%
   Discuss in detail the nursing care of a patient after tracheostomy.   60%

ALL ASPECTS OF NURSING CARE AND TREATMENT OF PATIENTS

January 1972

Morning Paper (3 hours and 5 questions)

1. An elderly man, who lives alone in a council flat, is admitted suffering from congestive heart failure. He is covered with flea bites and has a wallet containing £100
   in his pocket. Describe:

   (a) the management of this patient during the first twenty-four hours;
                                                                          60%
   (b) the care of his clothes and money;   15%
   (c) the social problems likely to arise when he leaves hospital.   25%

2. What are the factors governing the choice of a suitable diet in each of the following conditions and what are the difficulties associated with their provision:

   (a) obesity; $33\frac{1}{3}\%$
   (b) chronic renal failure; $33\frac{1}{3}\%$
   (c) coeliac disease? $33\frac{1}{3}\%$

3. Discuss the dangers of bed rest.   100%

4. A young man develops spontaneous pneumothorax.

   (a) Describe the probable signs and symptoms.   30%
   (b) What nursing care and observations would be required?   40%
   (c) What medical treatment is available?   30%

5. A young woman, recently returned from a holiday abroad, is admitted suffering
   from severe diarrhoea and pyrexia.

   (a) List the common causes of diarrhoea.   10%
   (b) What investigations may be carried out to establish this patient's
       diagnosis?   20%
   (c) Give an account of the nursing care she will require.   70%

6. A young long-distance lorry driver, with three children, develops diabetes
   mellitus and is admitted for stabilization.

   (a) What does the term 'stabilization' mean?   10%
   (b) Give an account of his management while in hospital.   70%
   (c) What advice should the nurse give to the patient and his wife when
       he leaves hospital?   20%

7. What advice and reassurance would you give if faced with the following situations:

   (a) A mother complains that her 10-year-old daughter has started to
       wet the bed at night. $33\frac{1}{3}\%$
   (b) A 40-year-old friend says that her periods are becoming more
       prolonged and heavy. $33\frac{1}{3}\%$
   (c) A first-year, unmarried, student nurse tells you that she may be
       pregnant. $33\frac{1}{3}\%$

ALL ASPECTS OF NURSING CARE AND TREATMENT OF PATIENTS

January 1972
Afternoon Paper (3 hours and 5 questions)

1. A 45-year-old patient is admitted with a history of recurring episodes of biliary colic.
    (a) Describe the condition during an attack.   20%
    (b) What investigations may be performed and how would the patient be prepared for them?   40%
    (c) Describe the care and management of the T tube if exploration of the common bile duct has been performed.   40%

2. A young man admitted after a motor accident has fractured ribs and a ruptured spleen.
    (a) What complications may occur after these injuries? $33\frac{1}{3}\%$
    (b) What surgical treatment may be required? $33\frac{1}{3}\%$
    (c) How should he be prepared for it? $33\frac{1}{3}\%$

3. An elderly patient is admitted with large bowel obstruction.
    (a) How should he be prepared for operation?   25%
    (b) Describe the nursing care which should be given if a colostomy has been performed.   50%
    (c) How can the patient be helped when he is ready for discharge from hospital?   25%

4. A six-year-old boy is brought from school to hospital with a perforated appendix.
    (a) Describe his condition on admission.   25%
    (b) Give an account of the management after appendicectomy.   50%
    (c) What complications may arise and how may your observations lead to their early detection?   25%

5. An elderly patient attends hospital complaining of pain and stiffness in an osteo-arthritic hip.
    (a) What non-operative measures can be used for the treatment?   30%
    (b) If an operation is performed what special postoperative care is required?   40%
    (c) Describe the complications which may occur.   30%

6. If you select this question answer ONLY A or B or C.
    (A) Give an account of the nursing observations and care during labour.   100%
    or
    (B) Describe the management and nursing care of a woman in the terminal stages of ovarian carcinoma.   100%
    or
    (C) An elderly man is admitted with acute retention of urine due to an enlarged prostate gland.
        (a) Describe the treatment on admission.   25%
        (b) What special tests may be performed?   25%
        (c) What operative treatment may be required?   10%
        (d) Describe the nursing care after any one of these operations.   40%

7. How would you explain to a junior nurse:

        (a) the causes of enlargement of the thyroid gland;   20%

        (b) the symptoms that may be produced by the enlargement;   20%

        (c) the special complications which may arise following partial thyroidectomy;   30%

        (d) the preparations made by the nurse to prevent or deal with these complications?   30%

Index

Notes

These pages have been included for the use of nurses who may wish to make individual notes on case histories, special procedures, etc.